MICROBIOLOGY

INTRODUCTION FOR HEALTH PROFESSIONALS

TO THE STUDENT

A Study Guide for the textbook is available through your college bookstore under the title Study Guide to accompany **MICROBIOLOGY: Introduction for Health Professionals** by **Paul A. Ketchum.**

The Study guide can help you with course material by acting as a tutorial, review and study aid. If the Study Guide is not in stock, ask the bookstore manager to order a copy for you.

MICROBIOLOGY

INTRODUCTION FOR HEALTH PROFESSIONALS

PAUL A. KETCHUM
Oakland University

JOHN WILEY & SONS
New York   Chichester   Brisbane   Toronto   Singapore

Library of Congress Cataloging in Publication Data

Ketchum, Paul A. (Paul Abbott), 1942–
     Microbiology.

     Includes index.
     1. Microbiology.   2. Medical microbiology.
3. Allied health personnel.   I. Title.

QR41.2.K47   1984   616'.01   82-23709
ISBN 0-471-06306-1

Printed in the United States of America

10 9 8 7 6 5 4 3 2

To my mother
Emily W. Ketchum
In memory of my father
Bostwick H. Ketchum
1912–1982

PREFACE

The knowledge generated from the study of micro-organisms has enriched virtually all segments of the biological sciences and established microbiology as a major scientific discipline. Microbiology is a broad discipline that covers a diversity of subject matter, ranging from the cell biology of immune systems to the molecular biology of viral infections. The work of many scientists with different perspectives concerning microorganisms has led to a tremendous body of knowledge. While microbiology has been undergoing its expansive development, more and more students have entered professional programs in the numerous health fields. Students enter these programs to learn the basic sciences and to receive training in the use of current technology. The programs designed for these health professionals continue to place pressure on the time available for and the content of the basic science curriculums. In response to these needs, many colleges and universities have modified existing courses or have developed specialized courses for students pursuing professional careers.

Microbiology is one of the basic sciences that comprise the foundations of our modern health care sys-

tem. I have written this textbook for use in introductory microbiology courses taken by first- and second-year college students who are preparing for careers in an allied health field or who are interested in health and infectious diseases. The subject matter covers the basic science of microbiology, with an emphasis on the application of this science to human health.

The material presented in Part One covers the fundamentals of microbiology needed to understand the biology of infectious diseases and the agents that cause them. The presentation is aimed at students who have had a high school exposure to chemistry; however, for students who lack this background, Chapter 2 reviews the chemical principles relevant to biology.

The major portion of the book is devoted to the discussion of infectious diseases. Part Two, "Host-Parasite Relationships," is an introduction to infectious diseases. The four chapters of Part Two cover the normal human flora, virulence and host resistance, immunology, and epidemiology. Part Three, "The Procaryotic Pathogens," is organized into seven chapters based on the taxonomic groupings of the bacteria. The advantages of the taxonomic approach to presenting the pathogenic bacteria are at least threefold: *(a)* each pathogen is discussed in one section of the book even when it causes diseases in more than one organ system; *(b)* the bacterial, viral, and eucaryotic pathogens are clearly differentiated; and *(c)* students who go on to study pathogenic bacteriology, which is universally presented by the taxonomic approach, will have an advantage. In addition, the taxonomic approach has enabled me to devote a major section of the book (Part Four) to the viruses. This emphasis on the viruses recognizes their impact on our health care system and on our everyday lives. Because the molecular classification of the viruses is cumbersome for an introductory textbook, the animal viruses are grouped according to the organ systems they infect. Part Five is devoted to the procaryotic pathogens and includes one chapter on the fungi and one chapter on the protozoa. Within the confines of a textbook designed for an introductory course, I have included discussions of all the major bacterial, viral, and mycotic infections of humans and an introduction to the protozoa, which includes a discussion of selected protozoan diseases.

Microbiology: Introduction for Health Professionals is first and foremost written for students. A number of features of the book are specifically designed to augment the learning process. Each chapter concludes with a concise summary. The chapters on infectious diseases also contain a summary table. The summary is followed by a series of review questions and topics for discussion. A list of references for further reading is included at the end of each chapter for students who want to do additional research on the topics covered.

Each new term is presented in boldface so that it can be referred to readily in the text. In addition, a comprehensive glossary is included at the end of the book. The glossary is supplemented by an appendix on the pronunciation of scientific names and terms. A separate study guide is available for students who would benefit from additional approaches to studying the material presented and from self-test questions.

Illustrations are extremely valuable for conveying biological and chemical concepts, mechanisms, and structures. I am grateful to all the scientists who have kindly permitted me to use their illustrations and micrographs. In addition, I am indebted to John Balbalis and the illustration department at Wiley for their excellent execution of the line drawings.

Many individuals provided invaluable help and guidance during the preparation, writing, and production of this book, and I thank them all. Selected chapters were read and critiqued by my colleagues (past and present) at Oakland University: William Forbes, Thomas Friedman, Esther Goudsmit, Charles Lindemann, Daphna Oliver, James Reynhout, Ann Sakai, Ruth Swarin, and R. Craig Taylor. I thank John B. Breznack (Michigan State University), James G. Cappuccino (Rockland Community College), William R. Clark (University of California at Los Angeles), Charles D. Cox (University of Massachusetts), Michael Danciger (Loyola Marymount University), Ruth Dass (Pontiac Osteopathic Hospital), James G. Garner (Long Island University), Haig H. Najarian (University of Southern Maine), Robert K. Nauman (University of Maryland Dental School at Baltimore), Elinor M. O'Brien (Boston College, The Senntag Institute for Cancer Research), Diane Cope Peabody (University of Massachusetts), Harry E. Peery (Freeville, New York), Paulette W. Royt (George Mason University), Natalie Sherman (Rockland Community College), Muriel H. Svec (Santa Monica College), Dwight E. Talburt (University of Arkansas), Jerry L. Tammen (Rochester Community College), Neil O. Thorpe (Augsburg College), William M. Todd (The University of Tennessee), and Ralph F. Wiseman (University of Kentucky) for reviewing major segments or all of the manuscript. I was helped in the production of the manuscript by my wife, Nancy, who proofread the entire manuscript at each stage of its development and offered invaluable support, advice, and criticism; Anne H. Lalas, who edited the manuscript at various stages of its preparation; and Ingrid McDermit, Susan Perlmutter, and Andrea Gentilcore, who typed various portions of the manuscript.

Paul A. Ketchum

CONTENTS

MICROBIOLOGY

INTRODUCTION FOR HEALTH PROFESSIONALS

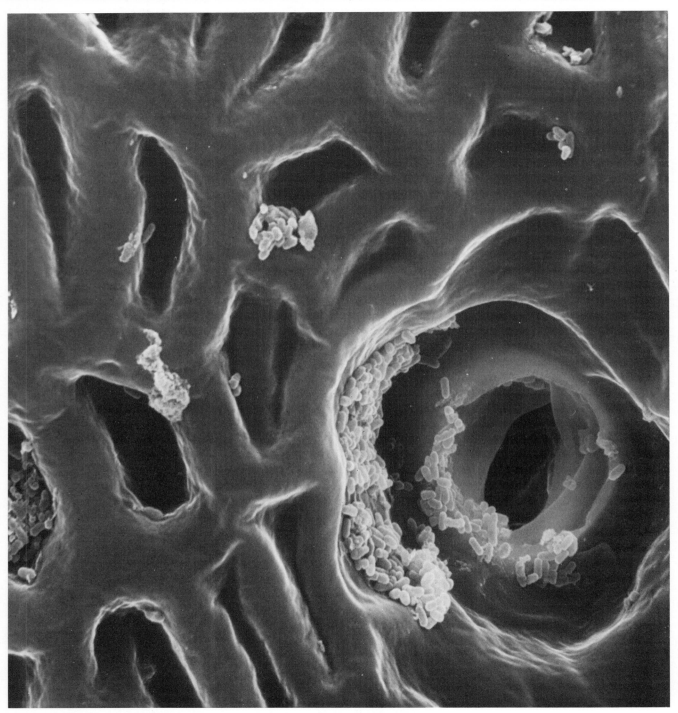

A scanning electron micrograph of bacteria associated with a stomate on the surface of a cucumber fermented by *Lactobacillus plantarum*. (Courtesy of M. A. Daeschel. From M. A. Daeschel and H. P. Fleming, *Applied Environ. Microbiol.,* 41:1111–1118, 1981.)

PART ONE

BASIC MICROBIOLOGY

1

MICROBIOLOGY

Microbiology is the study of small organisms. How small is small? Biologists have grouped together the organisms that cannot be seen with the unaided human eye and have designated them as "microorganisms." This definition includes those organisms that are less than one-tenth of a millimeter (0.1 mm) in size. Most microorganisms are single cells or clumps of cells with no discernible differentiation into tissues. This structural characteristic also sets microorganisms apart from the macroscopic (greater than 0.1 mm in size) animals and plants. Microorganisms include the viruses, bacteria, fungi, protozoa, and certain algae.

For most of recorded history, there were no devices capable of magnifying microorganisms sufficiently to make them visible to humans. Only since the middle of the 1600s have microscopes been available to observe microorganisms. The development of these microscopes and the discovery of microorganisms were remarkable events from both an historical and a scientific viewpoint.

DISCOVERY OF MICROORGANISMS

While Robert Hooke (1635–1703) was the curator of experiments for the Royal Society in London, he developed his first microscope. He spent many hours examining different materials under it and made a presentation to the Royal Society of his findings. The Society members were so impressed that they requested him to present a new microscopic observation at each subsequent meeting. They also encouraged him to publish his observations. Hooke published *Micrographia*, dedicating it to King Charles II, in November 1664. This book contains exquisite, detailed drawings of insects, insect larvae, seeds, eggs, feathers, hairs, rocks, cork, and microorganisms known as molds (Figure 1–1). Hooke described the molds as

long cylindrical transparent stalks, not exactly straight, but a little bended with the weight of a round white knob that grew on the top of each of them.

He compared the observed microscopic knobs to the tops of the common white mushroom. This is the first reported observation of molds. Hooke contributed greatly to knowledge through his observations of tissues and the compartmentalized structure of living things; however, he did not observe objects as small as bacteria. Credit for this discovery is given to Anton van Leeuwenhoek (1632–1723), a contemporary of Hooke's, who was born in and spent almost all of his life in Delft, Holland (Figure 1–2).

At the age of 16, Leeuwenhoek apprenticed to a linen draper in Amsterdam. He became proprietor of a draper's shop in Delft at about the time of his first marriage in 1654. Delft was a major center of commerce, and Leeuwenhoek did well in the draper's business. He was also a qualified surveyor. In 1660 he was appointed chamberlain to the chief judge, the sheriffs, and the law officers of the city of Delft;

FIGURE 1–1
Robert Hooke observed molds growing on the leather covering of a book. Hooke suggested that the morphological variation in the knobs (A, B, C, D, and E) were seed cases similar to those found on the tops of mushrooms. (Robert Hooke, *Micrographia*. Reprinted by Dover, New York, 1961.)

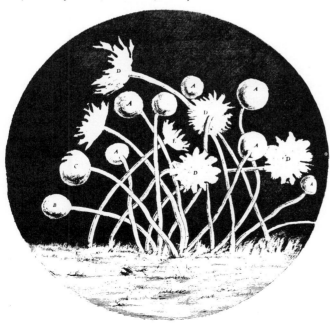

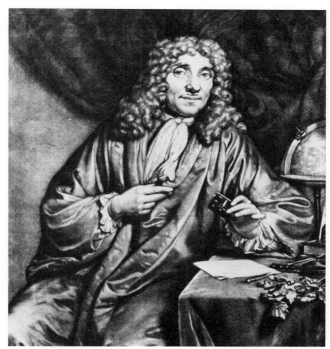

FIGURE 1–2
Anton van Leeuwenhoek (1632–1723) was the first person to see and describe bacteria. (The Bettmann Archive, Inc.)

he held this position for 39 years. He was successful, even though he had little formal education and could speak and write only in Dutch.

Leeuwenhoek developed the ability to grind lenses from glass and to mount them into brass contraptions (Figure 1–3) that he called microscopes. Samples placed on an adjustable needle were viewed from the opposite side by looking through the lens. This hobby fascinated Leeuwenhoek; he spent the greater part of his long life making microscopes, observing the microscopic world, and keeping detailed records of his observations in simple, unsophisticated language. When he was finally asked to communicate his observations to the Royal Society in London, he responded:

I have oft-times been besought by divers gentlemen, to set down on paper what I have beheld through my

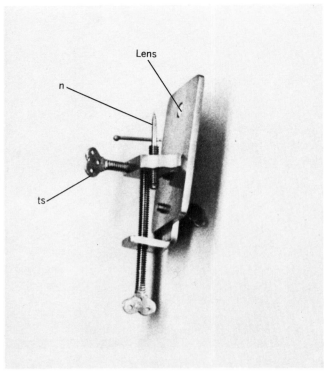

FIGURE 1—3

Anton van Leeuwenhoek ground his own lenses and mounted them in brass microscopes. Specimens are placed on the needle (n) and manipulated by the three thumbscrews (ts) of this replica of a Leeuwenhoek microscope.

newly invented microscopia: but I have generally declined; first because I have no style, or pen wherewith to express my thoughts properly; secondly, because I have not been brought up to languages or arts, but only to business, and in the third place, because I do not gladly suffer contradiction or censure from others. This resolve of mine however, I have now set aside at the entreaty of Dr. Reg. de Graaf and I gave him a memoir on what I have noticed about mould, the sting and sundry little limbs of the bee and also about the sting of the louse.

Leeuwenhoek attached this unsophisticated, humble message to his first communication to the Society. Many letters followed describing all kinds of microscopic things. The eighteenth letter, sent to the Society on October 9, 1676, is the famous "Letter on the Protozoa." It contains the first reported observations on protozoa and bacteria. Leeuwenhoek had looked at water samples from the freshwater river Maas, well water, rainwater, and seawater. He called the creatures that he observed under his microscope "animalcules" and compared their size to the eye of a louse or a grain of fine sand. His descriptions were so accurate that we can identify, among the animalcules he saw, *Daphnia* and *Vorticella*. In many of his observations he referred to organisms that were barely discernible, although he was able to describe them in remarkable detail.

Pepper infusions and the discovery of bacteria

Leeuwenhoek attempted to discover the reason for the hot taste of pepper. He mixed pepper grains with 3-year-old snow water and, at first, saw no living creatures. On the tenth day, he observed bacteria for the first time and commented:

I discovered very many exceedingly small animalcules. Their body seemed, to my eye, as long as broad. Their motion was very slow and oft times roundabout . . .

Nineteen days later, while observing the same pepper water, he wrote:

I saw still more of the oval animalcules and some of the most exceeding thin little tubes, which I had also seen many a time before this.

Here is an even later observation on the pepper water.

The same day, I discovered some very little round animalcules that were about 8 times as big as the smallest animalcules of all. These had so swift a motion before the eye, as they darted among the others that 'tis not to be believed.

Bacteria were discovered by the persistent and detailed observations of this remarkable Dutchman. For 50 years, Leeuwenhoek made scientific observations and reported them in writings to the Royal Society, of which he was made a full member in 1680 following his nomination by Robert Hooke. Among Leeuwenhoek's most publicized observations was the description of bacteria from the human mouth (Figure 1–4), contained in a letter dated in 1683. He described rod-shaped bacteria, sphere-shaped cocci, and spiral-shaped spirochetes.

Many of his observations went unconfirmed for years because no one was able to make microscopes of the quality needed to observe bacteria. Anton van Leeuwenhoek was very possessive of his microscopes and the technology needed to make them. Nobody was permitted to have one of his microscopes until just before his death, when he instructed his only child, Maria, to send 100 microscopes to the Royal Society in London. Apparently, nobody had the determination to follow in his shoes, and the science of microbiology was dormant for many years after his death.

FIGURE 1–4

Bacteria from the human mouth as sketched by Anton van Leeuwenhoek. (From Clifford Dobell, ed. and transl., *Antony Van Leeuwenhoek and His "Little Animals,"* 1932. Reissued with a new introduction by Cornelis B. van Niel, Russell & Russell, New York, 1958.)

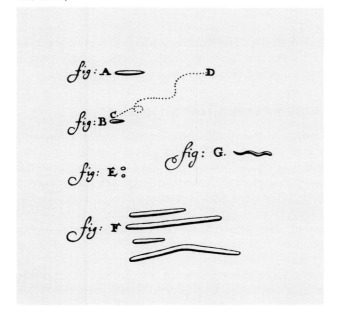

MICROBIOLOGY IN THE EIGHTEENTH CENTURY

Even though eighteenth-century biology was dominated by the struggle over the larger question of spontaneous generation (see next section), individuals did speculate on the relationship between microorganisms and disease. An Italian physician, M. A. Plenciz, proposed that all diseases were caused by microorganisms. Since no evidence was presented to support this theory, Plenciz's views were largely ignored. In 1720, Benjamin Martin published a book, *A New Theory of Consumptions: More Especially of Phthisis or Consumption of the Lungs,* which proposed that consumption (tuberculosis) was caused by animalcules transferred from infected people to others and then transmitted by blood to the lungs, that these animalcules were especially suited for growth in the lungs, and that other animalcules were responsible for other human illnesses, such as venereal disease. Clearly, Martin did not believe in spontaneous generation; on the contrary, he believed that all living creatures must be produced from an egg. Science has ignored the speculations of Martin and Plenciz mainly because they presented no evidence to support their theories. The experimental evidence needed to prove the infectious nature of certain diseases was not forthcoming for more than 100 years.

SPONTANEOUS GENERATION

Scientists and philosophers were in deep disagreement over the controversial concept of **spontaneous generation** (also known as **abiogenesis**). Many people living in the seventeenth and eighteenth centuries believed in the ability of living creatures to arise from nonliving matter such as dead animals, meats, or broths made from meats, hay, or gravy. Abiogenesis is not inconsistent with the biblical rendition of our earth's creation and was supported by many theologians. However, many experimentalists believed that living creatures originated only from ova or from living creatures.

Francesco Redi (1626–1697) was an Italian priest who pondered the question of abiogenesis. Redi was interested in how maggots develop in unprotected meat. He placed linen cloths over jars containing fresh pieces of meat and observed that flies, attracted to the meat, laid their eggs on the cloth. Maggots later developed on the cloth, but not in the meat. These simple experiments showed that maggots grow from fly eggs and are not able to develop spontaneously from meat.

Another Italian priest, Lazzaro Spallanzani (1729–1799), lived a century after Redi and was a contemporary of the devout English priest John Needham (1713–1781). These two individuals took opposite sides in the controversy over spontaneous generation.

Needham was a proponent of spontaneous generation and performed experiments to support his position. He first corked and then heated flasks of

FIGURE 1–5

Lazzara Spallanzani (1729–1799). (Courtesy of the National Library of Medicine.)

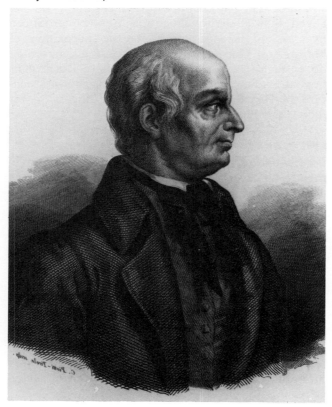

mutton gravy. The flasks were cooled and periodically observed microscopically for organisms. Needham observed microorganisms in all his flasks and claimed that they arose spontaneously from the mutton gravy.

Spallanzani (Figure 1–5) was deeply troubled by the inconsistency of Needham's and Redi's results and set out to do his own investigation. He set up two series of flasks: one was sealed at the top by melting the glass; the other was corked as Needham had done. The flasks were filled with seeds and vegetable matter and then heated for 1 hour before being sealed. Spallanzani set them aside for some time before he microscopically investigated their contents. The corked flasks contained a myriad of swimming animalcules, just as Needham had claimed. However, the flasks that were sealed with glass contained few animalcules. Spallanzani concluded that the animalcules in Needham's corked flasks entered from the air and that this would not happen if the flask was sealed by melting its glass top. Animalcules do not exist that can survive boiling for 1 hour, Spallanzani explained. This explanation did not satisfy the proponents of spontaneous generation, and some were quick to discredit Spallanzani's experiments. They charged that organisms need air to grow, so they were unable to grow in his sealed flasks. The controversy of abiogenesis lasted well into the middle of the 1800s, when Pasteur finally settled this basic biological question.

LOUIS PASTEUR (1822–1895)

Science in the nineteenth century was making great advances in chemistry and physics, and it was natural that Louis Pasteur (Figure 1–6) was educated in these disciplines. Pasteur entered school in Paris to study chemistry. His first major contribution was the discovery of optically different forms of organic molecules. His knowledge of organic molecules soon led him into discussions with Theodor Schwann. Schwann had elegantly demonstrated (1837) that yeasts were responsible for the formation of alcohol in wine and beer fermentations. This discovery was even more remarkable because it was contradictory to the chemical theory presented by Justin Liebig, a

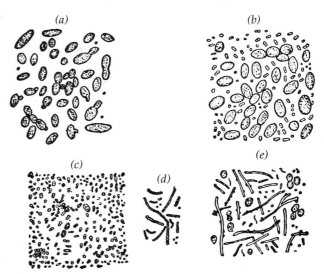

FIGURE 1—7
Diseases of wines. Pasteur observed different organisms in wines as they turned "bad": *(a)* yeast fermentation, *(b)* acid wine in an early stage, *(c)* acid wine in a later stage, *(d)* ropy wine, and *(e)* bitter wine. (From S. J. Holmes, *Louis Pasteur,* 1924, Dover, New York, reissued 1961.)

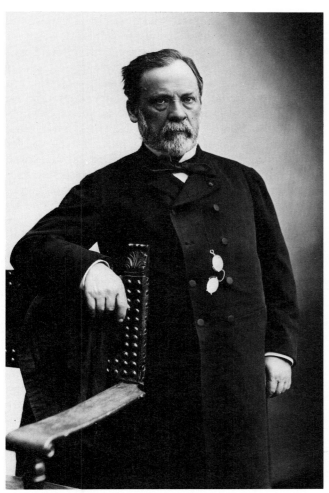

FIGURE 1—6
Louis Pasteur (1822—1895) was one of the great nineteenth-century microbiologists. (The Bettmann Archive, Inc.)

respected chemist. Liebig had proposed that fermentations were the result of the normal chemical decomposition of organic matter.

Pasteur was attracted to this controversy and investigated many different fermentations. He noticed that yeasts were present in all fermentations that resulted in the production of alcohol. When lactic acid or butyric acid was produced, the ferments contained organisms in addition to the yeasts (Figure 1–7). Even when wine turned "bad," rod-shaped or-

ganisms appeared in addition to the presence of the yeast. Pasteur concluded that the sugar of the ferment served as a food for the microorganisms. He professed that each ferment is caused by a specific organism that develops and grows only when the special requirements for its well-being are met. Pasteur set up a defined medium with sugar and salts and showed that the sugar was converted by the yeast into alcohol or cell material and that the nitrogen of the cells was derived from the ammonium salts. These remarkable conclusions supported Schwann's experiments (which had been largely ignored) and also laid the basis for the study of microbial physiology.

Aerobic and anaerobic growth

Aerobic is the term used to describe a process that takes place in the presence of oxygen. Since plants and animals require oxygen for growth, scientists in the middle of the nineteenth century assumed that microorganisms also require oxygen. However, observations of the organisms responsible for the butyric fermentation convinced Pasteur that life also exists and thrives in the absence of oxygen. Not only did these motile organisms lose their motility as they came into contact with air, but Pasteur demonstrated that their butyric fermentation was inhibited by oxygen. He coined the term **anaerobic** to describe organisms that grow in the absence of oxygen.

Pasteur's brilliance, combined with his knowledge of fermentation, catapulted him into the controversy of spontaneous generation. He reasoned that each ferment is caused by a given microbe; therefore, if you prevent the entrance of microbes into a flask of suitable broth, no growth should ensue provided that the broth was adequately heated. Pasteur heated flasks of broth and placed gun cotton on the tops of the flasks. This, he reasoned, would allow the free passage of air into the flask, a condition necessary to overcome Needham's criticisms of Spallanzani's experiments. Indeed, the flasks remained clear until the cotton was removed. Pasteur went a step further and invented the swan-necked flask (Figure 1–8). This flask allows the unencumbered passage of air into the flask while all dust particles and contaminants settle in the bend of the flask's neck. Heated flasks of this type remained clear and free of ferments until Pasteur broke the neck off. Flasks with broken necks turned cloudy within a few

FIGURE 1–8
Pasteur used swan-necked flasks to disprove the theory of spontaneous generation.

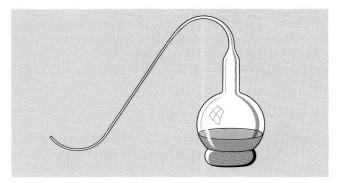

days. Pasteur explained that organisms capable of causing ferments exist in the air. When precautions were taken to prevent organisms from falling into a broth, ferments did not take place. By opening large numbers of flasks in different places—mountains, lakes, attics, cellars—and immediately resealing the flasks, Pasteur showed that the number of organisms in different air samples varied from place to place.

Pasteur's assumption that boiling broths for 1 hour would kill all living microbes was incorrect. This fact allowed proponents of spontaneous generation to attack Pasteur's experiments as they had attacked Spallanzani's experiments 100 years earlier. Indeed, some microbes in hay infusion were not killed by boiling the hay for 1 hour. For this reason, the beautiful experiments of Pasteur succeeded with yeast extract broths; they did not work with broths made from hay.

The English physicist John Tyndall was the first to explain this inconsistency. Tyndall recognized the presence of thermal-resistant, resting forms of bacteria that we call **spores.** Spores can change into growing forms when placed in an appropriate medium. Tyndall showed that by alternately heating and incubating hay infusion broths, all the spore forms change during incubation to growing forms of bacteria. The growing forms are killed during the heating process. Alternate cycles of heating and growth ultimately killed all forms of bacteria in the infusions; this is called **Tyndallization.**

The experiments of Tyndall and Pasteur laid to rest the theory of spontaneous generation. The concept that life could arise from inert material in a flask during a demonstrable period of time has not seriously been questioned since. Today there are theories concerning the origin of life in the universe that employ the concept of spontaneous generation. However, these theories propose the initiation of life as occurring under greatly different conditions from those that now exist on the earth. So the theory of spontaneous generation in organic infusions was conclusively disproved. This laid the groundwork for the discoveries of microorganisms as causative agents of diseases.

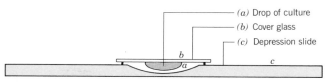

FIGURE 1–10
Robert Koch used the hanging drop technique to observe the growth of anthrax bacteria in fluid taken from the eye of an ox.

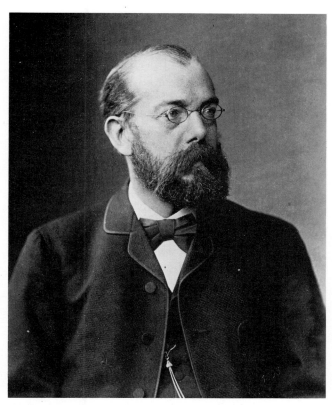

FIGURE 1–9
Robert Koch (1843–1910), the German microbiologist who experimentally demonstrated that anthrax is caused by a bacterium. (Culver Pictures.)

ROBERT KOCH AND ANTHRAX

Anthrax is a disease of sheep, cattle, and humans that caused extensive loss of life and property in the nineteenth century. Robert Koch (1843–1910) was a German country doctor who was intent on solving the problem of anthrax (Figure 1–9). Koch observed, in blood from sheep that died of anthrax, threads of rod-shaped organisms that were not present in healthy sheep. Desiring to study this disease and not having funds to purchase a flock of sheep, Koch injected the blood from the dead sheep into a mouse. The mouse died. The autopsy revealed diseased tissue and rods present in the mouse's blood. Koch tried to grow these rods in all types of broths.

Finally, he was able to grow them in a hanging drop slide (Figure 1–10) in the aqueous humor from an ox's eye. This amazing feat was the first time a disease organism was purposely cultivated outside of its host. Koch then took these organisms from the hanging drop and inoculated them into healthy mice. These mice also died. The dead mice again contained the rod-shaped bacteria. These experiments logically proved that microorganisms can cause infectious disease. Koch's classic experiment with anthrax is now summarized as **Koch's postulates:**

1. The microorganism must be demonstrable in all cases of the disease.
2. The microorganism must be isolated from the diseased animal and grown in pure culture.
3. The microorganism from this pure culture must cause the same disease when inoculated into a healthy animal.
4. The experimentally infected animal must contain the microorganism.

Robert Koch became the leader of the German School of Microbiology in Berlin. With his assistants, Loeffler and Gaffky, he discovered more bacteria that cause human disease and contributed greatly to the techniques of microbiology.

Pure cultures

Technical advances in obtaining pure cultures of bacteria rapidly followed Koch's work with anthrax. Koch noticed that the flat surface of an unrefrigerated boiled potato developed spots of different colors. Microscopic observation of material from these spots revealed the presence of bacteria. One spot contained **rods,** one was composed of the spherical cells known as **cocci,** and a third contained **spiral-shaped** cells. The chance physical separation of contaminating microbes on the potato surface permitted the growth of a single cell into a **colony** of many progeny cells. From these observations, techniques were developed that enabled microbe hunters to isolate pure cultures of microorganisms. Soon gelatin was used to solidify liquid media. In 1881, Dr. Walter Hesse and his wife Fanny Hesse introduced another solidifying agent. Fanny Hesse had used agar, a polysaccharide found in brown algae, to harden jelly. Agar turned out to be an ideal solidifying agent for microbiology media. By the middle of the 1880s, scientists were armed with the techniques of pure cultures and the concept of Koch's postulates. The search was on for the causative agents of disease.

MICROORGANISMS AND DISEASE

Many of the bacterial diseases that afflict humans were discovered between 1877 and 1900. A summary of these diseases is presented in Table 1–1. Note that the name of a microorganism is often derived from the name of its discoverer. For example, the human intestinal organism is called *Escherichia* after its discoverer Theodor Escherich. Not only were many of the causative agents of disease discovered during this time, but great strides were also made in preventing disease. Pasteur (1880) developed a method of attenuating the vibrio (comma-shaped organism) that caused cholera in chickens. He demonstrated that aged cultures of the cholera vibrio caused only a mild sickness in chickens. The same chickens subsequently resisted injections of disease-causing cholera organisms. Pasteur also developed a procedure for producing a vaccine against rabies. Elie Metchnikoff, in 1884, described the phagocytic action of blood cells engulfing foreign particles. During this period, Emil Roux discovered the **toxin** responsible for the symptoms of diphtheria, and he established that the toxin was produced by the bacterium *Corynebacterium diphtheriae*. Shortly after Roux's discovery, Emil A. Behring developed a means to inactivate the toxin. The inactivated toxin, called a **toxoid,** was used to immunize people against diphtheria. By the end of the nineteenth century, microbiology was an established science that had a great potential for helping humanity.

TABLE 1–1
Discovery of Major Bacteria Associated with Human Diseases

Disease	Organism	Discoverer	Year Reported
Anthrax	*Bacillus anthracis*	Robert Koch	1877
Gonorrhea	*Neisseria gonorrhoeae*	Albert Neisser	1879
Pyogenic infections	*Staphylococcus aureus*	Alexander Ogston	1881
Tuberculosis	*Mycobacterium tuberculosis*	Robert Koch	1882
Erysipelas	*Streptococcus pyogenes*	Friedrich Fehleisen	1882
Diphtheria	*Corynebacterium diphtheriae*	Theodor Klebs	1883
Tetanus	*Clostridium tetani*	Arthur Nicolaier	1884
Cholera	*Vibrio cholerae*	Robert Koch	1884
Typhoid fever	*Salmonella typhi*	Georg Gaffky	1884
Brucellosis	*Brucella melitensis*	David Bruce	1887
Gastroenteritis	*Salmonella enteritidis*	August Gaertner	1888
Gas gangrene	*Clostridium perfringens*	William Welch	1892
Bubonic plague	*Yersinia pestis*	Alexandre Yersin	1894
Botulism	*Clostridium botulinum*	Emile van Ermengem	1897
Dysentery	*Shigella dysenteriae*	Kiyoshi Shiga	1898

VIRAL DISEASES

Not all infectious diseases can be attributed to an invasion of free-living microorganisms. Some diseases resisted the approach of Koch because they are caused by viruses that are unable to grow on artificial media. **Viruses** are very small agents that are obligate intracellular parasites. Adolf Mayer was the first person to describe the infectious nature of a viral disease. He demonstrated (1886) that tobacco mosaic was an infectious viral disease. Another major breakthrough in virology occurred when D. Ivanovski discovered (1892) that tobacco mosaic virus (TMV) was a filterable agent. Loeffler and Frosch soon discovered that the causative agent of foot-and-mouth disease was also filterable. This was the first known animal virus to be described as passing through a filter. The ability to work with animal virus increased greatly following the development of tissue culture techniques during the 1950s (see Chapter 22).

CELL THEORY

Living systems are organized into the basic compartmentalized structure called a *cell*. Robert Hooke was the first to observe and describe compartments in biological material, and he is credited with naming them cells; this occurred before Leeuwenhoek's first letter was written to the Royal Society. Nevertheless, the theory that all living things are composed of cells was not presented until 1838, when Matthias Schleiden proposed that all plants are composed of cells. Theodor Schwann expanded the cell theory by suggesting that all animals are also composed of cells. Today we recognize that all organisms (with the exception of viruses) are organized into cells.* Although the basic structure of life is the cell, cells vary greatly in their morphology. The variations in cell morphology led early investigators to group cells according to their size and shape. These scientists were the first bacterial systematists. They developed

---

*Viruses are noncellular entities that replicate within susceptible living cells to produce a continuous lineage.

the protocol of classifying microorganisms along the classic hierarchy developed by Carolus Linnaeus.

THE BINOMIAL SYSTEM

Carolus Linnaeus (1707–1778) was the first person to develop a shorthand system of naming organisms. He classified plants by describing them and categorizing them into species. A **species** comprises those organisms that are morphologically the same and that can reproduce their own kind. Linnaeus's system described each organism with a latinized name consisting of two words. This binominal system is still in use today. The first word indicates the taxonomic group, or **genus** (pl., genera), to which a species belongs. The second word is the specific epithet (adjective or modifier) that defines a specific species of the genus. The proper name of a species is printed in italics, and the first letter of the genus is capitalized.

Vibrio cholerae is the name of the comma-shaped organism (vibrio) that causes cholera. The use of the generic name, *Vibrio,* refers to this and all other similar vibriod microorganisms. The epithet (cholerae) modifies the genus name and designates a specific type of *Vibrio,* namely, *Vibrio cholerae.* Note that the epithet (Table 1–1) can also be the name of a disease and that these names can vary in spelling: *B. anthracis,* anthrax; *Cl. tetani,* tetanus; *Cl. botulinum,* botulism. The binomial nomenclature enables microbiologists to name organisms and to define them in a systematic manner. *Bergey's Manual of Determinative Bacteriology* (8th edition) is the reference book for the classification of bacteria.

The study of systematics goes one step further and organizes all organisms into a hierarchy based on their interrelatedness. The earliest attempts to classify bacteria were published in 1786 by Otto F. Muller. From this early beginning, the systematics of bacteria continues as a dynamic field of endeavor in a constant state of change because of an increasing knowledge of bacteria and their relationships to other organisms (see Chapter 8 for a complete discussion). The major groups of microorganisms, however, appear to be well established, and it is appropriate to mention them here as a means of further introduction to the world of microorganisms.

THE MICROBIAL WORLD

Small cellular organisms and viruses comprise the microbial world. Systematists recognize five major groups among microorganisms: viruses, bacteria, protozoa, algae, and fungi. Viruses are the only noncellular living organisms. Bacteria, protozoa, algae, and fungi are cellular microorganisms that exist as single cells or as aggregates of undifferentiated cells.

Microscopists can readily distinguish between two types of cells: those that contain a nucleus and those that lack a nucleus (Figure 1–11). There appear to be only two major types of cells* on the earth. We call cells with a nucleus **eucaryotes** (*eu* means "true"; *karyon* means "nucleus") and cells without a nucleus, **procaryotes** (*pro* means "before"). All bacteria have the procaryotic cell structure. All other organisms have cell structures in the eucaryotic arrangement.

Eucaryotic and procaryotic cells differ in a number of distinctive characteristics (Table 1–2). Differences occur in the number and structure of chromosomes, the chemical structure of the cell wall, the mechanism of motility, the structure of the cytoplasm, and

*Methanogens may represent an exception (Chapter 3).

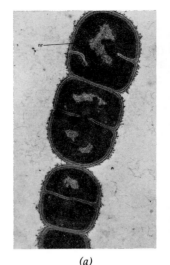
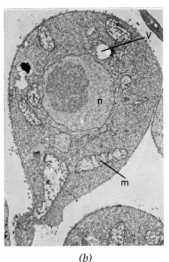

(a) *(b)*

FIGURE 1–11
Transmission electron micrographs of *(a)* a cross section of the bacterium *Caryophanon latum* showing the bacterial nuclear material localized in the nuclear region (nr). (Courtesy of Dr. R. K. Nauman.) *(b)* A cross section of the fungus *Blastocladiella emersonii* showing its membrane-bound nucleus (n), vacuoles (v), and mitochondria (m). (Courtesy of Dr. J. S. Lovett. From J. S. Lovett, *Bacteriol. Revs.*, 39:345–404, 1975, with permission of the American Society for Microbiology.)

the morphology of the membranes involved in respiration and photosynthesis. A more complete discussion of cytology is presented in Chapter 3.

TABLE 1–2
Organisms and Their Cell Type

Cell Type	Organisms	Distinctive Characteristics
Procaryotes	Bacteria (Cyanobacteria are considered to be bacteria)	Nuclear region, one chromosome, complex cell wall, simple flagella, division—binary fission or budding
Eucaryotes	(a) Algae, protozoa, fungi (microorganisms) (b) Plants and animals (macroorganisms containing differentiated tissue)	Membrane-bound nucleus, more than one chromosome, chloroplasts (plants only), mitochondria, complex flagella, chemically simple cell walls (when present), division—mitosis

Plants, animals, and many microorganisms have the eucaryotic cell structure. Most plants and animals are easily recognized as such and are classified in the kingdom **Planta** or **Animalia.** The eucaryotic microorganisms do not easily fit into these kingdoms because many of them share characteristics of both plants and animals. To deal with this perplexing problem, E. M. Haeckel proposed in 1866 that protozoa, algae, fungi, and bacteria be placed in a third kingdom, which he called **Protista.** Now that the bacteria are known to have a distinctive cell structure, they are separated from the other Protista and classified in a fourth kingdom, **Procaryotae.**

Procaryotae

Bacteria are the simplest cellular organisms known. They are greatly diversified in their size, shape, and means of gaining energy; yet they all have the procaryotic cell structure. Bacteria are distinctly unicellular organisms. Only rarely do bacteria aggregate in an organized manner. Recently, the procaryotic photosynthetic organisms that produce oxygen have been named the cyanobacteria (in *Bergey's Manual*) and grouped with the bacteria. Previously, they were called the *Cyanophyta* and were classified with the eucaryotic algae. Now all cells with the procaryotic cellular structure are classified as bacteria.

Protista

Protozoa are the eucaryotic unicellular animals. Protozoa are usually larger than bacteria and often feed on bacteria. Examples of protozoa are *Paramecium* and *Amoeba* (Figure 1–12). Some protozoa that cause disease in humans are described in Chapter 28.

Microorganisms with plantlike characteristics are divided into two groups: the nonphotosynthetic organisms are known as the **fungi,** and the photosynthetic organisms are known as **algae** (Figure 1–13). Fungi are a diversified group of nonphotosynthetic eucaryotic cells that are classified by their mode of sexual and asexual reproduction. Morphologically, this group is extremely diverse and includes such organisms as the yeasts—the organisms responsible for alcoholic fermentation—the mushrooms, and the

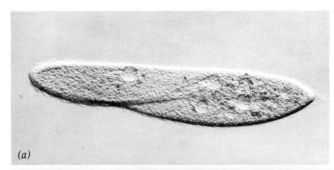

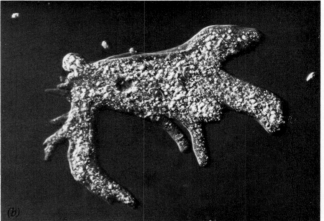

FIGURE 1–12
Micrographs of *(a) Paramecium* and *(b) Amoeba proteus,* two examples of unicellular, eucaryotic microorganisms. (Courtesy of Carolina Biological Supply Co.)

toadstools. The molds (Figure 1–1) seen by Hooke are also fungi. Certain fungi (as described in Chapter 27) cause disease in humans.

Algae are unicellular or multicellular eucaryotic cells. Nearly all algae are photosynthetic. Certain algae produce toxins that affect humans. The red tide dinoflagellate, *Gonyaulax catanella,* produces a potent nerve toxin that concentrates in shellfish and poisons humans who eat the shellfish. Most algae, however, are harmless to human health.

MICROSCOPY

Microscopy is just as important to modern microbiologists as it was to Anton van Leeuwenhoek. The

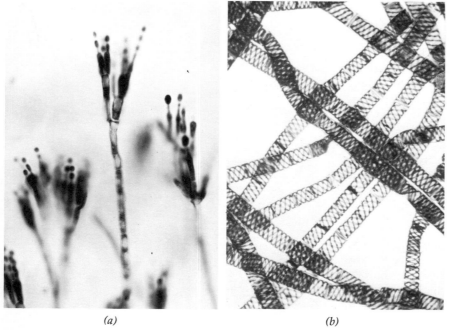

(a) *(b)*

FIGURE 1–13
Light micrographs of two eucaryotes: *(a)* the fungus *Penicillium,* and *(b)* the freshwater algae *Spirogyra. Penicillium* has spores at the tips of its hyphae; *Spirogyra* has spiral chloroplasts in each cell. (Photographs courtesy of *(a)* the Carolina Biological Supply Company, and *(b)* Hugh Spencer.)

development of new microscopes and of new microscopic techniques continues to expand the ability to visualize microbial structures.

Basic microscopy centers around the **light microscope** (Figure 1–14). The typical light microscope is composed of a condenser lens that collects the light rays and focuses them on the specimen; an objective lens that collects the light coming from the specimen; and an ocular lens that, together with the objective lens, magnifies the image. Such an instrument is called a **compound microscope,** since it is composed of multiple lenses. Each objective lens differs in its ability to magnify and in the degree to which it distorts the image of the specimen. Typical objectives are labeled as 20X, 40X, and 100X. When combined with a 10X ocular lens the total magnifications are 200X, 400X, and 1000X, respectively. Lenses can be specially ground to correct for **spherical aberration,** which is the inability to focus on the

entire field, and they can be corrected for color distortion, which is termed **chromatic aberration.**

Resolution is the ability of the human eye to distinguish two dots placed a specified distance apart. The resolving power of a microscope depends on the wavelength of light used and the **numerical aperture** (NA) of the objective lenses. The numerical aperture ($N \sin \theta$) is a measure of the ability of the objective lens to capture light. The larger the numerical aperture, the better (lower) the resolving power. These parameters are related by the mathematical definition of the resolving power (*d*)

$$d = \frac{0.5\,\lambda}{\text{numerical aperture}}$$

where λ is the wavelength of light. Scientists use the metric system for measuring distances and sizes. The wavelength of light is measured in nanometers

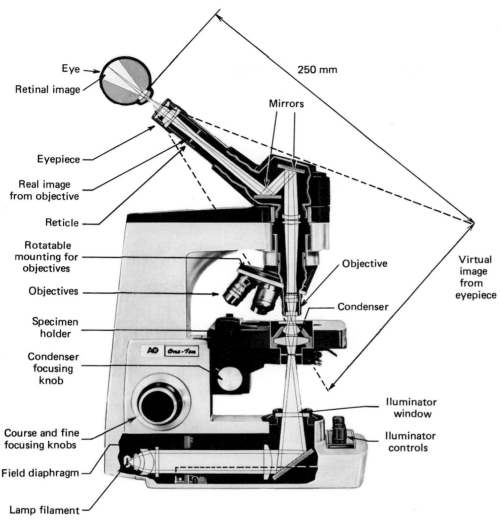

FIGURE 1–14
The light microscope is the basic tool of the microbiologist. Magnifications of up to 1000X and a resolution of 0.2 micrometers can be attained with the light microscope. (Courtesy of American Optical.)

(nm) (Table 1–3). Green light has a λ = 500 nm. Therefore, the limit of resolution using green light with an objective lens with a numerical aperture of 1.25 would be 200 nm (0.5 × 500 nm/1.25 = 200 nm). Note that 1000 nm is equal to 1 micrometer (μm); therefore, the resolution of the light microscope is 0.2 μm. Most bacteria have dimensions be-

tween 0.5 and 1.0 × 1 to 4 μm. The shapes of these bacteria (Figure 1–15) can be seen in the bright-field microscope. Bacteria are close to the limit of the resolving power of the light microscope, so few internal structures or appendages are visible without special stains. This is true even when a high power objective is used.

TABLE 1–3
Metric Units of Measure

Linear Measure[a] Metric	Relative Size
1 meter (m)	39.37 inches = 1 meter
1 centimeter (cm)	1/100 of a meter or 10^{-2} meters
1 millimeter (mm)	1/1000 of a meter or 10^{-3} meters
1 micrometer (μm)	1/1,000,000 of a meter or 10^{-6} meters
1 nanometer (nm)	1/1,000,000,000 of a meter or 10^{-9} meters
1 angstrom (Å)	1/10,000,000,000 of a meter or 10^{-10} meters

Volume Measure[b] Metric	Relative Capacity
1 liter (l)	0.2642 gallon
1 milliliter (ml)	1/1000 of a liter
1 microliter (μl)	1/1,000,000 of a liter

[a]Most microorganisms are measured in micrometers because their largest dimension is often only one millionth of a meter. One micrometer (sometimes called a micron) is near the limit of resolution by the light microscope. Transmission electron microscopy is capable of resolving structures that are 5 to 8 Å in size. Atoms and bond lengths between atoms are around 1 to 3 Å. Only the largest atoms have been seen in the electron microscope.

[b]The volume of a typical bacterial cell is estimated to be approximately 1 to 2×10^{-13} ml.

Modification of the light microscope has improved its usefulness to microbiologists. Inserting oil between the specimen and the objective lens increases the numerical aperture of the objective lens and allows the observer to see dots or points that are closer together. Most microscopes in microbiology laboratories contain one oil immersion lens which is designated 100X oil NA 1.25. Modification of the light passing to the specimen and thence into the objective lens can change the contrast but not the magnification or the resolution of the specimen. The simple light microscope can be used as a phase-

FIGURE 1–15
The light microscope can be used to distinguish bacterial cell shapes: *(a)* cocci, *(b)* rods, and *(c)* spirilla. (From R. Y. Stanier, *The Microbial World*, 3rd ed., Prentice-Hall, Englewood Cliffs, N.J., 1970.)

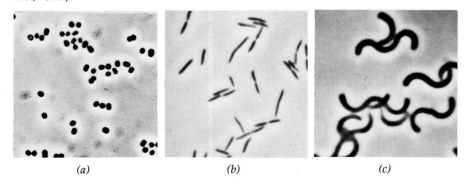

(a)   *(b)*   *(c)*

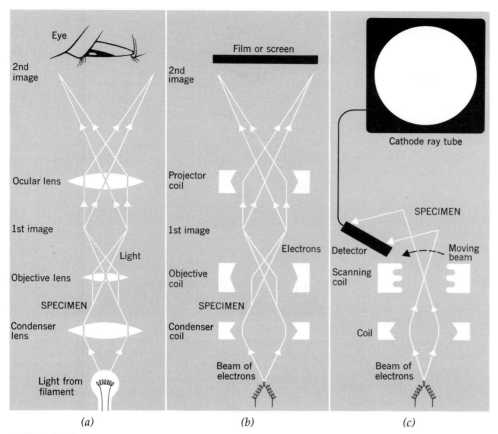

FIGURE 1–16

Diagrammatic comparison of *(a)* light microscope, *(b)* transmission electron microscope (TEM), and *(c)* scanning electron microscope (SEM). The light microscope uses glass lenses for focusing the light rays, which pass through a specimen, into a real image that can be seen by the human eye. The TEM *(b)* uses magnets to focus its electron beam. The electrons pass through the specimen before they are focused on an electron-sensitive plate to form an image that can be visualized or photographed. The SEM *(c)* scans the surface of a specimen with electron beams. Deflected electrons are collected by a detector, which sends signals to a cathode ray tube (television screen) on which an image is produced. (From G. Stephens and B. North, *Biology*, Wiley, New York, 1974.)

contrast microscope or as a dark-field microscope when the appropriate lenses and condensers are employed.

Electron microscopes use an electron beam as the source of energy for visualizing the specimen (Figure 1–16). An electron beam has a very small wavelength (0.04 nm), so the observer is able to resolve structures as small as 5 to 8 Å in size. This size is at the upper limit of large atoms that have only been visualized under extremely rare circumstances. However, it is possible to observe macromolecules such as proteins and nucleic acids using electron microscopy (Figures 2–9 and 5–8).

Living material cannot be viewed under the **transmission electron microscope**. The source of electrons in an electron microscope must be kept under low vacuum similar to the tungsten filament in a light bulb. All samples observed in an electron microscope must therefore be dried. Furthermore, it is necessary to stain samples placed in the electron microscope to increase the contrast. Specimens are prepared by fixing, staining, embedding, and then sectioning them on an ultramicrotome to obtain thin slices. The electron beam, after it passes through the thin section of the specimen, can be focused on a viewing screen. Transmission electron micrographs are made by exposing this electron image on a photographic plate (Figure 1–11).

Remarkable three-dimensional pictures of biological specimens (Figure 1–17) can now be obtained used **scanning electron microscopy** (SEM). The biological specimen is first coated with a thin layer of gold or silver. An electron probe scans the specimen in a standard pattern. Electronic devices collect the electrons emitted from the sample and then display the pattern on a cathode ray tube. This electronic collector picks up secondary electrons emitted from the sample. The topology of the sample is revealed in high contrast because the number of secondary electrons that reach the collector is proportional to the angle between the electron beam and the surface of the specimen. Scanning electron microscopy is used to visualize surfaces of the specimen. The degree of magnification is only 10 times greater than that obtained with the light microscope, so SEM is used to observe surface structures at low magnification.

Each microscope has its particular advantages. The light microscope can be used to observe living cells. Transmission electron microscopy has the best resolving power and is used to visualize subcellular structures and macromolecules. Scanning electron microscopy is used to observe surface structures. The ability to visualize the structure of microorganisms depends largely on microscopic techniques; whereas the ability to understand the function of those structures depends on a comprehension of basic chemical principles. Before we integrate the structural and functional features of microorganisms (Chapter 3), it is appropriate to review the basic concepts of chemistry relevant to biological systems (Chapter 2).

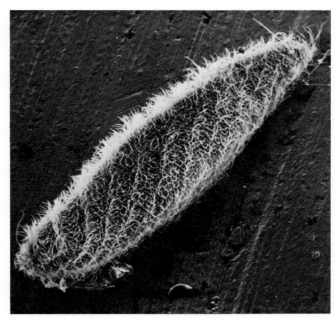

FIGURE 1–17

A scanning electron micrograph of *Paramecium* showing the numerous external cilia. (Photo by E. Vivier, from *Paramecium*, W. J. Wagtendonk, ed., Elsevier North-Holland Bio-Medical, New York, 1974.)

SUMMARY

Classical microbiology began in the middle of the 1600s when the English scientist Hooke and the Dutch draper Leeuwenhoek observed microorganisms through their homemade microscopes. Little progress was made in the field of microbiology during the eighteenth century because science turned its attention to physics and chemistry. Microbiology blossomed in the latter half of the nineteenth century. Pasteur, Koch, Tyndall, and many others laid the groundwork for the study of microbial physiology, pathogenic bacteriology, immunology, and virology. Most of the major bacterial diseases of the human race were discovered during the two decades beginning in 1880. These discoveries marked a turning point for microbiology and for the welfare of humanity. No scientific discipline develops in a vacuum, so it must be recognized that concepts in related sciences, and in technology, played a major role in the development of microbiology as a science. Classification and the binomial system of nomenclature came from botany; microscopy as a technical achievement developed from physical principles; and chemistry contributed a structured body of knowledge that helps us to define and understand life's physiological processes. By no means is the history of microbiology complete. Major advances in microbiology occur almost daily. The concepts presented in the following chapters will help you understand your relationship to microbes. This knowledge will enable you to control those microbes that hurt the human race and to cultivate those microbes that are helpful.

QUESTIONS AND TOPICS FOR STUDY AND DISCUSSION

Questions

1. How small are microorganisms?
2. Name two seventeenth-century microscopists and describe their contributions to microbiology.
3. When were human diseases first demonstrated to be caused by infectious agents? Explain.
4. How was the controversy over spontaneous generation resolved? How did spores enter into this controversy?
5. What is the binomial system of nomenclature? What is a species?
6. What are the major classification groups of microorganisms? Describe the characteristics of each group.
7. Explain the difference between resolution and magnification?
8. What part of a meter is a micrometer, an angstrom, a nanometer? What are the size ranges for bacteria and viruses?
9. Compare the limitations and uses of the scanning electron microscope to the transmission electron microscope.

Discussion

1. Why did microbiology not thrive during the 1700s?
2. What impact did the controversy over spontaneous generation have on microbiology as a science? Explain.

3. What scientific advances led to the discovery of a large number of bacterial diseases during the last 20 years of the nineteenth century?

FURTHER READINGS

Books

Brock, T. D. (ed.), *Milestones in Microbiology,* American Society for Microbiology, Washington, D.C., 1975. Translations and brief commentaries on selected scientific articles by famous microbiologists including Leeuwenhoek, Pasteur, and Koch.

DeKruif, P., *Microbe Hunters,* Harcourt, Brace, New York, 1953. A popularized history of microbiology that describes in a story format the major scientific contributions of a select group of important microbiologists.

Dobell, C., *Antony van Leeuwenhoek and His "Little Animals,"* Russell & Russell, New York, 1958. An introduction to the life and times of Leeuwenhoek. Dobell has translated and reprinted many of Leeuwenhoek's important letters to the Royal Society of London.

Dubos, R., *Louis Pasteur: Free Lance of Science,* Little, Brown, Boston, 1950. One of the better biographies of this famous microbiologist written by a widely respected microbiologist and scholar.

Grimstone, A. V., *The Electron Microscope in Biology,* 2nd ed., Edward Arnold, London, 1976. A short paperback that presents the basic techniques for and applications of the electron microscope.

Hooke, R., *Micrographia,* Royal Society London, 1665. Reproduced Dover, New York, 1961. Hooke's historic monograph that introduced science to the microscopic world.

Singleton, P., and D. Sainsbury, *Dictionary of Microbiology,* Wiley, New York, 1978. An important reference source for definitions and explanations of scientific terms and concepts used in microbiology. The current classification of many microorganisms is presented.

Articles and Reviews

Everhard, T. E., and T. L. Hayes, "The Scanning Electron Microscope," *Sci. Am.,* 226:54–69 (January 1972). An introduction to the technical design and experimental use of the scanning electron microscope.

2

REVIEW OF CHEMICAL PRINCIPLES RELEVANT TO BIOLOGY

Chemistry in the nineteenth century was a science of discovery. During this century scientists described most of the elements and arranged them into the periodic table proposed by Dmitri Mendeleyev, a Russian chemist. The identification of organic compounds kept pace with the discovery of the elements. This chemical information was directly applicable to the studies of microorganisms. The broad training of nineteenth-century biologists in chemistry and physics laid the groundwork for the classic experiments in microbiology. Our knowledge of microorganisms is still dependent on the concepts of physics and chemistry. An understanding of the important chemical principles and their significance to biological systems is an essential foundation for the study of microbiology.

CHEMICAL COMPOSITION

Microorganisms are composed of elements. Approximately 23 of the 92 naturally occurring elements are found in every organism. The elements are arranged into molecules and then into structures according to the laws of chemistry and physics.

The elements present in a typical bacterium are listed in Table 2–1. The major compound in cells is water, which accounts for the high amount of oxygen and hydrogen found in cells. Oxygen and hydrogen are also associated with carbon in molecules classified as **organic** compounds. All organic compounds contain carbon. Certain classes of organic molecules contain nitrogen, phosphorus, and sulfur in various combinations with carbon. Carbon, nitrogen, phosphorus, oxygen, and hydrogen make up more than 99 percent of the elemental composition of cells. Potassium, magnesium, iron, and calcium, and a group of **trace elements** are also found in cells, but their concentration is relatively small.

ATOMS AND MOLECULES

Elements are substances composed entirely of atoms having an invariant nucleus (isotopes are exceptions). Atoms that make up an element are composed of a nucleus surrounded by orbiting electrons (see Figure 2–1). An atomic nucleus is composed of a specific number of **protons,** which are positively charged particles, and a specific number of **neu-**

TABLE 2–1
Elements Found in a Typical Bacterial Cell

Element	Symbol	Atomic Weight	Percent of Cell's Wet Weight
Major Elements			
Oxygen	O	16.0	70.0
Carbon	C	12.0	13.0
Hydrogen	H	1.0	10.0
Nitrogen	N	14.0	5.5
Phosphorus	P	31.0	0.8
Sulfur	S	32.0	0.3
Potassium	K	39.1	0.3
Magnesium	Mg	24.3	0.05
Iron	Fe	55.8	0.01
Calcium	Ca	40.1	0.01
Trace Elements			
Boron	Bo	10.8	
Chlorine	Cl	35.5	
Cobalt	Co	58.9	
Copper	Cu	63.5	
Manganese	Mn	54.9	
Molybdenum	Mo	95.9	
Nickel	Ni	58.7	0.01% of cell's wet weight
Selenium	Se	79.0	
Silicon	Si	28.1	
Sodium	Na	23.0	
Vanadium	V	50.9	
Zinc	Zn	65.4	

trons, which are uncharged (neutral) particles. The **atomic number** is the number of protons in the nucleus. The **atomic weight** of an element is essentially equal to the combined number of protons and neutrons in the atom's nucleus. Electrons weigh $\frac{1}{1837}$ the weight of a proton or neutron, so they are not included in the typical weight calculations.

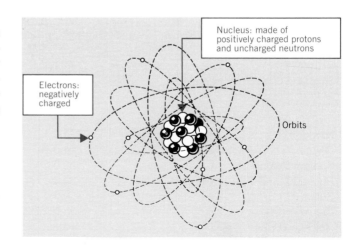

Nucleus: made of positively charged protons and uncharged neutrons

Electrons: negatively charged

Orbits

FIGURE 2–1
Neils Bohr proposed the planetary model of the atom in 1913. This schematic representation of the Bohr atomic model has electrons orbiting about a dense nucleus. The British physicist, Lord Rutherford, is given credit for the concept of the atomic nuclei.

Each element has an atomic weight (see Table 2–1). The element carbon, for example, has an atomic weight of 12. Addition of neutrons to the nucleus of an atom will change the atomic weight of an element. Atoms with the same number of protons, but with a different number of neutrons, are called **isotopes**. Carbon 14 (^{14}C) is an isotope of carbon that has six protons and eight neutrons.

Negatively charged electrons orbit around the positively charged nucleus. Each electron occupies a space referred to as the electron's **orbital**. The concept of electron orbitals was developed by Niels Bohr and can be visualized by comparing an atom to a solar system. The nucleus is the center of this system, which has electrons, analogous to planets, occupying the orbitals (Figure 2–1). Atoms of each element are neutral in charge; therefore, the number of electrons in an atom equals the number of protons.

Electron orbitals are described in mathematical terms, rather than in physical space, since it is impossible to describe the position of an electron at any given instant. Therefore, orbitals are described as the mathematical probability of an electron being found at a set distance from the nucleus. Each electron will possess a specific amount of energy depending on that electron's distance from the nucleus of the atom. Since the electron is restricted in its movement, it is said to occupy an **energy level**. The electron in the energy level closest to the nucleus

has the highest energy. It takes more energy to remove electrons from this first level than to remove electrons from any other level. Each energy level is limited in the number of electrons it can contain. The maximum number of electrons that can be in an energy level (n) is equal to $2 \cdot n^2$. According to this equation, the first level can contain two electrons ($2 \cdot 1^2$), the second level can contain eight ($2 \cdot 2^2$), the third level 18, and so on. The electronic configuration of some biologically important elements is shown in Table 2–2. The number of electrons in neutral atoms is equal to the number of protons in the atom's nucleus. What does this tell you about the nuclei of hydrogen and chlorine?

Ions

Each element tends to fill its outermost energy level with the maximum number of electrons. The reactivity of elements depends mainly on this principle. Some elements readily give up electrons from their outermost shell. Sodium and calcium become positively charged **cations** in solution when each gives up an electron. Sodium gives up an electron in level three to become Na^+, and calcium gives up two electrons in level four to become Ca^{2+}. Notice that the atom becomes positively charged when it loses the negatively charged electron. Other elements accept electrons in order to complete their outer level.

TABLE 2–2
Electronic Configuration of Some Biologically Important Elements

Element	Electro-negativity	Atomic[a] Number	Atomic Weight	Level Numbers, n 1	2	3	4
Hydrogen (H)	2.20	1	1.0	1			
Carbon (C)	2.50	6	12.0	2	4		
Nitrogen (N)	3.07	7	14.0	2	5		
Oxygen (O)	3.50	8	16.0	2	6		
Sodium (Na)	1.01	11	23.0	2	8	1	
Phosphorus (P)	2.06	15	31.0	2	8	5	
Sulfur (S)	2.44	16	32.0	2	8	6	
Chlorine (Cl)	2.83	17	35.0	2	8	7	
Calcium (Ca)	1.04	20	40.1	2	8	8	2

[a]Atomic number is equal to the total number of protons.

Chlorine can accept one electron to complete its outermost electron level with the eighth electron. Chlorine thus becomes a negatively charged ion (Cl^-) and is called an **anion.**

Ionic bonds

Objects with dissimilar charges attract each other. Na^+ and Cl^- ions in solutions will attract each other and, when present in appropriate concentrations, will form crystal structures of sodium chloride (NaCl). When Cl^- and Na^+ interact, the sodium donates an electron to the chloride atom leaving each atom with eight electrons in its outermost orbital. Sodium chloride is the simple molecule that you know as table salt. It is also referred to as an **ionic compound** because it is electrically neutral and is composed of an orderly array of oppositely charged ions. Other examples of ionic compounds are baking soda (sodium bicarbonate, $NaHCO_3$) and lye (sodium hydroxide, NaOH). The attracting force that holds the negatively and positively charged ions in a crystal structure is called an **ionic bond.** Ionic bonds also exist in macromolecules containing ions of opposite charge and are important to the functioning of many biomolecules.

Covalent bonds

Certain elements complete their outermost electron level by sharing electrons with either identical or dissimilar atoms. Chlorine, for example, will form chlorine gas (Cl_2), in which each atom shares one electron to complete the outside ring (Figure 2–2). Likewise, nitrogen atoms share three electrons to form the stable gas dinitrogen (N_2). When electrons

FIGURE 2–2
Covalent bonds are formed between atoms that share electrons. The Bohr model (1) accounts for all the electrons, whereas the electron dot model (2) shows only the outer shell electrons. The shared pair model (3) uses a bar to represent each covalent bond. The orbital model (4) shows the distribution of electrons around each atom.

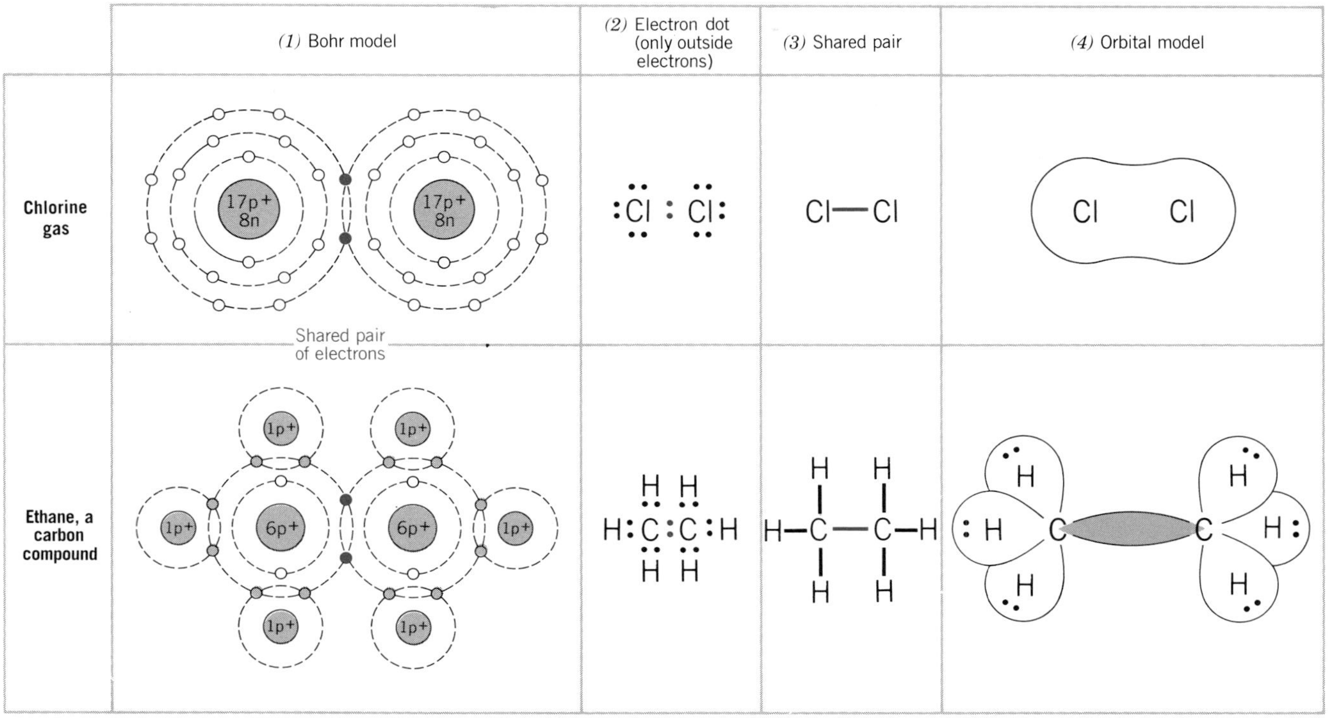

are shared by two atomic nuclei, the attractive force between the two nuclei is called a **covalent bond.** Each bond has a specific amount of energy that resides in the attractive forces between atoms. This bond energy is released when the bond is broken.

Carbon has an atomic number of six; two electrons are in the first energy level and four electrons are in the second energy level. To complete the second energy level's complement of eight electrons ($2n^2$), each carbon atom shares four electrons with other atoms. Stated another way, stable carbon atoms always form four covalent bonds. These bonds can be formed by sharing electrons with hydrogen and adjacent carbon atoms as shown in Figure 2–2. A carbon atom can form covalent bonds with oxygen, nitrogen, phosphorus, sulfur, and, of course, with other carbon atoms. The compounds formed with carbon are extremely varied because the number of possible combinations that result in the formation of stable compounds is immense. There are so many carbon-containing compounds that they are studied as a subdiscipline of chemistry called **organic chemistry.** Organic molecules play a major role in living systems.

Covalent bonds are relatively strong bonds. These bonds do not break down even when heated to the temperature of boiling water. If they did, the turkey placed in an oven at 177°C (350°F)* would break down into a mixture of atoms. Meats are composed of molecules held together by covalent bonds. Although the bond energies vary in strength, they will resist normal cooking temperatures. They will not resist the temperatures of a grease fire or of a wood fire. The charcoal on the end of a marshmallow results from the breaking of covalent bonds in the sugar molecule. The relative strength of the bond energy depends on the atoms involved and the number of covalent bonds formed between the two atoms.

The distance between the two atomic nuclei will

also vary, depending on the atom's attractive forces for electrons. The spacing between the atomic nuclei joined by covalent bonds are shown in Figure 2–3. Note that the distances are shown in nanometers. The strength of a covalent bond can be determined by calculating the amount of heat needed to break that bond. The heat is expressed as kilocalories per mole (kcal/mole) of substance. (A **kilocalorie** is the amount of heat required to raise 1 liter of water 1°C. A mole is the gram molecular weight of the substance in question.)

ELECTRONEGATIVITY

Chemists have developed the concept of electronegativity to explain certain chemical properties. **Electronegativity** is a measure of the ability of an atom in a compound to attract electrons to itself. Each atomic nucleus differentially attracts its own electrons depending on the number of protons in the nucleus and the arrangement of the electrons in their respective energy levels. Certain atoms easily give up electrons, whereas other atoms are more reluctant to give up electrons. An arbitrary scale from 0 to 4 has been established to express numerically this property of atoms called electronegativity. Unreactive elements such as helium are assigned a value of zero, whereas those elements that strongly attract electrons are assigned values near four.

To understand the properties of certain molecules, we can look at the electronegativity of the atoms involved (Table 2–2). In the molecule carbon dioxide (CO_2), oxygen is more electronegative than carbon, so we expect the shared electrons in the covalent bond to be closer to the oxygen atoms than to the carbon nuclei. Indeed this is the case, and we write O≦C≧O with arrows indicating the attractive force of the oxygen nuclei. Since carbon dioxide is a linear molecule, the attraction of the charged shared electrons in the molecule is canceled. Other covalently bound molecules, however, show an uneven distribution of charge; the resulting bonds are called **polar covalent bonds.** Nitrogen is more electronegative than hydrogen. These elements form a polar cova-

---

*Throughout this book we will use the centigrade scale, or Celsius. Conversion from centigrade to Fahrenheit can be approximated by doubling the centigrade number and adding 32. The exact formula for conversion is °F = ⅘ °C + 32.

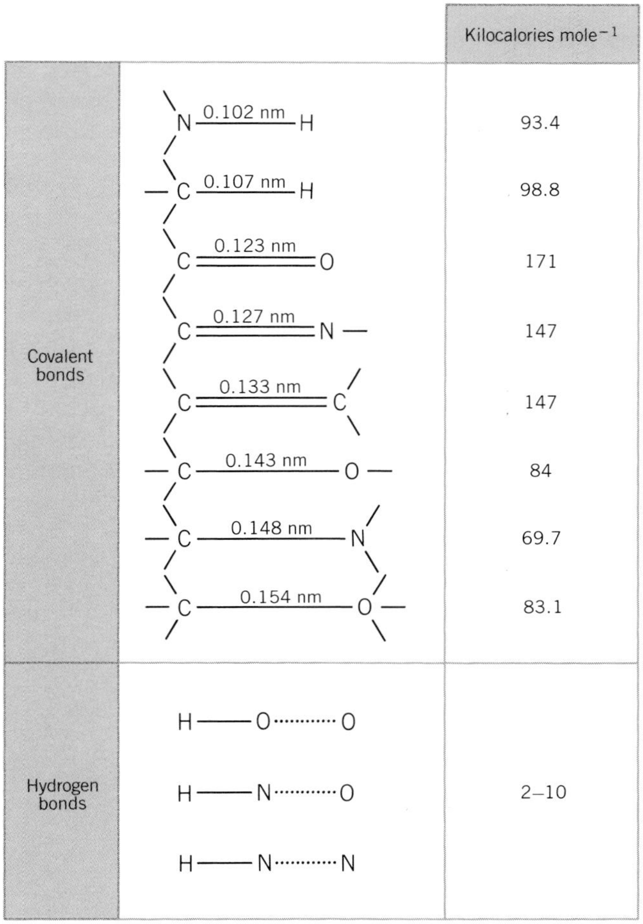

	Kilocalories mole^{-1}
Covalent bonds	
$\diagdown$N $\underline{0.102\text{ nm}}$ H	93.4
—C $\underline{0.107\text{ nm}}$ H	98.8
C $\underline{\overline{0.123\text{ nm}}}$ O	171
C $\underline{\overline{0.127\text{ nm}}}$ N —	147
C $\underline{0.133\text{ nm}}$ C	147
—C $\underline{0.143\text{ nm}}$ O —	84
—C $\underline{0.148\text{ nm}}$ N	69.7
C $\underline{0.154\text{ nm}}$ O —	83.1
Hydrogen bonds	
H —— O ·········· O	
H —— N ·········· O	2–10
H —— N ·········· N	

FIGURE 2–3

The distances between atomic nuclei joined by covalent bonds vary. The energy needed to break these covalent bonds depends on the atoms involved. Hydrogen bonds are significantly weaker than covalent bonds.

lent bond, $^-$N—H$^+$, such that the nitrogen atom is more negatively charged than the hydrogen atom. Oxygen atoms have a high electronegativity and form many polar covalent bonds: $^-$O—C$^+$, $^-$O—H$^+$, $^-$O—N$^+$. Elements that form bonds with themselves are, of course, nonpolar. The **nonpolar covalent** bonds (C—C—C) of long chain fatty acids are very important in making fats repel water.

WATER AND HYDROGEN BONDS

Water is the major component of all organisms, with the exception of endospores. Water is a polar molecule because of its molecular geometry and its polar covalent O—H bonds. Water is a nonlinear molecule. Therefore, the electronegativity of the oxygen atom attracts the shared electrons causing the hydrogen atoms to function as positively charged centers, whereas the oxygen atom functions as a negatively charged center. Water molecules readily interact with one another. When they do interact, the positively charged hydrogen protons on one water molecule are attracted to the negatively charged oxygen nucleus of a second water molecule. The attractive force between these two charged centers is called the **hydrogen bond**. Hydrogen bonds also play an important role in the structure of nucleic acids and proteins. In these molecules the bonding takes place between electronegative oxygen or nitrogen atoms and the positively charged hydrogen nucleus. Hydrogen bonds are weaker than covalent bonds and ionic bonds. It takes between 2 and 10 kcal to break hydrogen bonds. Hydrogen bonds are easily disrupted at the temperature of boiling water.

Water is an extremely good solvent because of its charged state. Almost all charged compounds are soluble in water. Charged compounds include the ions of salts as well as large proteins and carbohydrates. Most nonpolar compounds are insoluble in water. Examples include oil, gasoline, and fats and waxes found in biological materials. These are **hydrophobic** compounds because they dislike water. Compounds readily soluble in water are termed **hydrophilic** or water liking.

IONIZATION OF WATER

Water almost never exists in a pure molecular form. Water also contains ions that are the reaction products of water. When two water molecules collide, they can interact to form **hydroxide ions** (OH^-) and **hydronium ions** (H_3O^+).

$$H_2O + H_2O \rightleftharpoons H_3O^+ + OH^-$$

The concentration of hydronium ions in water is 10^{-7} moles/liter. For every hydronium ion in water there is also a hydroxide ion. We say that water is neutral, in an acid-base sense, because there is an equal number of hydronium ions and hydroxide ions.

If one adds to water a compound that will ionize to produce either a proton (H^+) or a hydroxide ion, the water will not be neutral. **Acids** are substances that increase the concentration of hydronium ions when added to water. **Bases** are substances that increase the hydroxide ion concentration when added to water. Acids release protons (H^+) that are, in fact, hydrogen ions (remember that a hydrogen atom is a proton and an electron). Strong acids completely ionize to form ions. An example is hydrochloric acid ($HCl \rightarrow H^+ + Cl^-$), which forms protons and chloride ions when added to water. The protons will react with water to form hydronium ions. Similarly, strong bases will completely ionize and will react with available hydronium ions.

The **pH scale** has been devised to keep track of hydronium ions in solutions. The scale is defined as the negative logarithm of the hydrogen ion concentration.

$$pH = -\log [H^+]$$

A neutral pH is defined as seven because this is the negative log of the hydrogen ion concentration (10^{-7}) of pure water. Values between pH 7 and pH 14 are termed **alkaline** and are obtained by adding a base to the solution. Values between pH 7 and 0 are termed **acidic** and are obtained by adding acids to the solution (Figure 2–4). Many common household products are noted for their ability to change the hydronium ion concentration. Some are listed in Figure 2–4.

Biological systems contain substances called **buff-**

FIGURE 2–4

The concentration of hydrogen ions [H^+] in solution is indicated numerically by the pH. The most basic and the most acidic pHs are rarely attained in aqueous systems. Living organisms are found in natural environments having pHs between 2.0 and 10.0.

The pH Scale

	pH		[H^+]	[OH^-]
	14	Basic	1×10^{-14}	1
	13		1×10^{-13}	1×10^{-1}
	12		1×10^{-12}	1×10^{-2}
	11		1×10^{-11}	1×10^{-3}
	10		1×10^{-10}	1×10^{-4}
Baking soda	9		1×10^{-9}	1×10^{-5}
Seawater	8		1×10^{-8}	1×10^{-6}
Human blood	7	Neutral	1×10^{-7}	1×10^{-7}
	6		1×10^{-6}	1×10^{-8}
Fungal growth	5		1×10^{-5}	1×10^{-9}
Tomato juice	4		1×10^{-4}	1×10^{-10}
Cola	3		1×10^{-3}	1×10^{-11}
Acid mine water	2	Acidic	1×10^{-2}	1×10^{-12}
	1		1×10^{-1}	1×10^{-13}
	0		1	1×10^{-14}

ers that chemically resist major changes in pH. Buffers are composed of compounds that react with and neutralize either acids or bases. Examples include the $HPO_4^{2-}/H_2PO_4^-$ (monohydrogen phosphate ion/dihydrogen phosphate ion) pair and the HCO_3^-/H_2CO_3 (bicarbonate ion/carbonic acid) pair. The phosphate system works as follows.

$$\text{Addition of base } H_2PO_4^- + OH^- \rightarrow HPO_4^{2-} + H_2O$$
$$\text{Addition of acid } HPO_4^{2-} + H^+ \rightarrow H_2PO_4^-$$

Note that the right-hand side of these reactions contain neither hydronium ions nor hydroxyl ions. Cells use these chemical mechanisms to maintain an optimal pH. Microbial cell growth is also very dependent on the pH of the environment, as will be seen in Chapter 7.

INORGANIC IONS AND GASES

Many of the essential components of microbial cells exist as soluble ions in aqueous solution. Ions that do not contain carbon are termed **inorganic** ions. Although carbonate salts contain carbon, we consider them to be inorganic compounds because their chemical properties are more like inorganic compounds. Almost all the biologically essential inorganic compounds exist as salts. When the salts are placed in water, they dissociate into their respective ions. For example, $CaCl_2$ is an ionic salt that dissociates in water to produce Ca^{2+} ions and Cl^- ions. We can express this interaction with the solvent (H_2O) by the following equation.

$$CaCl_{2(s)} \rightarrow Ca^{2+}_{(aq)} + 2Cl^-_{(aq)}$$

The designation (s) indicates a solid, and (aq) indicates aqueous solution. Inorganic ions that are important to microorganisms include potassium (K^+), calcium (Ca^{2+}), sodium (Na^+), phosphate (PO_4^{2-}), sulfate (SO_4^{2-}), sulfide (S^{2-}), nitrate (NO_3^-), nitrite (NO_2^-), ammonium (NH_4^+), carbonate (CO_3^{2-}), magnesium (Mg^{2+}), and manganese (Mn^{2+}). Essential **trace metals** are also available as inorganic ions, such as ferric iron (Fe^{3+}), or as metal-containing ions, such as molybdate (MoO_4^{2-}).

Certain nonpolar gases are used by microorganisms. Carbon dioxide (CO_2) is used by certain organisms as a source of carbon. Other organisms release this gas as a by-product of metabolism. Dinitrogen (N_2) is a gas that can be used by certain microorganisms as a nitrogen source. Seventy-eight percent (by volume) of our atmosphere is composed of dinitrogen. Methane-producing bacteria generate methane (CH_4) as a product of metabolism, whereas other bacteria oxidize methane as a source of energy. Many biological systems can use these gases as a source of nutrients.

ORGANIC MOLECULES

All organic compounds contain carbon. The carbon is often covalently bound to hydrogen as well as to adjacent carbon nuclei. In contrast, inorganic compounds almost never contain carbon. Although both organic and inorganic compounds are essential to biological systems, organic compounds exist in a great array of chemical formulations and serve a great diversity of functional roles in living systems.

Carbon is the major element in organic compounds and always forms four covalent bonds. These bonds join the carbon atom to oxygen, nitrogen, hydrogen, or another carbon atom. Organic chemists have named the **functional groups** formed by these interactions. Figure 2–5 shows some functional groups important to biological systems. Molecules can be manufactured by attaching these functional groups onto carbon backbones. The simplest formulation would be to join two methyl groups (H_3C—CH_3) to form the gas ethane. Or we could attach a carboxyl group to a methyl group

$$H_3C - \overset{\overset{\displaystyle O}{\|}}{C} - OH$$

to make acetic acid, the major component of vinegar. If we exchange the carboxyl group with an alcohol group, we now have ethanol (CH_3CH_2OH), which is the active ingredient of alcoholic beverages. Cells contain more than 700 different kinds of small organic molecules. It is not necessary to describe the

Functional Groups of Organic Compounds

Functional Group	Name	Where Found
$-CH_3$	Methyl	Attached to many classes of organic compounds
$-CH_2CH_3$	Ethyl	In compounds such as ethanol
$\overset{\displaystyle O}{\overset{\|}{-C}}-OH$	Carboxyl	Organic acids (gives up one proton, $-COO^- + H^+$)
$\overset{\displaystyle O}{\overset{\|}{-C}}-H$	Aldehyde	Sugars and aldehydes
$C=O$	Keto or carbonyl	Sugars and some organic acids
$\overset{\displaystyle O}{\overset{\|}{-C}}-O-$	Ester	Lipids
$-NH_2$	Amino	Amino acids, amino sugars
$-OH$	Hydroxyl	Sugars, alcohols
$-CH_2OH$	Alcohol	Glycerol, alcohols
$\overset{\displaystyle O}{\overset{\|}{-C}}-CH_3$	Acetyl	Organic compounds

FIGURE 2–5
Functional groups of organic compounds.

chemistry of all these different molecules; however, it is important to describe the major classes of bioorganic molecules.

MAJOR CLASSES OF BIOORGANIC MOLECULES

Four major groups of small organic molecules are important to biological systems because they are used in the manufacture of macromolecules. The four groups are fatty acids, carbohydrates, nitrogenous bases, and amino acids.

Amino acids are composed of the amino functional group attached to an organic acid (Figure 2–6). Organic acids can be recognized because they contain a carboxyl group. The 20 naturally occurring amino acids are shown in Appendix 1. Each amino acid differs in the structure of the "R" group. The symbol "R" is used to indicate that a number of different organic structures are possible. Amino acids will be discussed further when proteins are described.

Fatty acids contain a carboxyl group attached to a hydrocarbon chain (Figure 2–6). Fatty acids can vary in the number of carbons from 2 to more than 20. The short chain fatty acids, such as acetic acid, are soluble in water; whereas the long chain fatty acids, such as stearic acid, are insoluble in water because of their long nonpolar hydrophobic carbon chain. All

FIGURE 2–6

Representative organic molecules that are important in biology. The letter "R" indicates the portion of the molecule that can vary in structure.

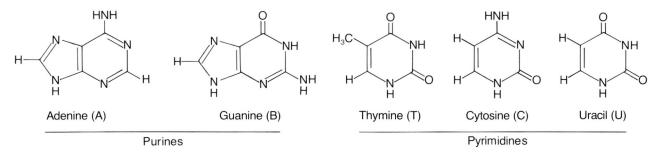

water-insoluble organic biomolecules that can be extracted from cells by nonpolar solvents are called **lipids.** Long chain fatty acids are used to build lipids, which in turn are the major component of membranes.

Carbohydrates are organic compounds that have the basic chemical formula $(CH_2O)_n$. These compounds are produced by plants through the fixation of carbon dioxide. Many living cells use carbohydrates as a primary source of carbon and energy. Carbohydrates are essential components of biological macromolecules. All cells use the carbohydrates ribose and deoxyribose to form their nucleic acids. Bacteria and plants use other carbohydrates in their cell walls.

Glucose is a common six carbon carbohydrate; its structure is shown in Figure 2–6. There are two ways to present the structure of carbohydrates; each way indicates the position of the hydrogens and hydroxyl groups in relation to the carbon atoms. In solution, glucose is a ring structure, so it is more appropriate to visualize it as the Haworth projection (Figure 2–6). Carbohydrates vary according to the number of carbon atoms present and the number and location of each hydroxyl group, aldehyde group, and keto group. Carbohydrates containing six carbons are termed **hexoses;** carbohydrates containing five carbons are termed **pentoses.** Polymers of carbohydrates are commonly found in biological systems.

Nitrogenous bases are the informational units of the genetic code. There are two main classes of nitrogenous bases: the **purines** and the **pyrimidines** (see Figure 2–6). Nitrogenous bases are heterocyclic ring structures that contain both nitrogen and carbon atoms. The double lines between two carbon atoms indicate a double covalent bond. The different nitrogenous bases are built from these basic structures to which are added oxygen, hydrogen, carbon, or nitrogen to make each nitrogenous base chemically distinct. These distinct nitrogenous bases are used by cells to encode macromolecular messages. The structures of the nitrogenous bases and the role they play in heredity are discussed in Chapters 5 and 6.

STRUCTURES OF MACROMOLECULES

Amino acids, sugars, and fatty acids can be made into large molecules that are used as the architectural building material of cells. Fatty acids are components of lipids found in membranes. Sugars combine to form the polysaccharides found in cell walls, and amino acids are the building blocks of the proteins. An understanding of cell structure and function requires a knowledge of the chemical properties of structural molecules.

Lipids

The biologically produced substances that are soluble in nonpolar solvents are the lipids. Lipids are organic molecules that are subclassified as waxes, steroids, neutral lipids, and phospholipids. Steroids are a diverse group of heterocyclic organic compounds that function as hormones in animals. Waxes are produced primarily by plants, animals, and insects. Beeswax is an example of this class of lipid that has many practical human applications. All cells produce and use the neutral triglycerides and the phospholipids as basic components of membranes.

When fatty acids are combined with a glycerol molecule, the complex is a neutral triglyceride (Figure 2–7). When they are combined with a glycerol phosphate molecule, a phospholipid is formed. These lipids are formed by the removal of water from the carboxyl group of the acid and the alcohol group of the glycerol, which are joined together by an ester bond.

$$R—OH + HO—\overset{\overset{\textstyle O}{\|}}{C}—R' \rightarrow R—O—\overset{\overset{\textstyle O}{\|}}{C}—R' + H_2O$$

This reaction results in a nonpolar molecule that is hydrophobic (insoluble in water). The triglycerides are neutral, but the phospholipids have a charge attributable to the phosphate ion. Phospholipids have a polar end, which interacts with water, and a nonpolar end (fatty acyl), which is hydrophobic. Triglycerides and phospholipids are ideal molecules for the construction of membranes because of their hydrophobicity (see Chapter 3).

Polysaccharides

Combinations of two sugar molecules are called **disaccharides;** combinations of three or more sugar molecules are called **polysaccharides.** Sucrose and lactose are disaccharides that are used as food sources by bacteria. Sucrose is formed by combining

FIGURE 2–7

Certain lipids are composed of long chain fatty acids and glycerol. Stearic acid and oleic acid are fatty acids. Phospholipids have a charged phosphate group; triglycerides are neutral.

Lipid Structure

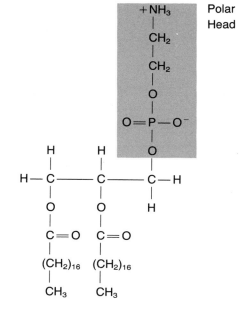

Fatty Acids

(a) Stearic acid (b) Oleic acid

(c) Triglyceride (1 myristoyldipalmitoyl glycerol)

(d) Phospholipid (phosphatidyl ethanolamine)

Disaccharide

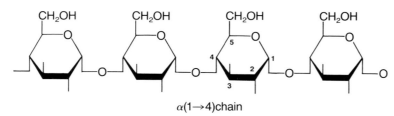

αGlucose   Fructose   Sucrose

Amino sugars

N-Acetylglucosamine

N-Acetylmuramic acid

Polysaccharide

α(1→4)chain

FIGURE 2–8
Sugars can be made into disaccharides or polysaccharides by forming a glycosidic bond
between two monosaccharides. Sucrose is a soluble disaccharide (common table sugar).
Cellulose is an insoluble polysaccharide (the major component of wood). The two amino
sugars shown are components of most bacterial cell walls.

the two hexoses, glucose and fructose, with a **gly-cosidic bond** (Figure 2–8). Lactose is also a disaccharide, but it is formed from glucose and galactose. Sugars can be modified by attaching noncarbohydrate groups to the basic sugar. Two modified car-

bohydrates are *N*-acetylglucosamine and *N*-acetylmuramic acid (Figure 2–8). These carbohydrates are components of most bacterial cell walls.

Long chains of sugar molecules held together by glycosidic bonds are called polysaccharides. Starch, glycogen, and cellulose are all polymers of glucose that vary in the specific carbons used to form the glycosidic bond and in the degree of branches formed. Starch and glycogen are examples of stored carbohydrate food reserves. Cellulose, also a polysaccharide, is used in the construction of cell walls of plants. Cellulose is the major component of wood.

Carbohydrates are often added to other polymers to make those polymers chemically different or to provide structural continuity. Deoxyribose is a five-carbon sugar that forms the backbone of the hereditary material DNA (*DeoxyriboNucleic Acid*). Ribose is a five-carbon sugar that forms the backbone of RNA (*RiboNucleic Acid*). Proteins modified by the covalent attachment of carbohydrates are known as **glycoproteins.** The carbohydrates that are attached to either serum proteins or sphingolipids in the membranes of red blood cells **(glycolipids)** are responsible for the differences between the A and B blood groups. Carbohydrate-peptide complexes are also involved in the structure of bacterial cell walls.

Proteins

Amino acids are the building blocks of proteins. There are 20 naturally occurring amino acids (Appendix 1). When two or more amino acids are joined, they form a peptide. The amino acid residues in a peptide are joined together by the peptide bond.

$$H_2N - \underset{\underset{H}{|}}{\overset{\overset{R}{|}}{C}} - \overset{\overset{O}{||}}{C} - OH \ + \ H_2N - \underset{\underset{H}{|}}{\overset{\overset{R'}{|}}{C}} - \overset{\overset{O}{||}}{C} - OH \ \rightarrow$$

Amino acid R   +   Amino acid R′   →

$$NH_2 - \underset{\underset{H}{|}}{\overset{\overset{R}{|}}{C}} - \overset{\overset{O}{||}}{C} - \underset{\underset{H}{|}}{N} - \underset{\underset{H}{|}}{\overset{\overset{R'}{|}}{C}} - \overset{\overset{O}{||}}{C} - OH \ + \ H_2O$$

Peptide   + Water

Key characteristics of this simple peptide include:

1. The peptide has two ends: an amino-terminal and a carboxyl-terminal end.

2. The R groups can be identical or they can characterize any one of the 20 amino acids.

3. The chemical properties of the peptide will depend on the sequence of the amino acids in the peptide.

Proteins are large peptides, or to say it another way, proteins have many amino acid residues. Proteins have molecular weights ranging from 6000 to 1,000,000 daltons (one dalton equals the mass of one hydrogen atom). If each amino acid residue averages a molecular weight of 100, then proteins would contain between 60 to 10,000 amino acid residues. Cells are remarkable in that they are able to make many copies of very large proteins all with the same amino acid sequence. To understand the complexities of proteins, it is necessary to look at their structure at different levels of organization.

The sequence of amino acid residues in a protein is called the **primary structure** of a protein. In most proteins this is dictated by the information encoded in the cell's gene for that protein; this will be discussed in Chapter 5. A given protein will always have the same amino-terminal end, the same carboxyl-terminal end, and the same sequence of amino acid residues in between. Once the primary sequence is established, the properties of the protein usually result from the chemical and physical interactions of these residues.

Proteins have a natural tendency to form hydrogen bonds. When proteins form hydrogen bonds between closely spaced residues, the peptide spirals to form an **alpha helix** (Figure 2–9). The hydrogen bonding between amino acid residues of a polypeptide chain is the **secondary structure** of the protein. Certain fibrous proteins, such as collagen, form hydrogen bonds between adjacent polypeptide chains. This type of structure leads to the formation of protein sheets, which are structural components of animal connective tissue.

Folding of the polypeptide on itself is called **tertiary structure.** Certain amino acid residues contain reactive groups that can interact with one another. These interactions can cause the polypeptide chain to fold back on itself. Interaction between hydrophobic R groups, between the sulfur groups on cysteine, and the ionic bonding between charged

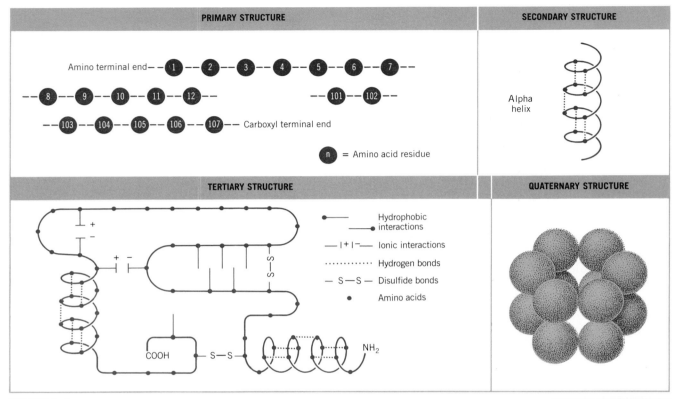

PRIMARY STRUCTURE	SECONDARY STRUCTURE

Amino terminal end —— ①—— ②—— ③—— ④—— ⑤—— ⑥—— ⑦——

——⑧——⑨——⑩——⑪——⑫——   ——⑩⑴——⑩⑵——

——⑩⑶——⑩⑷——⑩⑸——⑩⑹——⑩⑺—— Carboxyl terminal end

ⓝ = Amino acid residue

Alpha helix

TERTIARY STRUCTURE   QUATERNARY STRUCTURE

●—— Hydrophobic interactions
—|+|— Ionic interactions
·········· Hydrogen bonds
— S—S — Disulfide bonds
● Amino acids

COOH — S—S —   NH₂

FIGURE 2–9
Proteins are composed of amino acid residues joined by peptide bonds. This string of amino acids can interact within itself to form helices and can fold back on itself to form tight globular structures. Globular protein subunits can interact to form protein complexes. The electron micrograph and the diagram of glutamine synthetase shows the interaction of the 12 identical globular protein subunits of this enzyme. (Photo courtesy F. A. Eiserling and L. J. Wallace.)

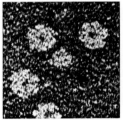

R groups stabilize the tertiary structure of protein (Figure 2–9).

The fourth level of protein structure results from the noncovalent interaction of either similar or dissimilar polypeptide chains. This protein organization, called **quaternary structure,** is important to structural proteins as well as to catalytic proteins. Protein viral coats, bacterial flagella, ribosomes, and many enzymes depend on quaternary interactions for their structure and function.

Proteins are obviously very complex chemicals, yet scientists have been able to analyze their structure and to determine how they function. Figure 2–10 shows space-filling models of yeast hexokinase before and after it has bound its substrate glucose. Like all proteins, this enzyme is composed of a linear sequence of amino acids. The active site of yeast hexokinase is located in the cleft created when the enzyme assumes its three-dimensional conformation. Note that the conformation of the enzyme

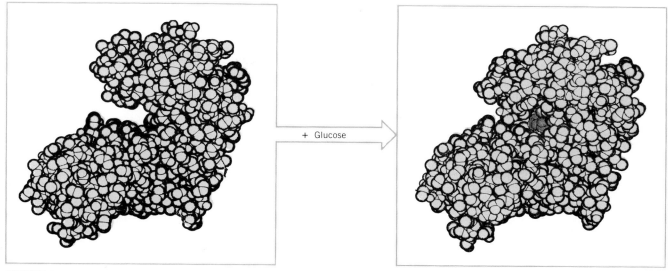

+ Glucose

FIGURE 2–10

Space-filling model of yeast hexokinase in the native state and after reacting with its substrate glucose. (Courtesy of Dr. T. A. Steitz. From C. M. Anderson, F. H. Zucker, and T. A. Steitz, *Science*, 240:375–380, 1979. Copyright © 1979 by the American Association for the Advancement of Science.)

changes after it has bound its substrate. Knowledge of the structure of proteins is an important aspect of understanding their function. The next two chapters will help to explain the role of proteins in the structure of cells and in cellular metabolism.

SUMMARY

Chemical principles underlie many aspects of the study of microbiology. Media preparation, diagnostic reactions, structure of the microbial cell, microscopic staining, and physiological reactions can all be understood on the basis of chemistry. Chemistry builds a body of knowledge based on the structure of atoms. Atoms interact to form molecules, which in turn can interact to form macromolecules. Atoms are bound together by specific types of bonds. Ionic bonding is found predominantly in inorganic compounds, whereas covalent bonding predominates in organic compounds. Hydrogen bonds, which are weaker than covalent bonds, are important in the structure of water and in the conformation of macromolecules such as proteins.

Approximately 15 different types of inorganic ions make up less than 2 percent of the wet weight of cells. These elements are essential to the functioning of the cell even though they are present in low quantities. On the other hand, organic compounds are extremely diverse in their nature; more than 700 different kinds of organic compounds are found in a cell. Carbon is the third most prevalent element in cells after hydrogen and oxygen. Carbon makes up 12 percent of a cell's wet weight and as much as 50 percent of a cell's dry weight. These organic compounds include the amino acids, carbohydrates, fatty acids, intermediates of metabolism, and, of course, the macromolecules. Polysaccharides, nucleic acids, and proteins are the major macromolecules found in microorganisms. These macromolecules are arranged into structures that in turn serve specific functions.

QUESTIONS AND TOPICS FOR STUDY AND DISCUSSION

Questions

1. In what biomolecules would you find carbon, oxygen, nitrogen, phosphorus, and sulphur?
2. Describe the atomic structure of hydrogen, carbon, nitrogen, and oxygen.
3. Define or explain the following terms.

atomic number	isotope
atomic weight	neutron
element	orbital
energy level	proton

4. Describe four kinds of chemical bonds, and write out examples of each.
5. What is the practical application of pH to biological systems? Describe a buffer, and name a common household acid and a base.
6. Write out the basic structure of an amino acid, a fatty acid, a carbohydrate, a purine, a pyrimidine, and label each functional group.
7. Write out the basic reaction for forming a lipid, a polypeptide, and a disaccharide.
8. Describe the four levels of organization in proteins.

Discussion

1. A polypeptide chain has an amino end and a carboxyl end. How does the directionality of the polypeptide structure influence the biological function of proteins?

2. Water is released when carbohydrates form disaccharides and when amino acids are joined to form a polypeptide. What chemical reactions do you envision being involved in the breakdown (hydrolysis) of these molecules?

FURTHER READINGS

Books

Callewaert, D., and J. Genyea, *Fundamentals of College Chemistry*, Worth, New York, 1980. A two-semester introductory textbook in college chemistry designed for students preparing for careers in allied health professions.

Holum, J. R., *Fundamentals of General, Organic, and Biological Chemistry*, Wiley, New York, 1978. A basic college chemistry textbook for students entering allied health professions.

Sackeim, G. I., *Introduction to Chemistry for Biology Students*, 2nd ed., Educational Methods, Chicago, 1977. A self-taught refresher course in chemistry for biology students.

Articles and Reviews

Luria, S. E., "The Bacterial Protoplasm: Composition and Organization," in I. C. Gunsalus and R. Y. Stanier (eds.), *The Bacteria*, vol. 1, pp. 1–34, Academic Press, New York, 1960. A classic paper on the chemical composition of bacteria.

3

CELLS: ORGANIZATION, STRUCTURE, AND FUNCTION

Cells are the organization unit of all living things except viruses. The cell unit was first recognized by Robert Hooke in 1665. Hooke's observations were not conceptualized until the middle of the 1800s, when Schleiden and Schwann developed the **cell theory,** which states that the cell is the basic unit of life. These early microscopists realized that cells vary greatly in size, shape, and appearance; and they were impressed with the diversity of life.

Electron microscopists were the first investigators to have a clear view of the subcellular structure of cells. The photographs they took revealed two basic cell types. Micrographs of plant and animal cells contained a true nucleus, whereas bacterial cells lacked a nucleus. Both cell types perform the same basic functions of growth and reproduction. These distinct cells are known as **eucaryotes** and **procaryotes.**

Bacteria* are defined as those organisms that have the structure of a procaryotic cell. Bacterial cells are distinct because they lack a membrane-limited nu-

clear region. Eucaryotic (Gr. *eu,* true; Gr. **karyon,** nucleus) cells contain a cell nucleus that in resting cells is bounded by a membrane. Eucaryotic cells are structurally more complex than procaryotic cells. All living systems other than bacteria and viruses are, or are composed of, cells of the eucaryotic structure. Extensive biochemical, genetic, and cytological studies have made it possible to correlate the biological and physiological function of each major cell structure in both the eucaryotic and the procaryotic cell type.

PROCARYOTIC CELLS

Procaryotic cells are structurally simple cells that contain a nuclear region in place of a true nucleus. Microscopists can observe the size and shape of procaryotic cells with the light microscope. The internal granules are sometimes visible by light microscopy, but the nuclear material is too fine a structure to be seen. To observe subcellular structure, such as the nuclear region, microscopists must use the electron microscope.

---

*Cyanobacteria, previously called the blue-green algae, are now classified as bacteria (see *Bergey's Manual*).

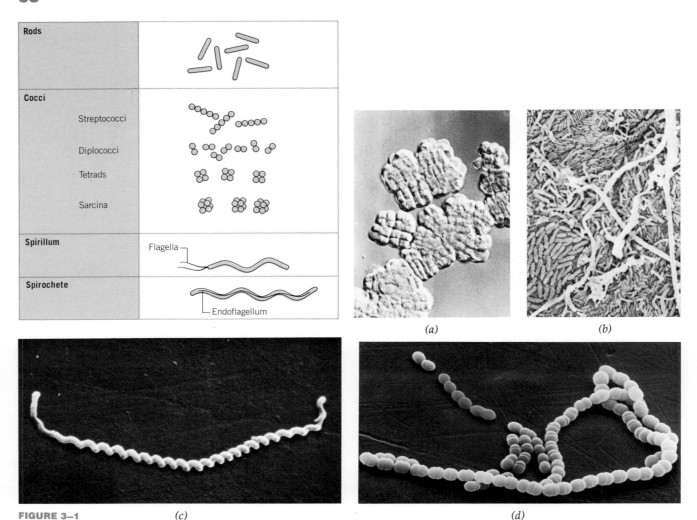

FIGURE 3–1

(a) *(b)* *(c)* *(d)*

The four basic shapes of bacteria. Phase contrast micrograph of *(a) Sarcina ventriculi,* which grows in packets of eight cells. Scanning electron micrographs *(b)* of rod-shaped bacteria in the gut of the termite. (Courtesy of Dr. J. A. Breznak. From J. A. Breznak and H. S. Pankratz, *Applied Environ. Microbiol.,* 33:406–426, 1977.) *(c)* A single spirochete. (Courtesy of Dr. N. Charon. From O. Carleton, N. Charon, P. Allender, and S. O'Brien, *J. Bacteriol.,* 137:1413–1416, 1979.) *(d)* Dividing streptococci. (Courtesy of Dr. G. D. Shockman. From D. L. Shungo, J. B. Cornett, and G. D. Shockman, *J. Bacteriol.,* 138:598–608, 1979.) *(b–d,* with permission of the American Society for Microbiology.)

Bacterial cytology

The shape and size of a bacterial cell is the first clue to its identification. Bacteria can have the basic shape of a sphere, a rod, a comma (vibrio), or a spiral. The shape of bacteria and their cellular arrangement in chains, clusters, tetrads, and so forth is important for bacterial identification and classification.

Bacteria often have names that indicate their

shape (Figure 3–1). Spherical cells, called **cocci** (sing., coccus), can be arranged as pairs, long chains, tetrads, or packets of eight, depending on whether the cell divides in one, two, or three planes. Bacteria generally divide by **binary fission,** which is a process of division that results in two equal daughter cells. When a coccus divides in one plane it forms a diplococcus; division at right angles to the first plane results in tetrad formation; and division in the third plane results in packets of eight cells known as sarcina.

Rod-shaped bacteria occur in various sizes and shapes ranging from football-shaped to long, slender filaments. Cross walls are often observable in these long filaments indicating the presence of individual cells. Some bacteria are **pleomorphic,** meaning that they can assume different shapes. Pleomorphism is a characteristic of specific bacterial genera that is more commonly observed in physiologically old cultures. For example, species of *Arthrobacter* change from rods to a spherical morphology during growth. Although most rods divide by binary fission, a few rod-shaped bacteria can also divide by **budding.** Cell division by budding results in daughter cells of unequal size. Each morphological characteristic of a rod helps to identify it since these characteristics are genetically passed to succeeding generations.

Bacterial cells with a helical or curved morphology are called spirilla or vibrios. **Spirilla** are long, curved or helix-shaped cells. **Vibrios** are short, comma-shaped cells. Movement of spirilla and vibrios is generated by polar flagellation. Helix-shaped cells containing endoflagella are called **spirochetes.** The endoflagella impart movement to these organisms.

Simple stains. Simple stains can be used to accentuate bacterial structures. Basic dyes, such as crystal violet, basic fuchsin, and methylene blue, stain the bacterial cytoplasm, whereas lipid-soluble dyes, such as sudan black, are used to stain lipid inclusions. Capsular material surrounding bacteria can be visualized when the background is stained with india ink (Figure 3–1). Bacterial capsules are important since they can prevent phagocytosis by white blood cells.

Differential stains. Differential stains demonstrate differences between two cell types or cell structures. These stains usually involve the application of more than one stain. The Gram stain and the acid-fast stain are examples of differential stains.

Gram stain. Hans Christian Gram developed his widely used differential staining procedure in 1884. Known as the **Gram stain,** this procedure distinguishes between cell types designated **Gram-negative** and **Gram-positive.**

The procedure is to fix the bacteria to the surface of a slide by heating the slide over a low flame. Crystal violet is then applied; the slide is washed with water, and then an iodine solution is applied. The iodine fixes the crystal violet inside Gram-positive cells. The slide is then washed with an organic solvent (alcohol or acetone), dried, and then counterstained with safranin. Gram-positive cells remain blue-violet throughout this procedure (Figure 3–2), since they retain the crystal violet stain (Color Plate 2). Gram-negative cells lose the crystal violet stain on washing with the organic solvent. When the col-

FIGURE 3–2
Steps in the Gram-stain procedure (shaded cells represent blue, colored cell appear red.)

Steps	Gram-negative Cell	Gram-positive Cell
1. Cells are heated to fix them to the slide. All cells stain blue with crystal violet (1 min).	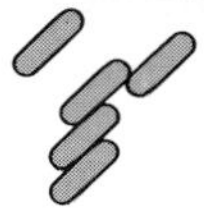	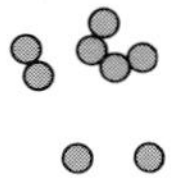
2. Iodine is applied (1 min), resulting in no color change.	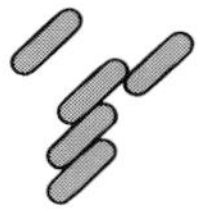	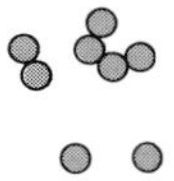
3. Cells are washed with alcohol. Gram⁻ cells are decolorized.	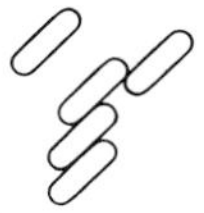	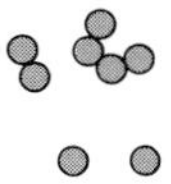
4. Cells are counterstained with safranin. The colorless Gram⁻ cells turn red.	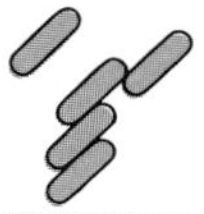	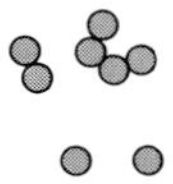

orless Gram-negative cells are counterstained with safranin, they stain red and are once again clearly visible under the light microscope.

The Gram stain must always be done with known controls on the same slide, since the actual staining technique varies among technicians. Moreover, cells can change their staining properties depending on their physiological state of growth; cells may be Gram-positive in vigorously growing cultures and then become Gram-negative in a later stage of growth called the **stationary phase.** Practice and judgment are necessary for the proper use and interpretation of the Gram stain. The Gram staining reaction is dependent on the structure of a bacterium's cell wall.

Acid-fast stain. A differential technique that is used in the identification of tubercule bacilli is the acid-fast stain. Acid-fast cells bind a primary stain tenaciously. In the Ziehl-Neelsen acid-fast stain, the cells are treated with carbolfuchsin and then decolorized with acidified alcohol. Acid-fast bacteria retain the stain, whereas non-acid fast bacteria are decolorized. The amount of lipid material in a cell has a direct bearing on its response to this differential stain.

The bacterial cytoplasm. A great amount of information concerning cell morphology has been gained from studies of living and stained cells observed in the light microscope. To understand the relationships between cell structure and functions, scientists had to do experiments at the subcellular level. These biochemical and electron microscopic studies on the subcellular structures of bacteria have resulted in a clear understanding of the structure and function of bacterial architecture.

Nuclear region. During reproduction, each cell replicates and transfers its genetic information to its progeny. The hereditary information of a cell is conserved in DNA, the macromolecule whose chemical name is **deoxyribonucleic acid.** The cell's DNA is seen in electron micrographs of the bacterial cytoplasm (Figure 3–3) as an electron-dense area. In procaryotic cells this is called the **nuclear region.** Bacte-

rial DNA exists as a closed circular macromolecule. We refer to this molecule as the **bacterial chromosome** since it contains all the genetic information necessary to perform the cell's life functions.

Bacteria contain only one chromosome. A given cell may contain either two or four copies of this chromosome if the cell replicates its chromosome once (two copies) or twice (four copies) before it divides. Associated with the chromosome are certain peptides, such as spermidine. **Spermidine** is a basic peptide that reacts with the acidic groups of the DNA molecule. Histones are basic proteins that function in a similar manner except that histones are found only in eucaryotic cells.

DNA from a bacterium can be isolated, stained, and viewed in the electron microscope (Figure 3–4). The approximate size of a bacterial DNA molecule is 10^6 nm (1 mm) in length with a molecular weight of 2.5×10^9. In rapidly growing cells, the DNA is constantly being replicated. The rather complex process of DNA replication will be presented in Chapter 5.

Inclusion bodies. Some bacteria generate granules that are deposited in their cytoplasm. Normally these granules are composed of carbohydrate or lipidlike substances that serve as a reserve source of energy. Polyhydroxybutyric acid (PHB) is made up of the four-carbon acid hydroxybutyric acid. PHB

FIGURE 3–3
Electron micrograph of a thin section through the bacterium *Escherichia coli.* (Courtesy of Dr. G. Cohen-Bazire.)

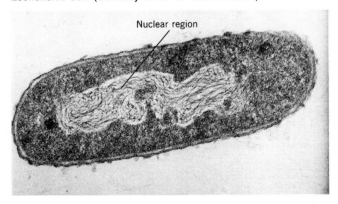

Nuclear region

stains with lipid stains such as sudan black. Granules composed of glycogen, a polymer of glucose, can be observed also in the bacterial cytoplasm.

Granules of PHB and glycogen are referred to as inclusion bodies since there is no discernible structure to these globules.

FIGURE 3—4

An electron micrograph of bacterial DNA released from a lysed cell of *Hemophilus.* The bacterial chromosome is a closed circular DNA molecule, approximately 1 mm long, that is packed into the cell's cytoplasm. [Micrograph courtesy of Dr. L. A. MacHattie. From L. A. MacHattie, K. I. Berns, and C. A. Thomas, Jr., *J. Mol. Biol.,* 11:648−649, 1965. Copyright © by Academic Press, Inc. (London) Ltd.]

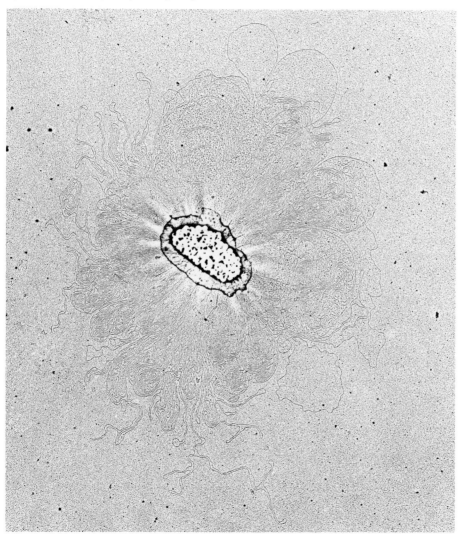

Bacteria can also accumulate and store phosphate as inclusion bodies. Cytologists have called these polyphosphate bodies volutin or metachromatic granules. The last term originates from the observation that polyphosphate granules change toluene blue to a reddish violet color (**metachromatic,** able to change color). Cytologists speculate that metachromatic granules function as a form of energy storage.

Gas vesicles are protein-surrounded cytoplasmic inclusions that are found in cyanobacteria. A protein coat surrounds each vesicle and allows the passage of gas into and out of the vesicle. The vesicles expand and collapse depending on the physiological state of the cell. Gas vesicles function to float nonmotile bacteria to a position in the water column where the appropriate light is available for photosynthesis.

Ribosomes. Protein synthesis occurs in the cytoplasm on structures called **ribosomes,** which are discrete cellular particles that are composed of protein (40 percent) and ribosomal ribonucleic acid (60 percent). Bacterial ribosomes are free in the cytoplasm, are not usually attached to membranes, and are easily isolated from lysed cells.

The size and shape of a ribosome can be determined by ultracentrifugation. Particles sediment at a given rate in a centrifugal field depending on their size and shape. The Svedberg unit (S) is a measure of the relative rate of the sedimentation of a particle in a centrifugal field. Bacterial ribosomes sediment as 70S particles and are composed of two subparticles that sediment at either 50S or 30S. Note that the Svedberg units are not arithmetically additive. This is because shape as well as size determines the value of the Svedberg unit. We shall see shortly that eucaryotic cells contain larger ribosomes that are structurally distinct from those found in bacteria.

Membranes, cell walls, and surface structures

One can think of the cytoplasm as a sac that contains both observable complex structures and small molecules that are too small to be seen. Among these small molecules are proteins, sugars, carbohydrates, and salts. The structure that encloses this sac is the cytoplasmic membrane.

Cytoplasmic membrane. Surrounding the cytoplasm is the plasma or **cytoplasmic membrane**; the membrane separates the interior of a cell from the cell's exterior. Electron micrographs reveal that the cytoplasmic membrane has a unit membrane structure (Figure 3–3). Unit membranes are approximately 8 nm in width and appear in transmission electron micrographs as a light band sandwiched between two dark bands. The cytoplasmic membrane is composed mainly of phospholipids and proteins. The hydrophobic ends of the lipid molecules interact in the center layers of the membrane, whereas the hydrophilic ends (charged groups) are aligned on the outside of the membrane (Figure 3–5).

Membranes are thought of as being fluid, that is, the proteins are able to float in the lipid layer just as an iceberg floats in the North Atlantic. Lipid and lipid-soluble molecules are chemically attracted to the fluid membrane and associate with the membrane as it grows. The membrane proteins confer sidedness to a membrane. A given portion of a protein will be exposed on only one surface of the membrane. This confers sidedness to a membrane, and the outside and the inside of the membrane can vary considerably in their function.

Signal hypothesis. What makes a membrane protein different from a cytoplasmic protein? One hypothesis suggests that membrane proteins have a unique N-terminal amino acid sequence that acts as a membrane translocation signal. The synthesis of these proteins is postulated to occur on membrane-bound ribosomes, so that synthesis and translocation occur simultaneously. One amino acid sequence signals translocation, and a later sequence functions

FIGURE 3–5
Diagram of a bacterial membrane showing membrane proteins responsible for transport and enzymatic reactions. (From Peter C. Hinkel and Richard E. McCarty, "How Cells Make ATP," *Sci. Am.,* 238:104–123, 1978, copyright © 1978 by Scientific American, Inc., All rights reserved.)

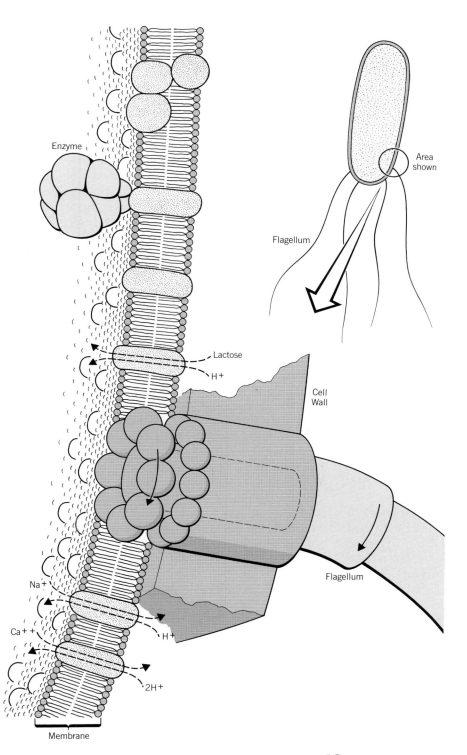

Enzyme

Lactose

H+

Cell
Wall

Na+

Ca++

H+

2H+

Membrane

Area
shown

Flagellum

Flagellum

to stop translocation. Under the signal hypothesis, proteins destined to function outside of the plasma membrane (see periplasmic space in the section on Cell Wall) would have the translocation signal, but they would lack the stop signal. Membrane proteins with a stop signal in the middle of their polypeptide chain would have their N-terminal end on the outside of the membrane and their carboxyl-terminal end on the inside. The signal hypothesis is one way to conceptualize how proteins synthesized in the cytoplasm can be found in membranes and in the periplasmic space.

Membrane permeability. Cytoplasmic membranes are semipermeable or selectively permeable barriers between the inside and the outside of the cell. Some molecules can cross the cytoplasmic membrane, whereas other molecules are excluded. **Diffusion** is the random movement of molecules from one location to another. This process does occur across cell membranes and is dependent on the mass of the molecule and on the temperature of the system. Only the smaller molecules enter cells by diffusion; larger molecules and charged molecules (sugars and amino acids) enter the cell by **mediated transport.** This process is specific for the compound being transported and has kinetic properties that are characteristic of protein substrate interactions. The two known types of mediated transport involve specific carrier proteins located on the membrane surface that bind the molecule being transported. **Facilitated diffusion** describes a carrier protein that mediates the transport process resulting in equal concentrations of the transported molecule on both sides of the membrane. **Active transport** also requires a carrier protein, but it results in a higher cellular concentration of the molecule being transported. Light energy, chemical energy, and/or electrical energy can each be coupled to the active transport process.

Membrane integrity. Any situation that results in the rupture of the cytoplasmic membrane destroys the cells. Normal bacterial cells contain a cell wall that confers shape and rigidity on the cell. Bacterial cells that lack a cell wall (protoplasts, L-forms) will tend to accumulate water unless they are placed in a medium of high solute concentration. The tendency to accumulate water when the concentration of solutes inside the cell is higher than the concentration of solutes outside the cell is called **osmosis.** This process will lead to a build-up of pressure inside the cell, a result of the increase in the number of water molecules. This force is called **osmotic pressure.** When the pressure becomes too great, the cell bursts, and we say that the cell has lysed. To counteract osmotic pressure, solutes can be added to the culture medium until water flows equally into and out of the cell across the semipermeable cytoplasmic membrane.

Mycoplasma are bacteria that are unable to synthesize cell walls and are always subject to lysis if they are not maintained in a medium with a high solute concentration. It is possible to grow bacteria under conditions that prevent cell wall synthesis or to remove cell walls from resting cells. A bacterium with its cell wall experimentally removed is called a **protoplast.** Certain antibiotics, such as penicillin, prevent the synthesis of bacterial cell walls. Protoplasts usually self-destroy by lysis because they are unable to resist the build-up of osmotic pressure.

Plasmolysis is the collapse of the cell due to an inordinately high solute concentration outside the cell. Under these conditions, water leaves the cell and the cell stops growing. Adding salt to red meat and fish and packing fruits in syrup preserves these foods. Because of plasmolysis, spoilage bacteria are unable to grow under these conditions.

Special membrane functions. The specialized metabolic functions of aerobic respiration and photosynthesis take place on bacterial membranes (Figure 3–6). Aerobic respiration is an energy-yielding process involving enzymes and components of the electron-transport system (see Chapter 4) that are localized in the bacterial cytoplasmic membrane. In the bacteria capable of photosynthesis, the photosynthetic pigments are always found associated with

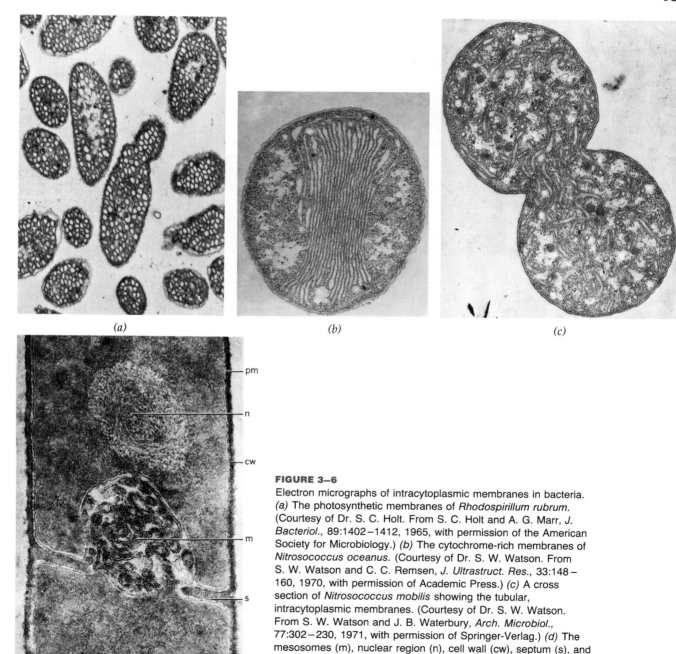

(a) *(b)* *(c)*

(d)

pm

n

cw

m

s

FIGURE 3–6

Electron micrographs of intracytoplasmic membranes in bacteria.
(a) The photosynthetic membranes of *Rhodospirillum rubrum.*
(Courtesy of Dr. S. C. Holt. From S. C. Holt and A. G. Marr, *J.
Bacteriol.,* 89:1402–1412, 1965, with permission of the American
Society for Microbiology.) *(b)* The cytochrome-rich membranes of
Nitrosococcus oceanus. (Courtesy of Dr. S. W. Watson. From
S. W. Watson and C. C. Remsen, *J. Ultrastruct. Res.,* 33:148–
160, 1970, with permission of Academic Press.) *(c)* A cross
section of *Nitrosococcus mobilis* showing the tubular,
intracytoplasmic membranes. (Courtesy of Dr. S. W. Watson.
From S. W. Watson and J. B. Waterbury, *Arch. Microbiol.,*
77:302–230, 1971, with permission of Springer-Verlag.) *(d)* The
mesosomes (m), nuclear region (n), cell wall (cw), septum (s), and
plasma membrane (pm) of *Bacillus subtilis.* (From P. Sheeler and
D. Bianchi, *Cell Biology,* Wiley, New York, 1980. Photo courtesy
of F. A. Eiserling.)

membranes. These membranes are called **bacterial thylakoid membranes** and can take the form of vesicles, lamellae, or disk-shaped membranes (Figure 3–6a). Thylakoid membranes are the site of the primary reaction of **photosynthesis,** the conversion of light into chemical energy.

Chemolithotrophs are bacteria that gain energy by oxidizing inorganic compounds. These specialized organisms often contain extensive intracytoplasmic membranes. These membranes (Figure 3–6b,c) are the location of the respiratory enzymes and components of the electron-transport chain, which are used to generate usable energy from inorganic compounds. The intracytoplasmic membranes in both photosynthetic bacteria and the chemolithotrophs normally develop as invaginations from the cytoplasmic membrane.

Mesosomes are specialized internal membranes that arise from the invagination of the cytoplasmic membrane. Mesosomes (when present) are associated with the cross wall formed by dividing bacteria (Figure 3–6d). It is thought that mesosomes function as a site of attachment for DNA during cell division. As the cell grows, the attached DNA may be physically placed in one of the two daughter cells.

Membranes function as a site for metabolic reactions, as a permeability barrier, and as a demarcation zone between the inside and the outside of the cell. Some bacteria contain no structures exterior to the cytoplasmic membrane, but these cells are the exception. Most bacterial cells contain a sequence of complex layers that confer rigidity to the cell's morphology and also serve as a penetration barrier for large molecules. These layers are referred to as the outer membrane or the cell wall.

Cell wall. Bacterial cell walls are chemically complex structures that are a continuous cell covering, lying exterior to the cytoplasmic membrane. The cell wall is rigid enough to define the cell's shape, protects the cell against osmotic pressure, and serves as the outside barrier to the environment. Procaryotic cells contain walls that are chemically complex and are distinctly different from the chemically simple

cell walls found in plant cells (animal cells do not have cell walls).

Cell walls of both Gram-negative and Gram-positive bacteria are composed of layers, the mucocomplex layer being common to both cell walls (Figure 3–7). **Peptidoglycan** is the basic building block of the mucocomplex layer. **Glycan** refers to the carbohydrate backbone of peptidoglycan and is made of N-acetylmuramic acid and N-acetylglucosamine (Figure 3–8). N-acetylmuramic acid is never found in eucaryotic cells. Attached to the glycan is a peptide that contains four or more amino acids including the rare D isomers of alanine and glutamic acid and one diamino amino acid, either **diaminopimelic acid** or **lysine.** The glycan backbones of this macromolecule are joined together by a peptide bond. These bonds join the diamino amino acid and the D-alanine residue that are located on opposite strands of the peptidoglycan. Sometimes the peptidoglycan macromolecules are joined by an intervening short peptide. These short peptides, or **interbridges** as they are called, are prevalent in the cell walls of Gram-positive bacteria.

The mucocomplex is a three-dimensional structure that forms a sac around the bacterium. The mucocomplex can be many layers thick or it can be only a few layers thick. Depending on its thickness, the mucocomplex layer acts as a sieve that prevents large molecules from passing through it. The thickness of the mucocomplex layer and its resulting filtering action are different in Gram-negative and Gram-positive bacteria.

Gram-positive. Gram-positive bacteria have a thick mucocomplex layer that extends from the cell membrane to the teichoic acid layer that coats the exterior of the cell (Figure 3–9). This mucocomplex layer is a three-dimensional structure with multiple layers of interconnecting peptidoglycan molecules. Attached to the surface of the mucocomplex layer are the negatively charged acidic polymers known as **teichoic acids** (Gr. *teichos,* wall). Teichoic acids are polymers of glycerol or ribitol connected by phosphate ester bonds. The exterior position of the teichoic acid layer is indicated by immunological studies; it is not visible in ordinary electron micrographs.

Gram-negative. Gram-negative cells have a very thin mucocomplex layer that is externally buttressed by a complex outer cell wall (Figure 3–10). The mucocomplex layer is composed of peptidoglycan that confers shape and rigidity on the cell. Both Gram-positive and Gram-negative bacterial cell walls contain chemically similar peptidoglycans. Adhering to the mucocomplex layer of the Gram-negative cell is the complex outer cell wall (also called the outer membrane) composed of polysaccharides, lipids, and proteins. These constituents of the outer wall are organized in the macromolecules known as **lipoprotein** and **lipopolysaccharide** (LPS). Isolated LPS from certain pathogenic bacteria can cause disease in humans. The chemical nature of the polysaccharide component of LPS varies greatly from strain to strain, creating many diverse surface structures

FIGURE 3–7

Diagrammatic representation of a Gram-positive and a Gram-negative cell wall. *(a)* Electron micrograph of a dividing cell of *Streptococcus faecalis.* Notice the thickness of the mucocomplex layer and the absence of a periplasmic space in this Gram-positive bacterium. (Courtesy of Dr. M. L. Higgins. From M. L. Higgins and L. Daneo-Moore, *J. Bacteriol.,* 141:938−945, 1980, with permission of the American Society for Microbiology.) *(b)* Electron micrograph of the cell wall complex of the Gram-negative bacterium, *Escherichia coli.* (Courtesy of Dr. G. Cohen-Bazire.)

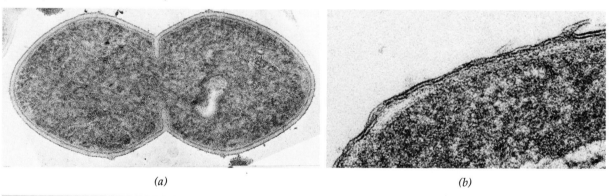

(a)   *(b)*

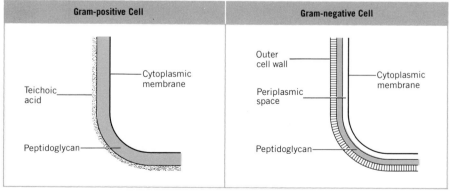

(c)

(a) Glycan

N-Acetylglucosamine (G)   N-Acetylmuramic acid (M)

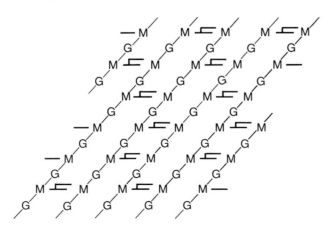

Lysozyme-sensitive bond

Peptide

(b) Peptide Bridges

—G—M—G— ——Glycan

L-Ala
D-Glu — Peptide
DAP —— Interbridge
D-Ala   D-Ala
             DAP
             D-Glu
             L-Ala
Glycan —G—M—G—

COOH
H$_2$N—CH
CH$_2$
CH$_2$
CH$_2$
H$_2$N—CH
COOH

Diaminopimelic Acid

COOH
H$_2$N—CH
CH$_2$
CH$_2$
CH$_2$
CH$_2$
NH$_2$

Lysine

(c) Peptidoglycan Layer

FIGURE 3–8
Chemical structure of peptidoglycan. *(a)* The glycan polymer of *N*-acetylglucosamine (G) and *N*-acetylmuramic acid (M). *(b)* The peptide bridges that connect the glycan polymer; the structures of diaminopimelic acid (DAP) and lysine. *(c)* Diagrammatic representation of the three-dimensional nature of peptidoglycan.

48

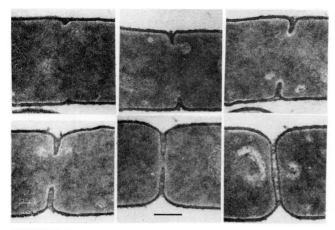

FIGURE 3—9
Cross-wall formation in *Bacillus subtilis*. The sequence begins at
the top left. The bar represents 0.2 μm. (Courtesy of Dr. N.
Nanniga. From N. Nanniga, L. H. Koppes, and F. C. deVries-
Tijssen, *Arch. Microbiol.*, 123:173–181, 1979, with permission of
Springer-Verlag.)

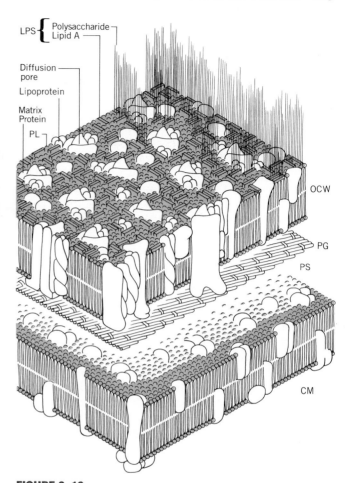

FIGURE 3—10
Cell wall of a Gram-negative bacterum: OCW, outer cell wall; PG,
peptidoglycan; PL, phospholipid; PS, periplasmic space; CM,
cytoplasmic membrane; and LPS, lipopolysaccharide.
(Reproduced with permission from the *Annual Review of
Biochemistry*, 47, copyright © 1978, Annual Reviews Inc.)

among the Gram-negative bacteria. These variations
in surface structure are evident in immunological reactions and in the interactions between cell surfaces
and viruses.

Between the cytoplasmic membrane and the
Gram-negative cell wall is the functionally defined
area known as the **periplasmic space.** This space
contains hydrolytic enzymes including phospha-
tases, nucleases, proteases, and lipases. Transport
enzymes for sugars and amino acids are also present. The hydrolytic enzymes in the periplasmic
space perform a role analogous to that of the eucaryotic lysosome. Macromolecules hydrolyzed by
these enzymes and their products are either excreted
or used as cell nutrients. The outer wall is selectively
permeable to nutrients on the basis of molecular
size; it prevents the passage of molecules having a
molecular weight greater than 900 daltons into the
cell. The periplasmic space is selective in that it contains enzymes capable of destroying macromolecules
while other enzymes transport nutrients on a selective
basis.

Not all bacteria contain peptidoglycan. Recently it
has been learned that the methanogens, *Halobacte-*

rium, Thermoplasma, and *Sulfolobus* have chemically
complex cell walls that lack peptidoglycan. Yeast
cells do not contain peptidoglycan, yet yeast cells
stain blue when subjected to the Gram-staining
procedure. This suggests that the Gram-stain reaction is not solely dependent on the presence of peptidoglycan.

Gram-stain theory. The differential staining characteristics of bacteria stained with the Gram-stain appear to be related to the differences in the structure of the cell wall. The crystal violet-iodine complex is rapidly removed only from the Gram-negative cells during the nonpolar solvent washing step. Since lipids are readily solubilized in nonpolar solvents, it is thought that this treatment destroys the outer wall of Gram-negative bacteria. The mucocomplex layer in Gram-negative bacteria is too thin to retain the blue crystal violet-iodine complex, so it is washed out with the nonpolar solvent. Gram-positive cell walls have a thick mucocomplex layer with pores (formed by cross-linkage) that are too small to permit the blue dye to be washed out. The result is that Gram-positive bacteria are stained blue, whereas Gram-negative bacteria are colorless until they turn red on counterstaining with safranin.

Capsules and slime layers.

Polymers of carbohydrates or amino acids are sometimes made by bacteria and deposited as a slime layer outside the outer cell wall. Material adhering to the wall with a uniform thickness (Figure 3–11) is referred to as a **capsule,** whereas a diffuse arrangement of these materials is termed a **slime layer.** Capsules can protect microorganisms from the destructive effects of white blood cells. In this sense capsules are virulence factors (see Chapter 12) that contribute to the ability of the microorganism to cause disease.

Motility

Movement of procaryotic cells can be mediated by simple flagella, by endoflagella, or by the flexible movement of the entire cell. Motility in bacteria and the mechanism of movement are readily determined and are often used in classification. The best-understood form of motility in bacteria is flagellar motility.

Flagella. Bacterial flagella (sing., flagellum) are external appendages (Figure 3–12) that can be located on one end of an organism **(monotrichous flagella),** on both ends **(amphitrichous flagella),** or dispersed

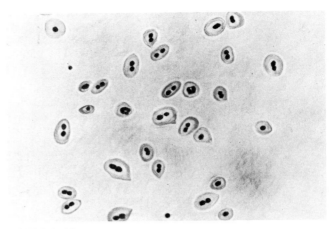

FIGURE 3–11

Capsules surround *Streptococcus pneumoniae*, which grows as a diplococcus. (Courtesy of the Centers for Disease Control.)

around the outside **(peritrichous flagella).** Bacteria that have polar tufts of flagella move by **lophotrichous flagella.** Flagella are thin, proteinaceous structures not visible in the light microscope unless they are first stained.

The flagella of Gram-negative bacteria contain multiple ring-shaped structures that anchor the flagellum to the complex outer membrane of the cell. The typical flagellum is composed of a **basal body,** a **hook** section, and a **filament** (Figure 3–13). The basal body is composed of paired rings. These rings are associated with the cytoplasmic membrane in a manner that allows them to rotate. In Gram-negative bacteria, there are additional disks that appear to be associated with the mucocomplex layer and the outer cell wall. The hook region is joined to the outermost disk and then forms a bend in the flagellum that quickly reduces in size to the slender hollow **flagellar filament. Flagellin** is the only protein found in the filaments. This protein self-assembles into the filament according to the forces governing quaternary protein structure (see Chapter 2). Flagella can be quickly regenerated by a growing bacterium as long as it contains a pool of flagellin.

Flagella generate movement through a rotary mo-

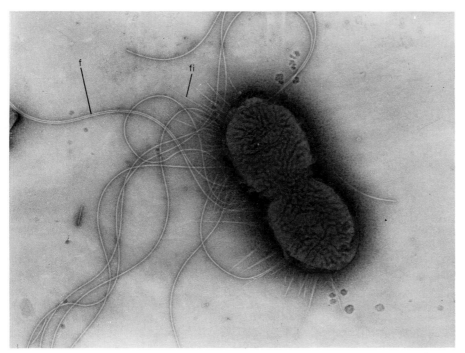

FIGURE 3—12

Electron micrograph of a negatively stained, dividing cell of *Proteus vulgaris* showing flagella (f) and short fimbriae (fi). (Courtesy of Dr. R. K. Nauman.)

FIGURE 3—13

(a) Diagram of a bacterial flagellum. (Courtesy of Drs. M. L. DePamphilis and J. Alder, *J. Bacteriol.,* 105:384–395, 1971, with permission of the American Society for Microbiology.) *(b)* Electron micrograph of flagella isolated from *Salmonella.* (Courtesy of Dr. K. Kutsukake. From K. Kutsukake, T. Suzuke, S. Yamaguchi, and T. Iino, *J. Bacteriol.,* 140:267–275, 1979, with permission of the American Society for Microbiology.)

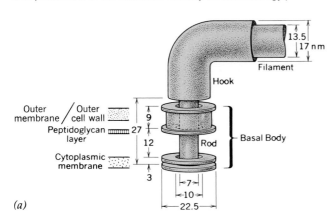

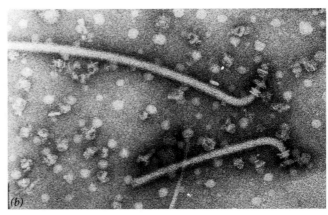

tion; they do not move with the whiplike motion observed in sperm motility. When polar flagella are attached to the surface of a slide, the bacterium spins in a circular motion. This rotational force is thought to be generated by the membrane-bound disks of the basal body (see Figure 3–5). The direction of motion depends on the direction of flagella rotation. In peritrichous flagellated bacteria, the direction of motion of the cell depends on which flagella are rotated.

Movement in bacteria is directional; that is, bacteria can respond to a chemical or a physical stimulus. **Chemotaxis** is the movement of bacteria toward chemical attractants or away from chemical repellents. **Phototaxis** is movement of bacteria in response to light. A photosynthetic organism's movement toward a light source depends on the wavelength of the light and on the intensity of the light.

Endoflagella. Spirochetes are propelled by two or more **endoflagella**. Each flagellum originates from an insertion point located at the end of a nondividing cell and extends toward the midpoint of the protoplasmic cylinder (Figure 3–14). Endoflagella lie on the cell surface beneath the spirochete's cell envelope. In some spirochetes as many as 100 flagella are wrapped around the cell's protoplasmic cylinder. In theory, endoflagella rotate around their insertion point, which in turn causes the spirochete to propel itself with a rotary motion.

Gliding motility. The cyanobacteria, the myxobacteria, and the cytophaga are able to glide on solid surfaces. Gliding bacteria appear to have flexible cell walls, but beyond this observation their means of motility is poorly understood.

Fimbriae and pili

Fimbriae (L. *fimbria,* fringe) are proteinaceous protrusions from the cell surface that help bacteria adhere to the surfaces of cells and teeth and to form pellicles on liquid surfaces. A cell can contain many of these short fimbriae (Figure 3–15). Some pathogenic bacteria use fimbriae to adhere to the tissue in which they cause disease. **Pili** (L. *pilus,* hair) are also proteinaceous protrusions from the cell surface; however, they are generally longer than fimbriae and are identified by their ability to bind certain bacterial viruses. Pili are the hollow structures thought to be involved in the exchange of genetic informa-

FIGURE 3–14
An electron micrograph of a spirochete, *Leptospira,* showing its endoflagella (E) and cell envelope (CE). (Courtesy of Dr. R. K. Nauman. From R. K. Nauman, S. C. Holt, and C. D. Cox, *J. Bacteriol.,* 98:264–280, 1969, with the permission of the American Society for Microbiology.)

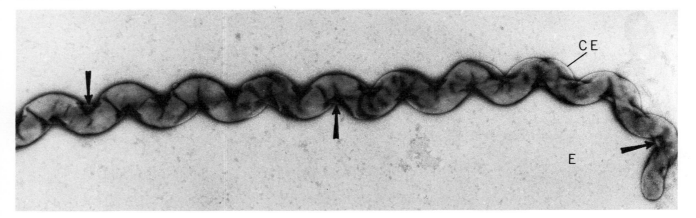

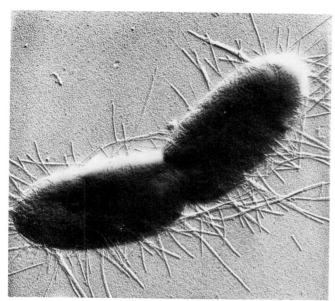

FIGURE 3–15
Fimbriae on the surface of a negatively stained preparation of *Escherichia coli.* The bar represents 0.5 μm. (Courtesy of Dr. D. C. Old. From S. Clegg and D. C. Old, *J. Bacteriol.,* 137:1008–1012, 1979, with permission of the American Society for Microbiology.)

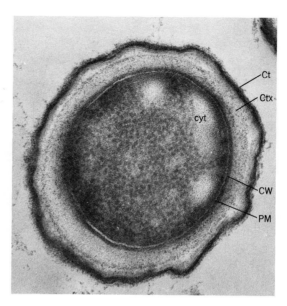

FIGURE 3–16
Electron micrograph of a thin section through an intact spore of *Bacillus megaterium* showing the spore coat (Ct), cortex (Ctx), core wall (CW), plasma membrane (PM), and cytoplasm (cyt). (Courtesy of Dr. P. C. Fitz-James. *J. Bacteriol.,* 105:1119–1136, 1971.)

tion during bacterial conjugation (see Chapter 6). The genes that code for pili are located on plasmids. Fimbriae and pili are distinct in their functions and in the chemistry of their protein subunits.

Spores and other resting forms of bacteria

When certain bacteria are subjected to adverse growth conditions, they change from actively growing cells to inactive resting forms called **spores** or **cysts.** Spores are often called **endospores** because they are formed within the vegetative cell. Bacterial cysts are different in that the entire vegetative cell becomes a cyst. As a general rule, bacterial spores are more resistant to heat, drying, radiation, and chemicals than are cysts or any other form of life.

Endospores are complex structures that form within a cell (Figure 3–16) during **sporogenesis.** As a culture of sporogenous cells enters the stationary phase of growth, a septum forms at one pole of the rod-shaped cell. This septum segregates a copy of the cell's DNA in the forespore. Instead of forming a cross wall, the membrane septum surrounds the forespore to separate it from the remaining parental cell's cytoplasm. The spore then matures by forming a **core wall** that surrounds the spore **protoplast.** Next, a spore cortex composed of a unique peptidoglycan and a spore coat composed largely of protein are formed outside of the core wall.

At some point during sporogenesis, the spore becomes refractile, and it develops a high resistance to heat. Experiments have shown that the spore first becomes refractile (Figure 3–17). The refractile spore then develops thermostability simultaneously with the deposition of dipicolinic acid and the accumulation of Ca^{2+} in the spore protoplast. The molar ratio of Ca^{2+} to dipicolinic acid in spores is equal, suggesting that the Ca^{2+} is chelated to dipicolinic acid.

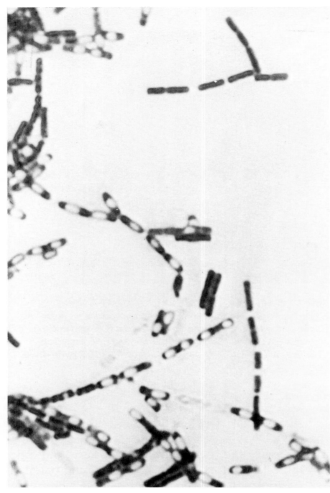

FIGURE 3–17
Micrograph of the endospores of *Bacillus anthracis*. (From
Schneierson's *Atlas of Diagnostic Microbioloby*, 7th ed., courtesy
of Abbott Laboratories.)

The final stage of sporogenesis is the autolysis of the
parent cell, which releases a free spore to the environment. These spores are highly dehydrated, have
no detectable metabolic activity, and are able to survive for years as a resting form of the cell.

Activated spores will undergo the process of **ger-
mination** when they are exposed to suitable growth
conditions. Spores can be activated by exposure to
heat (65°C), low pH, or strong oxidizing agents.

These treatments activate enzymes and initiate outgrowth from the spore state. During the stages of
initiation and outgrowth, the spore structures disin-
tegrate and the spore protoplast emerges as a growing vegetative cell.

Endospores are formed by five bacterial genera:
Clostridium, Bacillus, Sporolactobacillus, Sporosarcina,
and *Desulfotomaculum. Sporosarcina* is the only spore-
forming coccus known. Rod-shaped bacteria form
spores either in a central or in a terminal position in
the cell. Spores are refractile and have their own distinctive shape. Spore morphology is used to classify
organisms belonging to the spore-forming genera
(discussed in Chapter 15).

Certain bacteria can convert their entire cell to a
resting cell known as a **cyst.** Most cyst formers are
soil organisms such as *Azotobacter* and myxobacteria.
Cysts are more resistant to drying and desiccation
than their vegetative counterpart, but they are not
as resistant to these factors as the bacterial endospore. A number of protozoa produce cysts that enable these eucaryotic organisms to survive in adverse environments (see Chapter 28).

EUCARYOTIC CELLS

Bacteria make up only a part of the microbial world.
The protozoa, some fungi, and algae are also microorganisms by virtue of their size; however, they are
eucaryotes by virtue of their cell structure. Algae
and protozoa are simple eucaryotic organisms that
do not contain differentiated tissues. Certain fungi
also fit this description. In contrast, higher plants
and animals are macroorganisms that have differentiated tissues composed of eucaryotic cells.

The presence of a membrane-bound nucleus is the
major morphological feature of the eucaryotic cell. In
addition to the nucleus, eucaryotic cells contain a variety of membrane-bound cytoplasmic organelles
that perform specialized functions. The **cytoplasm** is
defined as the material in the resting eucaryotic cell
contained within the plasma membrane exclusive of
the nucleus. The **karyoplasm** is the material located
within the nuclear envelope (Figure 3–18). To develop an understanding of the structure and func-

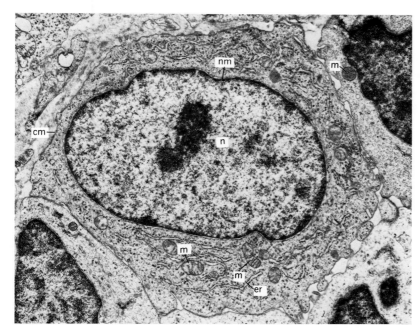

FIGURE 3–18
Electron micrograph of animal cells showing the nucleus (n), endoplasmic reticulum (er), mitochondria (m), the nuclear membrane (nm), and cytoplasmic membrane (cm). (From P. Sheeler and D. Bianchi, *Cell Biology*, Wiley, New York, 1980.)

tion of eucaryotic cells, let us first look at the nucleus.

Nucleus

The nucleus of a nondividing eucaryotic cell is contained within a double membrane referred to as the **nuclear envelope.** This nuclear envelope is perforated with pores. Products of synthetic reactions taking place in the karyoplasm flow through these pores into the cytoplasm. The nuclear envelope surrounds the cell's complement of DNA and the **nucleolus.** Nuclear DNA is the hereditary material of the cell and usually exists as a complex of DNA and histones (basic proteins). The DNA-histone complex appears as a mass of interwoven threads (Figure 3–18) and is known as **chromatin.** The nucleolus is the dark-staining region of the karyoplasm and is thought to contain precursors of ribosomes that are synthesized in the nucleus.

The amount of DNA present in the nucleus of a eucaryotic cell is relatively large (approximately 10^{-12} g/human sperm cell). This means that a eu-

caryotic cell can contain 100 times more DNA than is found in a typical bacterial cell. Whereas bacterial DNA is organized as a single closed circular macromolecule, the eucaryotic cell's DNA is present as many discrete molecules (always more than one and sometimes more than 100). These molecules of DNA, together with their associated proteins, are called **chromosomes.** Eucaryotic cells divide in a set series of stages known as the **cell cycle.**

Cell cycle. Eucaryotic cells intersperse periods of growth and synthesis between nuclear division. The eucaryotic cell cycle progresses (Figure 3–19) through a sequence of stages that includes mitosis (M), growth$_1$ (G$_1$), DNA synthesis (S), and growth$_2$ (G$_2$). The time involved in each stage is determined either microscopically (mitosis) or by measuring the rate of DNA synthesis. The period where neither mitosis nor DNA synthesis occurs is referred to as G$_1$ when it follows mitosis and G$_2$ when it follows synthesis. Interphase is the combined time of the G$_1$, S, and G$_2$ stages. These times vary from one eucaryotic cell to another. The cells of adult animals

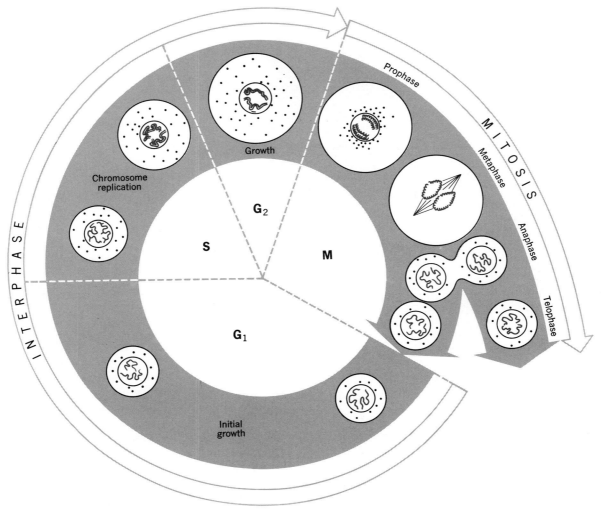

FIGURE 3-19
The cycle of growth and reproduction present in a typical
eucaryotic cell. (From P. Sheeler and D. Bianchi, *Cell Biology*,
Wiley, New York, 1980.)

may enter a nondividing stage after M. This stage is
more aptly referred to as G_0 since it has an indefinite
duration.

Mitosis. The orderly division and separation of
equal complements of nuclear DNA to daughter cells
is done by **mitosis** (Figure 3–20). Mitosis takes place
in four distinct phases that can be observed with the
light microscope (Figure 3–21). The DNA that was
replicated in the S stage of the cell cycle exists as
chromatin, which is composed of DNA bound to
histones. **Prophase,** the first and longest stage of
mitosis, takes about 60 percent of the total division
time. During prophase, the chromatin condenses to

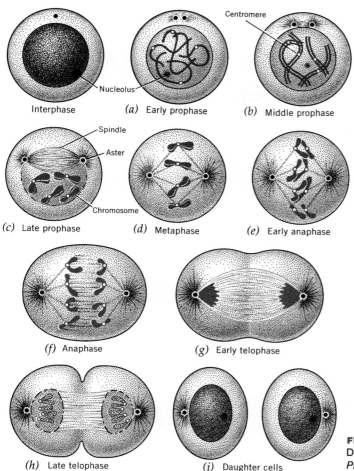

Interphase   *(a)* Early prophase   *(b)* Middle prophase

(c) Late prophase   *(d)* Metaphase   *(e)* Early anaphase

(f) Anaphase   *(g)* Early telophase

(h) Late telophase   *(i)* Daughter cells

FIGURE 3–20
Diagram of mitosis. (From E. J. Gardner and D. P. Snustad, *Principles of Genetics*, 6th ed., Wiley, New York, 1981.)

form the distinct structures known as **chromosomes,** the centrioles move to polar positions in the cell, and the nuclear envelope disappears. Prophase is followed by **metaphase.** The chromosomes line up in the middle of the cell during early metaphase and the spindle fibers, made up of microtubules, join the chromosomes to the centrioles. The duplicate copies of each chromosome (duplicated in interphase) move toward the centrioles during **anaphase.** Nuclear division is completed during **telophase** when a new membrane is formed around each separate complement of chromosomes. The distinct chromosomal structures unwind, and the DNA returns to the chromatin structure observed in interphase. Cell division, or cytokinesis, can proceed once the cell has two identical copies of the genetic material.

Eucaryotes require a complex form of nuclear division because it is necessary for them to partition a copy of each chromosome to a daughter cell or to their organelles. These cells do not continuously replicate themselves. Many eucaryotic cells have long resting stages where no replication occurs. This allows animal cells to grow rapidly during developmental periods after which some cells, such as nerve cells, do not divide. In contrast, bacteria have no complex division mechanisms and vegetative cells

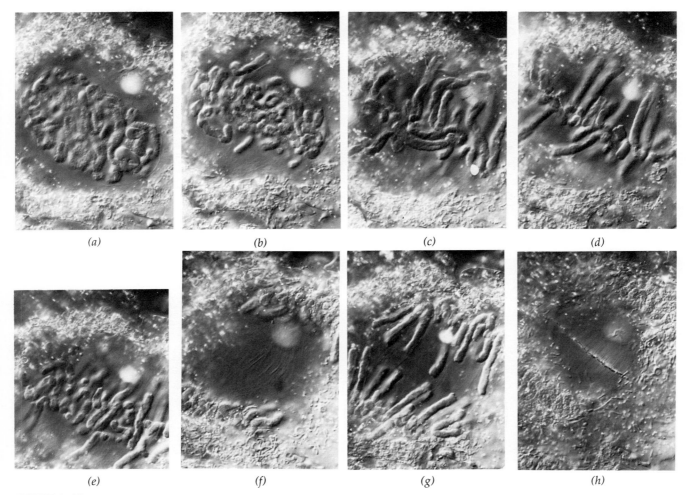

(a)   *(b)*   *(c)*   *(d)*

(e)   *(f)*   *(g)*   *(h)*

FIGURE 3–21
Photomicrographs from 16-mm time-lapse film taken of mitosis in the endosperm of
Haemanthus with Normarski optics. The time for the complete sequence was 160 minutes.
The letters correspond to the stages of mitosis diagramed in Figure 3–20. (Courtesy of Dr.
A. Bajer. From A. Bajer, *Chromosoma*, 24:384–417, 1968, copyright © 1968, Springer-
Verlag.)

appear to be constantly in the process of replicating
their nuclear material.

Cytoplasm

Outside the nuclear membrane are the components
of the cytoplasm. Major functions of the cytoplasm
include energy generation and biosynthetic reactions. Eucaryotic cells have distinctive structures involved in these processes. These structures help to
define the eucaryotic cell type and further empha-
size the differences between eucaryotic and procaryotic cells.

Mitochondria. Energy generation from respiration
takes place in mitochondria (sing., mitochondrion).

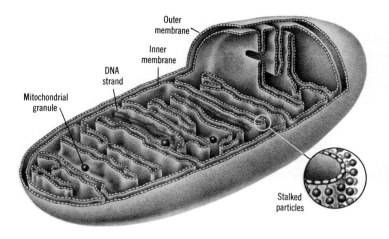

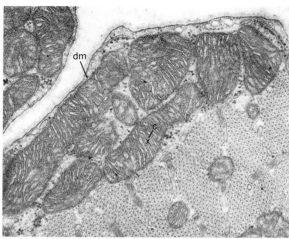

FIGURE 3–22

A diagram of a mitochondrion and an electron micrograph of skeletal muscle showing mitochondria possessing a double membrane (dm) and numerous internal cristae (c). (From E. J. Gardner and D. P. Snustad, *Principles of Genetics,* 6th ed., Wiley, New York, 1981. Electron micrograph courtesy of Dr. A. Nag.)

Mitochondria (Figure 3–22) are **organelles;** that is, they are distinct structures within the cell that can be purified from the cell as functionally and structurally intact units. Their role in the cell is to generate energy during aerobic respiration. Mitochondria are surrounded by a double membrane. The inner membrane contains specialized proteins and organic molecules involved in electron transport. This membrane consists of convoluted folds called **cristae** (Figure 3–22), which possess a large surface. The number of mitochondria in a given cell can vary greatly depending on the function of the cell. Muscle cells require large expenditures of energy and have many mitochondria; nerve cells have few mitochondria.

A mitochondrion is about the size of a typical bacterium. Biochemists have discovered that mitochondria contain DNA and ribosomes. This DNA is a closed circular macromolecule, and the mitochondrial ribosomes are 70S. These characteristics make mitochondria appear lifelike even though mitochondria are unable to divide outside of their cell. They can, however, divide within their host cell by fission.

Chloroplasts. Plant cells have two types of energy-generating organelles: mitochondria and chloroplasts. The organelle responsible for photosynthetic reactions in eucaryotic cells is the **chloroplast.** All the photosynthetic pigments of plant cells are contained in the **thylakoid membranes,** which are located in the interior of chloroplasts (Figure 3–23). These membranes are in turn surrounded by the double membrane that separates the chloroplast from the other components of the cytoplasm. Chloroplasts are similar to mitochondria in that they contain DNA and 70S ribosomes. Although chloroplasts develop and multiply within their cell's cytoplasm, they are unable to divide outside of that cell.

Ribosomes. Eucaryotic cells contain cytoplasmic ribosomes that are 80S in size. The 80S ribosome is composed of a 60S and a 40S component. Eucaryotic ribosomes are composed of RNA (60 percent) and protein (40 percent). The smaller ribosomes found in procaryotic cells, mitochondria, and chloroplasts are also composed of RNA (60 percent) and protein (40 percent). All ribosomes, regardless of size, function in protein synthesis. In eucaryotic cells the ribosomes are often attached to the intracytoplasmic membrane structure known as the **endoplasmic reticulum** (Figure 3–18).

Other Cytoplasmic Structures. Eucaryotic cells are large enough to contain a wide variety of cytoplasmic inclusions. Plant cells often contain food and water vacuoles. These structures are limited by a single membrane and can appear and disappear from the plant cell depending on environmental conditions. In mature plants, food material is often stored in the double-membrane-bound **leucoplast.** Another plant structure is the **chromoplast,** a cytoplasmic structure bound by a double membrane, which is responsible for the color of fruits and vegetables.

Animal cells also contain cytoplasmic structures known as **vesicles.** The **Golgi body** is a complex membrane folded into vesicles and sacs. This is an animal cell's packaging center. Enzymes and other cellular products are incorporated into vesicles that

FIGURE 3–23
An electron micrograph of a chloroplast in a green-plant cell. Chloroplasts are the photosynthetic organelles of plant cells. They contain membrane-bound chlorophyll and DNA. The enlarged drawing shows the DNA and the stacks of chlorophyll-containing membrane sacs known as grana. (From E. J. Gardner and D. P. Snustad, *Principles of Genetics,* 6th ed., Wiley, New York, 1981, micrograph courtesy of T. E. Weier.)

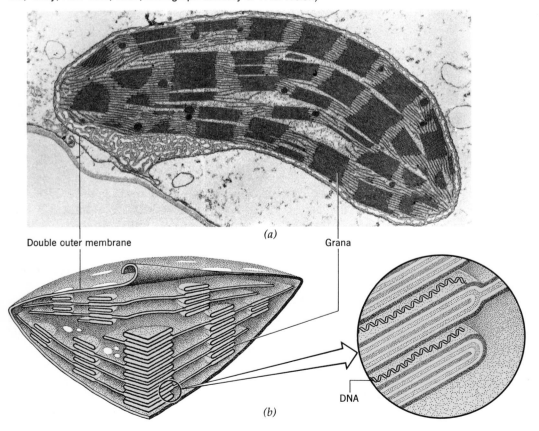

Double outer membrane

(a)

Grana

DNA

(b)

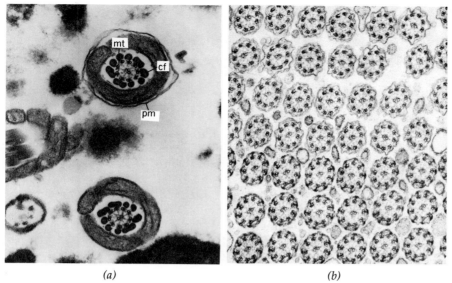

(a)   *(b)*

FIGURE 3–24

(a) Transmission electron micrograph of the cross section of bull sperm flagella showing the 9 pairs plus 2 arrangement of microtubules (mt); they form a circle inside the coarse fibers (cf). The entire flagellum is surrounded by a plasma membrane (pm). (Courtesy of Dr. C. Lindemann.) *(b)* Transmission electron micrograph of a cross section through the cilia of a ciliate showing their symmetrical arrangement and internal structure. (From P. Sheeler and D. Bianchi, *Cell Biology*, Wiley, New York, 1980.)

either remain within the cell or are excreted into the cell's environment. **Lysosomes** are vesicular structures that contain degradative enzymes and are important to host defense mechanisms. Lysosomes are an example of the type of vesicles formed by the Golgi body of animal cells.

Motility

Eucaryotic cells contain complex organs of movement called flagella or cilia. **Flagella** are organs of movement usually occurring as single structures, whereas **cilia** occur in groups and beat with a rhythmic motion. A flagellum is usually attached to the polar end of a eucaryotic cell; unlike bacterial flagella, it is easily observed in the light microscope. Mammalian sperm cells and many gametes from aquatic plants contain one or more flagella. Movement of these cells is generated by the whiplike ac-

tion of the flagellum. In many animals, cilia are found associated with mucous membranes. For example, cilia are present in the human tracheae and in human Fallopian tubes. Single-cell animals often use cilia for movement as well as for capturing food particles.

Cilia and flagella of eucaryotic cells have a common structure. The organ is composed of microtubules arranged in 9 pairs plus 2 configuration (Figure 3–24). The entire arrangement is surrounded by a membrane. **Microtubules** are found extensively in animal cells and appear to be formed from two types of proteins: α-tubulin and β-tubulin. These two types of tubulin molecules combine to form the long, hollow structures recognized as microtubules. The semicircular hook structures attached to the pairs of microtubules in flagella and cilia are dynein molecules. **Dynein** is the protein that has ATPase (an enzyme that releases energy from ATP) activity and is involved in the actual movement of flagella and cilia. At the base of the flagellum or cilium is a cylindrical structure called the **basal body.** The basal body extends into the cytoplasm and serves as the growth site for a flagellum or cilium.

Microtubules are also found inside animal cells. Microtubules are involved in spindle formation during mitosis. The centriole observed in many eucaryotic cells has the basic 9 pairs plus 2 structure, which indicates that it too is composed of microtubules. Microtubules have also been observed to interlace the cytoplasm of animal cells, suggesting that microtubules can play an architectural support role.

EVOLUTION OF EUCARYOTIC AND PROCARYOTIC CELLS

A summary of the structures of procaryotic and eucaryotic cells is presented in Table 3–1. Both cell types perform the functions basic to life, but the eucaryotic cell is structurally much more complex. Indeed, the organisms composed of eucaryotic cells are more varied in size, shape, and complexity than are the procaryotic cells. Still, there is a great diversity among the procaryotic cells, as will be seen shortly.

Biologists have tried to comprehend how two distinct cell types have come to exist in the earth's closed environment. If life originated from a single cell that in turn gave rise to all living systems, as the theory of evolution proposes, then the existence of two distinct cell types on the earth is a major dichotomy. Some biologists suggest that simple mutations in procaryotic cells, followed by natural selection, could give rise to all the characteristics of the eucaryotic cell type. Others suggest that a primitive eucaryotic cell joined forces with a procaryotic cell in a symbiotic relationship. This symbiotic relationship is postulated to have resulted in the development of a mitochondrion from an aerobic bacterium and in the development of a primitive chloroplast from a cyanobacterium. The development of these structures forms the basis of the **endosymbiotic theory** of cell type development. Even though the evolution of procaryotic and eucaryotic cell types is unresolved, these theories are a valuable starting point for thought and debate.

Are there other, yet to be characterized, cell types on the earth? Some scientists say yes. Recent experiments on the methane-producing bacteria suggest that these organisms may represent a third class of cells that is even more primitive than the pro-

TABLE 3–1
Procaryotic vs. Eucaryotic Cell Type

Characteristic	Procaryotic	Eucaryotic
DNA organization	Diffused in cytoplasm	Nucleus
Chromosome number	One	More than one
Cell wall	Complex, usually present	If present, of simple chemical structure
Movement	Flagella, simple structure	Complex 9 pairs plus 2 microtubule structure
Cytoplasmic structures		
Endoplasmic reticulum	Absent	Present
Vacuoles	Absent	Present
Ribosomes	70S, small ribosomes	80S, large ribosomes
Physiological Functions		
Site of photosynthesis	Membranes in cytoplasm	Membranes in chloroplast
Site of respiration	Cytoplasmic membranes	Mitochondria

caryotes. The methanogens have cell walls that lack peptidoglycan, they have different ribosomal RNAs, and they contain unique enzyme cofactors. Methanogens appear to be very primitive anaerobic organisms. Scientists have coined the term *Archaebacteria* to describe this group of primitive organisms.

Currently there are no concrete answers to the questions concerning the origin and the meaning of the various cell types. Yet, when we look at the basic cell functions, there is consistency among living things. By looking at the chemical mechanisms used by cells to perform cell functions, we realize that biological consistency is even greater. If cell structure represents a divergence in living systems, the biochemistry must represent the continuity of life.

SUMMARY

Microbiology is the study of microorganisms including the bacteria. All bacteria have the procaryotic cell structure. Procaryotic cells are relatively small and contain no membrane-limited, functional organelle smaller than the cell itself. Respiration and photosynthesis, when present in procaryotic cells, take place on the cytoplasmic membrane or on membrane structures derived from the cytoplasmic membrane. The cell's hereditary information is found in the cytoplasm in the nuclear region. This material consists of at least one copy of a closed circular DNA macromolecule that continually divides during growth. Ribosomes in bacterial cells are free in the cytoplasm and are smaller (70S) than ribosomes found in eucaryotic cells (80S). Procaryotic cells usually contain chemically complex cell walls. Peptidoglycan is the major component of the mucocomplex cell wall layer. This layer confers rigidity and shape on the bacterial cell. In addition, Gram-negative bacteria contain lipopolysaccharides in an outer cell wall. External proteinaceous appendages of bacteria include fimbriae, pili, and flagella, which are involved in cell attachment, genetic transfer, and motility, respectively.

Eucaryotic microorganisms include the fungi, algae, and protozoa. The major morphological feature of eucaryotic cells is the presence of a nucleus, the membrane-bound structure that contains the cell's complement of DNA. This DNA is organized into more than one chromosome and is divided and segregated to daughter cells by the process of mitosis. Eucaryotic cells contain organelles that perform specialized functions. Mitochondria are the cytoplasmic organelles responsible for respiration. The photosynthetic plant cells contain chloroplasts in addition to mitochondria. Both chloroplasts and mitochondria are surrounded by a double membrane, and both organelles possess 70S ribosomes and DNA. Nuclear-directed protein synthesis occurs on 80S cytoplasmic ribosomes. These 80S ribosomes are often attached to the membranes of the endoplasmic reticulum. If cell walls are present in eucaryotic cells, they are chemically simple structures. Motility in eucaryotic cells is mediated by cilia or flagella that are membrane-surrounded, complex structures containing microtubules arranged in a 9 pairs plus 2 pattern. Eucaryotic and procaryotic cells represent two distinct cell types. The eucaryotic microorganisms are distinct from higher plants and animals in that they do not contain differentiated tissue.

QUESTIONS AND TOPICS FOR STUDY AND DISCUSSION

Questions

1. Draw and label the known shapes of spherical bacteria.
2. Describe and compare a simple stain and a differential stain.
3. Compare the size, organization, and replication of a bacterial cell to an eucaryotic cell.
4. What is the size and cellular location of ribosomes in procaryotic and eucaryotic cells? What eucaryotic cell organelles have ribosomes?
5. Describe the structure and function of the cytoplasmic membrane. Which bacteria have specialized intracytoplasmic membranes and what function do these membranes perform?
6. Diagram the structure of the peptidoglycan found in bacterial walls. What is its function?
7. Compare the cell wall structure(s) of Gram-positive bacteria to those of Gram-negative bacteria.

8. Diagram the eucaryotic flagellum. How does this compare in structure and movement to the flagella found in procaryotic cells?
9. Define and explain the function of the following.

chloroplasts	endospores	mitosis
cilia	fimbriae	nucleolus
cysts	Golgi body	pili

Discussion

1. What evidence is there to support the endosymbiotic theory? Can you think of an argument against this theory?

FURTHER READINGS

Books

Dustin, P., *Microtubules*, Springer-Verlag, New York, 1978. A major book-length review of the biochemistry and biology of microtubules.

Gibbs, M. (ed.), *Structure and Function of Chloroplasts*, Springer-Verlag, Berlin, 1971. A collection of papers on chloroplasts.

Munn, E. A., *The Structure of Mitochondria*, Academic Press, New York, 1974. A major review of the structure and biochemical composition of the mitochondria.

Articles and Reviews

DiRienzo, J. M., K. Nakamura, and M. Inouye, "The Outer Membrane Proteins of Gram-negative Bacteria: Biosynthesis, Assembly, and Function," *Ann. Revs. Biochem.*, 47:481–532 (1978). An advanced biochemical review of these important proteins.

Dustin, P., "Microtubules," *Sci. Am.*, 243:66–76 (August 1980). A synopsis of the structure of microtubules and their function in nucleated cells.

Dworkin, M., "Spores, Cysts, and Stalks," in J. R. Sokatch and L. N. Ornston (eds.), *The Bacteria*, vol. 7, pp. 1–84, Academic Press, New York, 1979. A well-illustrated review of the structure and formation of bacterial spores, cysts, and stalks.

Goodenough, U. W., and R. P. Levine, "The Genetic Activity of Mitochondria and Chloroplasts," *Sci. Am.*, 223:22–29 (November 1970). The influence of mitochondria and chloroplast DNA on the structure and function of these organelles is discussed.

Margulis, L., "Symbiosis and Evolution," *Sci. Am.*, 225:48–57 (August 1971). Evidence supporting the endosymbiotic theory, which is one explanation of the evolutionary development of eucaryotic cells, is presented.

Racker, E., "The Membrane of the Mitochondrion," *Sci. Am.*, 218:32–39 (February 1968). A biochemist's approach to understanding mitochondria through the dissociation and reassociation of the mitochondrial membrane.

Satin, P., "How Cilia Move," *Sci. Am.*, 231:44–52 (October 1974). A detailed look at the structure and function of eucaryotic flagella.

Sokatch, J. R., "Roles of Appendages and Surface Layers in Adaptation of Bacteria to Their Environment," in J. R. Sokatch and L. N. Ornston (eds.), *The Bacteria*, vol. 7, pp. 229–289, Academic Press, New York, 1979. An illustrated review of bacterial flagella, pili, fimbriae, cell walls, and envelopes.

Stainer, R. Y., and C. B. van Neil, "The Concept of a Bacterium," *Archiv. fur Mikrobiologie*, 42:17–35 (1962). A classic paper that presents the arguments for recognizing the significance of the procaryotic cell structure.

4

MICROBIAL PHYSIOLOGY

Microbial physiology is the study of the chemical reactions used by microbes to grow and reproduce. These reactions are powered by the energy stored in chemical compounds or by the energy present in light from the sun. For almost every form of energy found in nature, there is a microorganism that can use it for growth. Although most microorganisms use organic compounds as a source of energy, there are bacteria that use inorganic compounds as their sole source of energy. Plants and some bacteria depend on light energy for growth and reproduction. All organisms, regardless of their energy source, can store energy in a form that powers their synthetic reactions.

Although microorganisms have diverse mechanisms for obtaining energy, many of the reactions they perform to synthesize cell components are common to all living systems. The basic building materials—the carbohydrates, the fatty acids, the amino acids, the nitrogenous bases—for all cells are similar, so it follows that the reactions used to manufacture these materials should be similar. For example, if we know the mechanism for the formation of glutamic acid in *Escherichia coli,* we can expect that a similar

mechanism will exist in humans, and indeed it does. This chapter discusses the energy-generating reactions that enable organisms to grow in diverse environments and the synthetic reactions that are common to these diverse organisms.

ENERGY

Matter and energy are the two fundamental components of the earth. **Energy** is the capacity to do work. Biological systems can use chemical and/or light energy to perform the work of manufacturing cell material to produce new cells. Sunlight is the ultimate biological source of energy and is converted to chemical energy through the process of **photosynthesis.** Organisms that use light energy include the green plants, the cyanobacteria, and a diverse group of purple and green photosynthetic bacteria. Organisms that convert light energy into chemical energy are known as **phototrophs.** The chemical energy generated during photosynthesis is stored in organic compounds and serves as the renewable source of chemical energy for nonphotosynthetic organisms.

Chemolithotrophs use the chemical energy in inorganic molecules to grow and reproduce, whereas **chemoorganotrophs** use the chemical energy in organic molecules to grow. The amount of energy released during chemical reactions is expressed as the **Gibb's free energy change, G.** ΔG represents the quantity of energy available to do useful work. When chemicals react or undergo a change from one form to another, energy is either lost to the surroundings or trapped in different compounds. Reactions that release energy are called **exergonic** reactions and have negative changes in free energy ($-\Delta G$). Reactions that consume energy are termed **endergonic** reactions and have positive changes in free energy ($+\Delta G$). An example of an exergonic reaction is the oxidation of glucose to carbon dioxide (CO_2) and water.

$$C_6H_{12}O_6 + 6 O_2 \rightarrow 6CO_2 + 6H_2O$$
Glucose   Oxygen   Carbon   Water
                          dioxide

$$\Delta G = -686 \text{ kcal mole}^{-1}$$

This reaction takes place in our bodies as well as in fireplaces where wood is oxidized to CO_2 and H_2. The oxidation of inorganic compounds can also be an exergonic reaction. Ammonium ion (NH_4^+) is oxidized to nitrate according to the equation

$$NH_4^+ + 2 O_2 \rightarrow NO_3^- + H_2O + 2H^+$$

$$\Delta G = -82.5 \text{ kcal mole}^{-1}$$

This reaction is an exergonic reaction because ΔG is negative.

Endergonic reactions include most of the synthetic reactions of biological systems; for example, protein synthesis is an endergonic reaction. The energy used in synthetic reactions can come directly from the breakdown of metabolites or indirectly from chemicals capable of energy storage. The amount of energy in these molecules is conventionally expressed as ΔG. Chemists usually report the free energy change of hydrolysis (or breakdown) because it is easier to determine this value than to determine the energy of formation. The ΔG of hydrolysis of certain biologically important compounds are reported in Table 4–1.

TABLE 4–1
Energy of Hydrolysis of Biologically Important Compounds[a]

Compound	$\Delta G^{\circ\prime}$ kcal mole^{-1}
Glucose-6-phosphate	−3.3
AMP	−3.4
ATP	−7.3
GTP	−7.3
CTP	−7.3
UTP	−7.3
Acetyl phosphate	−10.1
1,3-Diphosphoglyceric acid	−11.8
Phosphoenolpyruvic acid	−14.8

[a]These values are at standard conditions of 1 molar solutions, pH 7.0, and 30°C. Changes in these conditions can change the ΔG for a given hydrolysis.

Biological systems also use energy derived from the transfer of electrons (e^-). Certain biomolecules can act as transfer agents by accepting electrons and then passing them on to another biomolecule. When these molecules are arranged in a series, electrons travel from one molecule to the next. A compound that accepts an electron is said to be **reduced**. A compound that gives up an electron is said to be **oxidized**. These reactions can be written as half reactions.

$$H_2 \rightarrow 2H^+ + 2e^-$$
Hydrogen   Proton   Electron

$$O_2 + 1e^- \rightarrow O_2^-$$
Oxygen   Electron   Superoxide

Each half reaction is coupled to another half reaction in biological systems because electrons do not normally exist in the free state. Such a coupled reaction is called an **oxidation-reduction reaction**. Many oxidation-reduction reactions occur in biological systems.

The ability of a reduced compound, such as molecular hydrogen, to give up electrons can be measured electrically. The quantity measured is called the **oxidation potential** and is expressed in volts. The value obtained is the **electromotive force** and is indicated by E_0'. The more negative the E_0', the stronger is its reducing power. Energy is released

TABLE 4–2
Chemical Energy in Molecules[a]

I. Substrates

Compound	Reaction for Yielding Energy	Energy kcal mole^{-1}
Glucose	$C_6H_{12}O_6 + 6O_2 \rightarrow 6H_2O + 6CO_2$	-686
Lactic acid	$C_3H_6O_3 + 3O_2 \rightarrow 3H_2O + 3CO_2$	-318
Acetic acid	$C_2H_4O_2 + 2O_2 \rightarrow 2H_2O + 2CO_2$	-214
Adenosine triphosphate	$ATP + H_2O \rightarrow ADP + H_3PO_4$	-7.3

II. Coenzymes and Cytochromes

Compound	Half Reaction (Reduction)	Energy E_0' Volts
Pyridine nucleotide	$NAD^+ + 2H^+ + 2e^- \rightleftharpoons NADH + H^+$	-0.32
Ubiquinone	$Ubiquinone + 2H^+ + 2e^- \rightleftharpoons Ubiquinol$	$+0.10$
Cytochrome c	$2Cytochrome\ c_{ox} + 2e^- \rightarrow 2Cytochrome\ c_{red}$	$+0.25$
Oxygen	$2H^+ + 2e^- + \frac{1}{2}O_2 \rightarrow H_2O$	$+0.82$

[a]Energy in compounds can be released through oxidation. Since electrons ($2e^-$) do not exist as free atoms in biological material, we write half reactions for our convenience. The more negative an E_0', the more reduced the compound. A reduced compound can be oxidized by another compound that has a more positive E_0'. To calculate the energy generated from an oxidation-reduction reaction, use the equation: $\Delta G = nF(\Delta E_0')$, where n is the number of electrons, F is the faraday (23.058 kcal), and $\Delta E_0'$ is the difference in electromotive force between the reducing reaction and the oxidation reaction. When NAD_{red} is oxidized by oxygen in the electron-transport system, the theoretical energy generated is

$$\Delta G = -2(23.058\ \text{kcal})\ [-0.32-(+0.82)] = 52.5\ \text{kcal}$$

Since only three ATPs are made in this process, the efficiency of the process is $(3 \times 7.3\ \text{kcal})/52.5\ \text{kcal} \times 100 = 42\%$ efficient. The remainder of the energy in NAD_{red} is given off as heat.

when a reduced compound transfers electrons to an oxidized compound. Table 4–2 lists some biologically important compounds and the energy released when they undergo oxidation-reduction reactions.

Cells can transform the energy released during chemical reactions into other chemicals that serve as energy reservoirs. These reservoirs consist of energy transfer molecules (represented by X in Figure 4–1) and are found in all cells. Adenosine triphosphate (ATP) is a representative energy transfer molecule (Figure 4–2). It is composed of the nitrogenous base (adenine), a ribose molecule, and three phosphate molecules. ATP is formed from adenosine diphosphate (ADP) and inorganic phosphate in an endergonic reaction.

$$ADP + H_3PO_4 \rightarrow ATP + H_2O \qquad \Delta G = +7.3\ \text{kcal mole}^{-1}$$

The two terminal phosphate anhydride bonds in ATP are high-energy bonds. This has been experi-

mentally determined by measuring the amount of heat released during the hydrolysis of the terminal phosphate group from ATP. The value of 7.3 kcal mole^{-1} of ATP hydrolyzed to ADP and H_2O under standard conditions is routinely obtained and will be used in our discussion of energetics.

Another small molecule that transfers energy is nicotinamide adenine dinucleotide (NAD). NAD is made from adenine dinucleotide and the vitamin niacin (see Appendix 2 for formula). NAD is constructed such that it can exist in a reduced form (NAD_{red}) and in an oxidized form (NAD_{ox}). NAD_{ox} is converted to NAD_{red} when it gains two electrons and one proton.

$$NAD^+ + 2e^- + 2H^+ \rightarrow NADH + H^+$$
$$\text{Oxidized} \qquad\qquad \text{Reduced}$$

NAD is a metabolite that can transfer energy in the form of electrons. This molecule is involved in

FIGURE 4–1
Illustrative example of energy storage.

Energy is released (exergonic reaction) during the metabolism of substrate (S) to the product (P) as shown in reaction (1). A synthetic reaction, reaction (2), requires energy (endergonic reaction) to convert the metabolic intermediate (I) into a cellular constituent (C).

$$S \rightarrow P \qquad \Delta G = -10 \text{ kcal} \qquad (1)$$
$$I \rightarrow C \qquad \Delta G = + 5 \text{ kcal} \qquad (2)$$

Energy available from reaction (1) can be trapped in an energy transfer compound (X) such that X becomes energy rich (X_e).

$$X \rightarrow X_e \qquad \Delta G = +8 \text{ kcal} \qquad (3)$$

Reaction (3) is endergonic and will occur only when it is combined with an exergonic reaction such as reaction (1).

$$S + X \rightarrow P + X_e \qquad \Delta G = -2 \text{ kcal} \qquad (4)$$

Reaction (4) traps 8 kcal in X_e, leaving a net of minus 2 kcal, which are released as heat $[-10 + 8 = -2]$. Energy stored in X_e can now be used to drive the formation of C (2) as demonstrated in reaction (5).

$$I + X_e \rightarrow C + X \qquad \Delta G = -3 \text{ kcal} \qquad (5)$$

The combined change in free energy for reactions (4) and (5), ($\Delta G = -2 + -3 = -5$) is identical to the combined change in free energy for reactions (1) and (2).

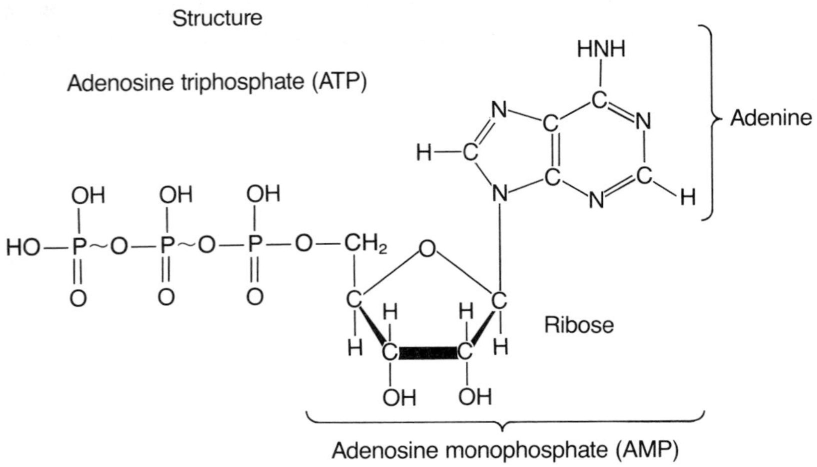

Structure

Adenosine triphosphate (ATP)

Adenine

Ribose

Adenosine monophosphate (AMP)

Reactions

$$ATP + H_2O \rightarrow ADP + H_3PO_4$$
$$ADP + H_2O \rightarrow AMP + H_3PO_4$$

FIGURE 4–2
Adenosine triphosphate contains energy-rich anhydride bonds ($\sim$) between the phosphate groups. Sequential hydrolysis of these two bonds yields adenosine diphosphate (ADP) and adenosine monophosphate (AMP) concomitantly with the release of 7.3 kcal mole^{-1} for each bond hydrolyzed.

many oxidation-reduction reactions in cells. Energy trapped in ATP and NADH is available for synthetic reactions which are catalyzed by enzymes. Enzymes are extremely important to cells. The amount and kinds of enzymes present in a cell determines the metabolic capability of that cell.

ENZYMES

Enzymes are proteins that function as catalysts; that is, they speed up the rate of a reaction without being changed in the process. As is true of proteins, most enzymes are inactivated by high temperatures and by extremes in pH. Most enzymes have a maximal catalytic activity between 30° and 37°C and within the pH range of 4.5 to 8.5. These are the ranges of temperature and pH routinely found in active biological systems.

Most chemical reactions proceed more slowly at room temperature than at elevated temperatures. For example, wood oxidizes very slowly at room temperature, yet it oxidizes very quickly when burned in a fireplace. Enzymes that function at the relatively low temperatures of biological systems speed up the rates of chemical reactions by having catalytic sites that specifically interact with the reactant (Figure 4–3). The reactant, called the substrate (S), combines with the enzyme (E) to form an enzyme-substrate complex, designated (ES). Because of its specialized structure, the enzyme places stress on the chemical bonds in the substrate molecule, resulting in breakage or rearrangement of chemical bonds. This results in the formation of a new compound called the product (P).

$$S + E \rightleftharpoons ES \rightleftharpoons E + P$$

This is the generalized reaction for an enzyme acting on a single substrate.

FIGURE 4–3

Diagrammatic representation of enzyme action. Enzymes bind reversibly with their substrate to form an enzyme substrate (ES) complex. The reaction is then catalyzed, converting the substrate (S) to the product (P). A noncompetitive inhibitor (I) can bind at a site other than the substrate site (active site). The inhibitor prevents the substrate from binding to the enzyme, so that no product is formed.

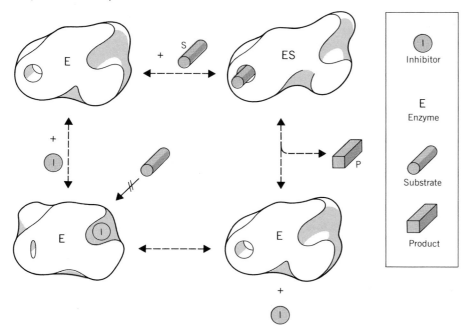

Enzymes are usually named after their substrate and the chemical action exerted on that substrate. The suffix -*ase* is used to designate enzymes. The enzymes protease, nuclease, and lipase conform to this convention.

Any given cell will have at least 1000 enzymes. Each one will belong to one of the six major enzyme classes. **Oxidoreductases** catalyze oxidation-reduction reactions. **Transferases** take a chemical group from one molecule and transfer it to another. **Hydrolases** cleave covalent bonds through the addition of a water molecule. This is in contrast to **lyases** that cleave covalent bonds without the addition of water and do so in the absence of oxidation-reduction reactions. Pyruvic acid decarboxylase is an example of a lyase. **Isomerases** catalyze geometric or structural changes within one molecule. Synthetic reactions are catalyzed by **ligases.** These enzymes catalyze the joining together of two molecules coupled to the hydrolysis of ATP.

An example of a specific enzymatic reaction is the decarboxylation of pyruvic acid, a reaction catalyzed by pyruvic acid decarboxylase.

$$CH_3 - \overset{\overset{O}{\|}}{C} - COOH \xrightarrow[\text{decarboxylase}]{\text{pyruvic acid}} CH_3 - \overset{\overset{O}{\|}}{C} - H + CO_2$$

Pyruvic acid   Acetaldehyde   Carbon dioxide

An enzyme usually catalyzes only one reaction. Enzymes are specific for the substrates they bind, so a cell must have a specific enzyme to catalyze each unique chemical reaction. In this example, the catalytic site of pyruvic acid decarboxylase binds only pyruvic acid.

Some enzymes have two substrates and catalyze a change in both molecules. Alcohol dehydrogenase is an example of this type of enzyme. The first substrate is the acetaldehyde molecule produced from pyruvic acid. The second substrate is NAD_{red}. NAD is not a part of the enzyme but exists in the cell as a small molecule that can participate in many different enzymatic reactions. Alcohol dehydrogenase catalyzes a reversible reaction that produces ethanol from acetaldehyde and oxidizes NAD_{red}.

$$CH_3 - \overset{\overset{O}{\|}}{C} - H + NAD_{red} \xrightarrow[\text{dehydrogenase}]{\text{alcohol}} CH_3CH_2OH + NAD_{ox}$$

Acetaldehyde   Ethanol

This is an example of an oxidation-reduction reaction, since NAD_{red} is oxidized to NAD_{ox} and acetaldehyde is reduced to ethanol.

NAD serves as a coenzyme in this reaction. **Coenzymes** are reusable organic molecules that play an accessory role in some enzyme-catalyzed reactions. Flavin adenine dinucleotide (FAD) and NAD are coenzymes that are made from vitamins, adenosine, and ribose. The vitamins, Table 4–3, are organic substances present in cells in trace amounts. Most of the vitamins are, or are used to manufacture, coenzymes. The reusable coenzymes can exist in two forms. FAD and NAD can exist in an oxidized and a reduced state. Other coenzymes accept and donate chemical groups. Since coenzymes are essential for growth, cells that are unable to manufacture coenzymes or their vitamin precursors must obtain them from their diet.

Enzymes and coenzymes are the workhorses of microbial physiology. The combined effect of all the enzyme-catalyzed reactions in a cell is to transform energy into cellular material, thereby allowing the cell to grow and reproduce.

AEROBIC RESPIRATION

Humans and many microorganisms obtain energy in aerobic environments. **Aerobic respiration** is the process of transforming chemical energy that uses oxygen as the terminal oxidizing agent. Glucose is oxidized by aerobic respiration to carbon dioxide and water. The oxidant (O_2) is reduced to H_2O, while the carbon atoms of glucose are oxidized to CO_2. The amount of energy released by the complete oxidation of glucose to $6CO_2$ and $6H_2O$ is 686 kcal mole^{-1} of glucose. Part of this energy is conserved as usable energy; some energy is always released as heat. The metabolism of glucose proceeds in a series of metabolic steps that include glycolysis, the tricarboxylic acid cycle, and the electron-transport chain.

TABLE 4–3
Vitamins and Their Function

Vitamin	Chemical Name	Coenzyme	Function
Niacin	Nicotinic acid	Pyridine nucleotides (NAD, NADP)	Oxidation-reduction reactions
Vitamin B_2	Riboflavin	Flavin nucleotides (FAD, FMN)	Oxidation-reduction reactions
Vitamin B_1	Thiamine	Thiamine pyrophosphate	Decarboxylations
Vitamin B_6	Pyridoxine	Pyridoxal phosphate	Amino acid metabolism, e.g., transamination
Pantothenic acid	Pantothenic acid	Coenzyme A	Keto acid oxidation, fatty acid metabolism
Folic acid	Folic acid	Tetrahydrofolic acid	One-carbon transfer
Biotin	Biotin	Biotin	CO_2 fixation, carboxyl transfer
Vitamin B_{12}	Cyanocobalamin	Cobamide	Molecular rearrangements

Glycolysis

Aerobic respiration combines the release of energy from glucose with the storage of energy in ATP. Glycolysis is the first sequence of reactions in glucose metabolism and results in the formation of 2 moles of pyruvic acid, 2 moles of NAD_{red}, and 2 moles of ATP. This metabolic pathway is shown as a sequential series of reactions in Figure 4–4 (see Appendix 3 for the chemical structures). In reality, all these reactions occur simultaneously in the cytoplasm of the cell. Each active cell will have many molecules of glucose and many molecules of each metabolite and each product all interacting with their respective enzymes. All the chemical reactions involved in glycolysis are presented in Appendix 3. This chapter is concerned with the reactions involved in the generation of ATP and in the reduction or oxidation of NAD.

Metabolism of glucose begins with the phosphorylation of glucose. One mole of ATP per mole of glucose is used (Figure 4–4), and one mole of glucose-6-phosphate and one mole of ADP are formed. The phosphate bond in glucose-6-phosphate retains some of the energy previously found in ATP. Glucose-6-phosphate is transformed to fructose 1,6-di-

phosphate by the transferral of a second phosphate group from ATP to glucose-6-phosphate. Next, fructose 1,6-diphosphate is enzymatically split in half, resulting in two 3-carbon sugars that are equivalent to glyceraldehyde-3-phosphate. A complex enzymatic reaction converts the two molecules of glyceraldehyde-3-phosphate to two molecules of 1,3-diphosphoglyceric acid and two molecules of NAD_{red}.

$$2 \text{ Glyceraldehyde-3-PO}_4 + 2H_3PO_4 + 2NAD_{ox}$$

$$\xrightarrow[\text{dehydrogenase}]{\text{glyceraldehyde-3-PO}_4}$$

$$2(1,3\text{-Diphosphoglyceric acid}) + 2NAD_{red}$$

Notice that inorganic phosphate (H_3PO_4) is combined with the glyceraldehyde molecule. This reaction results in **substrate level phosphorylation,** because the inorganic phosphate in 1,3-diphosphoglyceric acid (see Table 4–1) is now endowed with a high energy state.

The 2 moles of 1,3-diphosphoglyceric acid are metabolized to pyruvic acid in a series of reactions that remove 4 moles of phosphate from the carbohydrate while forming 4 moles of ATP in the process. Therefore, the net yield is 2 moles of ATP formed

Glycolysis

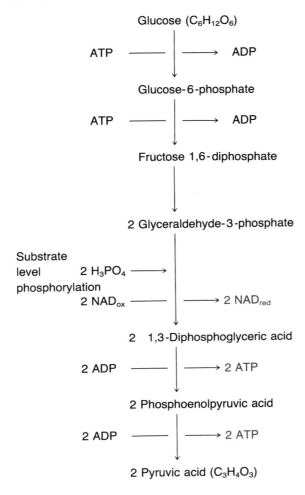

Overall

Glucose $\longrightarrow$ 2 Pyruvic acid + 2 ATP + 2 NAD$_{red}$

FERMENTATION

2 Pyruvic acid

2 NAD$_{red}$ $\longrightarrow$ $\longrightarrow$ 2 NAD$_{ox}$

2 Lactic acid (C$_3$H$_6$O$_3$)

FIGURE 4–4

Glycolysis is a sequence of enzymatic reactions that converts glucose to pyruvic acid. Only some of the reactions are shown. When this process operates in the absence of oxygen to produce lactic acid, it becomes the lactic acid fermentation.

$(4ATP − 2ATP_{used})$ for each mole of glucose metabolized to 2 moles of pyruvic acid. The overall reaction for glycolysis is

$$C_6H_{12}O_6 + 2H_3PO_4 + 2ADP + 2NAD_{ox} \rightarrow$$

$$\overset{\overset{\textstyle O}{\|}}{2CH_3 - C - COOH} + 2ATP + 2NAD_{red} + 2H_2O + 2H^+$$

Since pyruvic acid contains substantial amounts of energy, aerobic organisms metabolize pyruvic acid through the next sequence of reactions in aerobic respiration.

Tricarboxylic acid cycle

Aerobic respiration results in the complete oxidation of the organic substrate (glucose) to CO_2 and H_2O. All cells that are capable of aerobic respiration have the enzymes that make up the tricarboxylic acid (TCA) cycle.* The connecting link (Figure 4–5) between glycolysis and the TCA cycle is the decarboxylation of pyruvic acid. This end product of glycolysis is decarboxylated in the presence of coenzyme A to form acetyl-CoA, carbon dioxide, and NAD$_{red}$.

$$\overset{\overset{\textstyle O}{\|}}{2CH_3 - C - COOH} + 2NAD_{ox} + 2CoASH \xrightarrow[\text{dehydrogenase}]{\text{pyruvic acid}}$$

Pyruvic acid

$$\overset{\overset{\textstyle O}{\|}}{2CH_3 - C - SCoA} + 2NAD_{red} + 2CO_2$$

Acetyl-CoA

Carbon dioxide usually escapes to the environment as a gas. Acetyl-CoA combines with oxaloacetic acid to form the tricarboxylic acid, citric acid (Figure 4–5). The cyclical reformation of oxaloacetic acid

*The TCA cycle has also been called the Krebs cycle and/or the citric acid cycle.

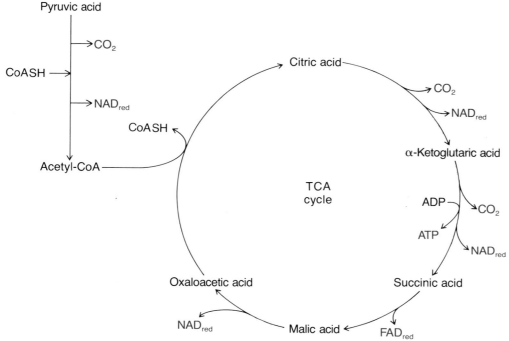

FIGURE 4–5

The tricarboxylic acid cycle is present in anaerobic cells. Acetyl-CoA, the substrate of this metabolic cycle, is derived from pyruvic acid produced in the glycolytic pathway. In the TCA cycle, each acetate is oxidized to two CO_2, three NAD_{red}, and one FAD_{red} with the formation of one ATP.

from citric acid by a series of enzymatic reactions produces 2 moles of CO_2, 1 mole of reduced flavin, 3 moles of NAD_{red}, and 1 mole of high-energy phosphate (ATP) per mole of acetyl-CoA entering the cycle. Therefore, the metabolism of the 2 moles of pyruvic acid produced in glycolysis results in the overall reaction

$$2CH_3 - \overset{\overset{\displaystyle O}{\|}}{C} - COOH + 8NAD_{ox} + 2flavin_{ox} + 2ADP + 2H_3PO_4 \rightarrow 6CO_2 + 2flavin_{red} + 8NAD_{red} + 2ATP$$

The cyclic nature of these reactions results in the regeneration of oxaloacetic acid. The cycle is then ready to begin again. As in glycolysis, one must envision all the reactions of the TCA cycle occurring simultaneously with many molecules of each intermediate and each enzyme in the cycle being present in the cell cytoplasm. The enzymes of the TCA cycle in eucaryotic cells are located in the innermost matrix of the mitochondria.

Electron-transport chain

Cells contain limited amounts of NAD. If all the NAD becomes reduced, then there is no oxidized NAD available to serve its role as a coenzyme. The machinery used to oxidize the reduced NAD generated by glycolysis and the TCA cycle is the electron-transport chain.

NAD_{red} and reduced flavins are oxidized by the membrane-bound electron-transport chain. In eucaryotic cells, the electron-transport chain is located in the inner mitochondrial membrane. Aerobic bacteria contain an electron-transport chain located either on their cytoplasmic membrane or on invaginated derivatives of the cytoplasmic membrane. The electron-transport chain is composed of a number of large molecules, such as cytochromes, flavoproteins, and iron sulfur proteins, and some small molecules, such as quinones. Each of these individual compounds can participate in an oxidation-reduction reaction.

The ability of these electron carriers to accept electrons from other compounds has been determined experimentally. The compound that will give up electrons to another compound will be the stronger reducing compound. The more reduced a compound is, the more energy it contains (Figure 4–6) and the more negative is its oxidation potential, E_0'. The diagram of the electrochemical gradient begins with the stronger reducing (more negative E_0') compounds of the electron-transport chain (NAD_{ox}/NAD_{red} = −0.32 volts) and progresses sequentially to oxygen, which is a strong oxidant with a positive E_0' (½ O_2/ H_2O = +0.816 volts). For simplicity, many of the electron carriers are omitted from Figure 4–6.

Electrons from NAD_{red} flow down this electrochemical gradient to oxygen as diagrammed in Figure 4–7. Oxygen in turn becomes reduced to water, hydrogen peroxide (H_2O_2), and superoxide (O_2^-). Overall, NAD_{red} is oxidized by the electron-transport chain to NAD_{ox} and O_2 is reduced to hydrogen peroxide (H_2O_2). Either the metabolically useful energy released in this oxidative process is converted to ATP by the three ATP synthetases found in the electron chain, or it is lost as heat.

Oxidative phosphorylation

Energy is released during the oxidation of NAD_{red} by the electron-transport chain (Figure 4–7). Oxidative phosphorylation is a process that forms ATP with the regeneration of oxidized NAD by an electron-transport chain that uses oxygen as the terminal electron acceptor. In mitochondria, the flow of electrons down the electrochemical gradient is coupled to phosphorylation at three specific sites that contain ATP synthetase. The first ATP synthetase site is between NAD and flavoproteins. The second and third sites are located between cytochromes (Figure 4–7). When the electrons in NAD_{red} are transferred to oxygen, 3 moles of ATP are formed per mole of NAD_{red}. Only 2 moles of ATP are formed when 1 mole of reduced flavin is oxidized. Since electrons from reduced flavins enter the electron-transport chain after site 1, transfer of electrons from the reduced flavin to oxygen only produce 2 moles of ATP per mole of reduced flavin. This is in contrast to the

FIGURE 4–6
Electrochemical gradient. Chemicals that can accept or donate electrons participate in coupled oxidation-reduction reactions. Electrons always flow downhill from a more reduced (high energy, more negative E_0') to a more oxidized (more positive E_0') compound.

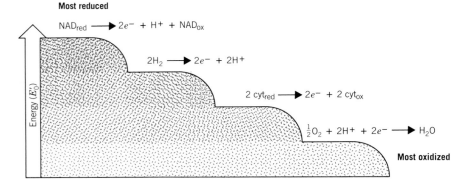

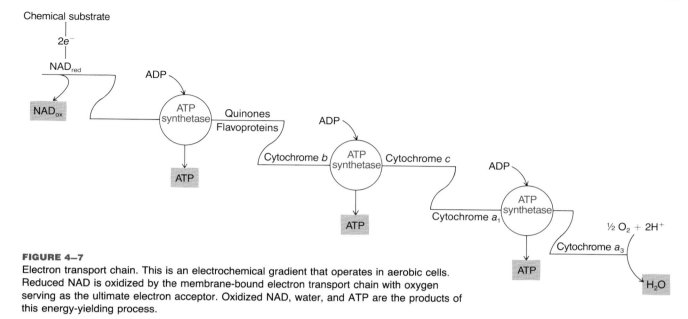

FIGURE 4–7
Electron transport chain. This is an electrochemical gradient that operates in aerobic cells. Reduced NAD is oxidized by the membrane-bound electron transport chain with oxygen serving as the ultimate electron acceptor. Oxidized NAD, water, and ATP are the products of this energy-yielding process.

3 moles of ATP produced when NAD_{red} is oxidized by the electron-transport chain.

Iron sulfur proteins, as well as the heme-containing cytochromes, are present in electron-transport chains. The active site of these proteins contains iron that undergoes a redox reaction enabling these proteins to function as electron carriers. Cytochrome *a* is called **cytochrome oxidase** since it is the terminal cytochrome and is directly oxidized by molecular oxygen. This reaction results in the formation of water together with some hydrogen peroxide (H_2O_2) and some superoxide (O_2^-). The superoxide radical is formed when oxygen is reduced by a single electron.

The NAD_{ox} molecules produced are reused by the enzymes in glycolysis and the TCA cycle. The small amounts of superoxide produced are converted by **superoxide dismutase** to hydrogen peroxide, which in turn is decomposed by **catalase**. Almost all aerobic cells contain catalase, which breaks down toxic hydrogen peroxide (H_2O_2) to the nontoxic products O_2 and H_2O.

$$2H_2O_2 \xrightarrow{\text{catalase}} 2H_2O + O_2$$

One can calculate (Table 4–2) that the total energy released from the oxidation of NAD_{red} by O_2 is 52.5 kcal/mole. A part of this energy is captured in the chemical bonds of ATP. For each mole of NAD_{red} that is oxidized by O_2, 3 moles of ATP are formed. Since each mole of ATP formed from ADP and H_3PO_4 captures 7.3 kcal, approximately 42 percent of the theoretical energy released from NAD_{red} is retained as chemical energy in the form of ATP. This energy is then used to synthesize compounds necessary for cellular growth and reproduction.

A major theory that describes a mechanism for coupling electron-transfer reactions to the formation of ATP is **chemiosmotic coupling**. Peter Mitchell received a Nobel Prize in 1978 for his contributions to developing this theory. The essence of chemiosmotic coupling is that the energy gained by transferring electrons in the electron-transport chain is used to establish a proton (H^+) gradient across a membrane. This gradient creates a potential that, combined with the membrane potential, is sufficient to remove water from ADP and H_3PO_4 to form ATP. Although the chemiosmotic coupling theory is widely supported,

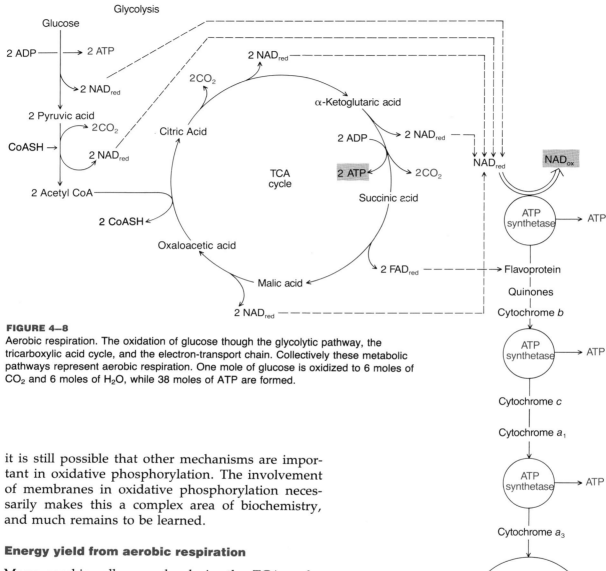

FIGURE 4-8

Aerobic respiration. The oxidation of glucose though the glycolytic pathway, the tricarboxylic acid cycle, and the electron-transport chain. Collectively these metabolic pathways represent aerobic respiration. One mole of glucose is oxidized to 6 moles of CO_2 and 6 moles of H_2O, while 38 moles of ATP are formed.

it is still possible that other mechanisms are important in oxidative phosphorylation. The involvement of membranes in oxidative phosphorylation necessarily makes this a complex area of biochemistry, and much remains to be learned.

Energy yield from aerobic respiration

Many aerobic cells use glycolysis, the TCA cycle, and the electron-transport chain to gain energy from the oxidation of glucose. Figure 4–8 is a composite diagram representing these processes that depicts the energy generated from them. A total of 38 moles of ATP can be formed from the complete oxidation of 1 mole of glucose to 6 moles of CO_2 and 6 moles of H_2O. When this theoretical yield is achieved, bi-

ological systems produce 277 kcal (38 moles ATP $\times$ 7.3 kcal mole^{-1} ATP = 277 kcal) per mole of glucose. Remember that the complete combustion of glucose yields 686 kcal mole^{-1}. Therefore, biological systems gain about 40 percent of the energy in glucose ($277/686 \times 100 = 40$ percent) when aerobic respiration is used.

ANAEROBIC ENERGY TRANSFORMATION

Certain biological systems can form ATP from carbohydrates in the absence of oxygen. Organisms that live in dark, anaerobic environments can produce ATP from carbohydrates using either fermentation or anaerobic respiration. Anaerobic environments exist throughout nature. Deep wells and the bottom of ponds are obvious anaerobic environments. Less obvious is the fact that the human intestine is often anaerobic enough to support the growth of anaerobic bacteria.

Anaerobic respiration

The energy-yielding process that uses an electron-transport system in which an inorganic compound, other than oxygen, serves as the terminal electron acceptor is **anaerobic respiration.** The electron-transport chain is similar or identical to that just described (Figure 4–7) except for the terminal oxidant. The two predominant electron acceptors involved in anaerobic respiration are nitrate (NO_3^-) and sulfate (SO_4^{2-}). *Escherichia coli* can grow anaerobically when glucose is oxidized, using nitrate as the terminal electron acceptor. Reduced products of nitrate, such as nitrite (NO_2^-) and nitrogen gas (N_2), are produced as the products of this type of anaerobic respiration. The ability of an organism to produce nitrite under anaerobic conditions is often used as a diagnostic tool in bacterial classification. *Desulfovibrio* grows by oxidizing organic compounds and reducing sulfate to sulfur (S) and hydrogen sulfide (H_2S). The hydrogen sulfide produced during sulfate reduction is responsible indirectly for the color of black mud and the color of the Black Sea. Hydrogen sulfide reacts with Fe^{2+} to form the black ferrous sulfide (FeS) compound. Even though H_2S has a disagreeable odor and is toxic, neither the sulfate-reducing bacteria nor their products play a major role in human disease.

Fermentation

Certain bacteria use the anaerobic process of fermentation to gain usable energy (Table 4–4). A **fermentation** is an anaerobic energy-yielding process in which a metabolic intermediate (derived from the substrate) is used as a terminal electron acceptor. The products of a fermentation are neither more oxidized nor more reduced than the substrate. In the glycolysis scheme, 1 mole of glucose is metabolized to 2 moles of pyruvic acid, 2 moles of NAD_{red}, and 2 moles of ATP. When pyruvic acid accepts electrons from NAD_{red} in the reaction catalyzed by lactic acid dehydrogenase

$$\underset{\text{Pyruvic acid}}{CH_3 - \overset{\overset{\textstyle O}{\|}}{C} - COOH} + NAD_{red} + \xrightarrow[\text{dehydrogenase}]{\text{lactic acid}}$$

$$\underset{\text{Lactic acid}}{CH_3 - \overset{\overset{\textstyle OH}{|}}{\underset{\underset{\textstyle H}{|}}{C}} - COOH} + NAD_{ox}$$

glycolysis becomes a fermentation. This process conforms to our definition of a fermentation because lactic acid ($C_3H_6O_3$) has the same basic formula $(CH_2O)_n$ as glucose ($C_6H_{12}O_6$); so lactic acid is neither more oxidized nor reduced than the substrate, glucose. Pyruvic acid is the intermediate derived from glucose that serves as the terminal electron acceptor. This process is called the **lactic acid fermentation** since lactic acid is the major product. Fermentations are usually self-contained processes in which no outside electron acceptor (such as O_2, NO_3^-, or SO_4^{2-}) is involved.

Usable energy is generated in fermentations by **substrate level phosphorylation.** In the lactic acid fermentation there is a net yield of 2 moles of ATP per mole of glucose metabolized (Figures 4–4). This overall process is exergonic.

Glucose → 2 lactic acid $\Delta G^\circ = -47$ kcal mole^{-1}

Since 2 moles of ATP are produced in the lactic acid

TABLE 4—4
Microbial Fermentations

Fermentation	Substrate	Products	Representative/Genera
Butyric acid	Glucose	Butyric acid, acetone, butanol, isopropanol, acetic acid	*Clostridium* (saccharolytic)
Lactic acid			
Homolactic	Glucose	Lactic acid	*Streptococcus*
Heterolactic	Glucose	Lactic acid, CO_2, ethanol	*Leuconostoc*
Propionic acid	Glucose or lactic acid	Propionic acid, CO_2, acetic acid	*Propionibacterium*
Mixed acid	Glucose	Acetic acid, formic acid, succinic acid, lactic acid, CO_2, H_2, 2,3-butanediol	*Escherichia coli* *Enterobacter*
Amino acid	Amino acids	CO_2, H_2, and organic compounds depending on amino acid(s) substrate	*Clostridium* (proteolytic)

fermentation per mole of glucose, the process is approximately 30 percent efficient (2×7.3 kcal mole^{-1}/47 kcal mole$^{-1} \times 100 = 31\%$). Organisms that cannot metabolize lactic acid excrete it into the environment, whereas organisms that grow on lactic acid use it as a substrate for growth.

Other fermentations either start with a different substrate or produce different products. Among the substrates that can be fermented are organic acids, amino acids, purines, and carbohydrates. The products of different fermentations vary and are often incorporated into the name of the fermentation (Table 4–4). Examples are the butyric acid fermentation, the propionic acid fermentation, the lactic acid fermentation, and the mixed acid fermentation.

People have used fermentations in the preparation of their food and beverages for centuries. The propionic fermentation is used in the manufacture of Swiss cheese, whereas the lactic acid fermentation is used in yogurt production. Ethanol is the major product of the yeast fermentation. Yeasts are eucaryotic fungi that can ferment the sugars found in fruit juice or in corn to ethanol and carbon dioxide. The yeast alcoholic fermentation has been used for thousands of years to produce alcoholic beverages and is now being used to produce automobile fuel.

AUTOTROPHY

Phototrophs

Photosynthetic bacteria can use sunlight as a source of energy. Except for the cyanobacteria, bacterial photosynthesis is an anaerobic process. Both the green sulfur bacteria, belonging to the family Chlorobiaceae, and the purple sulfur bacteria, belonging to the family Chromatiaceae, grow anaerobically in light using inorganic compounds as nutrients. The purple photosynthetic bacteria, belonging to the family Rhodospirillaceae, also grow anaerobically in the light, but they use organic nutrients. Reduced sulfur or reduced organic compounds serves as the primary reductant in the photosynthetic reactions of these bacteria. C. B. Van Neil worked out the following formula for bacterial photosynthesis by the Chlorobiaceae.

$$CO_2 + 2H_2S \xrightarrow{\text{light}} (CH_2O)_n + H_2O + 2S$$

When the sulfur photosynthetic bacteria photosynthesize, they produce elemental sulfur (S), which can be oxidized further to sulfate. The reducing compounds formed in this process (not shown) are used to reduce carbon dioxide to carbohydrate

(CH$_2$O). All photosynthetic organisms can form organic compounds by reducing CO$_2$ to carbohydrate. This process is called **CO$_2$ fixation.** Rhodospirillaceae use organic compounds (in place of H$_2$S) to generate reducing power.

Cyanobacteria and green plants produce oxygen during photosynthesis and are able to grow in aerobic environments. These phototrophs can split water to make a primary reductant that is used to reduce CO$_2$ to carbohydrate. Green-plant photosynthesis proceeds according to the equation.

$$CO_2 + 2H_2O \xrightarrow{\text{light}} (CH_2O)_n + H_2O + O_2$$

Notice that this equation is similar to the one for bacterial photosynthesis except that 2H$_2$O replaces 2H$_2$S as the reductant. This results in the formation of O$_2$ in place of 2S. Green plants and the cyanobacteria are the major biological generators of molecular oxygen on earth.

During photosynthesis, light energy is converted to ATP in the electron-transport chains found in the pigmented thylakoid membranes. Most photosynthetic organisms can grow using light as an energy source, either H$_2$S or H$_2$O as a source of reducing potential, and CO$_2$ as a carbon source. Carbon dioxide is fixed by a biochemical sequence referred to as the **Calvin pathway.** This series of reactions is also found in the chemolithotrophs: organisms that also fix CO$_2$.

Chemolithotrophs

Organisms that gain energy from the aerobic oxidation of inorganic compounds are called **chemolithotrophs.** These organisms are able to grow aerobically in completely inorganic media. Chemolithotrophs oxidize inorganic compounds such as ammonia (NH$_3$), nitrite (NO$_2^-$), and reduced sulfur compounds such as H$_2$S (Table 4–5). The source of carbon is CO$_2$. The chemolithotrophs are not able to grow in animal tissue, so they are not pathogenic to humans. They are beneficial to humanity because they participate in cycling inorganic nutrients that are necessary for the maintenance of an ecological balance on earth.

The majority of the bacteria are **chemoorganotrophs,** which are organisms that gain energy from the aerobic oxidation of organic compounds. We have already discussed their means for gaining energy, which can include glycolysis, the TCA cycle, and the electron-transport chain.

SYNTHESIS OF CELL CONSTITUENTS

Many microorganisms can synthesize all, or almost all, of their cellular constituents, if supplied with a source of energy, a source of carbon, a source of nitrogen, salts, and trace elements. As with the reactions involved in the breakdown of glucose, synthetic reactions are catalyzed by enzymes. Synthetic

TABLE 4–5
Oxidations by Chemolithotrophs[a]

Name	Reaction		Cycle	Representative Genera
Ammonia oxidation		NH$_3$ + ½O$_2$ → HNO$_2$ + H$_2$O	Nitrogen	*Nitrosomonas*
Nitrite oxidation		HNO$_2$ + ½O$_2$ → HNO$_3$	Nitrogen	*Nitrobacter*
Sulfur oxidation	(a)	H$_2$S + ½O$_2$ → S + H$_2$O	Sulfur	Sulfur photosynthetic bacteria
	(b)	S + 2O$_2$ → SO$_4^{2-}$	Sulfur	*Thiobacillus*
Hydrogen oxidation		2H$_2$ + O$_2$ → 2H$_2$O	None	*Hydrogenomonas*

[a]Chemolithotrophs gain their energy from the oxidation of inorganic compounds. Strict chemolithotrophs grow on media that contain only inorganic compounds. They make organic compounds by fixing CO$_2$ (like plants) supplied as Na$_2$CO$_3$. These bacteria are important in the cycling of inorganic nutrients, especially nitrogen and sulfur.

pathways need a supply of raw material and energy in the form of ATP. All the synthetic reactions take place inside the cell simultaneously with the reactions that generate energy, such as glycolysis and the TCA cycle. To simplify this complex metabolic process, we shall look at individual reactions.

Carbohydrates

Carbohydrates are used by cells to make cell walls, glycoproteins, glycolipids, nucleic acids, and capsules. The source of carbon for the various forms of carbohydrate usually originates from an organic food source (the substrate), which serves as both the carbon and energy source. An example of how a cell interconverts carbohydrates is the enzymatic conversion of a hexose (6-carbon sugar) to a pentose (5-carbon sugar). The hexose , glucose-6-phosphate, is converted to 6-phosphogluconic acid. The 6-phosphogluconic acid is then converted to the pentose ribulose-5-phosphate by the enzyme 6-phosphogluconic acid dehydrogenase.

$$
\begin{array}{l}
\text{COOH} \\
| \\
\text{HCOH} \\
| \\
\text{HOCH} + \text{NADP}_{ox} \quad \xrightarrow{\substack{\text{6-phosphogluconic acid} \\ \text{dehydrogenase}}} \\
| \\
\text{HCOH} \\
| \\
\text{HCOH} \\
| \\
\text{CH}_2\text{OPO}_3{}^{2-}
\end{array}
$$
6-Phosphogluconic acid

$$
\begin{array}{l}
\text{CH}_2\text{OH} \\
| \\
\text{C}=\text{O} + \text{CO}_2 + \text{NAD}_{red} \\
| \\
\text{HCOH} \\
| \\
\text{HCOH} \\
| \\
\text{CH}_2\text{OPO}_3{}^{2-}
\end{array}
$$
Ribulose-5-phosphate

Ribulose can then be converted to ribose or deoxyribose by enzymatic reactions.

Pentoses are found in nucleic acids. Ribose is the carbohydrate component of RNA, whereas deoxyribose is the carbohydrate component of DNA. NADP is the phosphorylated form of NAD and is used in the reaction just presented as well as in many other synthetic reactions. Although no energy in the form of ATP is utilized in this reaction, the energy present in the glucose molecule used for a structural role in the cell will not be metabolized through glycolysis to yield energy. This example demonstrates that organic molecules can be utilized either as a *carbon* or as an *energy* source.

Amino acids

Amino acids are the building blocks of proteins. There are 20 different amino acids commonly found in cells. Amino acids have the basic structure of

$$
\begin{array}{c}
\text{R} \\
| \\
\text{H}_2\text{N} - \text{C} - \text{COOH} \\
| \\
\text{H}
\end{array}
$$

where an amino group ($-\text{NH}_2$) and a carboxyl group ($-\text{COOH}$) are attached to an α-carbon atom. The R group can be any one of 20 different structures (Appendix 1), which transform this basic amino acid structure into one of the 20 different amino acids.

Amino acids are synthesized using metabolic intermediates and ammonia (NH_3). The syntheses of glutamic acid and aspartic acid are useful examples. The enzyme glutamic acid dehydrogenase takes ammonia and incorporates it into α-ketoglutaric acid, which is an organic intermediate of the TCA cycle (Figure 4–5). The reaction proceeds according to the following equation

$$
\begin{array}{l}
\text{COOH} \\
| \\
\text{CH}_2 \\
| \\
\text{CH}_2 + \text{NAD}_{red} + \text{NH}_3 \xrightarrow{\substack{\text{glutamic acid} \\ \text{dehydrogenase}}} \\
| \\
\text{C}=\text{O} \\
| \\
\text{COOH}
\end{array}
\qquad
\begin{array}{l}
\text{COOH} \\
| \\
\text{CH}_2 \\
| \\
\text{CH}_2 + \text{H}_2\text{O} + \text{NAD}_{ox} \\
| \\
\text{H}-\text{C}-\text{NH}_2 \\
| \\
\text{COOH}
\end{array}
$$
α-Ketoglutaric acid   Glutamic acid

Energy is expended in this reaction through the utilization of NAD_{red}.

Once glutamic acid is formed, it can be used to form other amino acids (Figure 4–9). The formation of aspartic acid uses another TCA cycle intermediate. Aspartic acid is formed by a transaminase that catalyzes the transfer of the amino group ($-NH_2$) from glutamic acid to oxaloacetic acid.

COOH   COOH
| |
CH$_2$ CH$_2$
| | glutamic oxaloacetic acid
C=O +   CH$_2$ $\xrightarrow{\text{transaminase}}$
| |
COOH   H—C—NH$_2$
            |
           COOH

Oxaloacetic   Glutamic
acid   acid

COOH   COOH
| |
CH$_2$ +   CH$_2$
| |
H—C—NH$_2$ CH$_2$
| |
COOH   C=O
          |
        COOH

Aspartic   α-Ketoglutaric
acid   acid

Cells that contain the appropriate enzymes can synthesize all of the 20 different amino acids from intermediates of cellular metabolism and ammonia.

Lipids

Cell membranes are composed of lipids and proteins. Lipoproteins give membranes their unique properties. Some lipids are composed of two parts; a carbohydrate portion, which is usually a derivative of glycerol, and a long chain fatty acid component. Glycerol is a 3-carbon alcohol that is formed from an intermediate in the glycolysis pathway.

Dihydroxy-acetone phosphate + NAD_{red} $\xrightarrow[\text{dehydrogenase}]{\text{glycerol-3-phosphate}}$

glycerol-3-phosphate + NAD_{ox}

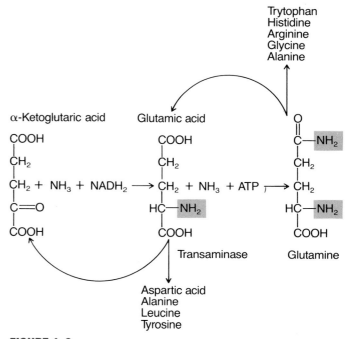

FIGURE 4–9
Amino acid synthesis. Inorganic nitrogen in the form of ammonia (NH_3) is used to form the amino acid glutamic acid or glutamine. These amino acids are then used to donate an amino group to enzymatic reactions that form the other amino acids.

Fatty acids are synthesized from acetyl-CoA in a complex series of reactions that can be illustrated by the following equation.

8Acetyl-CoA + 14NADP$_{red}$ + 7ATP + H$_2$O →
    Palmitic acid + 8CoA + 14NADP$_{ox}$ + 7ADP + 7H$_3$PO$_4$

Acetyl-CoA is the basic carbon unit used to form all long chain fatty acids and is produced from pyruvic acid (Figure 4–5). A large amount of energy is expended in this process. Note the use of both reduced NADP$_{red}$ and ATP as substrates. The fatty acetyl-CoA and glycerol-3-phosphate are combined in a third set of reactions to form the common type of phospholipid depicted in Figure 4–10.

The long chain hydrocarbon of the fatty acid repels water and is said to be hydrophobic. Therefore, the fatty acids attract each other on the inside of the membrane while the charged groups line up on the outside of the membrane. It is the hydrophobic nature of the fatty acid portion of lipids and the hydrophilic nature of the charged portion of lipids that confer stability on membrane structures.

Nucleotides

Nucleotides are the basic units found in nucleic acids. Some of them, such as ATP, can also be used for storing energy. ATP and dATP (deoxyadenosine triphosphate) are used by cells for synthesizing RNA and DNA, respectively. All nucleotides are composed of a nitrogenous base, a sugar, and a phosphate group (Figure 4–11). The sugar is either ribose, found in ribonucleic acid (RNA), or deoxyribose, found in deoxyribonucleic acid (DNA). The nitrogenous bases in DNA are adenine, thymine, guanine, and cytosine. Uracil replaces the nitrogenous base, thymine, in RNA.

Synthesis of nucleotides with their respective nitrogenous bases is a complex process. Nucleotides are synthesized with the ribose-5-phosphate portion of the molecule serving as the base plate. The purine or pyrimidine ring is formed and is attached to this structure by an enzymatic reaction. The use of nucleotides in the formation of DNA and RNA is discussed in the next chapter.

SUMMARY

Microorganisms gain energy by aerobic respiration, anaerobic respiration, fermentation, or photosyn-

FIGURE 4–10
Lipids are integral components of membranes. They are formed from glycerol and fatty acids; some also contain phosphate.

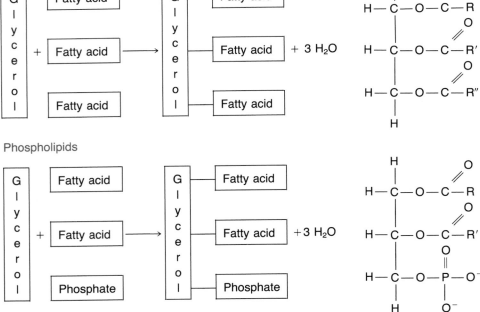

Components

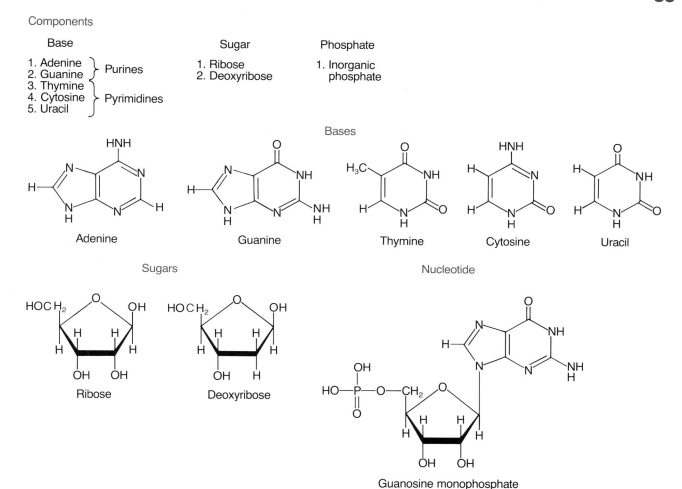

Base

1. Adenine ⎫
2. Guanine ⎬ Purines
3. Thymine ⎫
4. Cytosine ⎬ Pyrimidines
5. Uracil ⎭

Sugar

1. Ribose
2. Deoxyribose

Phosphate

1. Inorganic
   phosphate

Bases

Adenine Guanine Thymine Cytosine Uracil

Sugars

Ribose Deoxyribose

Nucleotide

Guanosine monophosphate

FIGURE 4–11
Nucleotides are composed of a nitrogenous base, a sugar, and phosphate.

thesis. Organisms are either chemoorganotrophs, chemolithotrophs, or phototrophs, depending on whether they use organic compounds, inorganic compounds, or light as a source of energy. The oxidation of glucose by aerobic respiration proceeds through the glycolytic pathway and then through the TCA cycle. Electrons generated by glucose oxidation are transferred to NAD and flavin, which in turn are oxidized by the electron-transport chain. As electrons are transferred in this chain, the energy of reduced NAD is used to form ATP in the process called oxidative phosphorylation. Oxygen serves as the terminal electron acceptor in aerobic respiration. Anaerobic respiration is similar to this process except that an inorganic compound, such as sulfate or nitrate, serves as the terminal electron acceptor in place of oxygen. Fermentations are another mechanism for generating energy under anaerobic conditions. Each different fermentation is characterized by the products that come from a fermentable substrate. Fermentations generate ATP by the mechanism of substrate-level phosphorylation.

Reproducing cells require the elements of life to form cellular constituents. Energy produced by cells is used to manufacture the cell materials needed for growth and reproduction. Among these materials are the amino acids, carbohydrates, vitamins, purines, pyrimidines, and lipids. The synthesis of each of these classes of compounds requires energy to convert environmental nutrients into cellular material. The cell products are organized into structures directed by enzymatic reaction, which in turn are formed under the direction of the genetic material.

QUESTIONS AND TOPICS FOR STUDY AND DISCUSSION

Questions

1. What is the role of ATP in metabolism?
2. Define or explain the following.

chemolithotroph	endergonic reaction
chemoorganotroph	exergonic reaction
coenzyme	oxidation-reduction reaction
enzyme	phototroph

3. Name the six major classes of enzymes and write out a reaction catalyzed by one enzyme in each class.
4. Diagram the key reactions of glycolysis. What products are formed when this pathway is used as a fermentation?
5. Describe what happens to pyruvic acid in aerobic bacteria. What is the mechanism for oxidizing reduced NAD?
6. What is the theoretical efficiency of aerobic respiration?
7. What are the major differences between anaerobic respiration and fermentation?
8. How is inorganic nitrogen used to form amino acids?
9. Draw the structure of a nucleotide and indicate the basic components that are used to build it.
10. Refer to Appendix 3 and Appendix 4 to determine the total number of NAD_{red}, $FADH_2$, and ATP produced in the aerobic metabolism of glucose through glycolysis and the TCA cycle.

Discussion

1. What is the environmental impact of having a wide diversity of energy-yielding pathways in bacteria?
2. What metabolic processes would you expect to encounter in disease-producing microbes? Which mechanism of energy metabolism would you not expect to find? Why?
3. Why have we omitted a discussion of viral metabolism?

FURTHER READINGS

Books

Doelle, H. W., *Bacterial Metabolism,* Academic Press, New York, 1975. An advanced text on microbial physiology that is an excellent reference source for bacterial metabolism.

Lehninger, A. L., *Principles of Biochemistry,* Worth, New York, 1982. An introductory textbook in biochemistry by an author who is highly regarded for his accuracy and writing style.

Articles and Reviews

Hinkle, P. C., and R. E. McCarty, "How Cells Make ATP," *Sci. Am.* 238:104–117 (March 1978). A description of the biomolecules involved in photosynthetic and oxidative phosphorylation followed by an explanation of the "chemiosmotic" theory of ATP formation.

Lehninger, A. L., "How Cells Transform Energy," *Sci. Am.,* 205:62–73 (September 1961). An elementary discussion of energy transformations in mitochondria and chloroplasts.

Philips, D., "The Three-dimensional Structure of Enzyme Molecules," *Sci. Am.,* 215:78–90 (November 1966). A detailed description of the experiments involved in discovering the three-dimensional structure of lysozyme.

Wood, W. A., "Fermentation of Carbohydrates and Related Compounds," in I. C. Gunsalus and R. Y. Stanier (eds.), *The Bacteria,* vol. 2, pp. 59–149, Academic Press, New York, 1961. A classic paper on the microbial metabolism of carbohydrates by fermentation mechanisms.

5

MACROMOLECULES

And into the ark with Noah went one pair, male and female, of all beasts
. . . of birds and everything that crawls on the ground two by two . . .

Gen. 7:8–9

Beasts beget beasts, birds beget birds, and crawly things beget things that crawl. For hundreds of years, humans have used this basic knowledge of life to improve animal breeds. We now have dogs that hunt and dogs that tend sheep; we have thoroughbred racing horses that are capable of great speeds and draft horses that pull heavy loads; we have beef cattle and cattle that are raised to produce milk. Many characteristics of animals are passed on to their progeny. A calf will possess traits inherited from both its parents. Similarly, since bacteria divide by binary fission, the traits of a bacterium are present in its daughter cells. Inherited bacterial traits can pass from parents to their progeny through thousands of generations. How can cells make exact replicas of themselves? They do so by replicating the macromolecule containing the chemical code for the design of the organism. The macromolecule is deoxyribonucleic acid (DNA); the sequence of nitrogenous bases in DNA is the chemical code.

DEOXYRIBONUCLEIC ACID

Friederich Miesher began a chemical analysis of cells in 1869 and discovered DNA in pus and salmon sperm. These cells contained DNA in their nuclei, and so DNA was originally called "nuclein." The significance of Miesher's discovery of DNA was not appreciated during his lifetime.

During 1928, Frederick Griffith investigated smooth colonies of *Streptococcus pneumoniae*, which caused pneumonia in mice, and rough colonies of *S. pneumoniae*, which did not. He found a "transforming principle" in cells from smooth colonies. This transforming principle converted avirulent cells taken from a rough colony into virulent cells that formed smooth colonies and caused pneumonia in mice. In 1943, this "transforming principle" was identified by Avery, MacLeod, and McCarty as a macromolecule with the chemical characteristics of DNA. This knowledge, in combination with the accumulated data on the composition and replication of bacterial DNA viruses, suggested that DNA was the hereditary material.

Discovery of the structure of DNA

Knowledge of the structure of DNA has had a profound impact on biology. The discovery of DNA structure can be compared to the discovery of atomic

85

structure and the development of quantum mechanics in chemistry. These discoveries provide a firm basis for understanding biological inheritance and chemical reactions.

Francis Crick and James Watson were central figures in the discovery of DNA structure. They met and worked together in the Cavendish Laboratory in Cambridge, England (Figure 5–1). They were both convinced that the components of DNA would fit together like a puzzle once they had all the pieces. The following pieces were known to Watson and Crick when they began to build their model for DNA.

1. DNA is composed of the sugar deoxyribose, phosphate, and four nitrogenous bases.

2. The nitrogenous bases in DNA are adenine (A), thymine (T), guanine (G), and cytosine (C). These bases are attached to deoxyribose, forming a compound called a **nucleoside**.*

3. X-ray diffraction studies of DNA, conducted by Wilkins and Franklin, indicated a double helical structure. Linus Pauling had previously shown that protein chains can form a helical structure stabilized by hydrogen bonds.

4. In a double-stranded DNA molecule, Chargaff showed that the quantity of adenine equaled the quantity of thymine and the quantity of guanine equaled the quantity of cytosine (A= T : G=C).

Using this information, Watson and Crick began building a model of DNA. The pieces of the puzzle fit together when (1) the sugar-phosphate backbone of the molecule took the shape of a helix and (2) the nitrogenous bases were paired with their counterparts (A with T, and G with C) located on an adjacent helix running in the opposite direction. The purines (A and G) paired with their respective pyrimidines (T and C) through the weak forces of hydrogen bonds.

Visualize this structure by thinking of a twisted ladder. The left sidepiece goes from the bottom to the top; the right sidepiece runs from the top to the bottom. The rungs represent the hydrogen bonding between nitrogenous base pairs. Now hold the bottom of the ladder and twist the top such that you put a *right-hand* twist in the ladder (Figure 5–2). This helical structure represents the structure of DNA. Double-stranded DNA exists as a right-hand double helix that is 20 Å wide and contains one complete turn of the helix every 34 Å (Figure 5–2). The ring structures of the purine and pyrimidine bases are stacked next to each other perpendicular to the helical axis. These nucleotide bases occupy the central core of the helix. The deoxyribose backbone has directionality because the joining of sugar molecules by phosphate-sugar linkages occurs sequentially

FIGURE 5–1
James Watson (left) and Francis Crick in front of the DNA model. (From J. D. Watson, *The Double Helix*, Antheneum, New York, p. 215, copyright © 1968, J. D. Watson, photo by A. C. Barrinton Brown.)

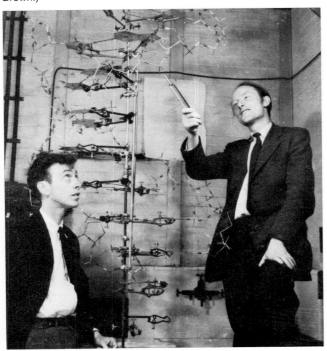

*A *nucleotide* is a nucleoside (nitrogenous base + sugar) attached to one or more phosphate groups.

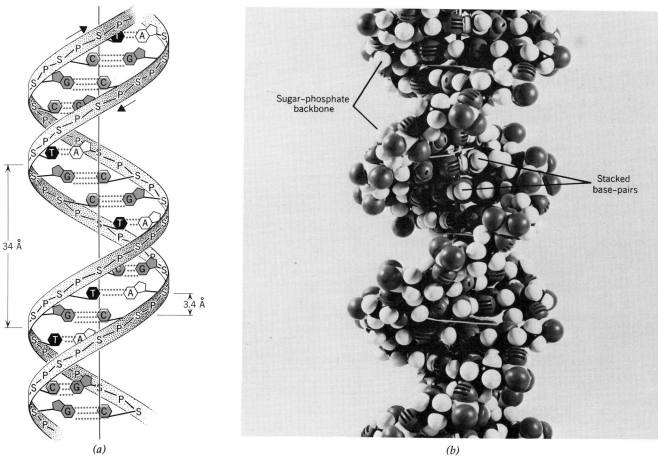

FIGURE 5-2
(a) Diagram of the Watson-Crick double helix model of DNA. A, T, G, and C represent adenine, thymine, guanine, and cytosine: S and P represent the sugar (deoxyribose) and phosphate. (From E. J. Gardner and D. P. Snustad, *Principles of Genetics,* 6th ed., Wiley, New York, 1981). *(b)* A photograph of a space-filling model of DNA showing the position of each atom. (Courtesy of the Ealing Corporation.)

through the oxygen atoms attached to the fifth carbon (5′) and the third carbon (3′) of deoxyribose. Therefore, one strand of the DNA molecule has a free 5′ end and proceeds to a free 3′ end; the complementary strand of the double helix begins at the 3′ end and proceeds to a free 5′ end. If you could cut the double helix at any given point, you would have two ends; one containing a 5′ end and the other a 3′ end (Figure 5–3).

Hydrogen bonding between nitrogenous bases. Hydrogen bonding occurs between the carboxyl groups and the hydrogen of amino groups ($-NH_2$) and between the hydrogen of a ring nitrogen and the ring nitrogen itself. Hydrogen bonding between adenine and thymine, and between guanine and cytosine, is shown in Figure 5–4. Hydrogen bonds are easier to break than are covalent bonds because hydrogen bonds contain less energy. At temperatures between 60° and 90°C, large portions of the two strands of DNA separate because of the rupture of the hydrogen bonds. The exact temperature at which the DNA strands separate depends on the proportion of purines (A and G) to pyrimidines (T and C). You can rejoin separated DNA strands by slowly cooling the solution in a process called **annealing of** *DNA* (Figure 5–5).

Double-stranded DNA always contains equal molar concentrations of adenine and thymine and of guanine and cytosine. However, the amount of guanine plus cytosine compared to the amount of adenine plus thymine can vary from one organism to the next (Table 5–1). To determine the variation among different samples of DNA, the number of moles of each nitrogenous base is measured for each preparation of DNA. The results are expressed as the ratio of the moles of guanine plus cytosine to the moles of guanine plus cytosine plus adenine plus thymine. This value is the **G + C moles percent.** Bacteria have values that vary from about 30 moles percent to more than 70 moles percent. The G + C moles percent among higher animals differ little. The composition of DNA is an important measure of the genetic relatedness between organisms and, because of its wide variation in bacteria, is used to differentiate these organisms.

FIGURE 5–3
A double break in a closed circular DNA molecule results in 5' and 3' ends.

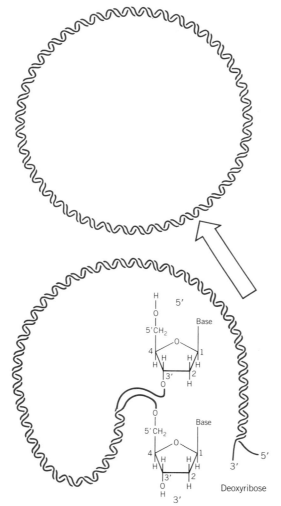

FIGURE 5–4
Base-pairing in DNA; adenine pairs with thymine and guanine pairs with cytosine. The nucleotides are joined by hydrogen bonds. The sugar molecule is deoxyribose (dR).

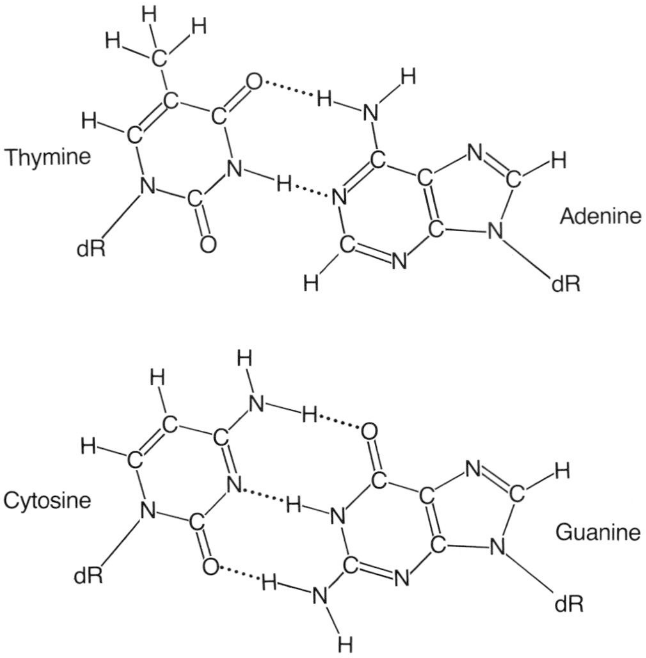

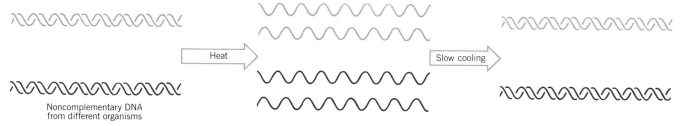

FIGURE 5–5

Elevated temperatures will break the hydrogen bonds of double-stranded DNA. The resulting single-stranded DNA molecules will anneal, if two strands with complementary base sequences come in contact with each other at an appropriate temperature.

DNA replication

If DNA is the biological molecule of inheritance, it must be able to make exact copies of itself. The double helix structure of DNA, base-pairing, and the ease with which DNA separates into single strands suggest a means of self-replication. Suppose that the two strands of DNA partially separate in the presence of the four nucleotides. One can envision insertion, by base-pairing of free nucleotides with bases on a separated DNA strand, in a manner that would preserve the nucleotide sequence of the DNA strand.

DNA strand separation. The Meselson-Stahl experiment provided solid evidence for DNA strand separation during bacterial replication (Figure 5–6). Bacteria were grown in a medium containing heavy nitrogen (^{15}N). The DNA formed in these cells synthesized DNA-^{15}N, making this DNA heavy. Normal cells grown in the regular nitrogen (^{14}N) formed DNA-^{14}N, which was light. The investigators, Meselson and Stahl, transferred the cells with heavy DNA to a medium containing ^{14}N and observed that the cells made an intermediate-weight DNA that

TABLE 5–1

Composition of DNA from Different Organisms

Source of DNA	G + C Content (moles %)[a]
Cytophaga johnsonae (bacterium)	33
Escherichia coli (bacterium)	50
Pseudomonas aeruginosa (bacterium)	67
Salmo trutta (brown trout)	43
Gallus domesticus (chicken)	42
Equus (horse)	43
Homo sapiens (human)	42
Triticum (wheat)	45
Saccharomyces cerevisiae (yeast)	36
Aspergillus niger (mold)	50
Paracentrotus (sea urchin)	35

[a]Moles percent G + C = $\dfrac{\text{moles G + moles C}}{\text{moles A + moles T + moles G + moles C}}$

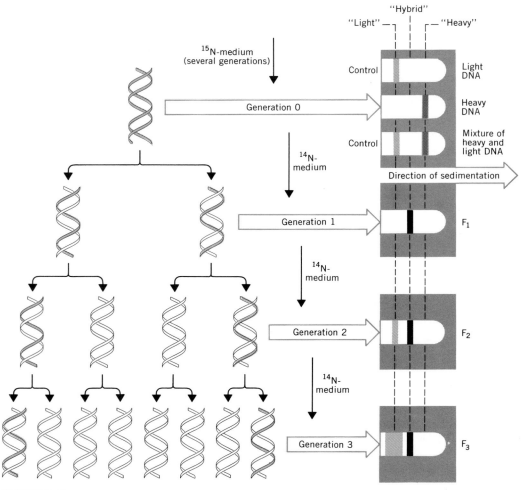

FIGURE 5–6

Bacteria replicate their DNA by a semiconservative mechanism (left), as was indicated by the Meselson-Stahl experiment (right). These researchers grew *E. coli* in a medium containing the heavy isotope of nitrogen (^{15}N). During growth, the bacteria produced heavy (density labeled) bacterial DNA. The cells were then transferred to medium containing normal nitrogen (^{14}N) and grown for varying periods of time (one generation, two generations, etc.). The presence of heavy, hybrid (equal quantities of heavy and light), and light DNA was measured in cesium chloride (CsCl) gradients centrifuged to equilibrium at ultrahigh speeds. The heavy DNA moved to the bottom of the centrifuge tube, while the light DNA stayed at the top of the tube: hybrid DNA was in between. After one generation, only hybrid DNA was present—these cells contained no light and no heavy DNA. Light DNA appeared after the second generation and increased in amount until the hybrid DNA became diluted out by the synthesis of light DNA. These results together with other studies have demonstrated that bacteria replicate their DNA by a semiconservative mechanism. (From E. J. Gardner and D. P. Snustad, *Principles of Genetics*, 6th ed., Wiley, New York, 1981. After M. Meselson and F. W. Stahl, *Proc. Natl. Acad. Sci., USA* 44:671, 1958.)

was half-heavy and half-light (DNA-^{15}N-^{14}N). When these cells divided, they produced one population of daughter cells containing the intermediate-weight DNA and another population of daughter cells containing light DNA (Figure 5–6). In order to form the intermediate DNA, the DNA strands had to separate during replication. In the normal medium, the new complementary strand of DNA was made with light nitrogen (^{14}N), which then paired with the existing strand of heavy DNA. This process is called **semi-** **conservative replication** since one of the strands of the DNA double helix is conserved in each new DNA molecule. The semiconservative replication of double-stranded DNA and the double helical structure of DNA are now firmly established concepts.

DNA superstructure. Bacterial DNA exists as a closed circular macromolecule that can twist back on itself to become **supercoiled DNA** (Figure 5–7). These coils are formed by twisting DNA in the op-

FIGURE 5–7

An electron micrograph of supercoiled DNA (left) and relaxed DNA (right). (Photo courtesy of Dr. Sam Kelly.)

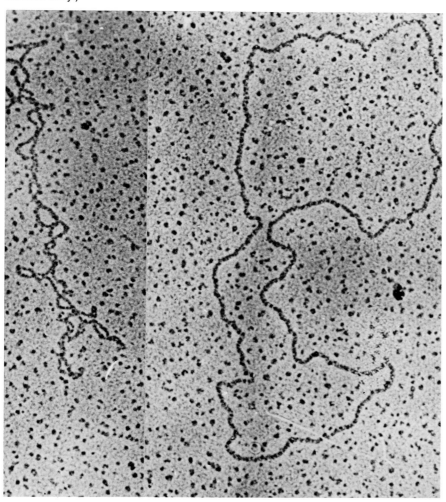

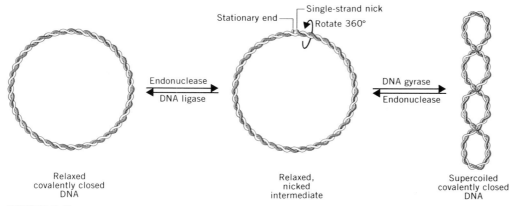

FIGURE 5—8

Relaxed covalently closed DNA is converted to supercoiled covalently closed DNA through a relaxed-nicked DNA intermediate. Covalently closed DNA will go to the relaxed form when endonuclease puts a nick in it. Nicked DNA can be converted into the supercoiled form by gyrase at the expense of ATP. Ligase repairs nicks in either form of DNA to form covalently closed DNA. (From E. J. Gardner and D. P. Snustad, *Principles of Genetics*, 6th ed., Wiley, New York, 1981).

posite direction to the twists of the DNA helix. One supercoil is found for every 15 helical twists in natural DNA. The supercoiled state is a strained or energized conformation that tends to unwind partially the helix of double-stranded DNA. This partially unwound state favors the binding of unwinding proteins that in turn promotes the further unwinding of DNA as required for DNA synthesis. The uncoiled state is referred to as **relaxed DNA**. Relaxed DNA is the energetically most stable state; supercoiled DNA energetically seeks the relaxed state. Conversion of relaxed DNA to supercoiled DNA requires the en-

zyme gyrase, endonuclease, and energy in the form of ATP (Figure 5–8). Gyrase puts the negative twists in double-stranded DNA.

Proteins of DNA replication. Many proteins are involved in the replication of DNA (Table 5–2). Unwinding proteins separate the strands of the double helix and bind to the resulting single strands. Once the first protein is in place, the second and subsequent unwinding proteins bind more readily (Figure 5–9). DNA contains a specific site for the initiation of DNA synthesis that is recognized by a DNA-di-

TABLE 5—2
Major Proteins Involved in DNA Synthesis

Protein	Substrate(s)	Function
DNA-directed RNA polymerase	Double-stranded DNA, ribonucleoside-5-triphosphates	Forms priming RNA
Unwinding proteins	Single-stranded DNA	Separates DNA helix
DNA polymerase (III + III*)	3′ end of priming RNA, deoxyribonucleoside-5-triphosphates	Forms DNA
Exonuclease (DNA polymerase?)	RNA-DNA hybrid	Removes priming RNA
DNA ligase	Single-stranded DNA fragments	Joins ends together

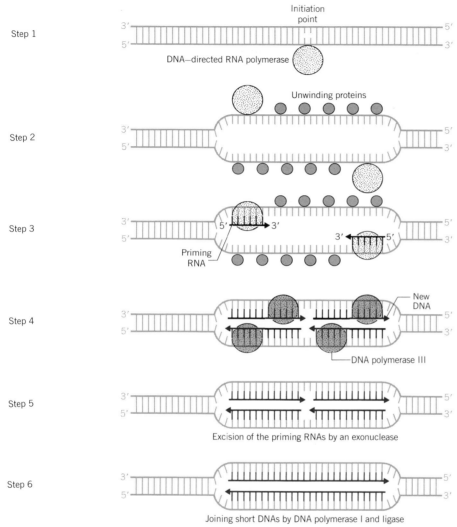

Step 1

Step 2

Step 3

Step 4

Step 5

Step 6

Initiation point

DNA–directed RNA polymerase

Unwinding proteins

Priming RNA

New DNA

DNA polymerase III

Excision of the priming RNAs by an exonuclease

Joining short DNAs by DNA polymerase I and ligase

FIGURE 5–9

DNA is synthesized in both directions as nucleotides are added to the 3′ end of the growing nucleic acid polymers. Unwinding proteins bind at the initiation site, which spreads the helix, enabling the DNA-directed RNA polymerase to bind. This enzyme synthesizes short RNA primer molecules. DNA polymerase III then attaches deoxynucleotides to the 3′ end of the primer to synthesize a new DNA strand complementary to the template. The RNA-primer molecules are excised by a nuclease activity, and the ends of the new DNA strands are joined by DNA polymerase I and lygase. (After A. Lehninger, *Biochemistry*, Worth, New York, 1975.)

rected RNA polymerase. This enzyme recognizes the initiation site on DNA and causes a mild disturbance by synthesizing short pieces of RNA. The unwind-

ing proteins take advantage of this disturbance and bind to the exposed single strands of DNA. The enzyme that synthesizes DNA, DNA polymerase, requires these short primer strands of RNA to begin DNA synthesis. DNA polymerase now binds and begins to make DNA on the ends of the RNA primer strands.

DNA-directed RNA polymerase uses ribonucleotides, whereas DNA polymerase uses deoxyribonucleotides as substrates. The specific nucleotides used depend on the enzyme and the DNA template. Hydrogen bonding aligns the purines with their complementary pyrimidine, and vice versa. The nucleotides are then sequentially joined and pyrophosphate (P—P) is released.

$$\text{DNA-3}' + \text{Nucleoside 5' triphosphate} \xrightarrow{\text{DNA polymerase III}}$$

dATP
dTTP
dGTP
dCTP

DNA-3'-5'-nucleotide-3' + Pyrophosphate

Synthesis of both DNA and RNA requires tremendous amounts of energy in the form of nucleoside triphosphates.

Increased tension within the closed circular DNA molecule is created as the DNA is unwound. To relieve this tension, gyrase breaks the DNA and then puts back just enough twists to maintain the DNA structure. Some investigators suggest that the energy in the supercoiled double helix drives DNA synthesis.

Direction of synthesis. Each DNA strand proceeds from a 5' to a 3' end, its complementary strand being antiparallel (Figure 5–2). DNA polymerase III can only add nucleotides to the 3' end of the growing nucleotide chain. So the synthesis of DNA proceeds on both strands in two directions (always from the 3' end to the 5' end of the growing strand) with the formation of short pieces of DNA (Figure 5–9). The short RNA primer molecules are cleaved off by a nuclease, leaving the short pieces of DNA known as **Okazaki fragments.** DNA polymerase I then fills in the gaps between the short strands of DNA (Figure 5–9), and ligase joins together the existing loose 5' and 3' ends, completing the DNA molecule.

This mechanism allows DNA to be synthesized in both directions starting at a single initiation point. Bidirectional synthesis continues until the entire chromosome is replicated. During replication, the bacterial chromosome is attached to the cytoplasmic membrane. This attachment enables the cell to separate mechanically one copy of the chromosome into each daughter cell.

Single-stranded DNA. Some bacterial viruses contain single-stranded DNA. This confused early investigators because the amount of adenine did not equal that of thymine, nor did guanine equal cytosine. The replication of single-stranded DNA (Figure 5–10) proceeds through an intermediate called the **replicative strand,** designated as " − ". This replicative strand is made directly from the single-stranded viral DNA. Synthesis of exact copies of the viral DNA or " + " strands takes place using the replicative strand as a template. DNA viruses are further discussed in Chapter 9.

FIGURE 5–10

Replication of single-stranded, viral DNA requires the formation of a replicative strand ("-"). The replicative strand is discarded after functioning as a template for viral (" + ") DNA synthesis.

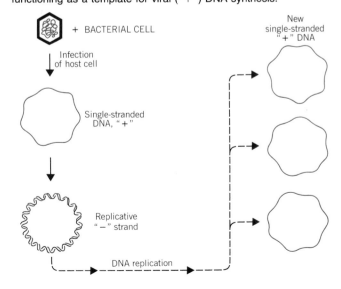

Heredity and DNA synthesis.   An organism's characteristics are passed from one generation to the next through the accurate replication of the cell's DNA. This DNA is organized in chromosomes. One complete copy of an organism's DNA is referred to as its **genome.** In bacteria, the genome is a single chromosome that contains the genetic information for the traits of that cell. The cellular characteristics that are observable are the cell's **phenotype.** While cells contain their hereditary information in their DNA (genotype), they express their phenotypes through protein synthesis.

PROTEIN SYNTHESIS

Proteins are polymers of amino acids, each arranged in an ordered sequence. The code for the sequence of amino acids in each protein is contained in DNA. However, there is no mechanism for the direct conversion of this code into a sequence of amino acids. The code in DNA must first be rewritten into a sequence of nucleotides in RNA. Rewriting the code in RNA is called **transcription.** The sequence of nucleotides in RNA is then decoded into a sequence of amino acids through the process of **translation,** which itself employs many different classes of protein and RNA molecules.

Structures of RNAs

RNA is different from DNA because RNA contains uridine and ribose rather than the thymine and deoxyribose that are found in DNA. RNA molecules are polymers of the ribonucleotides of adenine, uridine, guanine, and cytosine. Cells contain three types of RNA: ribosomal RNA (rRNA), transfer RNA (tRNA), and messenger RNA (mRNA). All cellular RNA molecules are thought to be coded for by cellular DNA. The DNA-dependent RNA polymerase reads the DNA code and inserts a uridine nucleotide into the newly formed RNA whenever adenine appears in the DNA.

Ribosomal RNA.   rRNA is found in both the 50S subunit and the 30S subunit of the bacterial ribosome. Ribosomal RNAs vary in size. The 30S subunit is composed of a 5S RNA, a 16S RNA, and 21 different proteins, whereas the 50S ribosomal subunit contains a 5S RNA, a 23S RNA, and 34 proteins. *Escherichia coli* ribosomes have been reconstituted from their component parts; however, the details of the structure and function of most of the individual components remain to be discovered. The rRNAs may provide recognition sites for other RNA molecules, but scientists do not think that rRNAs transfer information from DNA to proteins.

Messenger RNA.   DNA-directed RNA polymerase synthesizes single-stranded RNA directly from the DNA (Figure 5–11). The RNA that codes for the synthesis of specific proteins is called messenger RNA because it takes the code from DNA and carries it to the ribosomes, where it is translated into proteins.

FIGURE 5–11

Transcription (RNA formation) in *E. coli* of the large ribosomal RNA genes. The central strand is DNA; the dark objects are enzymes actively synthesizing RNA. (Courtesy of Dr. O. L. Miller. From O. L. Miller, B. A. Hamkalo, and C. A. Thomas, *Science,* 169:392–395, 1970, with permission of the American Society for the Advancement of Science.)

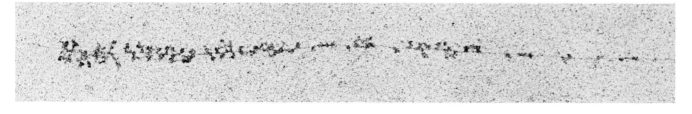

Proteins vary in size as do mRNA molecules. mRNA molecules in procaryotic cells have a half-life on the order of 2 minutes, indicating that they are rapidly metabolized. This is not the case in eucaryotic cells where the mRNA molecules are relatively stable. Procaryotic mRNAs are complementary to sections of the DNA, vary greatly in size, and are rapidly recycled by the cell.

Transfer RNAs. Every cell has a complement of transfer RNA molecules. These are small molecules containing between 73 and 93 nucleotide residues, some of which base-pair with each other to form a pseudo-cloverleaf structure (Figure 5–12). The structures of at least 50 tRNA molecules are known. At a specific site on each tRNA molecule there is a distinct sequence of three bases called the **anticodon.** The anticodon is complementary to the codon of mRNA. Also, each tRNA molecule binds a specific amino acid to its 3′ end. Attachment of an amino acid to its specific tRNA is catalyzed by a specific enzyme and requires energy in the form of ATP. Since there are 20 different amino acids in proteins, there must be at least 20 different tRNA molecules. In fact, there are more kinds of tRNA molecules in a cell than there are different kinds of amino acids. For a comparison of the characteristics of cellular RNAs, refer to Table 5–3.

The genetic code

Biological systems all use the universal triplicate codon-anticodon code. The need for a triplicate code can be rationally deduced. There must be at least 20 code words since there are 20 different amino acids in proteins. There are only four different bases in DNA. If one base coded for one amino acid, there would be four possible code words, 4^1. If two bases coded for each amino acid, there would be 16 possible code words, 4^2. This is not enough. Three is the minimum sequence of a four-base code that will provide sufficient code words for 20 amino acids. This triplicate code provides 64 possible code words, 4^3. The existence of the triplicate code has been substantiated experimentally.

The triplicate code is universal in the biological systems studied. The code is the same in human cells as it is in bacterial cells. The code is also redundant; that is, there is more than one code word for each of the amino acids except for tryptophan and methionine, which have only one each (Table 5–4). The code has been deciphered, and each possible triplicate sequence codes for an amino acid except the code words UAA, UAG, and UGA. These code words are signals to terminate the message.

In summary, the message is found in the mRNA. This message is coded for using uridine instead of

TABLE 5–3
Properties of Cellular RNAs

Type	Size	Half-life	Number of Kinds in Cell	Function
Ribosomal RNA (70S ribosomes)[a]	4×10^4, 5S 5×10^5, 16S 1×10^6, 23S	Stable	3	Serves a structural function in ribosomes
Messenger RNA	Variable	2 min in *E. coli*	1000	Carries code from DNA to proteins, binds to ribosomes
Transfer RNA	2.3 to 2.8 $\times 10^4$	Stable	Up to 61	Bridges codon on mRNA and amino acid

[a]The sizes of rRNA in the eucaryotic 80S ribosomes are different.

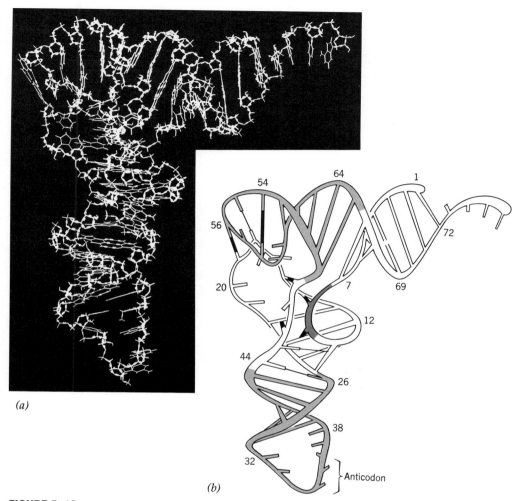

(a)

(b)

FIGURE 5–12

Photograph *(a)* and diagram *(b)* of a molecular model of the yeast phenylalanine tRNA showing its three-dimensional structure. The anticodon is at the bottom. (Photograph *(a)* reproduced with permission of Dr. S. H. Kim. From E. J. Gardner and D. P. Snustad, *Principles of Genetics*, 6th ed., Wiley, New York, 1981.)

thymine, which is found in DNA. The triplet code in the mRNA is called the **codon**, which is recognized by an anticodon on a tRNA molecule. Each cell contains many mRNAs of varying sizes, each coding for a specific protein or group of proteins. In addition, there are enough different tRNA molecules to read the 61 code words for amino acids (Table 5–4). Each tRNA molecule binds one specific amino acid and at the opposite end (Figure 5–12) contains a triplet sequence of bases called the anticodon. The message is read when the anticodon on the tRNA combines with the codon on the mRNA.

TABLE 5–4
The Genetic Code

First Position	Second Position				Third Position
5' End	U	C	A	G	3' End
U	UUU phe	UCU ser	UAU tyr	UGU cys	U
	UUC phe	UCC ser	UAC tyr	UGC cys	C
	UUA leu	UCA ser	UAA ter[a]	UGA ter	A
	UUG leu	UCG ser	UAG ter	UGG trp	G
C	CUU leu	CCU pro	CAU his	CGU arg	U
	CUC leu	CCC pro	CAC his	CGC arg	C
	CUA leu	CCA pro	CAA gln	CGA arg	A
	CUG leu	CCG pro	CAG gln	CGG arg	G
A	AUU ile	ACU thr	AAU asn	AGU ser	U
	AUC ile	ACC thr	AAC asn	AGC ser	C
	AUA ile	ACA thr	AAA lys	AGA arg	A
	AUG met	ACG thr	AAG lys	AGG arg	G
G	GUU val	GCU ala	GAU asp	GGU gly	U
	GUC val	GCC ala	GAC asp	GGC gly	C
	GUA val	GCA ala	GAA glu	GGA gly	A
	GUG val	GCG ala	GAG glu	GGG gly	G

[a]Chain termination.

Protein synthesis on ribosomes

When cells are growing rapidly, hundreds of proteins are being synthesized at any given instant. This entire process takes place in the bacterial cytoplasm. Messenger RNA is transcribed from DNA by DNA-dependent RNA polymerase. This mRNA then binds to the 30S ribosomal subunit at a specific site (Figure 5–13). At the same time, a N-formylmethionine tRNA binds to the 30S ribosome mRNA complex. This special tRNA is involved in the initiation of all polypeptide chain syntheses in procaryotic cells. A 50S ribosomal subunit attaches next, followed by the formation of polypeptide bonds.

Proteins are formed starting with the amino-terminal end and progressing toward the carboxyl-terminal end. The amino-terminal end is initially blocked by the insertion of N-formylmethionine as the first amino acid. This residue is eventually cleaved from the completed polypeptide. Certain protein initiation factors (not shown) and energy in the form of guanine triphosphate (GTP) are also required for translation. When these are present, mRNA is translated from the 5' to the 3' end. The message is read in only one direction.

Ribosomes have a complex structure that allows for the binding of two tRNA molecules (Figure 5–13) charged with amino acids (amino acyl tRNA). The amino acyl tRNAs interact with a protein elongation factor and GTP prior to binding at site B. The ribosomal tRNA site A is now occupied by fMet-tRNA. Ribosomal site B will then be occupied by the charged tRNA molecule that possesses an anticodon complementary to the codon on the mRNA positioned at site B. When both tRNA sites on the ribosome are filled, peptidyl transferase forms a peptide bond at the expense of GTP and the peptide chain

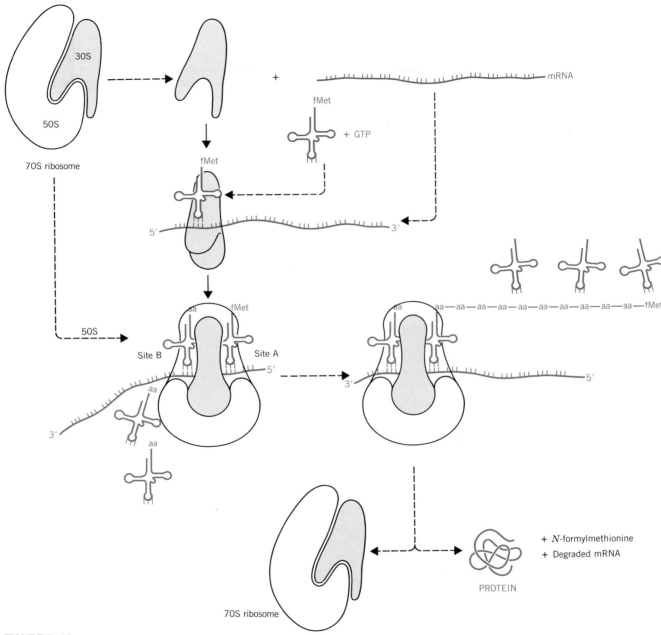

FIGURE 5–13
Diagrammatic representation of protein synthesis on a bacterial ribosome. Translation begins when the 30S ribosomal subunit binds mRNA and *N*-formylmethionine tRNA. The 50S ribosomal subunit then binds and aligns the charged tRNA molecules to enable peptide bond formation. The codons on the mRNA are read from the 5′ end to the 3′ end.

lengthens by one amino acid residue. The mRNA-tRNA complex now moves over one site to occupy site A, which leaves site B vacant. The uncharged tRNA that carried fMet leaves site A to be recharged in the cytoplasm. This process places the next codon in site B ready to be read. The protein remains attached to site A until the entire polypeptide chain is completed.

When more than one ribosome is attached to a single mRNA, the complex is called a **polyribosome** (Figure 5–14). Each ribosome serves as a site for protein synthesis. As a ribosome progresses from the 5′ to the 3′ end of the mRNA, the polypeptide chain increases in length. At the end of a message there is a termination or stop codon. This codon is read by proteins known as release factors.

Synthesis of a typical polypeptide containing 300–400 amino acid residues takes between 10 and 20 seconds in *E. coli*. The peptide immediately assumes much of its secondary and tertiary structure during chain elongation. In fact, the enzymatic activity of certain enzymes can be measured while they are still being synthesized on the ribosome.

Inhibition of protein synthesis

Cells are dependent on the continual synthesis of proteins for growth and reproduction. Irreversible inhibition of protein synthesis will kill a cell. Protein synthesis can be inhibited during either transcription or translation.

Actinomycin D is an antibiotic produced by the bacterium *Streptomyces*. Actinomycin D binds to DNA and prevents mRNA chain elongation. **Rifamycins** are a group of antibiotics that bind to DNA-directed RNA polymerase, preventing the initiation of mRNA formation. These antibiotics inhibit transcription.

Inhibitors of translation are useful drugs for treating animals with bacterial infections because these inhibitors often act on the 70S ribosomes of bacterial cells and do not inhibit protein synthesis on 80S eucaryotic ribosomes. **Tetracyclines** are antibiotics that block site B on the 70S ribosome and prevent the binding of charged tRNAs. Peptide chain elongation ceases in the presence of tetracycline. **Chloramphenicol** binds to the 50S ribosomal subunit and prevents

FIGURE 5–14

Electron micrograph of transcription and translation of *E. coli* genes. The mRNA is transcribed from one of the two DNA strands at the same time that ribosomes translate this RNA message into protein. (Courtesy of Dr. O. L. Miller. From O. L. Miller, B. A. Hamkalo, and C. A. Thomas, *Science, 169:* 392–395, 1970, with permission of the American Association for the Advancement of Science.)

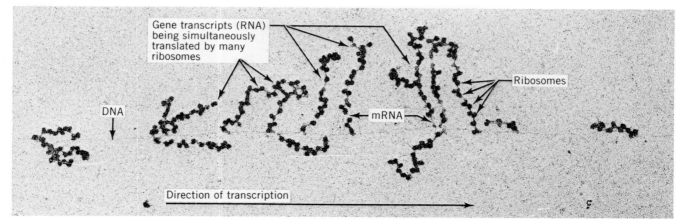

protein synthesis. This is by no means a complete presentation of inhibitors of protein synthesis (see Chapter 10 for more details), but it should be apparent that an understanding of protein synthesis is essential to the effective treatment of bacterial infections.

REGULATION

DNA contains all the information needed by a cell to grow and reproduce. Most cells contain additional information that is only expressed under certain conditions. This is obvious to us when we consider a fertilized egg (a zygote) of a frog. Even though the frog zygote appears round and egglike, we know that it will develop into a multicellular organism. All the DNA sequences present in the zygote are also present in each body cell of the frog, but only certain information is used by a given cell. We must conclude that there are regulatory processes controlling the expression of the code contained in DNA. Since the code is expressed through the synthesis of proteins, one can conclude that there is a regulatory system governing the synthesis of proteins.

Eucaryotic organisms are complex from a regulatory point of view. Bacteria contain fewer proteins, do not undergo development into complex tissues, and contain a single copy of the genetic information. Many current concepts pertaining to the regulation of protein synthesis have developed from the study of procaryotic cells.

Regulation of protein synthesis

Cells control the synthesis of certain proteins in response to the concentration of cellular metabolites. The genes for these proteins are organized in operons on the chromosome. An **operon** is a sequence of genes dealing with a single cellular function that is controlled by a regulator gene. The operon consists of a promotor and an operator sequence adjacent to the structural genes (Figure 5–15) and a regulator gene that can be located anywhere on the chromosome. The active form of the repressor protein binds to the operator region to prevent the transcription of the structural genes. The RNA polymerase involved in transcription only binds to the promotor region when the repressor protein is not bound to the operator.

There are two main control mechanisms for regulating procaryotic protein synthesis. **Enzyme induction** increases the cellular concentration of specific enzymes in response to the presence of substrate molecules called the **inducer.** **Feedback repression** stops the synthesis of specific enzymes in response to the accumulation of end products formed by that enzymatic pathway. The end-product metabolite responsible for the actual repression is called the corepressor. These two mechanisms of regulating protein synthesis operate at the level of transcription (DNA-RNA).

Enzyme induction.   Lactose metabolism is the classic example of enzyme induction (Figure 5–16). Lactose is a disaccharide of galactose linked to glucose

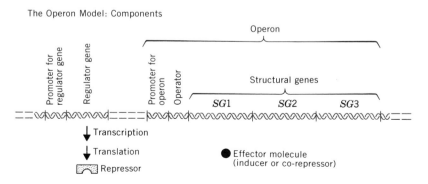

The Operon Model: Components

Transcription
Translation
Repressor

Effector molecule (inducer or co-repressor)

FIGURE 5–15
A diagrammatic representation of the operon model for gene regulation. An **operon** is a group of one or more structural genes (SG) together with the adjoining operator and promotor sequences. The **promotor for the operon** is the sequence to which RNA polymerase binds. The **operator** is the sequence that binds the **repressor protein.** The **regulator gene** and its promotor can be located anywhere on the genome. (From E. J. Gardner and D. P. Snustad, *Principles of Genetics,* 6th ed., Wiley, New York, 1981).

The Operon Model: Induction

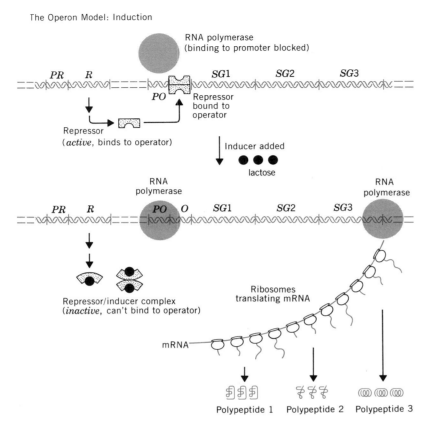

FIGURE 5—16

The *lac* operon: **induction.** The repressor protein formed by the lactose repressor gene (R) is **active;** when it binds to the operator (O), it prevents the transcription of mRNA from the DNA. The **inducer** (lactose) will combine with and inactivate the repressor to prevent it from binding to the operator. Under these conditions, RNA polymerase binds to the promotor (PO) and transcribes the structural genes into mRNA. Proteins are translated from these mRNAs. An inductive operon controls the synthesis of proteins required to metabolize specific substrates. (From E. J. Gardner and D. P. Snustad, *Principles of Genetics,* 6th ed., Wiley, New York, 1981).

through a β1-4 bond. β-galactosidase breaks the β1-4 glycosidic bond of lactose, producing one galactose and one glucose molecule. Two other enzymes are coded for by the lactose operon. They are galactoside permease, which transports lactose into the cell, and galactoside transacetylase, the importance of which is unknown. These three enzymes are induced in *E. coli* by the presence of lactose.

Escherichia coli will make the enzymes necessary to metabolize lactose when lactose is the only carbon substrate available. The genes that code for these proteins are located next to each other on the DNA (Figure 5–16). In front of these genes is an operator sequence that is preceded by the promotor region. This operon is called the **lac operon.** The regulator gene (Figure 5–16) continuously codes for the synthesis of an *active* repressor protein that binds to the DNA at the operator to prevent the initiation of mRNA synthesis. When lactose is present, the re-

pressor protein binds lactose and becomes inactive. It is now unable to bind to the operator. Transcription of the structural genes (SG1, SG2, and SG3) proceeds, and the resulting mRNAs are translated into proteins. The cell is now able to utilize lactose (the inducer) because the cell contains the necessary enzymes.

Escherichia coli will grow on lactose, but when glucose and lactose are both present, *E. coli* will use glucose preferentially over lactose. Many cells use glucose before they metabolize other suitable organic substrates. This happens because glucose represses the synthesis of the enzymes needed to metabolize many other substrates.

Cyclic AMP (a small nucleotide) appears to participate in the regulation of these inducible enzymes at the level of protein synthesis. When glucose is present, the concentration of cAMP in the cell decreases. In the absence of glucose, the concentration of cAMP in the cell increases. The induction of the *lac* operon requires, in addition to lactose, high concentrations of cAMP. The ability of glucose to repress the formation of metabolic enzymes is referred to as the **glucose effect** or **catabolic repression.**

Regulatory systems need not exist for all proteins. Many enzymes and structural proteins are constantly required by growing cells. The proteins synthesized continuously by cells are called **constitutive** proteins. The synthesis of constitutive proteins appears to be under little or no control other than the rate of growth of the cell itself.

Enzyme repression. When a cell contains excess amounts of an end product, the cell can decrease the amount of the synthetic enzymes in that pathway through a process called **feedback repression.** Many rapidly growing bacterial cells contain the enzymes necessary to manufacture all the amino acids. If large quantities of a given amino acid are added to the cell's environment, the cell can assimilate the amino acid directly, so that it no longer needs the enzymes required to produce it. Such an amino acid acts as a **corepressor** when it inhibits the synthesis of the enzymes used in its production.

Enzyme repression affects transcription from the DNA. Operons controlled by repression produce a repressor protein that is inactive until it combines with the corepressor (Figure 5–17). Reaction of the repressor protein with the corepressor activates the

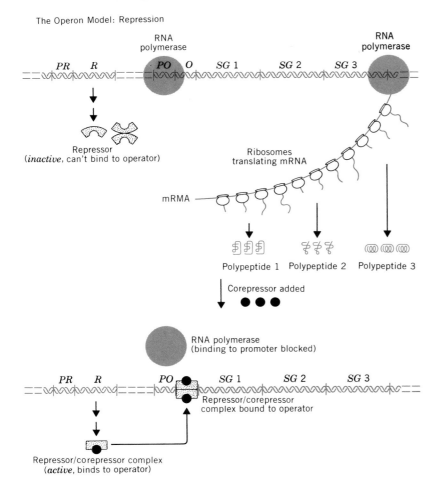

The Operon Model: Repression

FIGURE 5–17

The operon model: **repression.** Synthetic pathways are often controlled by repression. The repressor protein formed by the repressor gene is **inactive**—it will not bind to the operator (O). Under these conditions, the enzymes of the synthetic pathway are synthesized. The operon is turned off in the presence of the **corepressor,** which is usually the end product of the biosynthetic pathway controlled by the operon. The corepressor binds with the repressor protein to form an **active** repressor. The active repressor binds to the operator, which prevents the RNA polymerase from binding to the promotor. No transcription of the structural genes occurs in the presence of the corepressor. (From E. J. Gardner and D. P. Snustad, *Principles of Genetics*, 6th ed., Wiley, New York, 1981).

repressor protein, causing it to bind to the DNA at the operator site. This prevents the further transcription of the operon.

Enzyme induction and enzyme repression are mechanisms that regulate protein synthesis in response to environmental factors. Cells also regulate their cytoplasmic inventory of small molecules by controlling the rate of enzyme activity. This control is exerted on the enzymes as they participate in chemical reactions.

Regulation of enzyme activity

Allosteric enzymes. Enzymes strategically located in metabolic pathways often respond to the end product(s) of their pathway. The enzyme affected is usually the first enzyme (a) in a linear pathway or the enzyme (a') just prior to a branch point in a multiproduct pathway.

$$A \xrightarrow{a} B \xrightarrow{b} C \xrightarrow{c} D \xrightarrow{d} P \quad (1)$$

$$
\begin{array}{c}
A \xrightarrow{a'} B
\begin{array}{c}
\nearrow^{b'} C \xrightarrow{c'} D \xrightarrow{d'} P_1 \\
\searrow_{e'} E \xrightarrow{f'} F \xrightarrow{g'} P_2
\end{array}
\end{array}
\quad (2)
$$

Aspartate transcarbamylase is an example of a regulated enzyme. This enzyme combines aspartate and carbamyl phosphate to form *N*-carbamylaspartate, the first intermediate in the formation of cytidine triphosphate (CTP). CTP binds with aspartate transcarbamylase and inhibits its enzymatic activity. When enough CTP is present, the enzyme can be completely inactivated. This type of inactivation is reversible. The CTP binds at a site on aspartyl transcarbamylase that is separate and distinct from the catalytic site. This site is called an **allosteric site,** and aspartyl transcarbamylase is termed an **allosteric enzyme.** Regulation by this mechanism is termed **feedback inhibition.** When the concentration of CTP decreases in the cell, the enzyme again becomes active and synthesizes more CTP. Allosteric enzymes control the economy of small molecules within a linear or branched metabolic pathway.

Covalent modification. Key enzymes that serve as a central supply or as a major crossroad for multipathways can be under additional control. Certain key enzymes are covalently modified through the action of other enzymes that catalyze the covalent attachment of groups to the regulated enzyme. Covalent modification interconverts the enzyme between an active and an inactive state. This regulation is more permanent because reversal requires enzyme action.

Control at the cellular level

Biologists now know that cells are intricately controlled. The examples of control presented here are multiplied many times over within each cell. Control over transcription, translation, and enzymatic activity is used by cells to serve the immediate needs of that cell. Even when drastic changes in the cell's environment occur, the cell can respond almost immediately.

Regulation in eucaryotes. Multicellular organisms present more complex problems that require more elaborate regulatory systems. For example, these organisms possess hormones that simultaneously stimulate many cells to synthesize specific proteins. Multicellular organisms often go through complex developmental processes, many of which are poorly understood from the regulatory point of view. Recent evidence suggests that these cells modify the message transcribed from DNA. This opens up many theoretical possibilities for the explanation of complex regulatory phenomena.

The basic concepts of molecular biology have become firmly established during the years following the discovery of DNA structure. Much of our knowledge about heredity can now be explained by molecular biology. Molecular biology is leading us into an era of genetic engineering. Scientists are actually able to modify specifically DNA and the hereditary traits of an organism. We are now in an era when molecular biology and genetics can be combined to provide the world with new, rationally designed microorganisms that are capable of doing useful tasks for mankind. The next chapter discusses the basic concepts of bacterial genetics and the details of these new horizons of molecular biology.

SUMMARY

Cellular DNA is a double helix composed of two antiparallel deoxyribose phosphate polymers joined by hydrogen bonds between paired nitrogenous bases: adenine and thymine, guanine and cytosine. Bacterial DNA exists as a closed circular molecule and is often supercoiled. DNA is replicated by a semiconservative mechanism in both directions, beginning at an initiation point. DNA-dependent RNA polymerase produces short RNA chains on which DNA polymerase III adds deoxyribonucleotides to the 3′ end of the growing macromolecule. The short RNA initiation pieces are then cleaved off; DNA polymerase I fills in the gaps; finally, the short pieces of DNA are joined together by ligase. The completed double helix contains one old strand and one new strand of DNA.

Bacterial protein synthesis begins with the formation of a messenger RNA. mRNA is synthesized by DNA-dependent RNA polymerase in the process called transcription. mRNA binds to the small ribosomal subunit and fMet-tRNA. The larger ribosomal subunit then binds to the complex, and polypeptide chain elongation begins. The amino acyl-tRNAs read the codons in the mRNA through their specific triplicate anticodon. The code is a universal triplicate code containing 61 code words for 20 amino acids: the code is redundant. Enzymes, initiation factors, GTP, and ATP are required for protein synthesis. Amino acids are added to the carboxyl-terminal end of the growing peptide chain. A termination sequence in the mRNA ends the synthetic process. The peptide chain automatically assumes its tertiary structure and begins functioning. Ribosomes and tRNAs are reused in further protein synthesis; bac-

terial mRNA is used only a few times before it is degraded.

Cells regulate protein synthesis in response to environmental stimuli. Regulated enzymes in procaryotic cells are coded for by contiguous genes located next to an operator gene. The amount of induced enzyme is increased in response to the inducer. The inducer is a molecule that reacts with a specific repressor protein to form an inactive repressor. The genes are then transcribed into mRNA, and the mRNAs are translated into proteins. Repressible enzyme systems form inactive repressor molecules that become activated on combination with their corepressor. Corepressors are usually end products of a synthetic pathway, and they decrease the level of enzymes in that synthetic pathway.

Internal cellular control over the inventory of small molecules is also exerted directly on the enzymes. Allosteric enzymes contain a site, separate from the active site, that binds end products of the metabolic pathway. When this binding results in inhibition of enzymatic activity, it is called feedback inhibition. Covalent modification is a more permanent means for controlling enzymatic activity.

QUESTIONS AND TOPICS FOR STUDY AND DISCUSSION

Questions

1. What scientific evidence was available to Watson and Crick when they developed the double-helix model for DNA?
2. Define or explain the following.

antiparallel	feedback repression
base-pairing	genome
catabolic repression	Okazaki fragments
codon, anticodon	semiconservative replication
enzyme induction	supercoiled DNA

3. Name and describe the function of the enzymes involved in DNA synthesis.
4. What is meant by moles percent G + C? How is this value used in bacterial classification? Explain.

5. Describe the function of the three RNAs that participate in translation.
6. Trace the flow of information from a gene to a protein.
7. Describe the operon model for regulating protein synthesis.
8. Describe two methods for controlling the rate of an enzyme-catalyzed reaction.

Discussion

1. What are the implications of the universal genetic code to evolution and the replication of viruses?
2. Explain how some antibiotics inhibit bacterial protein synthesis without affecting eucaryotic cells. Would you expect a similar group of antibiotics to be effective against viral replication in animal cells?

FURTHER READINGS

Books

Haynes, R., and P. Hanawalt, *The Chemical Basis of Life— Readings from Scientific American*, Freeman, San Francisco, 1973. A compendium of readings from *Scientific American* that traces the historical development of the concept of the gene through the early 1970s.

Watson, James D., *The Double Helix*, Atheneum, New York, 1968. A personal account of the discovery of the double helix of DNA. This is probably the most significant discovery in biology during the twentieth century.

Watson, James D., *Molecular Biology of The Gene*, 3rd ed., Benjamin, Menlo Park, Calif., 1976. A well-written textbook in molecular biology that is widely recognized for its clear and informative illustrations.

Articles and Reviews

Bauer, W. R., F. H. C. Crick, and J. H. White, "Supercoiled DNA," *Sci. Am.*, 243:118–133 (July 1980). Physical models are presented to explain the molecular biology of supercoiled DNA.

Miller, O. L. Jr., "The Visualization of Genes in Action," *Sci. Am.*, 228:34–42 (March 1973). An article on the use of the electron microscope in studies of translation and transcription.

6

MICROBIAL GENETICS

Heredity is the passage of parental traits to offspring. **Genetics** is the study of heredity. Some of the most significant genetic work was done in the nineteenth century by Gregor Mendel (1822–1885). After failing his examinations for a teaching certificate, Mendel entered the Austrian monastery in Brunn (now Brno, Czechoslovakia). Here he worked in the monastery gardens and made detailed observations of plant heredity. Although his work concentrated on the inheritance of traits in the sweet pea, his contribution has significance in all biological systems. Mendel showed that traits, such as flower color and seed shape, are passed from parents to offspring in discrete units now known as genes. He demonstrated that plants carry pairs of genes that separate and independently assort during gamete formation. Mendel's work, published in 1865, was ahead of its time, and his contributions were not recognized until the year 1900. Geneticists now recognize that Mendel established the foundations for the study of heredity.

CONCEPT OF THE GENE

Molecular genetics had its foundations in the work of George Beadle and Edward Tatum, who investi-

gated the genetics of amino acid production in *Neurospora crassa*. This pink bread mold is an ideal organism for genetic studies. *Neurospora* can be grown in large quantities; and even though sexual reproduction does occur, *Neurospora* is haploid during most of its life cycle (Figure 6–1). Haploid (*n*) cells contain one copy of every gene; diploid (2*n*) cells contain two copies of every gene, one from the male and one from the female parent.

Beadle and Tatum began their experiments by using X rays to induce mutations in the asexual spores (conidia) of *Neurospora*. The irradiated conidia were then mated (Figure 6–1), and the resulting ascospores were isolated and grown on a complete medium. This assured the investigators that the mold cultures arising from the haploid ascospores were genetically pure. Next they isolated nutritional mutants that were unable to grow on a glucose-salts medium. These mutants required one or more essential nutrients; thus they grew only in a complete medium. Mutants unable to synthesize a particular amino acid were identified by their ability to grow on a glucose-salts medium supplemented with that amino acid. For example, mutants able to grow on glucose-salts plus the amino acid tryptophan were called tryptophan mutants. Wild type *Neurospora* can

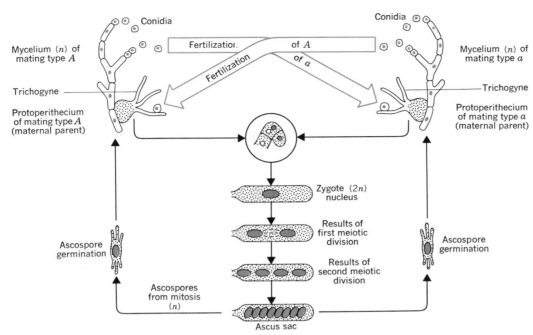

FIGURE 6—1

The life cycle of the pink bread mold, *Neurospora crassa*. Sexual reproduction occurs between conidia and protoperithecia of opposite mating types designated type *A* and type *a*. The resulting zygote (2n) undergoes two meiotic divisions to form 8 ascocpores (n) in an ascus. Each ascospore gives rise to a genetically pure strain of *Neurospora*. (From R. P. Wagner et al., *Introduction to Modern Genetics*, Wiley New York, 1980.)

grow on glucose-salts because it can produce all the amino acids.

One gene, one protein

From the experiments of Beadle and Tatum, it became apparent that the nutritional mutants required the presence of an amino acid in the growth medium because they were deficient in an enzyme necessary to synthesize that amino acid. These results led Beadle and Tatum to the conclusion that one gene codes for one enzyme. This was a major contribution to the understanding of genetics. Their contemporaries in biochemistry knew that enzymes were proteins, but they did not know how complex some enzymes are. We now know that many enzymes are composed of more than one polypeptide and that some

polypeptides, such as the peptide hormones and ribosomal proteins, have no enzymatic activity. Therefore, Beadle and Tatum's theory was modified to: one gene codes for one polypeptide. Genes also code for RNA, and some RNAs are not translated into polypeptides. Today we say that *a* **gene** *is a segment of DNA that is transcribed into RNA: most genes are translated into a polypeptide; however, the genes for rRNA and tRNA make only RNA molecules.*

MUTATIONS

Beadle and Tatum had exploited one of the key phenomena of genetics. Instead of looking for mutants in nature, they produced mutations in *Neurospora* with X rays. A **mutation** is an inheritable change in DNA. Only when a change occurs in the cell's DNA will it be passed to succeeding generations of cells. Alterations in a cell's RNA molecules do not qualify as mutations. Alterations in DNA can be caused by chemical or physical means, or they can occur spontaneously.

Types of mutations

DNA can be altered in a number of distinct ways (Figure 6–2). Addition of one or more nucleotides to the DNA will cause a mutation. Similarly, deletion of one or two nucleotides from the DNA sequence will cause a mutation. Both changes will result in a **frameshift** because the code words will now be improperly read. Substitution of certain bases will cause mutations; however, one must remember that the code is redundant; so not all substitutions will cause a change in the code (Table 5–4). For example, if the base sequence in DNA is *CAT*, then the code in mRNA is *GUA*, which codes for valine. Other DNA sequences that also code for valine are *CAC*, *CAA*, and *CAG*. Only an alteration in the first two bases (either C or A) would change the code.

Rate of mutation

Mutation of an individual gene occurs independently of mutations in other genes. The rate of mutation is a measure of the probability that permanent damage will occur to the DNA. If a mutation occurs once in 1 million divisions, the rate of mutation is 10^{-6} (1/1,000,000 divisions). The rate at which mutations occur in two separate genes is equal to the product of the individual rates. For example, assume that gene A normally mutates at a rate of 10^{-5} and gene B mutates at a rate of 10^{-8}. The formation of an organism containing mutations in both gene A and gene B will be one chance in 10 trillion divisions ($10^{-5} \times 10^{-8} = 10^{-13}$). Double mutations occur very rarely in nature except when cells are exposed to chemical and physical mutagens.

Chemically caused mutations

Mutagens are chemical or physical agents that increase the rate of mutation greatly above the natural or spontaneous level. Chemical mutagens directly

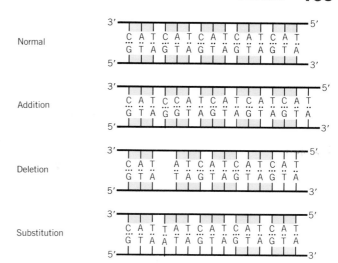

FIGURE 6–2
Mutations are inheritable alterations in DNA: they can result from additions, deletions, and/or substitutions. Any one of these events can alter the reading of the triplicate code.

alter the purine and/or pyrimidine bases in DNA. Mutagens can be either organic or inorganic compounds. Commonly used chemical mutagens include nitrous acid (HNO_2) and the alkylating agents—ethylmethyl sulfonate (EMS), mustard gas, and nitrosoguanidine.

Nitrous acid causes the deamination of bases in DNA, replacing the lost amino group with a keto ($\diagdown C=O$) group. Deamination of adenine by HNO_2 results in the formation of hypoxanthine (Figure 6–3a), which base-pairs with cytosine instead of thymine. Cytosine in DNA is converted to uracil by nitrous acid. This will cause the change in base-pairing from C≡G to U≡A.

Alkylating agents are the most potent group of chemical mutagens. They transfer the alkyl group to the carbonyl oxygen of a base. This chemical change alters the hydrogen-bonding capabilities of the base. Ethylmethyl sulfonate (EMS) chemically alters thymine to make it pair with guanine instead of adenine. Similarly, EMS chemically changes guanine to a compound that pairs with thymine instead of cytosine. Other alkylating agents include sulfur mus-

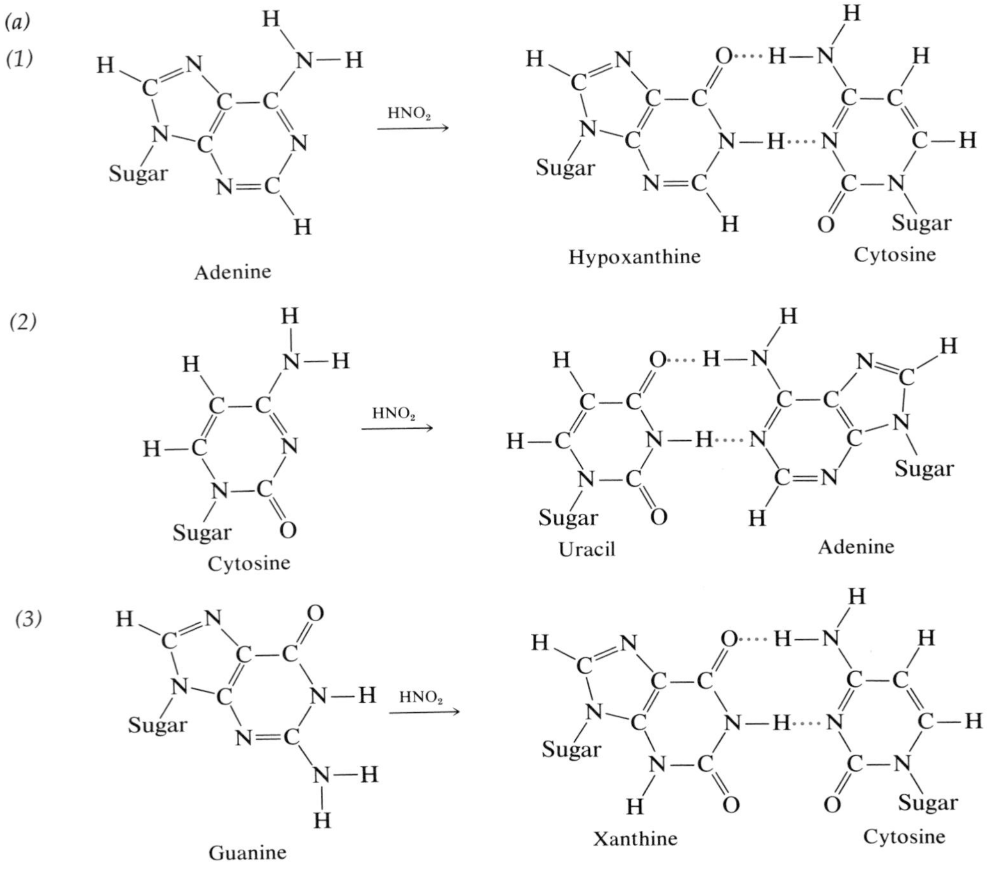

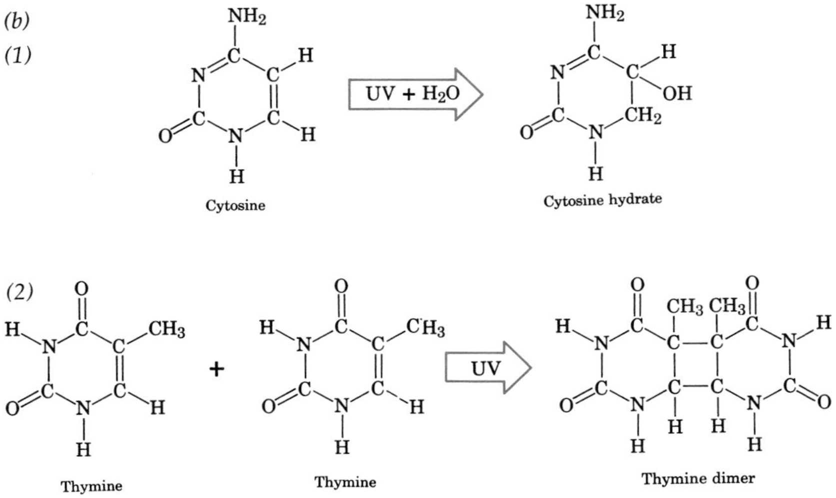

FIGURE 6–3
Chemical and physical mutagens. *(a)* Nitrous acid converts (1) adenine to hypoxanthine, which results in an AT → GC transition; (2) cytosine to uracil, which results in a CG → AT transition; and (3) guanine to xanthine, which is not directly mutagenic. *(b)* Ultraviolet irradiation can (1) cause the hydrolysis of cytosine to form the hydrate and (2) causes the formation of thymine dimers, which block replication. (Adapted from E. J. Gardner and D. P. Snustad, *Principles of Genetics*, 6th ed., Wiley, New York, 1981.)

tard and nitrosoguanidine. Even low concentrations of these compounds will cause mutations in biological systems.

Base analogues are compounds that are chemically similar to the natural compounds used to synthesize DNA. An analogue of thymine is 5-bromouracil. This compound is taken up by cells and base-pairs with adenine in place of thymine. When DNA is replicated on a strand containing 5-bromouracil, guanine base-pairs with it instead of adenine. This results in a base sequence change.

Physical causes of mutations

Ultraviolet light (UV) has sufficient energy to cause chemical changes in the pyrimidine bases of DNA. The formation of thymine dimers is the most common form of DNA damage caused by UV light. When adjacent thymine residues absorb UV light between 250 and 280 nm, they chemically join by covalent bonds (T=T) to form a dimer (Figure 6–3b and Figure 6–4). Thymine dimers cause errors to be made during DNA replications that lead to mutations.

FIGURE 6–4

(a) **Light-repair** mechanism of correcting thymine dimers in *E. coli* DNA. Thymine dimers are formed by UV irradiation. The enzyme involved in the light repair mechanism binds to the thymine dimer region of the DNA. In the presence of blue light, this enzyme cleaves the dimer cross-links. *(b)* The **dark-repair** mechanism requires a series of enzymes. The damaged area is excised by endonuclease and exonuclease activity. DNA polymerase and DNA ligase then combine to synthesize a new DNA strand complementary to the template. (From E. J. Gardner and D. P. Snustad, *Principles of Genetics,* 6th ed., Wiley, New York, 1981.)

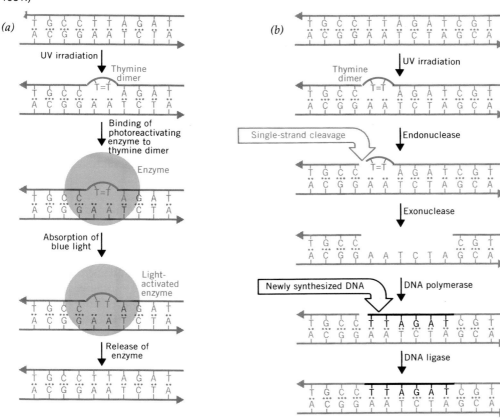

Cells are naturally exposed to the UV light that comes from the sun. Some cells have UV repair systems that cope with the mutations caused by this mutagen. For example, *Escherichia coli* possesses both a light-repair and a dark-repair mechanism (Figure 6–4). The **light repair** system involves a photoactivated enzyme that breaks the bonds between the thymine dimers. This protective mechanism is active only in visible light. Several enzymes are involved in the **"dark"-repair** mechanism that is independent of light. Endonuclease and exonuclease combine to excise the defective segment of DNA containing the thymine dimer. DNA polymerase and DNA ligase then patch the broken region by synthesizing a new DNA segment. The combination of the light and the dark-repair mechanisms enables *E. coli* to repair damage to their DNA that otherwise would cause lethal mutations.

Spontaneous mutations

Mutations that occur in the absence of all mutagenic agents are called **spontaneous mutations.** These normally occur at such a low rate that they are hard to detect. Some are observed by chance. For example, the pigment-producing bacterium *Serratia marcescens* spontaneously gives rise to nonpigmented strains. Spontaneous mutations can arise from the chemical effects of metabolic intermediates on the cell's own DNA. Nitrous acid is an example of a naturally produced metabolite that is mutagenic. Other causes of spontaneous mutations are not well documented.

Classes of mutants

Nutritional mutants. Mutations that alter an organism's ability to produce an essential metabolite are called nutritional mutants. Beadle and Tatum used nutritional mutants in their work on *Neurospora*. Mutants requiring a nutritional supplement in their growth medium are called **auxotrophs.** Wild type strains, or the parent from which a mutant strain is derived, are referred to as **prototrophs.** Wild

type strains of *E. coli* will grow on a glucose-salts medium without added nutritional supplements. Auxotrophs of *E. coli* will grow on glucose-salts medium provided that the medium also contains the appropriate nutritional supplements.

Methods are available to produce and to select for specific nutritional mutants (Figure 6–5). Millions of bacteria are exposed to a chemical or physical mutagen. From this mixture only 10 to 100 cells will contain the specific altered gene(s) desired. Several selection procedures can be used to isolate specific mutants. Most procedures manipulate the culture medium to kill the prototrophs. The experimenter selects against the parent strain, so that the mutants predominate in subsequent growth experiments. One technique used to select against the prototrophs is to transfer the mutagen-treated culture to a glucose-salts medium that contains penicillin. Penicillin is an antibiotic that kills only growing cells. Wild type cells will grow in the penicillin–glucose-salts medium and die. The nutritional mutants will be unable to grow in this medium, but they will survive.

Survivors are then grown on a complete medium without penicillin, and each mutant strain is given a number designation. To isolate all the nutritional mutants that require the amino acid tryptophan, each strain is inoculated into a glucose-salts medium containing tryptophan. Strains that grow in this medium and do not grow in a glucose-salts medium are tryptophan mutants (trp^-).* To isolate more complex genotypes and to expedite the screening process, Joshua and Esther Lederberg developed the **replica-plating technique.** A master plate is prepared (Figure 6–5) that contains between 10 and 100 mutant colonies. These mutant colonies are grown on a complete agar medium in a petri dish. A sterile velvet pad on a transfer block is then used to inoculate each of the colonies from the master plate onto plates containing glucose-salts medium plus one or more nutritional supplements (Figure 6–5). Each strain is scored for growth on the supplements cho-

---

*Geneticists use ($+$) to indicate that a gene is functional and ($-$) to indicate that the gene is inoperative or absent.

FIGURE 6–5

Nutritional mutants are isolated and characterized by replica plating. After mutating the culture, mutants are isolated and grown on a master plate. The master plate shown contains the nine mutant colonies that are replica-plated on four separate media. Isolate 5 is a revertant to wild type because it grows on glucose-salts medium. Isolates 1, 3, and 6 are tryptophan auxotrophs *(try⁻)* because they grow on glucose salts plus tryptophan, but not on glucose salts alone. Similarly, isolates 7 and 8 are arginine auxotrophs *(arg⁻)*. Isolates 2, 4, and 9 are double auxotrophs *(try⁻, arg⁻)* because they grow only on media containing both tryptophan and arginine.

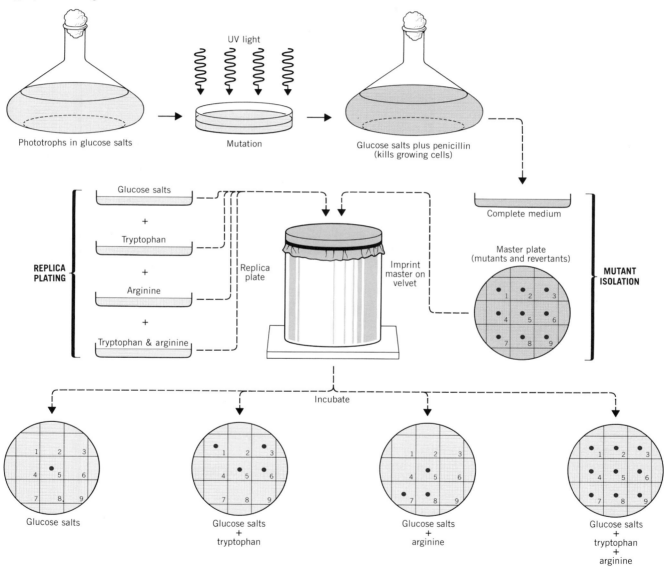

sen by the investigator. Suppose that a strain grew on glucose salts plus tryptophan and arginine but did not grow on glucose salts plus tryptophan or on glucose salts plus arginine (Figure 6–5, strains 2, 4, and 9). This strain is a double mutant with the genotype *trp⁻*, *arg⁻*. The study of bacterial genetics relies on the investigator's ability to isolate and analyze different mutants. The replica-plating technique greatly facilitates this process.

Mutations and cancer

Many chemical mutagens are also carcinogens. **Carcinogens** are compounds that cause cancer in animals. The U.S. Federal Drug Administration (FDA) is under congressional order to remove all carcinogens from consumable goods. To prove that a chemical is, or is not, a carcinogen requires that it be given to thousands of animals in a testing procedure that takes considerable time and costs hundreds of thousands of dollars. To test more compounds for less cost and in less time, Bruce Ames developed a bacterial test for carcinogens. The **Ames test** determines if a compound can mutate cultures of *Salmonella*. This is a screening test that indicates if a compound is a potential carcinogen. Animal tests are still required to prove carcinogenicity.

Ames test. Histidine auxotrophs of *Salmonella typhimurium* are grown in a minimal medium without histidine. Histidine auxotrophs have a very low rate of reverse mutation to the wild type (prototrophs). However, when these bacteria are grown in the presence of a mutagen, their rate of reverse mutation to wild type increases. Compounds that increase the rate of mutation are called mutagens. Since only prototrophs can grow on the medium used in the Ames test, the mutagenicity of the compound on the filter disk (Figure 6–6) is directly related to the number of colonies that surround the disk. There appears to be a strong correlation between the mutagenicity of a compound and its known carcinogenic properties (Table 6–1). In the reported experiments, 88 percent of the known carcinogens proved to be bacterial mutagens. Similarly, 86 percent of the compounds known as noncarcino-

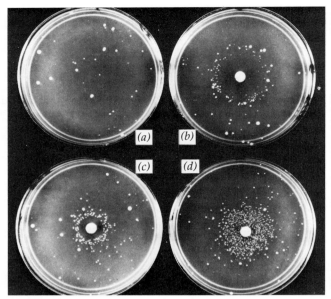

FIGURE 6–6
Results of an Ames spot test for mutagens. A culture of the histidine auxotroph (TA98) of *Salmonella* was plated on minimal medium. Only the *Salmonella* that have reverted to wild type are able to grow on minimal medium. Chemical mutagens increase the number of revertants. Mutagens were applied to filter paper disks (6 mm) that were then placed on plates *b, c,* and *d* (plate A is the control): *(a)* spontaneous revertants, *(b)* furylfuramide (1 μg), *(c)* aflatoxin B₁ (1 μg), and *(d)* 2-aminofluorene (10 μg). Mutagen-induced rerevertants appear as a ring of colonies around each disk. (Courtesy of Dr. B. Ames. From B. Ames, J. McCann, and E. Yamasake, *Mutation Research*, 31:347–364, 1975, copyright © 1975, Elsevier Scientific Publishing Company.)

gens were not mutagenic in the Ames test. Refinements in the Ames test have increased the sensitivity of this test, making it an important screening test for carcinogenic compounds.

BACTERIAL GENETICS

Bacteria are ideal organisms for genetic study. They are so easy to handle that an investigator can maintain hundreds of strains in a single refrigerator-size incubator. Bacteria grow rapidly, which enables investigators to analyze the results of a genetic experiment within 48 hours. Moreover, procaryotes are

TABLE 6-1
Ames Test Results

Group of Compounds	Carcinogens Mutagens/Total Tested	Noncarcinogens Mutagens/Total Tested
Aromatic amines	23/25	2/12
Alkyl halides	17/20	2/3
Polycyclic aromatics	26/27	2/9
Esters, epoxides, carbamates	13/18	4/9
Nitro aromatics and heterocycles	28/28	3/4
Miscellaneous organics	1/6	0/13
Nitrosamines	20/21	0/2
Fungal toxins and antibiotics	8/9	0/5
Cigarette smoke concentrate	1/1	0/0
Azo dyes and diazo compounds	11/11	1/3

Source: J. McCann, E. Choi, E. Yamasaki, and B. N. Ames, *Proc. Natl. Acad. Sci. USA*, 72:5135 (1975).

haploid (*n*) organisms during their entire life. Even with all these superb traits, not all bacteria are ideal genetic tools because not all bacteria can exchange genetic information.

Among bacteria, there are three mechanisms of genetic transfer. **Transformation** is the transfer of naked DNA from the environment to a competent recipient cell. **Conjugation** is the transfer of genetic information from a donor cell to a recipient cell when the two cells are physically joined together. **Transduction** is the viral-mediated genetic transfer of markers from a host cell to a recipient cell. It is described in Chapter 9. To demonstrate genetic transfer, marker genes in the transferred DNA must be expressed in a recipient cell. In many instances genetic transfer and expression are rare events, but the small size of bacteria and the selective techniques available allow geneticists to screen billions of cells for the desired few.

Transformation

The earliest reported observations of genetic transfer in bacteria were made by F. Griffith in 1928 during his investigations of pneumococcal infections in mice (Figure 6–7). Disease-causing strains of *Streptococcus*

pneumoniae, a bacterium that causes pneumonia in humans, have a distinctive capsule and form smooth, mucoid colonies (called the S strain). This strain spontaneously reverts to a noncapsulated strain that forms rough colonies (called the R strain). Only the capsulated S strain will cause pneumonia in animals.

When Griffith injected mice with cultures of the R strain, all the mice lived. Mice injected with heat-killed S strain also lived. When Griffith injected mice with cultures of the R strain combined with heat-killed cultures of the S strain, the mice died (Figure 6–7). From these dead mice he isolated capsulated cells that produced smooth colonies. Griffith postulated that a "transforming principle" was released by the heat-killed S strain and then taken up by the viable R strain. The transforming principle converted the R strain into an S strain. These experiments were later reproduced in the test tube. In 1944, Avery, MacLeod, and McCarty purified the transforming principle and proved that it was DNA.

Transformation has now been demonstrated in *Hemophilus, Neisseria, Escherichia, Bacillus,* and *Streptococcus*. A great amount of our knowledge of transformation comes from work on *Hemophilus* and *Streptococcus*.

Transformation is the uptake of free DNA by a competent cell. Transformation is prevented by DNAase because this enzyme breaks down unprotected (free) DNA. Recipient cells must be competent. This physiological state is not well understood, but protein synthesis is required for cells to become competent. An enzymelike factor is synthesized in exponentially growing cells that can confer competency on noncompetent cells. Competency probably involves a change in cell-wall structure that enables the cell to bind the extracellular DNA.

Once donor DNA has attached to the cell surface, it is cleaved by one or more nucleases into short pieces (average molecular weight of 4 to 5 $\times$ 10^6 daltons). In *Streptococcus*, one strand of the DNA is degraded while the other strand of DNA is transported into the cell in an energy-dependent process. *Hemophilus* takes up only double-stranded homologous

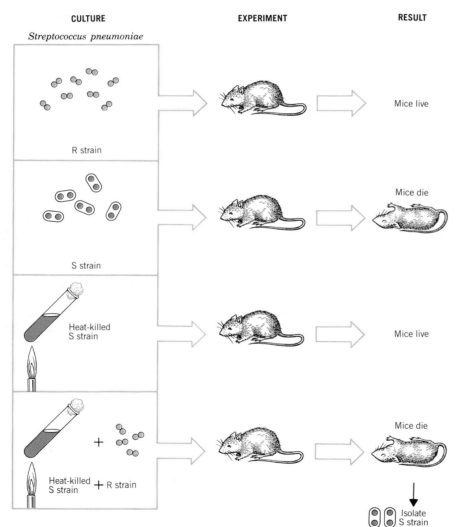

CULTURE   EXPERIMENT   RESULT

Streptococcus pneumoniae

R strain — Mice live

S strain — Mice die

Heat-killed S strain — Mice live

Heat-killed S strain + R strain — Mice die

Isolate S strain

FIGURE 6–7
Griffith's transformation experiment with *Streptococcus pneumoniae*. Type S (S for smooth colony formation) capsulated pneumococci kill mice. However, when heat-killed type S pneumococci were injected into mice, the mice survived. Similarly, mice survived when they were injected with living *noncapsulated* pneumococci type R (designated R for rough colony formation). Injection of either living type S or a mixture of nonliving type S and living type R resulted in severe pneumonia and death. Only type S pneumococci could be isolated from the dead mice. These experiments suggested that the noncapsulated rough strain acquires a "transforming principle" from the smooth strain that then converts them into smooth pneumococci. (Modified from E. J. Gardner and D. P. Snustad, *Principles of Genetics*, 6th ed., Wiley, New York, 1981.)

(from the same genera) DNA. Integration of DNA into the host chromosome takes place very rapidly in both genera. Transformation is a limited tool for genetic analysis because the assimilated pieces of DNA are randomly selected by the cell and because these pieces carry few genetic markers. Nevertheless, transformation is an important concept, and it is the only method of genetic analysis in some bacteria.

Conjugation

Transfer of genetic information from a donor bacterium to a recipient bacterium through cell-to-cell contact (Figure 6–8) is called **conjugation**. This process was discovered in 1946 by Joshua Lederberg and Edward Tatum, who were working with the now famous K-12 strain of *E. coli*. They produced mutations in *E. coli* and then isolated an auxotroph that required both biotin and methionine for growth (bio^-, met^-, thr^+, leu^+). Another *E. coli* auxotroph that required both threonine and leucine (bio^+, met^+, thr^-, leu^-) for growth was also isolated. Lederberg and Tatum mixed these strains together and then selected recombinants that had the wild type genotype (bio^+, met^+, thr^+, leu^+) by growing them on glucose-salts medium. Approximately 200 colonies developed on glucose-salts medium when 10^8 cells of each strain were mixed together. This result indicated that genetic transfer occurred between these strains: the transfer event was not phage-mediated, it was insensitive to DNAase, and it required

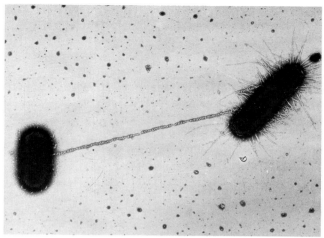

FIGURE 6–8

Bacterial conjugation between an Hfr and an F⁻ strain of *E. coli*. The bacterial cell with numerous appendages is the donor cell, which is connected to the smooth-surfaced recipient cell by a sex or F pilus. DNA from the donor cell is transferred through the F pilus to the recipient cell. In this electron micrograph, small virus particles are bound to the F pilus to differentiate it from the fimbriae located on the surface of the donor cell. The viruses are not involved in conjugation. (Courtesy of Dr. C. Brinton, Jr. and J. Carnahan.)

cell-to-cell contact (Table 6–2). Further investigations revealed that the necessary cell-to-cell contact occurs when the donor cell contains a **sex pilus** (pl., pili) on its cell surface. The pilus is a hollow proteinaceous extension found only on donor cells. The pilus

TABLE 6–2

Characteristics of Bacterial Genetic Transfer

| Characteristic | Genetic Process | | |
	Transformation	Transduction	Conjugation
DNAase sensitive	+	−	−
Bacteriophage required	−	+	−
Cell-to-cell contact	−	−	+
Transfer of small DNA molecules	+	+	+
Transfer of large DNA molecules	−	−	+

shortens when it contacts an appropriate cell to bring the two cells together. This physical contact is a major characteristic that separates conjugation from the other types of bacterial genetic transfer.

Plasmids. Bacterial conjugation is intimately linked with the presence of plasmids in bacteria. **Plasmids** are self-replicating, extrachromosomal, circular DNA molecules. Their presence in cells can be detected by both genetic and physical techniques. Since plasmids are extrachromosomal, they usually code for dispensible information. When a cell loses its plasmid, it is said to be cured. Curing is irreversible, and it can be expedited by chemical treatment. Acridine orange prevents plasmid replication at concentrations that do not affect cell replication. When the replication of a plasmid is prevented (Figure 6–9), the progeny cells that lack the plasmid also lack the

FIGURE 6–9

(a) Replication of plasmids in untreated cells occurs independently of chromosomal replication. (b) Acridine orange preferentially prevents plasmid replication resulting in curing cells of their plasmids.

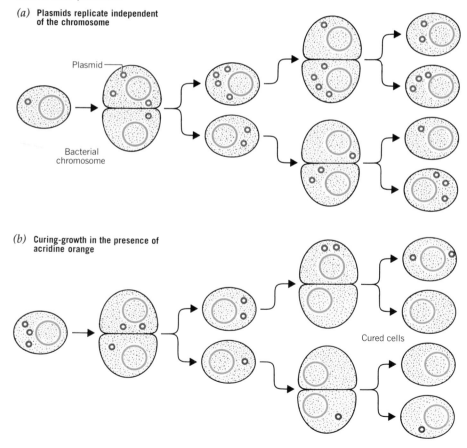

(a) Plasmids replicate independent of the chromosome

Plasmid

Bacterial chromosome

(b) Curing-growth in the presence of acridine orange

Cured cells

genetic traits coded for by the plasmid DNA. The irreversible loss of a trait or a group of traits under nonmutating conditions is genetic evidence for the loss of a plasmid. This loss can be confirmed by physical data.

Plasmids are closed, circular, double-stranded DNA molecules that can be separated from chromosomal DNA by physical and chemical techniques. They vary in size from small molecules, which code for only a few genes, to molecules with molecular weights of 5×10^7 daltons, which code for as many as 100 genes. Often the G + C moles percent of the plasmid varies from that of the chromosomal DNA. The size, structure, and base composition of plasmids enable them to be isolated by ultracentrifugation (Figure 6–10). Agarose gel electrophoresis is another technique used to separate and identify plasmids. This technique is also used to demonstrate supercoiling in plasmid DNA molecules. Supercoiling is clearly demonstrated by electron microscopy (see Figure 5–7).

Plasmids replicate independently of the bacterial chromosome, and they replicate more quickly because of their small size. These DNA molecules are replicated by the cells' enzymes. **Conjugative plasmids** can be transferred from one cell to another. During the transfer of a conjugative plasmid, a single strand (5′ end) of DNA is transferred; and the recipient cell synthesizes the complementary strand using the transferred strand as a template. The remaining strand in the donor cell maintains its circular structure and serves as a template for the synthesis of a complementary strand. Both the donor and the recipient cell end up with a complete double-stranded plasmid.

Fertility plasmids. Conjugation in bacteria always proceeds from the male donor cell to the female recipient cell. Maleness is coded for by the **fertility plasmid**. Cells containing this plasmid are designated F^+ cells; cells without the fertility plasmid are designated F^- cells. When F^+ cells conjugate with F^- female cells, all the recipients become F^+ cells, demonstrating that the male traits are genetically

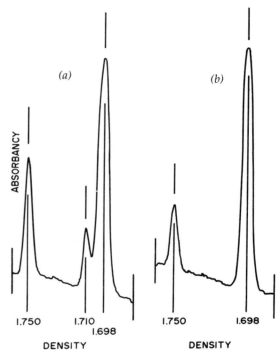

FIGURE 6–10
Density gradient (CsC1) centrifugation separates plasmid DNA from chromosomal DNA. The tracings (ultraviolet light absorption) show the distribution of nucleic acid in the centrifuge tubes at equilibrium. The band of DNA at 1.750 g/cm³ is a standard. (a) DNA extracted from *Proteus mirabilis* infected with a plasmid. The plasmid DNA bands at a density of 1.710 g/cm³. (b) DNA extracted from a *Proteus mirabilis* strain that did not contain a plasmid. (Courtesy of Dr. S. Falkow. From S. Falkow, J. A. Wohlhieter, R. V. Citarella, and L. S. Baron, *J. Bacteriol.*, 87:209–219, 1964, with permission of the American Society for Microbiology.)

transferred during conjugation. Fertility plasmids code for the genes needed to produce the pili and for the enzymes involved in the actual transfer of the plasmid. F plasmids normally do not code for chromosomal (essential) genes.

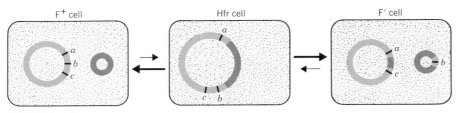

FIGURE 6–11

The integration of an F plasmid into the host chromosome converts an F$^+$ cell into an Hfr cell. The Hfr cell readily reverts to an F$^+$ cell through the excision of the F plasmid. When one or more chromosomal genes are excised with the F plasmid, the resulting cell is termed an F′ cell.

The Lederberg and Tatum experiment is an example of the transfer of chromosomal markers by conjugation. Transfer of chromosomal markers by the fertility plasmids can occur by two distinct mechanisms: transfer from an Hfr cell and transfer from an F′ cell.

Formation of an Hfr cell. The fertility factor (F) can be integrated into the host chromosome in a manner similar to the insertion of lambda phage (see Chapter 9). The *E. coli* chromosome contains at least 15 insertion sites. These sites have DNA sequences that are homologous to those on the F plasmid. Insertion of an F factor into a cell's genome (Figure 6–11) converts an F$^+$ cell to an Hfr cell. Hfr cells actively transfer genetic information to F$^-$ recipient cells, resulting in a **high frequency of recombination** (Hfr). Plasmids that can exist in an autonomous self-replicating state as well as in an integrated part of the host cell's chromosome are termed **episomes**.

Formation of F′ cells. When an F factor is excised from the chromosome of an Hfr strain (Figure 6–11), the F factor can pick up chromosomal genes. Cells that have F plasmids carrying chromosomal genes are termed F′ cells. The plasmid in an F′ cell is self-replicating, and sometimes it is indispensible because it contains chromosomal genes. The specific genes involved depend on the insertion site occupied by the F factor in the Hfr strain. The excision of

an F′ plasmid from an Hfr strain (Hfr ⇌ F′) occurs about once for every 10 cell divisions. The formation of an Hfr strain (F$^+$ → Hfr) is a rare event that occurs only once in every 10^5 cell divisions.

Conjugation with an Hfr donor. The integrated fertility factor in the Hfr strain is capable of mediating genetic transfer to an F$^-$ cell. When Hfr cells are mixed with F$^-$ cells, they interact with each other through the F pilus contact point. Once contact is established, genetic transfer begins (Figure 6–12). At any given time after mixing, the conjugation can be stopped by physically disrupting the cell-to-cell contact. This is done by mixing the suspension in a blender-type mixer.

Recombinants for different genetic loci form at different rates in the recipient cell because there is a sequential transfer of genetic information (Figure 6–12). The chromosome breaks in the middle of the F factor and is transferred in one direction to the F$^-$ cell. In *E. coli* at 37°C, complete transfer of the chromosome takes about 90 min. Complete transfer is a rare event, but when it does occur, the F$^-$ recipient cell can be converted to an F$^+$ or an Hfr cell.

An actual conjugation experiment is shown in Figure 6–13. Since the conjugation pairs between Hfr and F$^-$ cells do not all form simultaneously, the actual data for a given marker forms a straight line with time. Extrapolation of this data back to the first recombinational event provides a measure of that

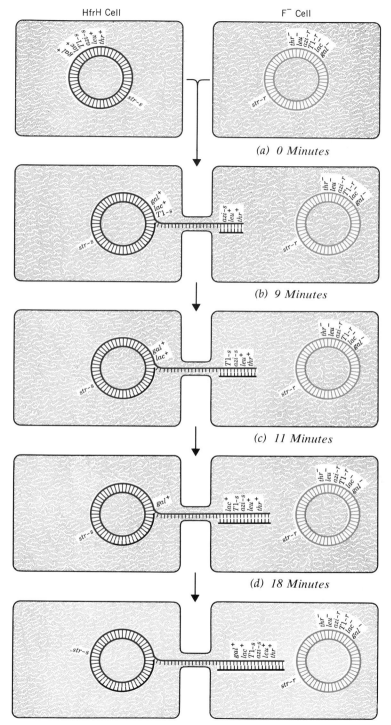

HfrH Cell   F⁻ Cell

(a) 0 Minutes

(b) 9 Minutes

(c) 11 Minutes

(d) 18 Minutes

(e) 25 Minutes

FIGURE 6–12

Conjugation between an Hfr and a F⁻ bacterium. Only one strand of the DNA is transferred into the recipient cell. The recipient cell forms the complementary strand of DNA to make the double helix. The minutes indicate the interval following initiation of conjugation. The genetic elements are not drawn to scale: only about one-fourth of the Hfr chromosome has been transferred during the 25 minutes of conjugation. (From E. J. Gardner and D. P. Snustad, *Principles of Genetics,* 6th ed., Wiley, New York, 1981.)

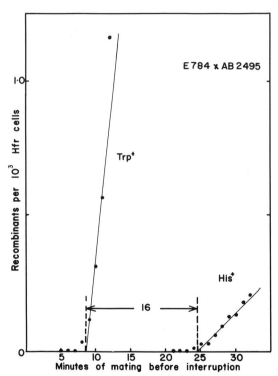

FIGURE 6–13

Interrupted mating curves for *Escherichia coli* Hfr donor strain (E784) and *E. coli* recipient strain (AB2495). The F⁻ recipient cell requires tryptophan *(trp⁻)* and histidine *(his⁻)*. At intervals, mating was interrupted by vigorous mixing, and then the number or recombinants *(trp⁺)* and *his⁺)* were determined. This experiment shows that the *trp* gene and the *his* gene are located 16 minutes apart on the chromosome. (Courtesy of Dr. B. J. Bachmann. From B. J. Bachmann, K. B. Low, and A. L. Taylor, *Bacteriol. Reviews,* 40:116–167, 1976, with permission of the American Society for Microbiology.)

gene's position in relation to the other genes that are being transferred. The distance between genes is expressed in minutes. In the experiment shown, the tryptophan and histidine genes are located 16 minutes apart. This map covers about one-fifth of the *E. coli* chromosome. By choosing different markers and by using different Hfr strains, a relatively complete map of a chromosome can be attained. The map of the *E. coli* chromosome (Figure 6–14) summarizes the genetic data of many investigators, including the experiments of Lederberg and Tatum.

Conjugation with F$^+$ and F' strains. Transfer of the autonomous dispensible F$^+$ plasmid to an F$^-$ cell occurs through conjugation. The entire replicated strand of the plasmid is usually transferred so that the recipient cell is converted to an F$^+$ cell. When F' cells mate with F$^-$ cells, the entire plasmid is transferred, forming another F' cell, called a secondary F' cell. A secondary F' cell has two copies of select genes and is now a partial diploid. These are examples of conjugative plasmids, that is, plasmids that can be transferred from one cell to another.

Major groups of plasmids

Plasmids have special significance for the control of bacterial disease in humans. During a Japanese epidemic of dysentery in 1955, a strain of *Shigella dysenteriae* was isolated that was resistant to four antibiotics: chloramphenicol, streptomycin, sulfanilamide, and tetracycline. By 1965, 50 percent of all *S. dysenteriae* isolated in Japan's hospitals showed multiple drug resistance. Now we know that many organisms possess resistance to multiple drugs and that this resistance can be genetically transferred by conjugation. The genes for multiple-drug resistance are contained in a DNA plasmid called the **r-determinant**. This DNA can be mobilized by the **resistance transfer factor** (RTF) and transferred to other bacteria (Figure 6–15). The r-determinant plasmid is not by itself conjugative, but becomes conjugative when it combines with the RTF. The two molecules together are called the **R factor**. R factors are found in staphylococci and in the enteric bacteria. Rapid dissemi-

nation of drug resistance among bacteria is a serious health problem.

Bacteriocins are toxic bacterial proteins that kill closely related strains of bacteria. There are many different bacteriocins, and their genes are found on plasmids. These plasmids in *E. coli* are termed *Col* plasmids; some are conjugative, some are not. The *Col* plasmids that are nonconjugative, such as *Col* E$_1$ and *Col* E$_2$, can be mobilized by the fertility plasmid to become conjugative (refer to Figure 6–15).

Pseudomonads are capable of metabolizing a large group of organic compounds and can be considered the organic compound scavengers of the microbial world. Enzymes for this extensive metabolic machinery are not needed for normal growth. A number of the genes required for these enzymes are found on **degradative plasmids**. For example, the enzymes for octane degradation are contained in a plasmid in *Pseudomonas putida*. In addition to the plasmids just mentioned, some bacteria have plasmid DNA of undetermined function. These plasmids, which are detected by physical techniques, are called **cryptic plasmids.**

Genetic engineering

Bacterial genetics has led the human race almost full circle: from the descriptive genetics of the plant and animal breeders, through three decades of molecular biology, and now back to applied genetics in the form of genetic engineering. Through our knowledge of molecular biology, humans can now manipulate genes to produce organisms beneficial to humanity. Gene manipulation is generally referred to as **genetic engineering**, and it involves recombinant DNA.

Recombinant DNA. Genetic engineering is the process of producing an organism that contains a gene or genes not naturally present in that organism. This gene may then be expressed in its adopted home, because the genetic code is universal. When human genes are placed in a bacterium, they will code for the human protein just as if they were in a human cell. To place a gene from one organism into

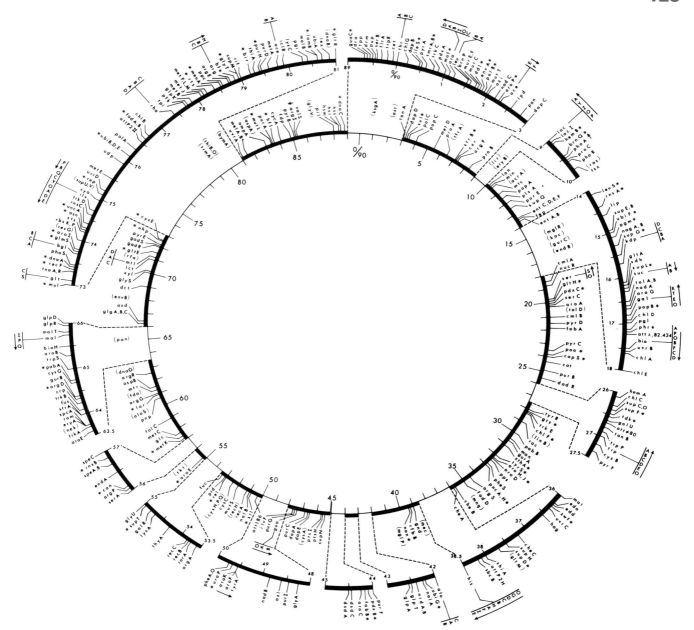

FIGURE 6–14

The genetic map of *Escherichia coli* K-12. The map is divided into minutes with the zero point arbitrarily set at the *thr A* locus. (Courtesy of Dr. A. L. Taylor. From A. L. Taylor and C. D. Trotter, *Bacteriol. Reviews,* 36:504–524, 1972, with permission of the American Society for Microbiology.)

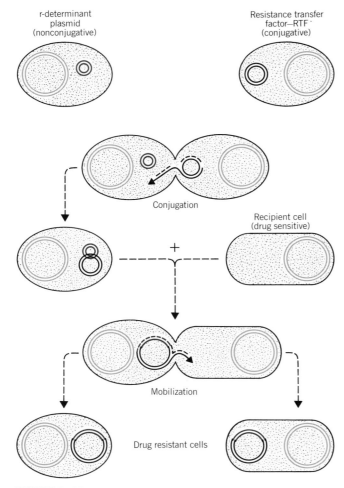

r-determinant
plasmid
(nonconjugative)

Resistance transfer
factor—RTF
(conjugative)

Conjugation

Recipient cell
(drug sensitive)

+

Mobilization

Drug resistant cells

FIGURE 6–15
Plasmid mobilization. Multiple-drug resistance is coded for by a nonconjugative r-determinant plasmid. This plasmid is mobilized when it combines with the resistance transfer factor (RTF). Together they can be transferred to other cells.

an entirely different organism uses the techniques of recombinant DNA.

Production of a clone of recombinant DNA requires the steps portrayed in Figure 6–16. The important steps are

1. A gene is isolated from a donating organism.

2. The gene is inserted into a DNA carrier molecule.
3. The carrier molecule is then transferred to a cell.
4. The cell replicates the recombinant DNA, creating a clone of cells.
5. Conditions are created to ensure expression of the gene.

Each step can now be accomplished using the techniques of bacterial genetics and molecular biology.

Genes can be isolated randomly. For certain types of recombinant DNA work this is an appropriate approach, but success normally depends on the investigator's ability to select, or to probe for, the specific DNA or gene desired. A second approach is to make a copy of the gene from isolated mRNA. Certain animal cells produce predominantly one protein. An example is the production of egg albumin (egg white) by the chicken oviduct. Albumin mRNA can be isolated from these cells, and the DNA gene can be made in vitro using RNA-directed DNA polymerase (see Chapter 22). A third approach is to make a theoretical gene using the techniques of organic chemistry and the known sequence of amino acids in the protein. All three techniques have their applications, and all have been used.

Insertion of the gene into the DNA carrier molecule is done with **restriction endonucleases**. These enzymes are present in bacteria and naturally function to protect against invading DNA molecules. Each restriction endonuclease cleaves DNA at a specific site that usually contains at least six bases. The E. coli enzyme EcoR1 recognizes the base sequence GAATTC (Figure 6–16). Cleavage is between G and A, resulting in a linear molecule that contains sticky ends composed of single-stranded AATT. Other bacteria contain other restriction endonucleases that recognize different sequences.

A carrier molecule must be small, should have a single site at which the restriction endonuclease can act, and must be replicative once it is back in the cell. Plasmids are ideal carrier molecules. To form a recombinant DNA molecule, both the plasmid and the DNA molecule containing the desired gene are treated with the restriction endonuclease to create sticky ends on both molecules. When mixed together in the presence of ligase, these molecules

form a closed circular recombinant DNA molecule (Figure 6–16).

Cells are now treated so that they will take up the recombinant DNA plasmid. Plasmids containing the

FIGURE 6—16

Genetic engineering. Foreign DNA is incorporated into a bacterial plasmid vector. The breaks in the DNA are made with a specific endonuclease (EcoR1), which creates sticky ends (T-T-A-A). These sticky ends anneal to form recombinant DNA, which can be taken into a bacterium by transformation. The transformed cells are resistant to tetracycline, so they are selected for using media containing this antibiotic. These cells, together with their recombinant DNA, replicate to form a clone of cells; each cell contains one or more copies of the new genetic information.

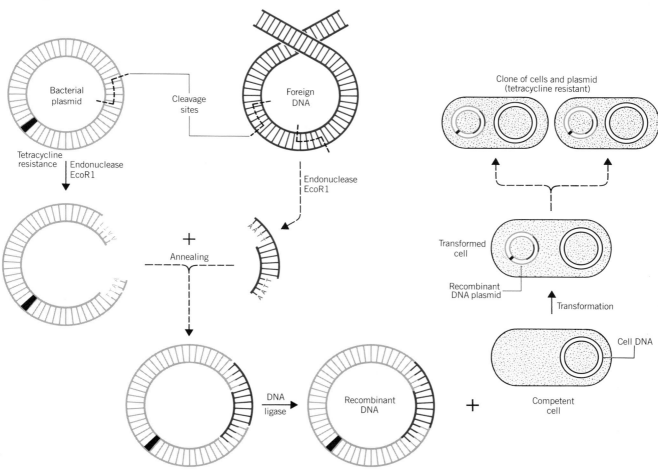

tetracycline resistance marker are used because this marker is easily selected for. Only transformed recipient cells will be able to grow in the tetracycline-containing medium. The cells and the plasmids they contain replicate and produce a clone of the gene. The final aspect of genetic engineering is to entice the cell to express the recombinant gene. This is often difficult, but it is not impossible. The discussion of regulation in Chapter 5 should give you a good understanding of this problem.

The potential of genetic engineering is just becoming evident. Companies are already talking about the commercial production of insulin, human growth hormone, and interferons by genetically engineered bacteria. Genetic engineering is destined to play an important role in our future economic and physical health.

Current concept of the gene

Exciting new concepts of the gene have evolved during the last decade from work with the small bacteriophage φX174. The gene is still considered to be the basic unit of inheritance, but we must modify our concept of the gene as being a discrete, linear sequence of DNA.

The small DNA bacteriophage φX174 has a small genome that codes for nine proteins. The amino acid sequence of all nine proteins was known when Frederick Sanger (Nobel laureate in 1980) determined the nucleotide sequence of φX174 in 1977. He realized that there were not enough nucleotides to code for the nine proteins by using a linear sequential code. Sanger and colleagues solved this dilemma by discovering that a linear sequence of nucleotide bases can code for more than one polypeptide if a reading frameshift occurs (Figure 6–17). Proteins E and D are coded for by the same sequence of DNA; their amino acid sequences are different because the code is shifted by one nucleotide. One sequence of nucleotides can, at least in φX174, code for more than one polypeptide.

SUMMARY

Genetics is the study of the inheritance of biological traits. Each trait is coded for by a sequence of nucleotides in the DNA called a gene. Genes are transcribed into RNA, and most genes are translated into polypeptides. The genes for rRNA and tRNA make only RNA molecules. Inheritable alterations in a cell's DNA are mutations. These changes can be caused by chemical and physical mutagens. Often carcinogens are also mutagens. The Ames test screens for potential carcinogens by determining if a compound is mutagenic. Mutations have been extensively used to understand biochemical and genetic processes.

Bacterial genetic information can be transferred by transformation, transduction, or conjugation. Naked DNA is assimilated during transformation, and the process is inhibited by DNAase. Bacterial conjugation is the transfer of genes between cells in contact with each other. Genetic transfer during conjugation is directional and is mediated by plasmids. Conjugation can be used to construct a circular map of a bacterial chromosome.

FIGURE 6–17
The bacteriophage φX174 has a single-stranded DNA molecule composed of 5375 nucleotides. This genome codes for nine proteins, which in total contain more than 1800 amino acids. Assuming a triplicate code, there are insufficient code words in the linear genome to code for the proteins. Therefore, the viral DNA sequence must code for *overlapping* genes.

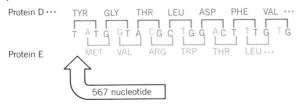

Plasmids are autonomous, self-replicating, extra-chromosomal, circular DNA molecules. F (fertility) plasmids code for F pili and are transferred during conjugation. F^+ male cells transfer the F plasmid to F^- recipient cells. Integration of the F plasmid into the bacterial chromosome creates an Hfr cell. These cells transfer genes at a high frequency and are capable of transferring the entire bacterial chromosome. Excision of the F factor from an Hfr strain can form an F' cell. The F' plasmid often contains chromosomal genes and is transferred to F^- cells in $F' \rightarrow F^-$ crosses. F plasmids are one type of bacterial plasmid; others include drug resistance factors, *Col* plasmids, and degradative plasmids.

The techniques of genetic engineering are used in altering the capabilities of organisms by the insertion of new genes. Recombinant DNA is formed using restriction endonucleases. A bacterial cell is then transformed with the recombinant DNA plasmid. The clone of the gene is produced when the bacterium and its plasmid replicate.

QUESTIONS AND TOPICS FOR STUDY AND DISCUSSION

Questions

1. What is the current concept of a gene?
2. What is a mutation? What techniques are used by bacterial geneticists to isolate specific mutants?
3. If carcinogens are mutagens, explain how the Ames test is used to detect potential carcinogens.
4. Define or explain the following.

bacterial conjugation	Hfr cell
bacterial transformation	plasmid
transduction	R plasmids
F' cell	bacteriocins

5. How are the plasmids involved in the transfer of genetic information between bacteria?
6. Name four plasmid types and explain the advantages or disadvantages accorded the cell possessing them.
7. How is conjugation used to map the bacterial chromosome?
8. Diagram the essential steps in producing recombinant DNA.

Discussion

1. What practical implications do you foresee for the application of genetic engineering?
2. What is the significance of the overlapping genes discovered in φX174?
3. Why are many known carcinogens mutagenic?

FURTHER READINGS

Books

Hayes, W., *The Genetics of Bacteria and Their Viruses*, 2nd ed., Wiley, New York, 1968. A classic textbook in bacterial genetics that describes many of the initial experiments that led to our modern concepts of molecular genetics.

Gardner, E. J., and D. P. Snustad, *Principles of Genetics*, 6th ed., Wiley, New York, 1981. A beginning college-level genetics textbook that is both current and readable.

Articles and Reviews

Brown, D. D., "The Isolation of Genes," *Sci. Am.*, 229:20–29 (August 1973). The application of molecular hybridization to the isolation of the ribosomal RNA genes from the frog *Xenopus*.

Campbell, A. M., "How Viruses Insert Their DNA into the DNA of the Host Cell," *Sci. Am.*, 235:102–113 (December 1976). The biochemical basis for specialized transduction is reviewed with the lambda/*E. coli* system as a model.

Clowes, R. C., "The Molecule of Infectious Drug Resistance," *Sci. Am.*, 228:18–27 (April 1973). An article on the role of bacterial plasmids in the transfer of antibiotic resistance between bacteria.

Cohen, S. N., "The Manipulation of Genes," *Sci. Am.*, 233:24–33 (July 1975). The use of a restriction endonuclease to insert DNA fragments into a plasmid is described and illustrated. This article also describes the basic concepts of cloning.

Cohen, S. N., and J. A. Shapiro, "Transposable Genetic Elements," *Sci. Am.*, 242:40–49 (February 1980). An introduction to the history of transposons followed by a detailed discussion of the significance of these genetic elements.

Gilbert, W., and L. Villa-Komaroff, "Useful Proteins from Recombinant Bacteria," *Sci. Am.*, 242:74–94 (April 1980). The authors describe genetic engineering methods used in the bacterial cloning of the human genes for insulin and interferon.

Novick, R. P., "Plasmids," *Sci. Am.*, 243:103–127 (December 1980). A brief review of the biochemistry and genetics of extrachromosomal bacterial DNA. The author raises penetrating questions concerning the ultimate biological role of bacterial plasmids.

7

MICROBIAL GROWTH

Cultivating microorganisms is a routine activity of every microbiological laboratory. Diagnostic laboratories grow microbes to identify them and to test their sensitivity to antibiotics. Industrial microbiologists produce alcohol and antibiotics as by-products of microbial growth. Microbial geneticists cultivate microbes to produce and isolate mutants and to analyze the results of genetic experiments. Microbial physiologists grow microbes to study their chemistry.

Microorganisms are also used to study population dynamics. Microbes are so small and grow so rapidly that the growth of an entire population, containing billions of cells, can be studied in a small flask in a reasonable amount of time. Moreover, microbial growth environments are easily established and manipulated by the investigator. This chapter explores the techniques used to obtain pure cultures, the physical and chemical factors that affect growth, and the dynamics of growing microbial populations.

PURE CULTURES

Microbiologists usually work with pure cultures of microoganisms because pure cultures facilitate the interpretation of experimental results. Robert Koch developed some of the important techniques used to obtain pure cultures. He obtained essentially pure cultures of the anthrax bacillus by cultivating them in hanging drops of the aqueous humor of the ox's eye. He later developed the technique of growing bacteria on media solidified with gelatin and then with agar. **Agar** is a polysaccharide of seaweeds and was once used to solidify jelly. It is soluble in boiling aqueous solutions and can be added to any liquid medium. A hot agar solution remains liquid until it cools to about 44°C and solidifies. Once solid, agar will remain a gel until it is reheated to 100°C. Koch initiated the use of this solidifying agent during the 1880s; it is still used to solidify microbiological media.

Isolation techniques. Individual bacterial cells will grow into colonies when they are provided with a proper growth medium. The **streak plate** is extensively used to separate bacteria so that a colony has a high probability of arising from a single cell (Figure 7–1). Streak plates are inoculated with a wire loop that has been sterilized by heat. Successive back-and-forth streaking motions with the wire loop sep-

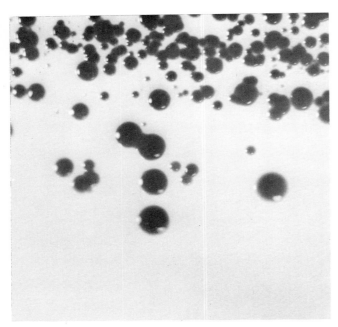

FIGURE 7—1
Colonies on streak plates appear visible when they contain one million or more cells.

arate the bacteria on the agar surface. Bacterial cells that are sufficiently separated by the streaking process will grow into isolated colonies. A culture is said to be pure if only one colony type results from streaking the culture on two successive plates. Theoretically, a pure culture is a group of organisms that grew from a single cell. For most practical purposes, all the cells in a colony are genetically identical.

Every bacterial species has an inheritable **colony morphology** for a given set of growth conditions. These morphologies can be described as small, large, mucoid, rough, raised, flat, filamentous, or spreading. A colony must contain around 1 million cells before it is visible to the human eye. Colony morphology is a distinguishing characteristic of microorganisms and is used in their classification.

Shake-dilution tubes (Figure 7–2) are also used to isolate bacteria. To prepare a series of shake-dilution tubes, a bacterial culture is diluted in a liquid agar

medium, the agar is allowed to solidify, and then the tubes are incubated at an appropriate temperature. Tubes of the higher dilutions contain a small number of physically separated cells that develop into isolated colonies. To obtain pure cultures, the shake-dilution tube procedure is repeated until only one colony type is present. Removing a colony from the solidified agar in the shake tube is often tricky. A procedure that bypasses this problem is the **pour plate** technique in which the contents of each shake-dilution tube is poured into a petri dish before the agar solidifies. Anaerobic and aerotolerant organisms will grow within the agar while aerobes will grow on the surface. Facultative anaerobes will grow in both environments. Colonies developing within the agar are usually smaller than the colonies growing on the agar surface.

Physical factors affecting growth

Temperature. Microbes are able to grow over a wide range of the temperatures found on earth. Some microorganisms grow in the oceans where the average temperature is 5°C; others grow in hot springs where the average temperature can hover around 90°C. Microbes can grow over a 30°C span of temperatures; however, a given microbe will have a narrow temperature range for optimum growth.

Soil organisms and human pathogens usually grow at temperatures between 20° and 50°C. These microbes are termed **mesophiles**. As a general rule, human pathogens grow well at 37°C (the temperature of healthy humans) and soil microbes grow well at 30°C. Each mesophile has an optimum temperature, and many grow poorly or not at all at the extremes of the mesophilic temperature range. The ability to grow at specific temperatures is used in the identification of bacteria.

Thermophiles are organisms that require temperatures above 45°C to grow. Some thermophiles even grow in hot springs at temperatures above 90°C. These organisms have specialized enzymes, proteins, and membranes that are stable at these high temperatures. At the low temperature extreme are the **psychrophiles,** which grow at temperatures of less than 20°C. They are found in cold marine environments and at the poles of the earth. Some psychrophiles grow at temperatures as low as −5°C.

Temperature affects the rate of microbial growth. In general, microorganisms grow more slowly at lower temperatures. An organism might grow into a visible colony at 37°C in 12 hours, but take 48 hours to produce a colony of the same size at 23°C. Cultures are grown at specific temperatures in incubators that maintain the temperature within ±0.5°C. A microbiology laboratory will often have two or three incubators set at different temperatures to deal with the temperature requirements of the microbes being cultivated.

Hydrostatic pressure. Barophilic organisms grow optimally at high pressures. Until recently, the very existence of barophilic bacteria has been a controversial topic. Deep-sea bacteria live at extreme hydrostatic pressures due to the weight of the overlaying water column. Now a marine bacterium has been isolated from a depth of 5700 meters. This organism grows optimally between 2 and 4°C and is a true **barophile** because it grows preferentially at high hydrostatic pressures. These extremes in pressure are difficult to reproduce in the laboratory, thus the study of barophiles is limited to specialized laboratories that deal with marine microbiology.

Osmotic pressure. Cells possess a semipermeable membrane that separates the cell's cytoplasm from its extracellular environment. **Osmosis** is the movement of water from a less concentrated solution to a more concentrated solution across a semipermeable membrane. This migration of water across a membrane can be prevented by exerting a force, equal to

FIGURE 7–2

Shake dilution tubes are used to isolate bacteria under anaerobic growth conditions. In this example a culture of photosynthetic bacteria was diluted in liquid agar, the agar solidified, and then the tubes were incubated in the light. The colonies develop in the agar in proportion to the number of bacteria present. The tube on the right is the highest dilution: therefore it has the smallest number of colonies.

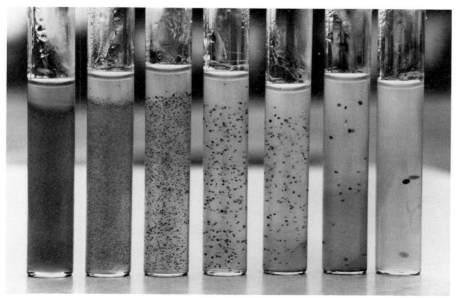

the **osmotic pressure**, in the opposite direction. Osmosis is directly proportional to the concentration of solute* particles and is independent of their nature. The rigidity of the bacterial cell wall resists the normal outward pressure from osmosis. Protoplasts and cells that lack cell walls must be protected against osmotic pressure to prevent them from bursting. This protection can be provided in the laboratory setting by increasing the solute concentration of the extracellular medium.

Plasmolysis occurs when the solute concentration of the environment is in great excess over the solute concentration in the cytoplasm. Under these conditions, water leaves the cells, causing the cells to collapse. This causes damage to the cell membrane, and the cells are unable to grow normally. Preserving fruits with syrup uses this phenomenon to prevent bacterial growth.

Osmophiles are organisms that grow in conditions of high osmotic pressure. **Osmophiles** are able to grow in environments with a high solute concentration; whereas **halophiles** are osmophiles that require concentrations of 12 percent or more NaCl to grow. Halophilic bacteria can be found in the Great Salt Lake in Utah and in meat products preserved with salt; salted codfish is an example. The solute or NaCl concentration of a growth medium is a factor that can be used to select for, or against, a bacterial species.

Chemical factors affecting growth

Each microbe must assimilate or manufacture all of its cellular components before it can reproduce. Some heterotrophs can do this from a simple salts medium containing glucose; others require complex nutritional supplements. All organisms require a supply of the essential elements: nitrogen, phosphorus, sulfur, carbon, inorganic salts, and trace metals. The specific compounds that a microbe uses to meet these elemental requirements are used in classification.

Defined media. Media composed of known concentrations of known chemicals are referred to as **defined media**. Glucose-salts medium (Table 7–1) is a defined medium in which certain bacteria can grow by manufacturing all their organic compounds from glucose. Ammonia is the source of nitrogen, sulfate is the source of sulfur, and potassium phosphate is the source of phosphorus. Other essential components are supplied as salts (Mg^{2+}, K^+) or as trace elements (see Table 2–1).

Adding a vitamin or an amino acid to this medium does not change its defined nature, because the investigator still knows the chemical composition of the medium. In contrast, there are a number of commercially available microbiological growth media that are chemically ill defined. These include yeast extract, peptone (an hydrolysate of meat), trypticase soy broth, and casitone (a digest of milk). These poorly defined substances are used to make **complex media** (Table 7–2). Many bacteria thrive on complex media that often provide the spectrum of essential amino acids and vitamins.

Hydrogen ion concentration. Each bacterial species grows preferentially in a narrow pH range. pH is the negative log of the hydrogen ion concentration. The range of pH in nature extends from about 1.0 to a pH of 11. Acid mine waters have a low pH as does the human stomach. Marine environments are alkaline; they have a pH around 8.4. Soils can be either acidic

TABLE 7–1

Glucose-Salts Medium for *Escherichia coli*

Ingredient	Amount
Glucose	5.0 g
Dipotassium phosphate (K_2HPO_4)	7.0 g
Monopotassium phosphate (KH_2PO_4)	2.0 g
Magnesium sulfate ($MgSO_4$)	0.008 g
Ammonium chloride (NH_4Cl)	1.0 g
Trace elements	1.0 ml
Distilled water	999 ml

Solid medium can be prepared by adding 15 g of agar per 1000 ml of medium.

---

*A *solute* is any substance dissolved in a liquid.

TABLE 7–2
Complex Medium (MacConkey Agar)[a]

Ingredient	Grams per liter H$_2$O
Peptone	17.0
Proteose peptone	3.0
Lactose	10.0
Bile salts	1.5
Sodium chloride	5.0
Agar	13.5
Neutral red	0.03
Crystal violet	0.001

[a]MacConkey broth is prepared by omitting the agar. This medium is commercially available.

(pH <7), neutral (pH = 7), or alkaline (pH >7). Plants are similar to bacteria in that they grow well at specific pHs. Farmers use lime to raise the pH of an acid soil and crushed sulfur to lower the pH of an alkaline soil.

Bacteria often alter the pH of their environment by excreting metabolic by-products. Lactic acid, produced during the lactic acid fermentation, decreases the pH of the culture medium. The metabolism of urea (H$_2$N—$\overset{\overset{\textstyle O}{\|}}{C}$—NH$_2$) to CO$_2$ and NH$_3$ makes a neutral medium alkaline by increasing the pH. Ac-

cumulation of too much acid or alkali will change the pH and can prevent the growth of an organism. Buffers work to prevent extreme changes in pH. Potassium phosphate (K$_2$HPO$_4$/KH$_2$PO$_4$) and amino acids are examples of compounds that function as buffers. A buffer resists changes in pH by accepting hydrogen ions or a hydroxyl group. Buffering compounds are often added to microbiological media (Table 7–1) to stabilize the pH during growth.

Oxygen. Aerobic organisms require oxygen for growth. Air is the major source of oxygen on the earth and is composed of 76 percent nitrogen and 23 percent oxygen. The oxygen content in liquid cultures can be increased by shaking the cultures. Also, tubes of agar can be tilted (slants) to produce a large surface area exposed to air. Microbes that grow in low concentrations of oxygen are termed **microaerotolerant** or **microaerophilic**. These organisms grow in aerobic environments, but they grow more slowly than an aerobe would. **Anaerobes** can be grown in agar slab cultures or in anaerobic growth chambers designed to remove the oxygen. **Strict anaerobes** are killed by oxygen, whereas **facultative anaerobes** are able to grow either with or without oxygen. Growth tests (Figure 7–3) can be used to analyze an organism's ability to use oxygen.

FIGURE 7–3
Growth response of different microbes to oxygen when grown in a semisolid medium or in a solid culture (1.5% agar). The highest concentration of oxygen is present at the top of the tube, whereas the lowest concentration of oxygen is at the bottom of the tube.

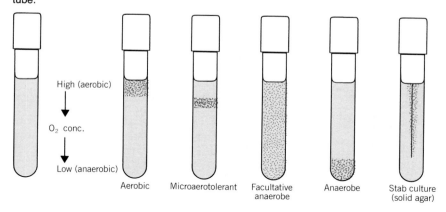

High (aerobic) ↓ O$_2$ conc. ↓ Low (anaerobic)

Aerobic   Microaerotolerant   Facultative anaerobe   Anaerobe   Stab culture (solid agar)

The killing of strict anaerobes by oxygen is at least partially due to the accumulation of superoxide (O_2^-). This free-radical is a potent cytotoxic agent that is produced metabolically in aerobic environments. Aerobic and aerotolerant organisms have the enzyme superoxide dismutase, which metabolizes superoxide to hydrogen peroxide (H_2O_2). When strict anaerobes are grown in the presence of oxygen, superoxide accumulates and kills them because they lack superoxide dismutase.

Hydrogen peroxide is also toxic to cells. Aerobic cells usually contain catalase, which metabolizes hydrogen peroxide to H_2O and O_2. The absence of catalase in many anaerobes also contributes to their oxygen sensitivity.

Selective enrichments. Different species of microorganisms abound in natural environments. To isolate a specific microbe from this milieu, a growth enrichment of the organism is made. **Selective enrichments** establish conditions under which the desired organisms can outgrow the competing organisms present in the inoculum. The physiological characteristics of the desired organism dictate the composition of the medium in the selective enrichment as well as the conditions of incubation. Some of these conditions are obvious. For example, a strict aerobe will require oxygen for growth, whereas a strict anaerobe will not grow in the presence of oxygen.

An organism's resistance to heat can also be used to select for bacteria. Spore-forming bacteria can be isolated from soil by first boiling the soil to kill vegetative cells. The heated soil can then be inoculated into an appropriate medium for the growth of the spore-forming organisms. Species of *Bacillus* are aerobic spore-formers that can be selected for in this manner and then grown with oxygen present. Species of *Clostridium* are anaerobic spore-formers, and as such, grow in the absence of oxygen. These selective enrichments combine the use of heat with the chemical composition of the medium to isolate a given species. The theory of selective enrichment is based on the premise that each organism survives in nature because it has its own ecological niche. Simulation of this niche in the laboratory enriches the microbial population with the organism of interest. Isolation techniques can then be used to obtain pure cultures.

Selective versus differential media. Selective media are commercially available for isolating many bacteria. These media can select against a group of organisms as well as for a desired organism. **Differential media** distinguish between a variety of microorganisms capable of growing on that medium. MacConkey agar (Table 7–2) is both a selective and a differential medium. It contains lactose, peptone, neutral red, crystal violet, and bile salts and is used to differentiate among the Gram-negative enteric bacteria. The bile salts and the crystal violet inhibit Gram-positive organisms, making this a selective medium for the enteric bacteria (see Chapter 15). Among the enteric bacteria are both lactose fermenters and lactose nonfermenters. The lactose-fermenting enteric bacteria change the neutral-red dye from colorless to red (Color Plate 10), and they also precipitate the bile salts (Figure 7–4). Other enterics, including *Salmonella enteritidis*, and most strains of *Shigella* do not ferment lactose and do not cause these changes. MacConkey agar is therefore a differential medium by virtue of its ability to distinguish between these two types of enteric bacteria. Differen-

FIGURE 7–4

MacConkey agar is a selective medium for Gram-negative organisms. Lactose fermenters grow as dark red colonies. (Photograph by Oxoid Limited, Basingstoke, Hampshire, England).

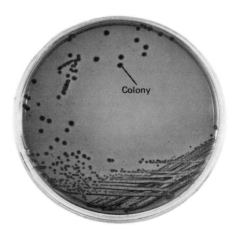

Colony

tial and selective media are widely used in diagnostic microbiology.

Stock cultures

Once a pure culture is obtained, it can be maintained in a stock culture. Stock cultures can be stored in a refrigerator at +4°C as long as they are transferred to a fresh medium every couple of months. Each laboratory maintains stock cultures of the strains they use on a routine basis.

The American Type Culture Collection (ATCC) maintains stock cultures of most known microbes and many viruses. Teachers and researchers can obtain these stock cultures from ATCC for a modest fee. Each culture is maintained in a preferred medium and is usually stored in a dormant state. Two major techniques—lyophilization and storage in liquid nitrogen—are used to maintain dormant stock cultures of bacteria.

Lyophilization. Cells frozen in an appropriate medium can be dried by subliming off the water in a vacuum. This process is called **lyophilization** and is easily done in a special apparatus. Freeze-dried foods are prepared in a similar manner, and taxidermists are now using this technique to preserve small fish and mammals. Lyophilized bacterial cultures remain viable for years, they are convenient to store and to mail, and they are easily prepared and regenerated.

Liquid nitrogen. Dewar flasks containing liquid nitrogen (−196°C) can be used to store frozen microbial cultures (Figure 7–5). Microbes suspended in a supportive medium such as 20 percent glycerol are placed in vials and cooled at a rate of −1°C/minute to a final temperature of −196°C. These frozen cultures can remain viable for months or years when stored at −196°C. To activate a culture, the vial is placed in water at room temperature and then the thawed culture is transferred to a suitable growth medium. Cultures of sperm, mammalian cell cultures, and many bacteria can be maintained in liquid nitrogen.

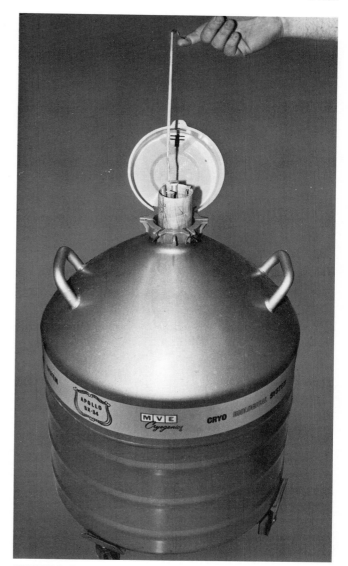

FIGURE 7–5
Stock cultures can be stored in vials attached to a holder immersed in a dewar flask containing liquid nitrogen (−196°C).

Methods of measuring growth

Often it is important to measure the size of a microbial population. Such measurements can be based on the number of cells present or on the mass of the cells in a given volume of culture. Each technique for measuring microbial populations has its advantages and disadvantages.

Cell number. The number of cells in a liquid culture can be determined microscopically. The Petroff-Hausser counting chamber (Figure 7–6) consists of a glass slide marked in small squares. The volume occupied by the liquid above the small squares is known. The number of bacteria per milliliter can be determined by counting the bacteria visible in a number of squares and dividing that number by the volume of liquid above those squares. At least 10^6 cells per milliliter are required before they are abundant enough to be seen in the microscopic field. Microscopic counts determine the total number of cells present, including both living and dead cells. An advantage of this technique is that the cell count can be done in a few minutes. Electronic counters are also available for determining cell number.

Viable cell count. Differentiating between viable (living) and dead cells can be done by *plate counting*. An appropriate dilution of the culture is made, and then a known volume of the dilution is plated onto a suitable medium in a petri dish. After incubation of the plates for 12 to 48 hours, the average number of colonies on duplicate plates is determined. To determine the number of bacteria per milliliter of the initial culture, the average plate count is multiplied by the reciprocal of the dilution and then by 1/plating volume (in milliliters). This calculation determines the number of viable cells per milliliter of the culture. The viable cell count is invariably less than the total cell count. This is an accurate means of determining the viable cell population, but it takes at least 24 hours to obtain results.

Cell mass. Cell mass can be determined in a few minutes by using a **spectrophotometer** (Figure 7–7), which is a device used to measure the amount of light passing through a solution that is read on a scale of absorbance or percent transmittance. The wavelength of light used is controlled by a prism or a diffraction grating. Light that passes through the sample strikes a phototube, which converts light energy into electrical energy. This electric current is registered on a scale of transmittance or absorbance and is a function of the optical density of the sample.

Turbid solutions contain particles (such as cells) that scatter light and prevent it from passing through the solution. Solutions with greater turbidity have a greater optical density. Light scattering is directly proportional to the size and number of particles, so light scattering is a measure of the cell mass in a culture.

To measure turbidity, culture samples are placed in a cuvette (an optically clean glass tube), 1 cm thick, and placed in the spectrophotometer. The optical density at a given wavelength, such as 600 nm, can be read directly and then corrected for the optical density of an uninoculated control. The optical density of a given culture is a measure of cell mass and can be related to cell number or dry weight by constructing a suitable standard curve. Measuring cell mass at different times is a rapid and accurate method of measuring growth. The disadvantages of this technique are that at least 10^6 cells per milliliter

FIGURE 7–6
Diagram of a Petroff-Hauser bacterial counting chamber. The chamber is used to count the total number of bacteria in liquid samples.

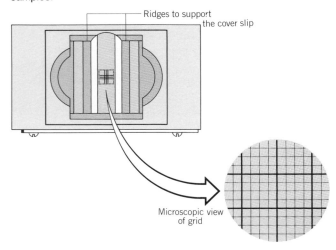

Ridges to support the cover slip

Microscopic view of grid

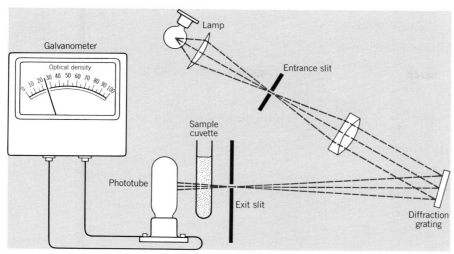

FIGURE 7–7
Diagram of a spectrophotometer. Spectrophotometers, such as the Bausch & Lomb
Spectronic 20, are used to measure the optical density of bacterial cultures.

are required before a reading can be obtained, large cells contribute more to the optical density than do small cells, and both nonliving and living cells are measured.

Equipment used for growing microorganisms.
Many different types of shakers are available for aerating liquid cultures of microbes (Figure 7–8a). **Shakers** provide a convenient means of growing aerobic microbes without the sterility problems posed by aerating a culture with compressed air. Anaerobic cultures can be grown under an atmosphere of an inert gas (argon or nitrogen) in a special growth chamber or in anaerobic jars that chemically remove the oxygen (Figure 7–8b). Large-scale growth chambers, called **fermenters,** have controls for maintaining the temperature, adding gases, stirring, and maintaining the pH. Very large fermenters are used in the commercial production of antibiotics and in the brewing industry. The growth dynamics of microbial cultures are economically important to the fermentation industry; moreover, they tell us a great deal about the growth of populations in general.

BACTERIAL GROWTH DYNAMICS

Bacterial growth is the orderly increase in cell constituents that results in an increase in the number of cells through the mechanism of binary fission. Bacterial cells divide in half to form two daughter cells. Growth of individual cells must precede cell division, otherwise the daughter cells would get progressively smaller. Microorganisms will grow and divide, given the appropriate environment. This environment must provide the essential nutrients and physical conditions needed for the growth of the specific microbe. Once these conditions are met, the population growth dynamics of any given culture will follow a repeatable growth pattern.

Growth curve

Bacteria have generation times that range from 12 minutes to many hours. **Generation time** is the interval between divisions of a growing microorganism. In microbiology it is determined as the time required for the population of cells in a culture to double, since each organism usually produces two

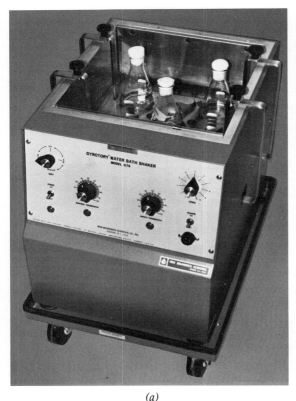
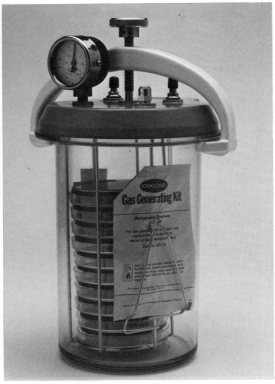

(a)   (b)

FIGURE 7–8
(a) A New Brunswick temperature controlled shaker that is used to grow aerobic cultures, and (b) an anaerobic jar that is used to grow anaerobic bacteria on plates. The foil contains chemicals that remove oxygen after the jar is sealed. (Photograph for b supplied by Oxoid Limited, Basingstoke, Hampshire, England.)

offspring per generation. A population of growing bacteria increases as a geometric progression. The generation time of a bacterial culture is not constant with time but changes as the composition of the culture medium changes. Generation time is also dependent on the initial medium, its pH, and the temperature at which the culture is grown.

If a single bacterium began unrestricted growth with a generation time of 20 minutes, in 48 hours it would produce 2.2×10^{43} cells. Since each bacterium weighs about 10^{-13} grams, the cells in this culture would have a weight of 2.2×10^{30} grams, which is about 400 times the weight of the earth. Obviously, bacteria do not grow in a completely unrestricted fashion.

A growth study of *Escherichia coli* in a closed environment can be initiated by inoculating a pure culture of *E. coli* into a sterile glucose-salts medium. Growth of this culture can be measured with time by determining (1) the cell mass of the culture, (2) the total number of cells, or (3) the number of viable cells over the lifetime of the culture (Figure 7–9). The culture will develop and decline through distinctive phases.

Lag phase. The cells of a culture, inoculated into fresh medium, experience an adjustment period called the **lag phase.** No detectable growth occurs during this time. These cells are physiologically active as they adjust to the new medium by making

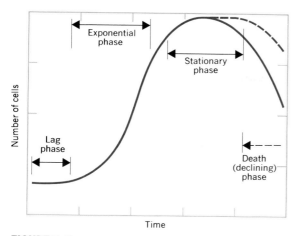

FIGURE 7-9
A typical bacterial growth curve for a liquid culture; the dashed line is the total number of cells, and the solid line is the number of viable cells.

TABLE 7-3
Mathematics of Unrestricted Bacterial Growth

Number of Generations (n)	Number of Bacteria (N)	Log₂N	Log₁₀N
0	1	0	0.000
1	2	1	0.301
2	4	2	0.602
3	8	3	0.903
4	16	4	1.204
5	32	5	1.505
6	64	6	1.806
7	128	7	2.107
8	256	8	2.408
9	512	9	2.709
10	1024	10	3.010

the needed enzymes and by accumulating cellular materials. New cell constituents are then manufactured, and the cells begin to grow and reproduce. The lag period ends when the culture establishes a constant generation time.

Exponential phase. Each time a bacterial cell divides it produces two daughter cells. This is mathematically expressed as $2N$ where N is the number of cells in the culture. When the cells in a culture are dividing at a constant rate, the number of cells in the culture expands exponentially. This phase of growth is termed the **exponential** or **logarithmic growth phase.** The increase in the number of cells through 10 divisions beginning with a single cell is shown in Table 7–3. Plotting this data on an arithmetic graph results in a curved line (Figure 7–10a). Plotting the same data on a semilogarithmic graph (Figure 7–10b) results in a straight line, which is another way of demonstrating that bacterial growth during this

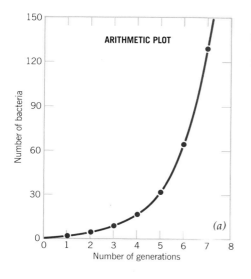

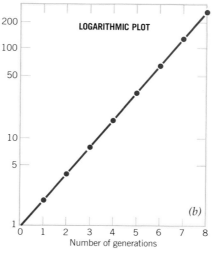

FIGURE 7-10
The (a) arithmetic and the (b) logarithmic plot of the data in Table 7–3 showing that populations of bacteria increase exponentially.

phase can be represented as an exponential function. During exponential growth, all cells in the culture are physiologically identical for all practical purposes. If all the individual components (proteins, DNA, etc.) of these cells are changing at the same constant rate, the cells are said to be in **balanced growth**. Exponential growth cannot continue for an indefinite time because closed cultures run out of essential nutrients, and the cells produce by-products that retard growth. This leads to a reduction in the growth rate of the culture.

Stationary phase.   Bacteria reach a population density that is maximum for a given growth environment. Some cells continue to divide, albeit more slowly, whereas other cells die. The net change in the number of cells in the population becomes zero. This is called the **stationary phase.** The culture has now accumulated enough metabolic by-products and toxic products released during cell lysis to change significantly the chemistry of the medium.

Decline or death phase.   The number of viable cells in the culture now begins to decrease, and very few cells are able to reproduce. The nutrients become depleted, and the level of toxic products increases, creating an environment where the cells are unable to maintain their essential functions. These cells die. The number of viable cells decreases more rapidly than the total number of cells, which includes viable cells and unlysed dead cells (Figure 7–9). Certain cells can form resting stages that overcome these adverse environmental conditions. Cells that form endospores and those that form cysts enter a dormant state following the stationary phase of growth and do not die.

Mathematical expression of growth

Bacterial growth is balanced during the exponential growth phase. The following mathematical expressions of growth are applicable only to the exponential phase where the culture expands with a constant generation time. The symbols are

g = Generation time
N_0 = Number of cells at time zero
N_t = Number of cells at time t
t_0 = Zero time
t = A time after t_0
n = Number of generations

Generation time (g) is the time required for the mass or the number of cells in the culture to double. Because bacteria divide by binary fission, the number of cells (N_t) at time t is equal to the number of cells at zero time (N_0) times 2 raised to the nth power, or

$$N_t = N_0 \cdot 2^n$$

where n is the number of generations (Table 7–3). By taking the logarithm* of each side, this equation becomes

$$\log_{10}N_t = \log_{10}N_0 + n \cdot \log_{10}2$$

which can be rewritten as

$$n \cdot \log_{10}2 = \log_{10}N_t - \log_{10}N_0$$

The $\log_{10}2 = 0.301$ (Table 7–3), and so the equation becomes

$$n = \frac{\log_{10}N_t - \log_{10}N_0}{0.301}$$

The number of generations (n) can also be defined as $(t - t_0)/g$; therefore

$$n = \frac{t - t_0}{g} \text{ and } \frac{t - t_0}{g} = \frac{\log_{10}N_t - \log_{10}N_0}{0.301}$$

which can be arranged as follows

$$g = \frac{0.301(t - t_0)}{\log_{10}N_t - \log_{10}N_0}$$

This equation can be used to determine the generation time of a bacterial culture during exponential growth.

---

*Basic logarithmic functions include: if $N = a^b$ then $\log_a N = b$; $\log_a a^x - \log_a a^y = x - y$; $\log_a N^x = x \log_a N$; $\log_a (x \cdot y) = \log_a x + \log_a y$.

Bacteria and aging

A bacterium divides by binary fission to form two daughter cells, each of which represents one half of the parent cell. Since bacteria do not progress through a life cycle, there is no concept of age that can be attributed to a bacterial cell. Bacterial cells either die, or they continue to reproduce. On the other hand, bacterial cultures change from a rapidly growing state, to a static state, to a state of decline. Microbiologists obtain bacteria from cultures in balanced growth when their work requires a physiologically constant population of cells. This enables investigators to repeat their experimental results.

SUMMARY

Microbiologists deal with the practical aspects of microbial growth on a daily basis, so a knowledge of the parameters affecting growth is essential. Microbial growth is influenced by osmotic pressure, the pH, and the temperature of the medium. Most organisms are intolerant of high osmotic pressure and plasmolyze in media of high solute concentration. Halophiles are different because they require high concentrations of salt for growth. Thermophiles grow at high temperatures, whereas psychrophiles grow at low temperatures. Most microbes are mesophiles and grow between 20° and 50°C. Each microbe requires a source of carbon, nitrogen, sulfur, phosphorus, salts, and trace elements. Some organisms grow on a chemically defined medium such as glucose-salts, whereas others require a complex medium containing compounds such as vitamins and amino acids. The pH of the medium and the availability of oxygen also influence growth.

Bacterial growth is the orderly increase in cell constituents that results in an increase in cell numbers through the mechanism of binary fission. Bacteria growing on a solid medium will divide many times to reproduce a colony of cells. Bacterial cultures that are provided with the nutrients and physical conditions needed for growth will follow a distinctive growth pattern. Cells inoculated into a fresh medium adapt during the lag phase of growth. The cells next enter the exponential growth phase as they attain a constant generation time. This rapid rate of growth soon depletes the available nutrients, and the population enters the stationary phase, where there is no net change in the size of the population. Finally, cells lyse and die at an accelerated rate during the death phase of the culture. The growth of a bacterial population in the exponential phase can be described in simple mathematical terms. These expressions are used to analyze and to control microbial growth.

QUESTIONS AND TOPICS FOR STUDY AND DISCUSSION

Questions

1. Describe three techniques for isolating colonies in agar media.
2. How do the pH, salt concentration, and temperature of a medium affect bacterial growth? In what range of pH, salt, and temperature will most pathogenic bacteria have optimal growth rates?
3. Define or explain the following.

barophiles	microaerotolerant
defined media	psychrophiles
facultative anaerobe	selective enrichment
halophile	strict anaerobe
mesophile	thermophiles

4. Describe three methods of maintaining bacterial stock cultures.
5. What are the advantages/disadvantages of using the viable cell count versus the cell number or cell mass as an indicator of a bacterial population?
6. Diagram the normal bacterial growth curve and describe the phases of growth.
7. A bacterial culture containing 100 cells increases in population to 1 billion cells in 10 hours. What is the generation time of this culture in minutes?
8. A bacterial culture containing 100 cells has a generation time of 15 minutes. How long will it take for this culture to reach a population of 1 million cells?

Discussion

1. What factors prevent bacteria from continuous exponential growth? Do similar factors influence the human population?

FURTHER READINGS

Books

Finegold, S. M., and W. J. Martin, *Baily and Scott's Diagnostic Microbiology*, 6th ed., Mosby, St. Louis, 1982. A detailed reference source or advanced textbook that covers the techniques used in diagnostic microbiology.

Stanier, R. Y., E. A. Adelberg, and J. Ingraham, *The Microbial World*, 4th ed., Prentice-Hall, Englewood Cliffs, N.J., 1976. An advanced microbiology textbook that has two excellent chapters on the growth of microorganisms.

Manuals

Difco Manual of Dehydrated Culture Media and Reagents for Microbiological and Clinical Laboratory Procedures, 9th ed., 1971, Difco Laboratories, Detroit. This manual contains the composition of and the uses for this manufacturer's bacteriological media and reagents. It is used as a reference source for these widely used microbiological media.

Articles and Reviews

Van Niel, C. B., "Natural Selection in the Microbial World," *J. Gen. Microbiol.*, 13:201–217 (1955). A classic article on the environmental influence over the growth and selection of microbial species.

8

CLASSIFICATION

The characteristics of biological systems vary greatly among organisms. Taxonomists are the scientists who study the diversity of living systems and classify organisms into biologically related groups. The classification scheme that we are using separates organisms into four kingdoms. The first three kingdoms contain organisms with eucaryotic cell structure. Plants are classified in the kingdom **Plantae;** animals are classified in the kingdom **Animalia.** The eucaryotic microorganisms are grouped in the **Protista.** Some taxonomists create a separate kingdom for the fungi; however, for convenience we will consider the fungi as eucaryotic microorganisms and will classify them with the Protista.

Taxonomists have long debated the proper positioning of bacteria among living things. All bacteria were formerly classified as plants, and as such were the responsibility of botanists. But bacteria are not truly plants. Like animals, many bacteria are motile; like plants, purple and green bacteria and cyanobacteria utilize light energy. Now taxonomists recognize the remarkable cytological distinctions between procaryotes and eucaryotes. This has led to the proposal and the acceptance of **Procaryotae** as the fourth

kingdom of organisms. Viruses are noncellular entities, which are classified separately (see Chapter 9).

REASONS FOR CLASSIFICATION

Classification of organisms is important to biologists because it systematically defines and names organisms. Taxonomists attempt to describe and name each kind of organism in a fashion that distinguishes it from all other known kinds. The description must be exact enough to enable an investigator to identify an unknown isolate, if indeed the organism has been previously classified. Organisms are then organized into an artificial classification scheme based on the similarities and differences between them, or they are arranged into a phylogenetic scheme based on evolutionary relationships and lines of common descent. Bacteria are organized only into an artificial classification scheme.

Naming organisms

Each organism is given a name to facilitate the communication of ideas, concepts, and experimental results pertaining to that organism. Early in the history of taxonomy, each organism was described by cumbersome, latinized prose. This was the practice when Carolus Linnaeus began his detailed study of plants during the eighteenth century. He soon found that his Latin margin notes served as suitable names for these organisms. This led Linnaeus to develop the binomial system of nomenclature whereby each species was assigned two latinized names. Remember that a **species** comprises those organisms that are morphologically the same and that can reproduce their own kind. The first name in the binomial is the **genus** (pl., genera), which describes a group of closely related species. The second name is the specific epithet that modifies the genus name and defines the specific species of the genus. Together, these two names comprise the **binomial system of nomenclature.** All organisms are given a latinized binomial, and, by convention, the first letter of a genus name is capitalized and the entire binomial name is printed in italics.

Species of bacteria can be further defined by strain or variety designations. *Bacillus cereus* is a common rod-shaped soil bacterium that grows into distinct colonies on solid media. This organism is differentiated from an apparently identical species that grows into swirling, rhizoid colonies (Figure 8–1). The cells of this second organism grow in this fashion because of unequal cell division and therefore are assigned to a **variety:** *Bacillus cereus* var. *mycoides.* The **strain** name is used to designate a specific isolate of a given species. An example is *Escherichia coli* strain K12, which can be abbreviated as *E. coli* K12.

Identification

When you see a cat you can immediately identify it as a domestic cat, *Felis catus*. You recognize the sleek shape, the small size (at least in comparison to a lion), the fur, the whiskers, and the long tail. Recognizing a bacterium is not quite so easy; therefore special tests must be performed to describe each one accurately. Descriptions of bacteria are catalogued in a master index called *Bergey's Manual of Determinative Bacteriology.* Published under the editorial direction of the Bergey's Manual Trust, it is revised on a reg-

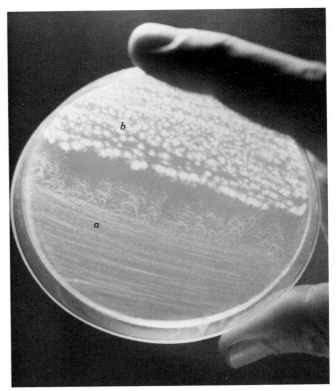

FIGURE 8–1

The bacteria known as *(a) Bacillus cereus* and *(b) Bacillus cereus* var. *mycoides* appear to be identical except for their colony morphology. *Bacillus cereus* var. *mycoides* forms rhizoid colonies because of the unequal nature of its cellular division.

ular basis. This compendium contains a description of each recognized bacterium (except the cyanobacteria). Specific traits of an unknown bacterium can be used in its identification by following the procedures set forth in the introductory essays for *Bergey's Manual.* The manual also contains a ''Key to Genera of the Manual'' written by V. B. D. Skerman. *Bergey's Manual of Determinative Bacteriology* is the authoritative work on the classification and identification of bacteria.

Bacterial classification schemes are devised to facilitate the identification of microorganisms. Bacterial **systematics**, the ordering of bacteria according to their evolutionary relationships, is a difficult task, considering our current knowledge of bacteria. Bacteria apparently evolved into their diverse forms so long ago that there are few remaining vestiges of their evolutionary development. The fact that bacteria do not interbreed further complicates this task, so bacterial classification relies heavily on subjective judgments.

Species concept in bacterial classification

Plant and animal taxonomists distinguish a species by grouping together those organisms that interbreed. Domestic cats mate with domestic cats, but are hardly able to mate with cougars. The cougar and the domestic cat are classified as distinct species and are given different species names. However, they share many common characteristics, so they are given the same genus name, *Felis*. We even think of these animals as being in the same family and as having a common ancestry. Taxonomists have acknowledged the evolutionary relatedness of cats by placing them in the same genus, family, and kingdom.

Bacteria do not breed. Thus the concept that species are distinct breeding groups is not applicable to bacterial classification. Each bacterium is given a species name, but this name is assigned on an artificial basis. The taxonomists must make a judgment as to the similarity of the organisms' characteristics and then make a decision where to combine groups of bacteria into a single species and where to create new species.

BACTERIAL CLASSIFICATION

The kingdom Procaryotae* is divided into two divisions. The cyanobacteria comprise division I, which contains all the oxygenic (O_2-producing) photosynthetic procaryotes. These cells are usually nonmotile (except for gliding motility), unicellular or filamentous organisms that are widely distributed on the earth. There is currently no compendium describing

*This book will use the classification scheme adopted by *Bergey's Manual*, 8th edition.

these organisms, partly because of the incomplete nature of our knowledge of the cyanobacteria. Reports on these organisms appear periodically in microbial and botanical literature.

Bacteria comprise division II of the kingdom Procaryotae. This division includes all the procaryotes, except those that form oxygen during photosynthesis. Purple and green bacteria are photosynthetic; however, these procaryotes grow only under anaerobic conditions. The bacteria are divided into nineteen parts, each comprising a group of closely related organisms. Among the criteria used to establish the parts are morphology of the cells, Gram-stain reaction, energy-generating metabolism, motility, formation of metabolic products, spore formation, and obligate intracellular growth.

Certain parts are subdivided into families of genera. For example, Enterobacteriaceae is the family that encompasses the enteric bacteria and includes the genera *Escherichia* and *Shigella*. Most of the major parts of division II are firmly established; however, some parts could undergo changes as more data become available.

Tools of the taxonomists: classic techniques

The major parts of division II were established with classic microbiological data. Classic taxonomy obtains information by using the tools and techniques available in a basic microbiology laboratory. Classic criteria include cell morphology, culture characteristics, and metabolic traits.

Morphology. Microscopic observations of living and stained bacterial preparations reveal information that is descriptive of these cells. Eucaryotic cells are readily distinguished by the presence of a visible nucleus. Procaryotic cells lack a nucleus, but they can be characterized according to their size, shape, presence of spores, and often their motility, by observation of them in a living state (wet mount preparations). The Gram-stain reaction, the acid-fast reaction, and the presence of capsules and flagella (Figure 8–2) can be observed in stained preparations. Morphological traits are the primary characteristics used to identify many microorganisms.

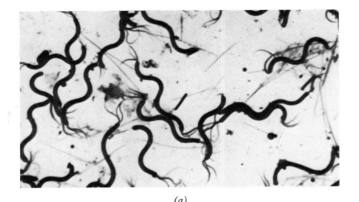

(a)

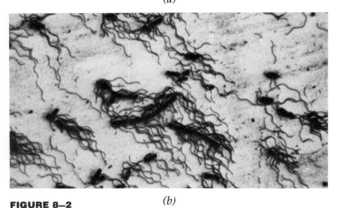

(b)

FIGURE 8–2

The presence and distribution of flagella on the surface of bacteria are inherited characteristics used in classification. Light micrographs of flagella-stained cells of *(a) Spirillum volutans* and *(b) Salmonella typhosa.* (Courtesy of General Biological Supply House, Inc. Chicago.)

Culture characteristics. An investigator able to grow a microorganism already knows a lot about it. Does the organism grow as an aerobe, an anaerobe, or a facultative anaerobe? What substrate does it grow on? Does it require nutritional supplements? Is light required for growth and can the microorganism grow on an inorganic medium? These questions can be answered by simple growth experiments with pure cultures of the organism in question.

Metabolic traits. Cells produce easily detectable by-products of metabolism and enzymes that are used in their classification. Metabolic by-products can be used to group organisms into genera, or to differentiate between species belonging to a single genus. A major criterion for grouping organisms in the genus *Propionibacterium* is the production of propionic acid as a major fermentation product. The individual species belonging to the genus *Clostridium* are in part differentiated on the basis of their fermentation products, which include acetone, isopropanol, butanol, butyric acid, and acetic acid. Fermentation products are used as a major criterion for classification because they represent the end products of multienzyme pathways.

Cellular production of detectable enzymes and toxins is important in determining the differences between species, or between closely related genera. Among these proteins are urease, coagulase, and hemolysins (Table 8–1). Urease is easily detected using whole cells; it is present in most species of *Proteus*, but is absent in other genera of the Enterobacteriaceae including *Escherichia*, *Salmonella*, and *Shigella*. The enzyme coagulase is produced by *Staphylococcus aureus* and distinguishes it from the other staphylococci. Toxins that lyse red blood cells (hemolysins) are easily detected on blood agar plates and are used to distinguish between different species of *Streptococcus*. *Streptococcus pyogenes* produces β-hemolysin, which lyses red blood cells; whereas *Streptococcus salivarius* does not produce any hemolysins.

Metabolic tests are also used to differentiate between two closely related members of the Enterobacteriaceae. Members of the genus *Enterobacter* produce 2,3-butanediol from glucose, but they do not produce indole from tryptophan (Figure 8–3). Species of *Escherichia* produce indole from tryptophan, but they do not produce 2,3-butanediol as a product of glucose fermentation. A combination of biochemical, metabolic, and morphological traits, similar to those described here, is routinely used in the classification and identification of microorganisms.

Other classification tools. Techniques are available to define bacteria in greater detail. Some bacteria that have a major impact on the health or economic well-being of humans are further classified by more discerning techniques. Some species of *Salmonella* can cause typhoid fever and other diseases in hu-

TABLE 8-1
Enzymes and Toxins Important in Bacterial Classification

Enzyme	Assay Results	Group or Organism
Coagulase	Coagulation of plasma	*Staphylococcus*
Tryptophanase	Indole production from tryptophan	Many bacteria
Urease	Alkaline medium from urea	*Proteus*
Gelatinase	Protein hydrolysis	Many bacteria
Amylase	Starch hydrolysis	Many bacteria
Catalase	Oxygen evolution from H_2O_2	Aerobes
Oxidase	Ability to oxidize a dye	*Neisseria* and *Pseudomonas*
Toxins		
β-Hemolysin	Clear lysis of red blood cells	*Streptococcus pyogenes* and other pathogens
α-Hemolysin	Partial (green) lysis of red blood cells	*Streptococcus* and other genera

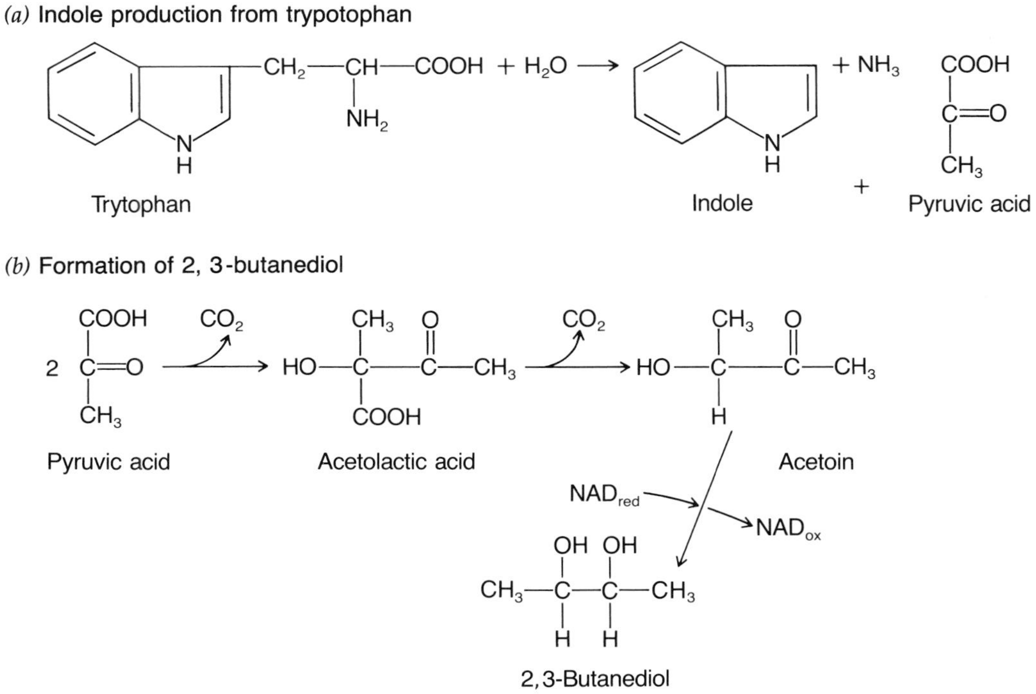

(*a*) Indole production from trypotophan

(*b*) Formation of 2, 3-butanediol

FIGURE 8-3
Metabolic by-products: (a) Indole is produced by the enzyme tryptophanase and is detected by adding Kovac's reagent to the medium; (b) the pathway for producing 2, 3-butanediol is detected by measuring acetoin production with the Voges-Proskauer test.

mans. These organisms infect humans through the consumption of food or water contaminated by human feces (see Chapter 16). To prevent the spread of these organisms, it is necessary to identify the human carriers. Immunological techniques have been used to identify the more than 1500 serotypes of *Salmonella* that are listed in *Bergey's Manual*. Serotyping determines the surface structure differences between isolates by measuring the presence or absence of specific antigenic determinants (see Chapter 13). Investigators are then able to study the dissemination of the diseases caused by the *Salmonella*.

Bacteriophages are specific in their interactions with the bacterial cell surface and can be used to define types of bacteria. Phage-typing is done by determining which of a series of bacteriophages will lyse a bacterial isolate. Phage-typing is used as an epidemiological tool to characterize human isolates of coagulase positive staphylococci (see Chapter 18).

Resistance or susceptibility to antimicrobial agents is also used to differentiate bacteria. Susceptibility to certain dyes is dependent on the cell structure. For example, eosin inhibits the growth of Gram-positive bacteria, but it does not inhibit the growth of Gram-negative bacteria. Antibiotics selectively inhibit some groups, genera, or strains, and not others.

Numerical taxonomy

Each of the criteria just presented can be used to define a microorganism. To the casual observer, some criteria appear to be more important than others. Is the ability to form spores a more significant trait than the presence of flagellar motility? Taxonomists have answered affirmatively to this question; all the bacteria that form endospores are now grouped in part 15 of division II, whereas motile organisms are widely dispersed in the classification scheme.

Another approach to taxonomy is to weigh each trait equally and to avoid the biased judgment of the observer. **Numerical taxonomy** attempts to do this by using as many characteristics as possible and by giving them all equal weight. Organisms that share similar traits are classified together; the more traits they share, the more tightly they are grouped. Numerical taxonomy is not yet extensively used in the classification of bacteria, but it certainly has applicability.

Tools of the taxonomists: molecular techniques

Molecular biology has provided taxonomists with sophisticated tools to analyze the genetic relationships between microorganisms. Since the traits of an organism are dictated by the genes of each cell's DNA, the amount of similarity between the base sequence in the DNAs of two cells is a measure of their evolutionary relatedness. Organisms sharing evolutionary ancestry will also share DNA base sequences.

Moles percent G + C. DNA can vary in its base composition from one group of organisms to the next. This variation can be measured as the moles percent of guanine plus cytosine (percent G + C) in the cellular DNA. The percent G + C in bacterial DNA ranges from 21 to 75. If two organisms have significantly different percent G + C values, taxonomists can conclude that they are not related to each other. If two organisms have the same percent G + C, then no conclusion can be drawn because both unrelated and closely related organisms can have the same G + C value. For example, many bacteria have a percent G + C value of 42, which is identical to the percent G + C value of human DNA. Obviously, bacteria are not closely related to humans. So there must be a significant difference in the percent G + C values before they are useful in classification. At least one pseudomonad has a percent G + C of 70 (Table 8–2), which is clearly far removed from the 42 percent G + C of human DNA. In this case, the percent G + C is good evidence that these organisms are different.

Bacterial taxonomists use this technique to identify the evolutionary relationships between major groups of bacteria. At one time, both the fruiting myxobacteria and the nonfruiting myxobacteria were grouped together because they all have gliding motility. Now it has been discovered that the nonfruiting group (cytophaga) possesses a low percent G + C, whereas the fruiting myxobacteria (myxobacteria) have a high percent G + C (Table 8–2). These organisms are evolutionarily far apart and are now classified in separate orders under part 2, the gliding bacteria. The apparent relatedness of the genera *Micrococcus* and *Staphylococcus* has also been questioned

TABLE 8–2
Moles Percent G + C of Selected Bacteria

Organism or Group	Moles Percent G + C
Clostridium hemolyticum	21
Clostridia	21 – 28
Sarcina maxima	29
Bacillus sp.	32 – 62
Staphylococcus sp.	30 – 40
Cytophaga	34 – 43
Treponema	32 – 50
Proteus sp.	39 – 42
Escherichia sp.	50 – 53
Bacteroides sp.	40 – 55
Pseudomonas sp.	58 – 70
Rhodospirillum sp.	62 – 66
Micrococcus sp.	66 – 75
Fruiting Myxobacteria	68 – 71

Source: Data was obtained from R. E. Buchanan and N. E. Gibbons (eds.), *Bergey's Manual of Determinative Bacteriology,* 8th ed., Williams & Wilkins, Baltimore, 1974.

on the basis of percent G + C values. Members of these genera are aerobic, Gram-positive, nonmotile, nonspore-forming cocci, yet they have vastly different percent G + C values (Table 8–2). On evolutionary grounds (based on percent G + C) they appear to be distantly related. Regardless of this fact, they are still classified in the same family for the purpose of identification because of their morphological similarities.

Hybridization of DNA. Double-stranded DNA dissociates upon heating into single strands. Under appropriate conditions, slow cooling will reestablish the hydrogen bonding between the complementary strands to re-form double-stranded DNA. This process is called **annealing of nucleic acids.** When single strands of DNA from different organisms are mixed together and allowed to anneal, the extent of double-stranded DNA formation depends on the degree of base sequence similarity between the unlike DNAs (Figure 8–4). Double-stranded DNA containing one strand of DNA from two separate organisms

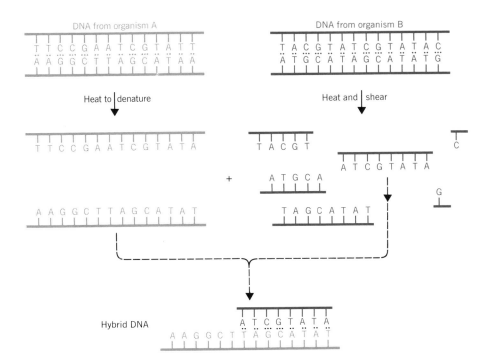

FIGURE 8–4
DNA hybrids are formed by annealing complementary pieces of single-stranded DNA obtained from different organisms.

is called a hybrid, and the process of forming hybrids is called **DNA hybridization.** This is a technique that has been used to demonstrate the relatedness of organisms.

DNA hybridization experiments can be performed using ^{32}P labeled DNA and a filtration technique (Figure 8–5). Results from this type of experiment using the DNAs obtained from the Enterobacteriaceae are reported in Table 8–3. The control organism is *Escherichia coli*, which shows 88 to 100 percent binding with its own DNA. This is established when single-stranded *E. coli* DNA is mixed with single-stranded ^{32}P labeled DNA from *E. coli* under conditions that promote annealing. The amount of radioactivity in the hybrid DNA that binds to the filter is determined by radioactive count.

Next, single-stranded DNA from other genera is prepared and mixed with the ^{32}P labeled DNA from *E. coli*. The amount of radioactive DNA from *E. coli* that forms hybrids with the single-stranded DNA from each organism is determined. This value is a measure of the base sequence similarity between the species tested and is always less than 100 percent. *Shigella flexneri* shares more base sequences with *E. coli* than does *Salmonella typhimurium*. *Proteus mirabilis* is even less related to *E. coli* than the *S. typhimurium* on the basis of these DNA hybridization tests (Table 8–3). This form of molecular analysis can provide important information on the taxonomy of closely related genera and species.

Protein sequencing. It is now possible to determine the amino acid sequences of small proteins isolated from phylogenetically different organisms. Closely related organisms will have essentially identical amino acid sequences in a given protein. A change in the amino acid sequence is indicative of a change in the gene coding for that polypeptide. The more closely related two organisms are, the fewer changes taxonomists expect from evolutionary pressure. This type of analysis has been done using cytochrome *c* isolated from many different organisms. The evolutionary relationships between these organisms have been correlated with the amino acid sequence changes in this protein. Based on these data,

TABLE 8–3
Percent Relatedness of DNA from Bacterial Sources

Source of Unlabeled DNA	Percent Relatedness[a,b]
Escherichia coli K12	88–100
Shigella flexneri	84–85
Citrobacter freundii	50
Salmonella typhimurium	45
Klebsiella pneumoniae	38
Enterobacter aerogenes	37
Serratia marcescens	24
Proteus mirabilis	6

Source: The data was derived from Kenneth E. Sanderson, "Genetic Relatedness in the Family Enterobacteriaceae," *Ann. Rev. Microbiol.*, 30:327–349 (1976).
[a]Source of labeled DNA is *Escherichia coli* K12.
[b]Percent relatedness =
$$\frac{E.\ coli\ DNA\ ^{32}P\ that\ binds\ to\ unlabeled\ DNA \times 100}{E.\ coli\ DNA\ ^{32}P\ that\ binds\ to\ unlabeled\ E.\ coli\ DNA}$$

a progression from the simple bacterial cells to humans has been constructed using the minimum changes or mutational distances required to bring about the observed change. The importance of this approach to bacterial classification is limited because many bacteria do not contain cytochrome *c*, and the analysis is costly and time-consuming. Although the percent G + C, DNA hybridization, and protein sequencing are important in defining the evolutionary relationships between bacteria, these procedures play no practical role in the identification of bacteria.

The tools of molecular biology have given taxonomists a new perspective on bacterial classification. Over a period of time, microbiologists will use these data to organize bacteria into schemes that demonstrate the evolutionary relationships between the species of bacteria. For the present, the classic techniques will still be used in the everyday identification of bacteria and will remain the major criteria used in bacterial classification.

BACTERIAL DIVERSITY

Bacteria comprise division II of the Procaryotae, which is divided into 19 parts. This artificial classification scheme was arrived at by the board of trustees of the Bergey Manual Trust following consulta-

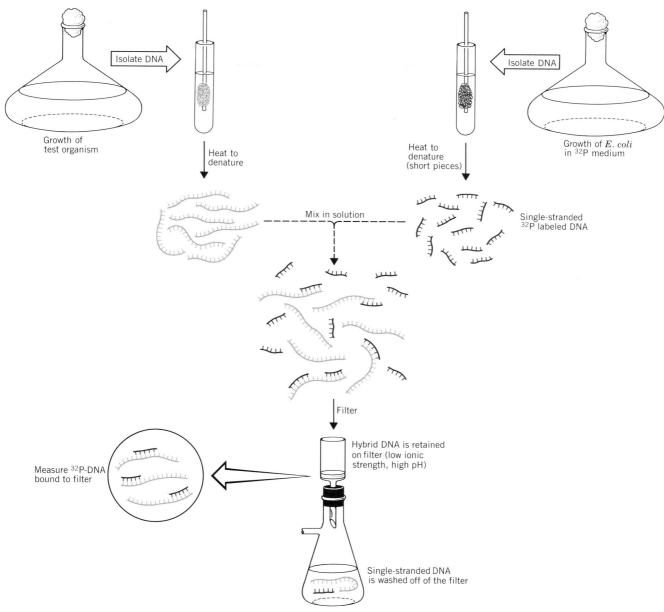

FIGURE 8–5

DNA hybridization. Double-stranded DNA is isolated from suspensions of lysed cells by twirling the DNA onto a glass rod. The DNA is then purified and heat-denatured into single strands. On mixing, homologous DNA sequences anneal to form hybrids composed of double-stranded DNA. These hybrids bind to nitrocelluose filters at low ionic strength and high pH, whereas the single-stranded DNA molecules wash off the filter. In the illustrated example, the DNA from *Escherichia coli* is labeled with ^{32}P, while the DNA of the test organism is unlabeled. The amount of homology between the DNAs from these organisms is indicated by the amount of ^{32}P label retained on the filter. Alternative methods of separating DNA hybrids from single-stranded DNA include ultracentrifugation and column chromatography.

151

tions with 14 advisory committees. The scheme does not imply evolutionary relationships, nor does it imply lines of common descent between the 19 parts. A brief description of each of the 19 parts is included here to demonstrate the wide diversity among bacteria.

Kingdom Procaryotae: division II, the bacteria

Part 1, phototrophic bacteria. Representatives are predominantly aquatic, Gram-negative, anaerobic bacteria that use light as a source of energy. All the photolithotrophs and the photoorganotrophs that do not produce oxygen are included and are called the purple and green bacteria.

Part 2, gliding bacteria. These are unicellular, Gram-negative rods or filaments, typically embedded in a slime layer, that are capable of slow, gliding movement. Some form fruiting bodies. They are widely dispersed in terrestrial environments, and some marine forms are known.

Part 3, sheathed bacteria. This is a small group of organisms that can form a sheath around a chain of growing cells. Some are free-living; others are attached to the substratum by a holdfast.

Part 4, budding and/or appendaged bacteria. Reproduction in budding bacteria results in unequal daughter cells. Bacteria exhibiting appendages or holdfasts are also grouped here.

Part 5, spirochetes. These cells are coiled, unicellular bacteria with one or more complete turns in their helix. Each cell is constructed of a protoplasmic cylinder enclosed by an outer envelope. The outer envelope surrounds endoflagella that function in cell motility.

Part 6, spiral and curved bacteria. These cells are curved rods or helical cells with less than one to many complete turns to their helix. Movement is generated by one or more polar flagella that impart straight-line motion in a corkscrew fashion. All members of this group are chemoorganotrophs that grow under aerobic and/or anaerobic conditions.

Part 7, Gram-negative aerobic rods and cocci. These chemoorganotrophic, rod-shaped bacteria are widely dispersed in nature. Some members of this group can fix atmospheric nitrogen. Some cause disease in humans (see Chapter 21).

Part 8, Gram-negative facultatively anaerobic rods. A large group comprised of the nonspore-forming, chemoorganotrophic rods. A number of these genera are pathogenic for humans and animals. Classification within this group relies heavily on biochemical characteristics that are further discussed in Chapters 16.

Part 9, Gram-negative anaerobic bacteria. All obligate chemoorganotrophic, nonspore-forming, anaerobic bacteria that are normal inhabitants of the natural cavities of humans, animals, and insects are included.

Part 10, Gram-negative cocci and coccobacilli. This is a small group of aerobic, nonmotile, spherical cells that grow in pairs or short chains. Some members of the genus *Neisseria* (see Chapter 18) are pathogenic to humans.

Part 11, Gram-negative anaerobic cocci. This group includes four species of bacteria that are not easily classified with others.

Part 12, Gram-negative chemolithotrophs. This group contains cells of diverse morphologies that can grow on completely inorganic media. They are widely distributed in nature and are important to the cycling of inorganic compounds. These organisms do not cause disease in animals or plants and do not form endospores.

Part 13, methane-producing bacteria. These organisms are strictly anaerobic rods or cocci, with or without motility. They produce methane (CH_4) gas as a major metabolic product by reducing carbon dioxide or carbon monoxide, or by fermenting acetate or methanol to methane. These organisms are important to the natural production of methane gas.

Part 14, Gram-positive cocci. The spherical cells that divide in one, two, or three planes are included. Anaerobic and aerobic genera are represented. Some of these organisms cause human disease (see Chapter 18).

Part 15, endospore-forming rods and cocci. These are the cells that grow aerobically and/or anaerobically and form heat-resistant endospores. Only one species of spore-forming cocci is known. Some endospore-forming rods can cause disease in humans (see Chapter 15).

Part 16, Gram-positive, nonsporing, rod-shaped bacteria. This group includes the straight or curved nonmotile rods that ferment carbohydrates. *Lactobacillus*, the major genus, is found in fermenting animal and plant products. Pathogenicity is unusual in this group. The taxonomic criteria for dividing Part 16 and Part 17 is arbitrary.

Part 17, actinomycetes and related organisms. The largest group of bacteria, it is composed of Gram-positive organisms capable of pleomorphic or mycelial growth. Some form spores at the tips of their aerial mycelia. Some members of this group produce antibiotics, and some cause disease in humans (see Chapter 17).

Part 18, rickettsias. The bacteria classified here are strict intracellular parasites. This group is composed of small, nonmotile, Gram-negative cells that are often pleomorphic. Many cause disease in humans; some have insect vectors (see Chapter 20).

Part 19, mycoplasmas. Bacteria that lack a true cell wall and are pleomorphic, nonmotile, facultative anaerobes are placed in this part. Some require sterols for growth. Many species inhabit or are pathogens of cattle, birds, and/or humans (see Chapter 21).

Bacteria are morphologically diverse. They are capable of a broad spectrum of metabolic activities, and they are ubiquitous on the earth. It is important to realize that only a small number of bacterial species cause disease in humans and animals. The number of bacteria that are helpful to humans far exceeds the number involved in human disease. For example, the natural cycling of organic matter, inorganic nitrogen, and inorganic sulfur results largely from the activities of bacteria. The remainder of this book will concentrate on those microorganisms and viruses that cause disease in humans. Other microbes are equally significant to the well-being of the human race, but do not come within the scope of this book. The material contained in the reading list supplements this short description of bacterial diversity and is highly recommended as a source of additional information.

SUMMARY

Bacteria are classified in the kingdom Procaryotae, whereas the eucaryotic microorganisms are classified in Protista. Viruses are noncellular and are organized separately. Taxonomists classify organisms to name them, to define them, and to provide an organizational scheme that demonstrates their evolutionary relationships and serves as an identification guide. Each species is assigned a binomial name consisting of a genus name and a specific epithet. At the time of compilation, all recognized bacterial species are described in *Bergey's Manual*. This manual divides the Procaryotae into two divisions: the cyanobacteria are placed in division I and the bacteria are placed in division II. Division II is further divided, under the criteria of classic taxonomy, into 19 parts. Classic criteria include morphology, growth characteristics, and biochemical traits. More recently, bacteria have been analyzed with techniques developed by molecular biologists. These techniques include moles percent G + C, DNA hybridization, and amino acid sequencing of small proteins. Both the classic and the molecular techniques have been applied to bacterial classification. Microbiologists recognize the great diversity among bacteria and are continuously involved in improving bacterial classification. The classification scheme presented in the latest edition of *Bergey's Manual* is used as the standard guide to the identification and naming of bacteria.

QUESTIONS AND TOPICS FOR STUDY AND DISCUSSION

Questions

1. Why do scientists classify microorganisms?
2. What is the concept of species in bacterial classification? How does this concept differ from the concept of an animal species?
3. Name three classic techniques used to classify bacteria. How can the data obtained from these techniques be applied to numerical taxonomy?
4. The use of DNA hybridization and moles percent G + C in classification is based on what principles of molecular biology?
5. Choose five bacteria described in parts 1 through 19 and describe the ecological niche where one would expect to find them.

Discussion

1. Discuss the problems faced by microbiologists who attempt to devise one absolute classification scheme for the bacteria.
2. Discuss the implications of the continued changes in the classification of bacteria on students and the medical establishment.

FURTHER READINGS

Books

Brock, T. D., *Biology of Microorganisms*, 3rd ed., Prentice-Hall, Englewood Cliffs, N.J., 1979. A highly regarded college textbook that has an extensive chapter on the biology of the different bacterial groups.

Buchanan, R. E., and N. E. Gibbons (eds.), *Bergey's Manual of Determinative Bacteriology*, 8th ed., Williams & Wilkins, Baltimore, 1974. This volume is the main reference book for bacterial classification. Each known bacterium is described, and electron micrographs are included to illustrate many species. The manual also contains a key for identifying bacteria and an extensive bibliography of the early literature.

Stanier, R. Y., E. A. Adelberg, and J. L. Ingraham, *The Microbial World*, 4th ed., Prentice-Hall, Englewood Cliffs, N.J., 1976. A highly regarded advanced-level textbook that has extensive chapters on the characteristics and classification of the bacteria.

Manuals

BBL Manual of Products and Laboratory Procedures, 5th ed., 1968, Becton, Dickerson & Co., Cockeysville, Md. This manual contains the composition of and the uses for this manufacturer's bacteriological media and reagents. It is an important reference book for these media, which are widely used in microbiology.

Difco Manual of Dehydrated Cultured Media and Reagents, 9th ed., 1971, Difco Laboratories, Detroit. This manual contains the composition of and the uses for this manufacturer's bacteriological media and reagents. It is an important reference book for these media, which are widely used in microbiology.

Lennette, E. H., A. Balows, W. J. Hausler, and J. P. Truant, *Manual of Clinical Microbiology*, 3rd ed., 1980, American Society for Microbiology, Bethesda, Md. This is a current manual that contains instructions and discussions of the major microbiological and immunological assays used to identify microorganisms in the clinical laboratory.

Skerman, V. B. D., *A Guide to the Identification of Genera of Bacteria*, 1967, Williams & Wilkins, Baltimore. An abridged form of *Bergey's Manual* that is a useful key for the identification of bacteria.

Articles and Reviews

Dickerson, R. E., "Cytochrome *c* and the Evolution of Energy Metabolism," *Sci. Am.*, 242:136–153 (March 1980). The amino acid sequences of cytochrome *c*, isolated from many bacteria, are presented and analyzed from an evolutionary perspective. The author constructs a phylogenic tree for the bacteria based on the amino acid sequences in bacterial cytochromes.

9

INTRODUCTION TO VIROLOGY

Viruses are complex macromolecular forms of life that use their own genetic information, encoded in DNA or RNA, to produce replicas of themselves. They do this by commandeering the biosynthetic machinery of their host cell for their own reproductive purposes. Viruses are composed of one type of nucleic acid (either DNA or RNA but never both) surrounded by a protective protein coat known as a **capsid.** All viruses lack a cell structure, so they are described as noncellular forms of life.

The status of viruses as organisms is still a topic of scientific debate. Viruses are self-contained, reproductive entities that produce a continuous lineage; as such they are similar to organisms. On the other hand, viruses are noncellular. The question of how and when viruses originated is still unanswered. These characteristics make it impossible to interrelate viruses with the evolutionary and taxonomic schemes of cellular organisms. Viruses, however, are considered to be microbes because of their small size, their unique composition, and their ability to propagate. **Virology,** the study of viruses, historically developed as an integral part of microbiology.

HISTORY OF VIROLOGY

Dimitri I. Ivanovski discovered that the causative agent of tobacco mosaic disease passed through bacterial filters. His report of these findings, published in 1892, is acknowledged to be the discovery of the filterable nature of viruses. Unaware of Ivanovski's work, Martinus W. Beijerinck reported the same findings in 1898. He described the phenomenon as a *contagium vivum fluidum.* Beijerinck further proposed that these infectious agents replicate inside the tobacco leaves.

Discovery of animal viruses

In 1898, Friedrich J. Loeffler and Paul Frosch described the filterable nature of foot-and-mouth disease (Table 9–1). They transferred this cattle disease by injecting small amounts of filtered lymph into healthy calves. The filtering technique of Loeffler and Frosch was soon used to demonstrate the filterability of a number of infectious animal diseases. By 1911, the infectious agents responsible for yellow fever, rabies, poliomyelitis, measles, and chicken sarcoma had been reported (Table 9–1) as filterable.

TABLE 9–1
Historical Events in Virology

Year	Scientist	Event
1798	Edward Jenner	Developed a smallpox vaccine
1892	Dimitri I. Ivanovski	Discovered filterability of TMV
1898	Friedrich J. Loeffler and Paul Frosch	Discovered filterability of foot-and-mouth disease (animal virus)
1898	Martinus W. Beijerinck	Discovered intracellular reproduction of TMV
1901	Walter Reed and colleagues	Discovered yellow fever virus
1903	P. Remlinger and Riffat-Bey	Discovered the rabies virus
1907	P. M. Asburn and C. F. Craig	Discovered the virus of dengue fever
1908	V. Ellerman and O. Bang	Transferred chicken leukemia
1909	S. Flexner and P. A. Lewis	Discovered poliomyelitis virus
1911	J. Goldberger and J. F. Anderson	Discovered the measles virus
1911	Peyton Rous	Transferred chicken sarcoma (cancer) by means of a cell-free filtrate
1915	Frederick W. Twort	Discovered bacterial viruses
1917	Felix d'Herelle	Rediscovered bacterial viruses, named them bacteriophages
1921	Jules Bordet and M. Ciuca	Described lysogeny
1934	C. D. Johnson and E. W. Goodpasture	Discovered the mumps virus
1935	Wendell M. Stanley	Crystallized tobacco mosaic virus
1936	Martin Schlesinger	Discovered phage nucleic acids
1938	Y. Hiroals and S. Tasaka	Discovered the rubella virus
1939	G. A. Kausche, E. Pfankuch, and H. Ruska	Used electron microscopy to visualize virus
1949	John H. Enders, T. H. Weller, and F. C. Robbins	Cultivated polio virus in nonneuronal tissue culture
1951	D. Hershey and M. Chase	Discovered that bacteriophage DNA enters cell
1952	Norton D. Zinder and Joshua Leaderberg	Described transduction in *Salmonella*
1953	James D. Watson and Francis H. C. Crick	Proposed double-helix model of DNA
1957	A. Isaacs and J. Lindenmann	Discovered interferon
1970	David Baltimore; Howard Temin and Satoshi Mizutaki	Independently discovered RNA-directed DNA polymerase

Discovery of bacterial viruses

Frederick W. Twort (Figure 9–1) spent his early professional career studying the nutritional growth requirements of bacteria. As a logical extension of his work, Twort attempted to grow filter-passing viruses on artificial media. His attempts resulted in failure; however, during these experiments he isolated a bacterium that appeared to be diseased. Colonies of this micrococcus became watery, and some of these colonies could not be subcultured. When these colonies were kept for a long time, they gradually turned glassy and transparent. Twort was able to transfer this diseased state to other micrococcal colonies, even after filtering the affected cultures through a Chamberland candle. In 1915, Twort concluded that *this disease of the micrococcus was caused by a filterable infectious agent that multiplied within the micrococci and caused them to lyse.*

Felix d'Herelle (Figure 9–2), a well-traveled Canadian microbiologist, rediscovered bacterial viruses in 1917. Unfortunately, he was unaware of Twort's earlier publication, and for 4 years he was acknowledged as the discoverer of bacterial viruses.

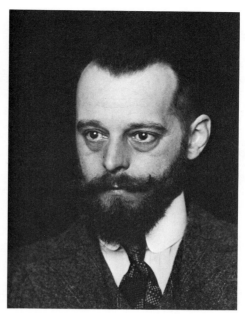

FIGURE 9–2
Felix d'Herelle (1873–1949), one of the first microbiologists to work with bacterial viruses. (Pasteur Institute Museum.)

FIGURE 9–1
Frederick W. Twort (1877–1950), who reported the glassy transformation of micrococcus. (Godfrey Argent Studio, London.)

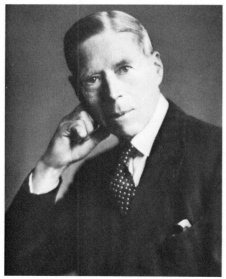

D'Herelle was working in Paris when he discovered a filterable virus that lysed a dysentery bacillus. He isolated the bacillus from a dysentery patient's stools shortly after the patient was admitted to the hospital of the Pasteur Institute. For 4 consecutive days d'Herelle filtered the patient's stools and added the filtrates to broth cultures of the dysentery bacillus. For 3 days the cultures grew normally. On the fourth day, however, the filtrate-inoculated culture of bacillus turned perfectly clear. D'Herelle soon found that this filterable agent could be transferred to other cultures of Shiga dysentery bacilli. He named these viruses **bacteriophages** (phages for short), which essentially means bacteria-eating.

D'Herelle's discovery stimulated scientists to investigate the ability of bacteriophages to cure infectious diseases. This approach to treating infectious diseases never proved effective, but the concept led to a great amount of work in bacterial virology. In 1921, Jules Bordet reintroduced Twort's work and challenged the priority of d'Herelle's discovery. In-

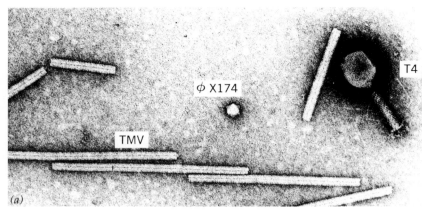

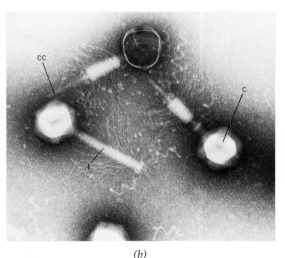

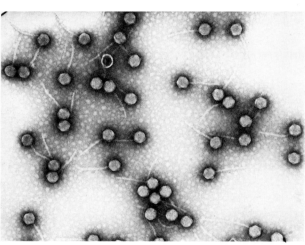

FIGURE 9-3
Viruses. (*a*) Transmission electron micrograph of a mixture of tobacco mosaic virus (TMV), T₄ bacteriophage and φX174 bacteriophage. (Courtesy of Dr. F. A. Eiserling.) (*b*) Electron micrograph of *Bacillus* bacterophages, 100,000 ×. The virus with the dark capsid (c) has lost its DNA. One virion has an extended tail, while the tails of two of the virions have contracted tails (t) and an exposed central core (cc). (Courtesy of Dr. R. K. Nauman.) (*c*) The lambda bacteriophage has a flexible tail that terminates in a single tail fiber. (Courtesy Prof. J. T. Finch, MRC Laboratory of Molecular Biology, Cambridge.)

(*a*) (*b*) (*c*)

deed, there is still a controversy over who deserves credit for discovering bacterial viruses.

Viruses and the development of molecular biology

Bacteriophages were an enigma to biologists, who had a difficult time understanding the basic nature of these invisible, infectious agents. A major turning point occurred in 1935 when Wendell M. Stanley crystallized tobacco mosaic virus (TMV). He was able to purify TMV using techniques of protein purification and crystallization. Stanley obtained nee-

dle-shaped crystals of TMV that were infectious even after a 1 billionfold dilution. He concluded that tobacco mosaic virus was an "autocatalytic protein" that replicated in living tobacco cells.

Stanley's hypothesis was not entirely correct. Martin Schlesinger soon purified a bacteriophage and found that it contained nucleic acid in addition to protein. Virologists soon realized that all viruses are composed of nucleic acid (either RNA or DNA) surrounded by a protein capsid. The diverse morphology of viruses (Figure 9-3) was only realized after the development of the electron microscope in the late 1930s.

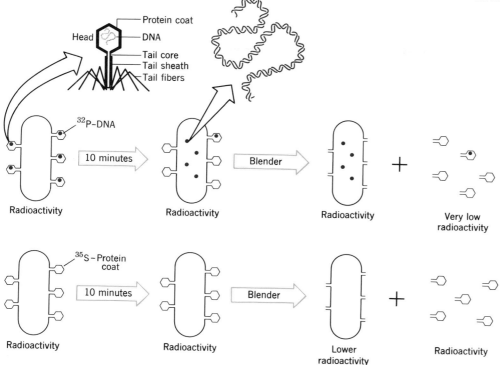

FIGURE 9–4

The Hershy-Chase experiment. T_4 bacteriophages whose DNA had been labeled with the isotope ^{32}P were used to infect *Escherichia coli*. Ten minutes later, the infected bacteria were placed in a blender and the bacteriophage capsids, which remained attached to the bacterial cell wall, were sheered off. After centrifugation, the ^{32}P labeled DNA was associated with the bacterial cells found in the pellet. When T_4 bacteriophages whose protein had been labeled with the isotope ^{35}S were used, the label was found in the supernatant solution. This experiment provided early evidence for the role of DNA in heredity. (From E. J. Gardner and D. P. Snustad, *Principles of Genetics,* 6th ed., Wiley, New York, 1981.)

Many virologists work with bacteriophages because the bacteria they infect are easily cultured under controlled conditions. Experiments have demonstrated that bacteriophages reproduce in an assembly-line fashion—not by growth and binary fission. The component parts of a bacteriophage are produced inside the infected bacterium during a short latent period. The virus is then assembled into a complete infective virion. When enough virus particles are present, the cell lyses and releases the bacteriophages into the environment.

Studies of the DNA bacteriophages contributed to the identification of DNA as the molecule of heredity (Figure 9–4). D. Hershey and Martha Chase (1951) grew bacteriophages such that their DNA was labeled with ^{32}P and their protein was labeled with ^{35}S. With this experiment they demonstrated that the ^{35}S-labeled protein stayed outside the cell, whereas the ^{32}P-labeled DNA entered the cell during bacteriophage infection and replication. Since the bacteriophages faithfully reproduced themselves inside cells, Hershey and Chase concluded that the in-

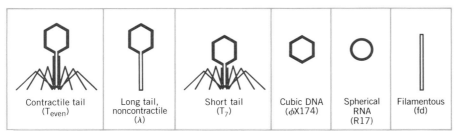

FIGURE 9–5
Bacteriophage morphology is used in the classification of these viruses.

formation required for virus propagation must be present on the bacteriophage DNA. Shortly after these experiments, James Watson and Francis Crick proposed their model of DNA, which ushered in the age of molecular biology.

BACTERIOPHAGES

Current concepts in virology rely heavily on our knowledge of bacteriophages. The previous chapters on bacteriology provide an appropriate foundation for our discussion of bacterial virology. A discussion of animal virology is presented in Chapter 22.

Classification

Chemical composition and morphology are the major criteria used in bacteriophage classification. Viral nucleic acid is either DNA or RNA, and it is either single-stranded, double-stranded, linear (two free ends), or closed. Surrounding the nucleic acid is a protein capsid that can be symmetrical or helical. Additional proteins can be present in the bacteriophage tail assembly; however, not all bacteriophages have tails (Figure 9–5). Indeed, bacteriophage morphology can be described as cubic, filamentous, pleomorphic, or tailed. Viral morphology and nucleic acid composition are used to define the major groups of bacteriophages (Table 9–2).

Some bacteriophage groups contain hundreds of individual viruses, whereas others contain only one. Therefore, chemical composition and morphology cannot be used as the sole criteria to identify and

classify bacteriophages. The other criteria that are used include the viral particle size, shape, structure, weight, buoyant density, together with the type of nucleic acid and its molecular weight.

Isolation of bacteriophages

Bacteriophages are present in almost all natural environments. They can be isolated by filtering mixtures of natural material suspended in water. During filtration, the bacteriophages pass through the filter, while the filter retains the debris and any bacteria that are present. The filtrate is then mixed with a growing culture of the host bacterium. The bacteriophages reproduce in their host cells and are released into the medium. Clones of individual bacteriophages can then be isolated from this medium following their growth on a lawn of host cells.

Plaque assay. Bacteriophages can produce distinct clones when infected bacteria are sown over the surface of an agar plate. The bacteria grow as a continuous lawn except where the viruses have lysed the bacteria to produce a clear area (Figure 9–6). The clear spots in the bacterial lawn are **plaques**, which contain thousands of invisible (too small for the naked eye to see) bacteriophages.

The plaque assay is a means of counting bacteriophages since the number of plaques is directly proportional to the number of infected bacteria present. A plaque assay is performed by mixing a sample of bacteriophages containing 10 to 200 virions with approximately 10^8 cells of the host bacterium suspended in sloppy agar (0.8% agar). The mixture is

TABLE 9–2
Classification of Bacteriophages

Shape	Nucleic Acid	Example	Characteristics	Number Known
Tailed	ds DNA, L	T_2	Contractile tail	450
	ds DNA, L	Lambda	Long, noncontractile tail	800
	ds DNA, L	T_7	Short tail	300
Cubic	ss DNA, C	ϕX174	Large, knoblike capsomeres	25
	ds DNA, C	PM2	Lipid-containing capsid	2?
	ds DNA, L	PRD1	Double coat, lipids, pseudotail	4?
	ss RNA, L	R17	———	35
	ds RNA, L	ϕ6	Lipid-containing envelope	1
Filamentous	ss DNA, C	fd	Long rods	17
	ss DNA, C	MV-L1	Short rods	10
Pleomorphic	ds DNA, C	MV-L2	Lipid-containing envelope	3?

Source: Adapted from Hans-W. Akerman et al., "Guidelines for Bacteriophage Classification," in M. A. Lauffer, F. B. Bang, K. Maramorosch, and K. M. Smith (eds.), *Advances in Viral Research,* Academic Press, New York, 23:1–24 (1978).
Key: ss, single-stranded; ds, double-stranded; C, circular; L, linear.

FIGURE 9–6
Plaques of T_4 bacteriophage growing on a lawn of *Escherichia coli* B. The number of plaques is directly proportional to the concentration of virions in the sample plated on the lawn of bacteria. Petri dish *(a)* contains approximately 10 times more plaques than does petri dish *(b).* (Courtesy of Dr. L. D. Simon.)

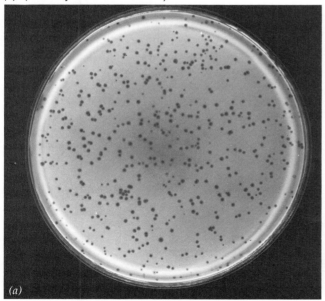
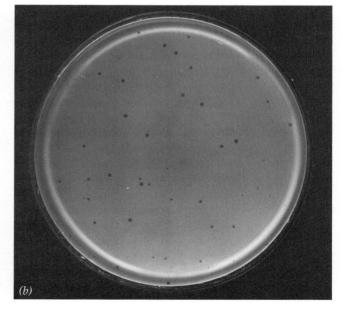

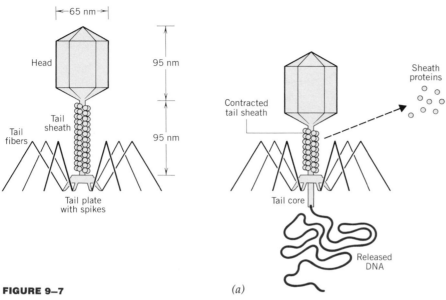

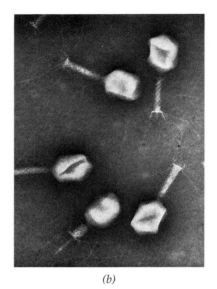

FIGURE 9—7

(*a*)

(*b*)

(*a*) Diagram of T-even bacteriophages; one with an extended tail sheath and one with a contracted tail sheath. Proteins are lost from the tail sheath during tail contraction. (*b*) Electron micrograph of negatively stained T$_4$ bacteriophages showing the complex morphology of the tail. (Photo courtesy of Dr. E. Boy de la Tour and E. Kellenberger.)

FIGURE 9—8

The T$_2$ bacteriophage capsid contains a single linear DNA molecule (note the two ends) about 500,000 Å long. The DNA has been released from the bacteriophage head (center) by gentle lysis. (Photo courtesy of Dr. A. K. Kleinschmidt, *Biochem. Biophys. Acta*, 61:861, 1962.)

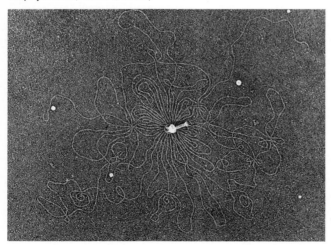

then dispersed over a solid layer of nutrient agar. Each viral-infected bacterium will produce progeny viruses, which in turn will cause a plaque to form on the plate. Each plaque arises from a single virus-infected bacterium, so *the number of plaques on a plate is equivalent to the number of bacteriophages in the sample plated.*

DNA bacteriophages

The T-bacteriophages are double-stranded DNA viruses that infect *Escherichia coli.* They are designated by numbers, T$_1$ through T$_7$. Morphologically, the T-even bacteriophages (T$_2$, T$_4$, and T$_6$) are composed of a head, a tail, and a tail plate with tail fibers (Figure 9–7). The head is composed of capsomeres surrounding a compartment that contains the DNA (Figure 9–8). Their DNA is a linear molecule (1.2 × 10^8 daltons) that is protected against degradation by environmental nucleases because of its location inside the bacteriophage head. Protruding from the head is a tail core surrounded by the tail sheath. The sheath is attached to a tail plate. The tail plate has spikes and tail fibers that specifically react with receptor sites on the outer membrane of the bacterial cell wall. Following adsorption to the host cell, the tail sheath loses proteins in a process that shortens the sheath and propels the tail core through the cell wall (Figure 9–7). At this time the DNA is extruded out of the bacteriophage head and into the cell's cytoplasm.

Lytic cycle. The presence of the bacteriophage DNA in the cell's cytoplasm initiates the **lytic cycle** of bacteriophage replication. This growth cycle is demonstrated by the one-step growth experiment using *E. coli* and T_4 (Figure 9–9). In this experiment, the number of infective centers was measured as a function of time. The **latent period** lasts for 23 minutes, during which time no increase in the number of infective centers is observed. During the next 10 minutes, the number of infective units increases one-hundredfold. This second time interval is referred to as the **rise period**. The difference between the initial and the final number of infective centers (100) is the **burst size**. The lytic cycle of bacteriophage reproduction is initiated by infection and culminates with the release of progeny viruses into the environment by the lysis of the host cell.

Do the bacteriophages divide inside the cytoplasm during the latent period? Experiments show that they do not. If the cells are experimentally lysed during the first 11 minutes of the lytic cycle, no bacteriophages are recovered from the cell lysate. Following this 11-minute **eclipse** period, increasing numbers of infective bacteriophage particles are present inside the cell until their numbers plateau off at the maximum burst size.

Phage replication is similar to an assembly line. The product is not visible during the time that the workers are making the parts; however, once the parts are available for assembly, they are joined in a sequential fashion to form the desired product. Bacteriophages are produced in an assembly-line fash-

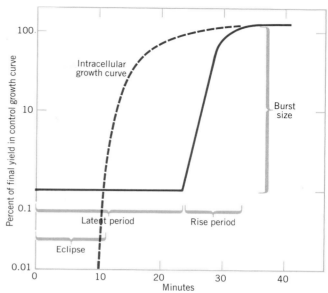

FIGURE 9–9

One-step growth curve of a bacteriophage (T_1) grown on *Escherichia coli*. The growth experiment was started with 10^5 infective units per ml of culture. The dashed line represents the production of infective centers within the cell as observed following the artificial lysis of culture samples at sequential intervals. (Modified from A. H. Doermann, *J. Gen. Physiol.*, 35:645–656, 1952, with permission.)

ion, with completed bacteriophages being self-assembled from their component parts.

Replication of a T-even bacteriophage. The replication of bacteriophage T_4 in *Escherichia coli* has been chosen to demonstrate the principles of viral replication. The intracellular development of bacteriophage T_4 in *E. coli* is shown in Figure 9–10 in a series of electron micrographs. The individual steps in the replicative process are diagrammed in Figure 9–11.

Adsorption. Bacteriophage T_4 adsorbs to a specific lipopolysaccharide receptor on the outer membrane of the *E. coli* cell (Figure 9–12). The tail fibers help to position the bacteriophage over the cell's receptor in the initial steps of binding. Not all *E. coli* cells possess this lipopolysaccharide: cells that do not are resistant to T_4 infection.

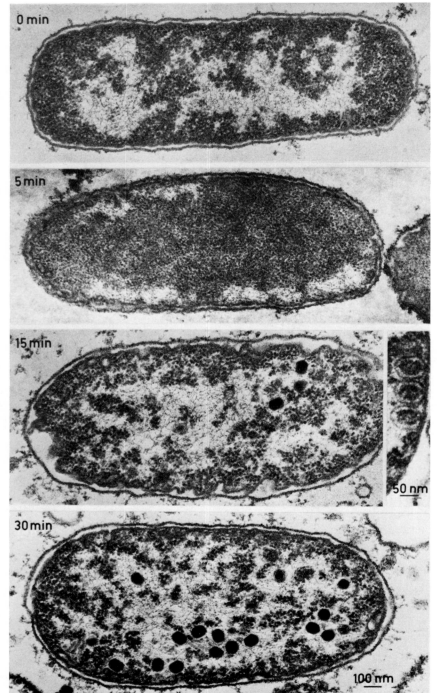

FIGURE 9—10

Intracellular development of bacteriophage T$_4$ in *Escherichia coli*. **Time 0′:** This cell has the morphology of an uninfected cell with the typical nuclear region of a cell in exponential growth. The infection starts after adsorbtion of the phage, partial penetration of the central core of the tail, and injection of the DNA. **Time 5′:** The bacteriophage infection results in "nuclear disruption" caused by the viral directed hydrolysis of the host's DNA. The DNA and its breakdown products are found in marginal vacuoles. The nucleotides from the host DNA are later used by the bacteriophage to synthesize its own DNA. **Time 15′:** About 8 minutes after infection, the synthesis of the structural proteins used for assembling the maturing bacteriophages begins. A few minutes later, the first infective viruses appear and continue to mature at a rate of 5 per minute. It is generally thought that a prehead with no or only a little DNA is made first (insert). The fine fibrillar material ressembling the bacterial nucleus is the "vegetative bacteriophage." **Time 30′:** A later stage of bacteriophage development showing increasing amounts of finished heads. The amount of virion particles per section is about one-twentieth of the total number per cell. (The electron micrographs and the legend were kindly provided by Beate Menge, Jacomina v. d. Broek, H. Wunderli, K. Lickfeld, M. Wurtz, and E. Kellenberger.)

Other bacteriophages use other cell surface receptors. Bacteriophage receptors include the pili of *E. coli*, the Vi-antigen of *Salmonella*, glucosylated teichoic acid of *B. subtilis*, and portions of the outer membrane of Gram-negative bacteria. Because adsorption is a specific biochemical reaction, bacteriophages can infect only certain host cells. This adsorption is so specific that it can be used to classify bacteria within a given species. Strains having the same bacteriophage receptors are classified together just as bacteria possessing the same surface antigens are classified together.

Penetration. Tailed bacteriophages have a "contractile" mechanism that propels the central tail core through the cell wall and into the bacterium's cytoplasmic membrane. The T_4 tail sheath shortens by a displacement of one-half its tail sheath proteins. The DNA in the T_4 capsid then passes through the central tail core into the host cell's cytoplasm, while the empty protein capsid remains attached to the cell surface (Figure 9–12). Shortly after penetration, superinfections by other bacteriophages are prevented by a complex process involving newly synthesized bacteriophage protein.

Early protein synthesis. Bacteriophage proteins are translated on the host cell's ribosomes using

FIGURE 9–11

Reproduction of a DNA bacteriophage. (Modified from P. Sheeler and D. E. Bianchi, *Cell Biology*, copyright © 1980, Wiley.)

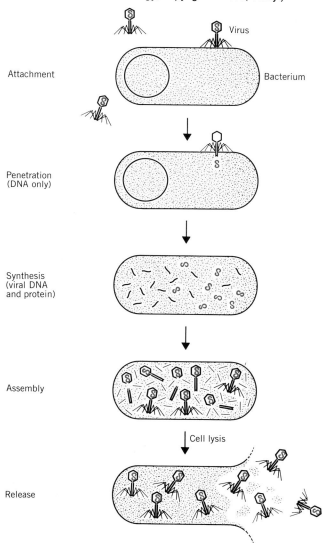

FIGURE 9–12

An electron micrograph of T_4 bacteriophages adsorbed to an *Escherichia coli* B cell. (Courtesy of Dr. L. D. Simon. From L. D. Simon and T. F. Anderson, *Virology*, 32:279–295, 1967.)

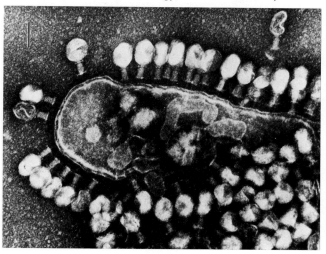

mRNAs transcribed from the bacteriophage's DNA. mRNAs that code for early protein are transcribed by the bacterium's DNA-directed RNA polymerase. This cellular enzyme can work on only a small portion of the bacteriophage genome because the promotor region in T_4 DNA limits the genes that it can transcribe. These early mRNAs are then translated on the cell's ribosomes into "early" proteins.

Early proteins are involved in commandeering the host's cellular machinery and in manufacturing progeny bacteriophages. Early proteins include nucleases, synthetic enzymes, and polymerases. These bacteriophage **nucleases** specifically hydrolyze bacterial DNA and thereby destroy the cell's ability to replicate. Bacteriophages also make enzymes that are involved in the biosynthesis of the precursors used to synthesize bacteriophage DNA. The actual synthesis of phage DNA is done by a viral DNA polymerase that is formed early in the replication cycle. This enzyme makes the copies of bacteriophage DNA used in the final assembly of the virions. Some bacteriophages also make an RNA polymerase that synthesizes the mRNA used in late protein synthesis.

Late protein synthesis. Toward the end of the replication cycle, T_4 synthesizes **late proteins.** These include the structural proteins necessary for virion self-assembly, the enzymes involved in maturation, and the proteins used in the release of bacteriophages from the cell. Bacteriophage DNA is synthesized in the cell's cytoplasm at the same time that the viral structural proteins are being synthesized on the host's ribosomes. At this stage of the replication cycle, the cell becomes a repository for pools of all the bacteriophage proteins and copies of its DNA.

Bacteriophages mature through a sequential process of self-assembly that is governed in part by the laws of quaternary protein structure. The head protein capsomeres join to form bacteriophage capsids (heads); at the same time they are filled with bacteriophage DNA (Figure 9–10). Concomitantly, the tails are formed from their component parts. The DNA-containing capsids combine with the tails, and then the tail fibers attach to complete the process of phage maturation.

Release. Infective T_4 bacteriophages are released into the surrounding environment when their host cells lyse. Release is mediated by lysozyme and another viral protein that damages the cell membrane. The viral lysozyme specifically breaks down the peptidoglycan of the host's cell wall. The combined actions of these enzymes lyse the host cell, thus causing the release of the progeny virions.

Transduction

Viral infections do not always result in lysis of the host cell. Infections can result in defective bacteriophages that can sometimes transfer bacterial genes. **Transduction** is the bacteriophage-mediated transfer of bacterial genes from a donor cell to a recipient bacterium. Transduction can occur by two basic mechanisms: (1) **generalized transduction,** in which random pieces of bacterial DNA are transferred; and (2) **specialized transduction,** in which only a limited group of genes can be transferred.

Generalized transduction. During the normal lytic cycle of phage infection, host-cell DNA is broken down into small pieces. This host-cell DNA can be incorporated accidentally into new phage particles in place of some or all of the phage DNA (Figure 9–13). These new phage particles are defective because they lack a full complement of their own DNA. When these defective phages infect a bacterial cell, they inject bacterial DNA (from the donor cell) instead of phage DNA. Once in the cell, the genes from the donor cell can recombine with the host cell's DNA to become a part of the host-cell genome. This process is known as generalized transduction because the phage can pick up any piece of host-cell DNA, so that any gene on the host chromosome can be transferred. Generalized transduction can be used to perform genetic mapping; however, its applicability is limited by the small pieces of DNA that are transferred.

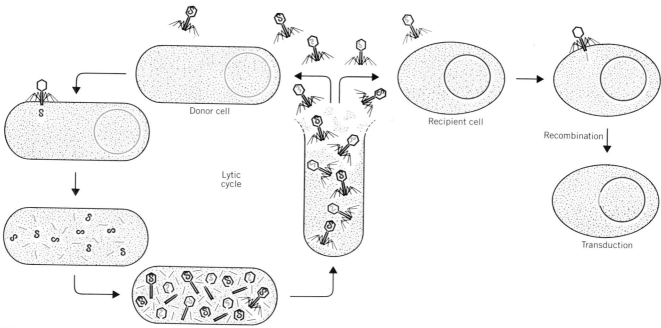

FIGURE 9–13

Generalized transduction. During the normal lytic cycle of phage reproduction, defective bacteriophage are formed that have taken up host-cell DNA in place of phage DNA. Any piece of host-cell DNA can be incorporated into the bacteriophage. These defective bacteriophages will transfer the bacterial DNA to the next bacterial cell they infect. This form of bacteriophage-mediated transfer of bacterial DNA is known as generalized transduction.

Specialized transduction. The DNA of certain bacteriophages can exist in two distinct states: as a replicative form in the cytoplasm of its host cell (as just described) or as a segment of DNA integrated into the host genome. A phage that can exist in both states is called a **temperate** phage. When the DNA of a temperate phage is integrated into the host chromosome, the phage is referred to as a **prophage** (Figure 9–14).

Lambda (λ) is a temperate DNA phage that infects *E. coli*. It can exist as a replicative form in the cytoplasm or it can be integrated into the *E. coli* chromosome through the covalent binding of the phage DNA to the bacterial DNA. The infection of *E. coli* by lambda can be manipulated to produce a lytic cycle or to produce the prophage state (Figure 9–14).

A cell carrying a prophage is termed a **lysogenic cell;** the process of producing a lysogenic cell is termed **lysogeny.**

Lysogeny occurs when lambda DNA is integrated into a specific site on the *E. coli* chromosome. The site of integration contains base sequences similar to those found in lambda DNA. Following integration, *E. coli* proceeds to multiply as if nothing has happened. Every time the *E. coli* chromosome is replicated, lambda DNA is also replicated.

The lytic replicative cycle of lambda can occur spontaneously, or it can be stimulated by inducing the lysogenic *E. coli* cells. **Viral induction** can be caused by many factors: UV light is commonly used to induce lambda to enter the lytic cycle. During induction, the lambda DNA is usually excised from the bacterial chromosome in its entirety and then replicated. Replication under these conditions results in a lytic cycle, during which virulent lambda phages are released to the environment following cell lysis. Another possible outcome of induction is that a part of the lambda DNA remains attached to a piece of the bacterial chromosome during excision (Figure 9–15). When this occurs, the bacterial DNA can be transferred to the next cell the phage infects. The phage, however, will not be able to replicate in its new host because it lacks essential phage genes and therefore is defective.

Lambda always integrates into the bacterial DNA at a specific site between the genes for galactose (*gal*)

FIGURE 9–14
Replication and lysogeny caused by a temperate bacteriophage. After the genome of a temperate bacteriophage enters the host cell, the virus can progress through a lytic cycle to generate multiple progeny virions or it can be integrated into the bacterial genome as a prophage. The prophage is prevented from replicating when a viral repressor protein, formed in the cell, prevents transcription of the viral genome. Occasionally, the prophage is induced (the repressor is inactivated) and produces infective virions. The virus then can enter a lytic replicative cycle.

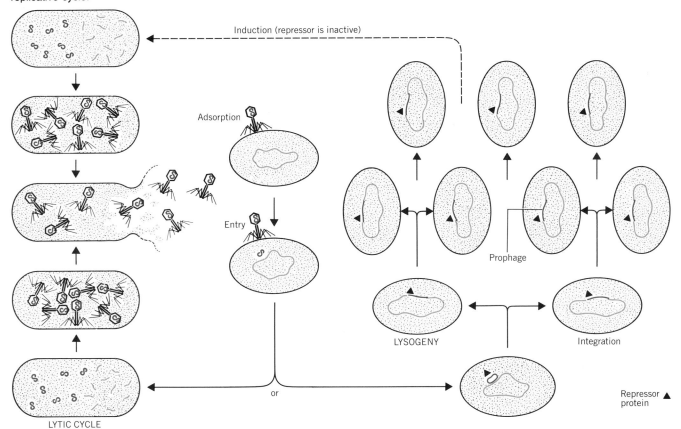

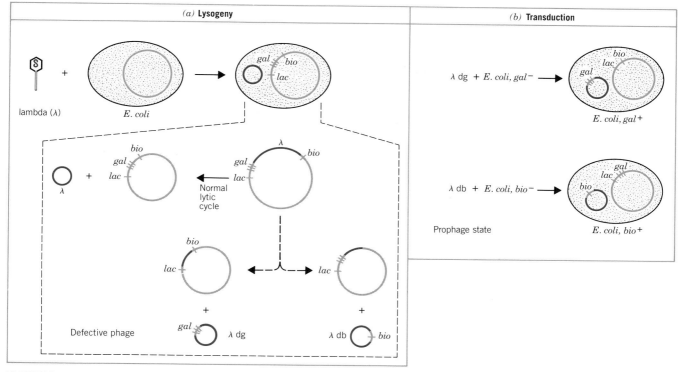

FIGURE 9–15

Specialized transduction by lambda bacteriophage. (a) Lambda is a temperate bacteriophage that always integrates into the host chromosome at a specific point. Mistakes in excision can lead to the formation of an incomplete lambda genome that carries host-cell genes (*gal* or *bio*). (b) Specialized transduction occurs when these host-cell genes are transferred to a recipient cell.

and biotin *(bio)*. When a defective lambda phage is produced, it picks up either the *gal* or the *bio* gene— never both. When a lambda-dg or a lambda-db infects an *E. coli* cell that is auxotrophic for either galactose or biotin *(gal⁻, bio⁺ or gal⁺, bio⁻)*, recombination can occur to form prototrophs *(gal⁺, bio⁺)*. This is an example of **specialized transduction.** Only special genes can be transferred by specialized transduction: they are the genes adjacent to the lambda attachment site on the bacterial chromosome.

Molecular biology of lysogeny

Lysogeny is a common natural state. Many lysogenic bacteria have been isolated from nature. Moreover,

there are certain diseases, including diphtheria and certain forms of botulism, that are caused only by lysogenized bacteria. The process that dictates if an infection by a temperate phage will enter a lytic cycle or a lysogenic cycle is not completely understood. We do know that the lysogenic state caused by lambda is maintained by a repressor protein synthesized at the direction of the lambda genome.

The lambda repressor protein. The viral genes necessary for lambda reproduction are not transcribed in lysogenic cells. Only the short segment of the lambda genome that codes for the repressor protein is transcribed. This repressor protein accumulates in the cell, and it prevents the transcription of the remainder of the lambda genome. The lambda repressor acts in an analogous manner to the repressor protein of the lactose operon (see Chapter 5). As long as the repressor is bound to the lambda DNA, transcription does not occur; and the prophage is passed to all bacterial progeny.

The lysogenic state can be disrupted when the repressor mechanism is inhibited. In some strains, the repressor is thermolabile and can be destroyed by heating at 43°C. When the repressor protein is destroyed, the bacteriophage genome is transcribed and infective lambda particles are produced. Exposure of lysogenic cells to UV light is a more general means of reversing this repression. These techniques **induce** the prophage to form infective bacteriophages.

Integration of lambda genome. Lambda DNA is double-stranded except for a short 12-base sequence at the 5' end of each strand (Figure 9–16). These single-stranded tails are complementary, so lambda DNA can spontaneously form a nicked ring structure.

Lambda DNA is integrated into the host genome at a specific site on the host DNA by the viral enzyme **integrase.** Integrase is formed from the time of infection until the repressor protein is formed. Because integrase breaks both the host and the viral DNA at specific sites, lambda DNA is always integrated at the same site on the bacterial chromosome (Figure 9–16). Therefore, integrated lambda DNA is always present in the same sequential order between specific host genes.

Excision of lambda genome. Excision is normally a precise process that results in a replicative form of lambda. Excision is catalyzed by the enzyme **exciginase.** Imprecise excision can result in an incomplete bacteriophage genome attached to a few host cell genes. Such bacteriophages are defective in that they cannot reproduce; but they can transfer their genome, containing host-cell genes, to a recipient cell—the process of specialized transduction. Lysogenized cells can be cured of their prophage if the prophage is improperly excised from its bacterial genome. These incomplete bacteriophage genomes cannot replicate, so they are not passed on to progeny cells.

Phage conversion

Many bacteria exist in the lysogenic state; that is, they carry genetic information in their chromosome that is part of a viral genome. These viruses are taking a free ride and are being replicated in the prophage state each time the cell replicates. **Phage conversion** is an alteration of the phenotype of a lysogenized cell caused by the expression of a prophage gene. The prophage genes of special interest to medical microbiologists are those that code for toxins.

Lysogenized strains of *Corynebacterium diphtheriae* produce diphtheria toxin, which causes the symptoms of diphtheria in humans. Diphtheria toxin is a protein that is coded for by a beta-phage gene. Only cultures of *Corynebacterium diphtheriae* carrying the beta prophage can cause diphtheria. Similarly, protein toxins produced by certain streptococci and by some strains of *Clostridium botulinum* are coded for by prophage genes. When the lysogenized cells lose their prophage, they also lose the ability to produce the toxin.

Host-range modification

A constant war rages between the viruses, which possess the propensity to commandeer their host cell for replicative purposes, and the host cell, which wants to prevent viral infection. The weapons of this war are nucleases that attack DNA; the defense mechanisms are other enzymes that shield DNA from the attacking nucleases.

Restriction endonucleases. Bacteria produce restriction endonucleases, which cleave double-stranded DNA at specific sites. (**Endonucleases** cleave bonds within the DNA molecules, whereas **exonucleases** act only on free ends of single- or double-stranded DNA.) Restriction endonucleases limit the type of

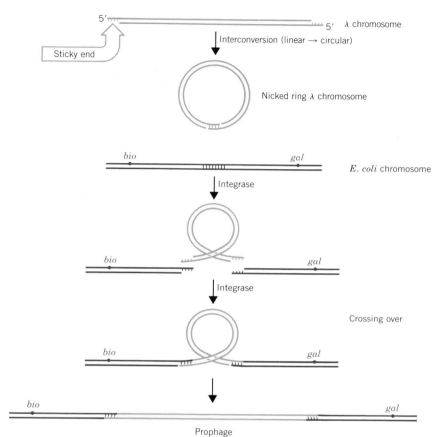

5' λ chromosome

Sticky end

Interconversion (linear → circular)

Nicked ring λ chromosome

bio *gal* E. coli chromosome

Integrase

bio *gal*

Integrase

Crossing over

bio *gal*

bio *gal*

Prophage

FIGURE 9–16
Integration of lambda bacteriophage into the *Escherichia coli* genome. Single-stranded, lambda DNA spontaneously forms a closed nicked ring prior to being joined with the *E. coli* chromosome by integrase.

DNA that can be replicated within a cell. They recognize 4- to 6-base sequences that are symmetrical about a central point (Table 9–3). EcoRI is an endonuclease that cleaves DNA in two places.

$$
\begin{array}{c}
-\text{G}-\text{A}-\text{A}-\text{T}-\text{T}-\text{C}- \\
\ \ |\quad\ |\quad\ |\quad\ |\quad\ |\quad\ | \\
-\text{C}-\text{T}-\text{T}-\text{A}-\text{A}-\text{G}-
\end{array}
\rightarrow
$$

$$
\begin{array}{c}
-\text{G} \\
| \\
-\text{C}-\text{T}-\text{T}-\text{A}-\text{A}-
\end{array}
+
\begin{array}{c}
-\text{A}-\text{A}-\text{T}-\text{T}-\text{C}- \\
\qquad\qquad\qquad\qquad| \\
\text{G}
\end{array}
$$

The resulting single-stranded ends are attacked by exonucleases that cleave off the A—A—T—T ends,

thus preventing reannealing. Other normal cellular nucleases then degrade the remaining double-stranded DNA.

Since all DNAs have some G—A—A—T—T—C sequences, the bacterial cell must protect its own DNA from degradation by its own restriction endonuclease. Cells do this by enzymatically modifying their DNA. *E. coli* protects itself from EcoRII (Table 9–3) by methylating the first cytosine present in the DNA sequence —mC—C—A—G—G—. EcoRII will not act on —mC—C—A—G—G—. Many bacteria have specific exonucleases and specific modifying enzymes that prevent foreign DNA from invading their cytoplasm.

Viruses counterattack by modifying their own DNA. T₄ bacteriophages use hydroxymethyl cytosine and glucosylated hydroxymethyl cytosine in their DNA. The presence of these nitrogenous bases renders their DNA resistant to most endonucleases. The host-range of a given bacteriophage depends on the ability of its DNA to resist the cell's endonucleases.

Restriction endonucleases are essential for the procedures used in genetic engineering. Genetic engineers use restriction endonucleases to make fragments of DNA that can be incorporated into a plasmid vector (see Chapter 6). Because restriction endonucleases make specific breaks in DNA, they can make reproducible fragments of specific DNA molecules. These DNA fragments are small enough to be sequenced chemically. These techniques were used in determining the complete nucleotide sequence of ϕX174 DNA.

Replication of single-stranded DNA bacteriophages

Viruses with single-stranded DNA are either filamentous (F1) or cubic (ϕX174) viruses. The filamentous bacteriophages attach to the pili of the cell. Either they are pulled into the cytoplasm or their DNA travels down the pilus to the cytoplasm. ϕX174 is a cubic bacteriophage that attaches to the lipopolysaccharide of the outer membrane of E. coli. The single-stranded DNA, accompanied by one of the spikes on the surface of ϕX174, then penetrates into the cell's cytoplasm.

TABLE 9–3
Restriction Endonucleases

Organism	Enzyme	Recognition Sequence
Escherichia coli	EcoRI	—G—A—A—T—T—C— / —C—T—T—A—A—G—
	EcoRII	—N—C—C—A—G—G—N— / —N—G—G—T—C—C—N—
Hemophilus influenzae	Hind II	—G—T—Py—Pu—A—C— / —C—A—Py—Pu—T—G—
	Hind III	—A—A—G—C—T—T— / —T—T—C—G—A—A—

Key: A, adenine; G, guanine; C, cytosine; T, thymine; Py, any pyrimidine; Pu, any purine; N, any nucleotide.

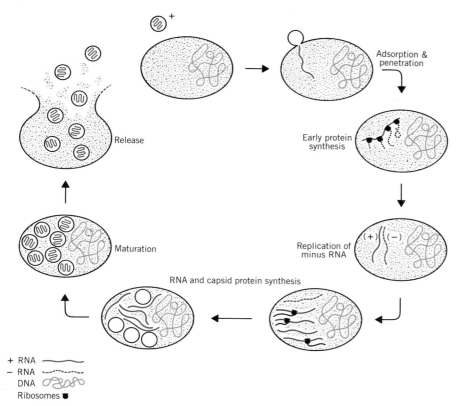

+ RNA ————
− RNA -------------
DNA
Ribosomes

FIGURE 9–17

Replication of a plus RNA bacteriophage. The infective RNA strand (positive strand) is used as a message (mRNA) to make early proteins. These proteins make a replicative (minus RNA) strand that is used as a template to make viral plus RNA.

The entering single-stranded DNA, the plus strand, serves as a template for synthesis of a minus strand. The cell's DNA polymerase is used in this process since no transcription of the plus strand occurs. The resulting double-stranded DNA is the replicative form from which multiple copies of the plus strand are synthesized.

Replication of RNA bacteriophages. RNA bacteriophages are the simplest of the known viruses. The single-stranded RNA viruses contain only three genes and reproduce between 5000 and 10,000 progeny bacteriophages in a 30- to 60-minute replication cycle. These viruses do not have tails, but they ad-sorb specifically to pili on the cell's surface. All RNA bacteriophages except one* contain single-stranded RNA. Since the RNA of single-stranded plus RNA bacteriophages can serve as mRNA, transcription is not a prerequisite to bacteriophage protein synthesis (Figure 9–17). A specific replicase, in conjunction with host-cell translation factors (Tu and TS), replicates the viral plus RNA to form a minus RNA strand. The minus strand then is used to form many plus RNA strands, which combine with coat protein to form infectious virions. RNA bacteriophages can be extruded from the cell without causing cell lysis.

*φ6 infects *Pseudomonas* and is the only known double-stranded RNA bacteriophage.

SUMMARY

Viruses are complex macromolecular forms of life with their own genetic information encoded in either DNA or RNA. The nucleic acid of a virus is either single-stranded or double-stranded, linear or circular. Bacteriophages are classified according to their nucleic acid composition, structure, morphology, size, and shape. They are specific for their host bacterium. Bacteriophages can be counted by determining the number of plaques produced on a lawn of host bacteria.

Progeny bacteriophages are produced within their bacterial host during a lytic cycle. Most DNA bacteriophages adsorb irreversibly to the outer membrane of their host cell and then inject their DNA into its cytoplasm. Viral proteins are translated on the cell's ribosomes using mRNA transcribed from the bacteriophage DNA. The T_4 bacteriophage DNA codes for nucleases, DNA polymerase, synthetic enzymes involved in DNA precursor formation, the bacteriophage structural proteins, lysozyme, and a bacteriophage protein that destroys the cell's membrane. Bacteriophages self-assemble from precursor pools of their constituent components. Progeny virions are released into the environment when the host cell lyses.

Transduction is the phage-mediated transfer of host-cell genes. This occurs by generalized transduction, where any host-cell gene can be transferred, or by specialized transduction, where only certain genes are transferred. Temperate bacteriophages can enter a lytic cycle to produce progeny bacteriophages, or they can become prophages. A prophage exists in a lysogenic bacterium as a sequence of bacteriophage genes that are integrated into the host cell's genome. When defective phage particles are produced, they can carry bacterial genes to their next host cell. Phage conversion is the phenotypic alteration of a bacterium's phenotype caused by the expression of a prophage gene. In both forms of transduction, the phages are defective and do not replicate by a lytic cycle.

Restriction endonucleases are produced by bacterial cells to destroy invading bacteriophage DNA.

Bacteriophages respond by chemically modifying their DNA to make it resistant to the endonucleases. The host range of a given bacteriophage depends on the ability of its DNA to resist the endonucleases made by that host. Restriction endonucleases are used for genetic engineering.

Nontailed RNA bacteriophages infect host cells by attaching to a cell's pilus. The nucleic acid or the entire virion is transposed down the pilus into the cytoplasm, where it replicates. The nucleic acid of most single-stranded RNA viruses serves as the mRNA for protein synthesis. Using this plus RNA strand, a viral RNA polymerase makes a minus RNA strand that is used to replicate more viral RNA.

QUESTIONS AND TOPICS FOR STUDY AND DISCUSSION

Questions

1. Why were bacteriophages important to the development of virology? Explain.
2. Describe the plaque method for counting bacteriophages. How can this technique be adapted to count plant and animal viruses?
3. Compare the biology of bacteriophage reproduction to the multiplication of a bacterium.
4. Define or explain the following.

lytic cycle	generalized transduction
burst size	temperate bacteriophage
eclipse period	viral induction
adsorption	lysogeny
specialized transduction	phage conversion

5. What is the function of the lambda repressor in lysogeny?
6. Why do bacteria produce restriction endonuclease?
7. What special problems are encountered by single-stranded RNA and single-stranded DNA bacteriophages during their replication cycle?
8. What mechanisms are used by bacteriophages to infect their host cells?

Discussion

1. Felix d'Herelle envisioned using bacteriophages to treat and cure patients with infectious bacterial diseases.

Discuss why this has not come to be. Are there reasons why viruses were discovered when they were?

2. What is the impact of the molecular biology of lysogeny on human health?

FURTHER READINGS

Books

Cairns, J., G. S. Stent, and J. Watson, *Phage and the Origins of Molecular Biology: Essays,* Cold Spring Harbor Symposium, Cold Spring Harbor, N.Y., 1966. A collection of articles about the beginnings of molecular biology as told by the scientists who participated in its development.

Luria, S. E., J. E. Darnell Jr., D. Baltimore, and A. Campbell, *General Virology,* 3rd ed., Wiley, New York, 1978. An advanced, detailed textbook that covers all groups of viruses.

Stent, G. S., *Molecular Biology of Bacterial Viruses,* Freeman, San Francisco, 1963. A well-written introduction to the bacteriophages that approaches the subject from a historical perspective.

Watson, J. D., *The Molecular Biology of the Gene,* 3rd ed., Benjamin, California, 1976. One of the best textbooks on the molecular aspects of biological systems. This book covers the molecular biology of viruses, bacteria, and eucaryotic cells.

Articles and Reviews

Duckworth, D. H., "Who Discovered Bacteriophages?" *Bacteriol. Revs.,* 40:793–802 (1976). An interesting essay on the roles of Twort and d'Herelle in the discovery of bacteriophages.

Fenner, F., "The Classification of Viruses: Why, When, and How," *Austral. J. Exp. Bio. Med. Sci.,* 52:223–240 (1974). A description of the beginnings of the International Committee on Nomenclature of Viruses (ICNV) and the status of the classification of viruses at the committee's inception.

Fiddes, J. C., "The Nucleotide Sequence of a Viral DNA," *Sci. Am.,* 237:54–67 (December 1977). The discovery of overlapping genes in the genome of ϕX174 is described together with the complete nucleotide sequence of this single-stranded DNA bacteriophage.

Maniatis, T., and M. Ptashne, "A DNA Operon-repressor System," *Sci. Am.,* 234:64–76 (January 1976). A detailed description of the lambda bacteriophage repressor system.

Studier, W. F., "Bacteriophage T_7," *Science,* 176:367–375 (1972). A review of the genetics and the biochemistry of this *E. coli* bacteriophage.

10

CONTROL OF MICROORGANISMS

Many microbes are detrimental to human welfare. The destructive effects of these microbes can be controlled by killing them or by preventing their growth. Microbiologists have developed chemical and physical techniques that are widely used to control microorganisms. Many toxic chemicals kill microbes, but they are also toxic to humans and are therefore used only on fomites (inanimate objects). Other chemicals have selective toxicity against microorganisms. Physical techniques of controlling microorganisms also have their advantages and disadvantages. This chapter describes the appropriate use of the physical and chemical techniques for controlling the detrimental effects of microorganisms.

KILLING MICROBES

Microbiologists use the word **sterile** to describe an object or place that is devoid of all life including microbes, spores, and viruses. **Sterilization** is the process used to free completely a substance or object of all living things. A flask or a tube of media can be sterilized by heating it at an appropriate temperature for an appropriate period of time. Aseptic techniques can then be used to inoculate this sterile medium. Microbiologists use the term **aseptic** to mean in the absence of contaminating organisms and/or infectious agents.

The control of microorganisms can be accomplished by physically removing them, by killing them, or by preventing their growth and reproduction. **Bacteriostatic** agents, such as the antibiotic tetracycline, prevent bacterial growth (Figure 10–1) without killing them. In contrast, penicillin causes the lysis of growing cells of susceptible bacteria, so it is called a **bacteriolytic** antibiotic. Methods of killing bacteria other than cell lysis are referred to as **bactericidal** (Figure 10–1). Killing in this sense is the irreversible loss of the ability of the cell to reproduce.

Theory of sterilization

Practical sterilization procedures are devised to assure that the probability of a single cell surviving the process is infinitesimally small. Cells die exponentially (Figure 10–2) during sterilization; they do not all die at once. The logarithm of the number of surviving bacteria per milliliter is a straight-line function of the duration of exposure to a lethal agent. This

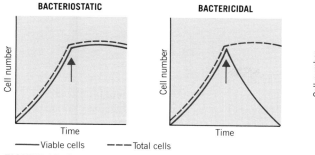
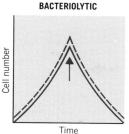

FIGURE 10–1

The growth of bacterial cultures can be inhibited by agents that prevent growth (bacteriostatic), that kill the cells (bactericidal), or that lyse the cells (bacteriolytic). The solid line indicates viable cells; the dashed line indicates total cells.

means that the majority of the cells die quickly, but that some cells are more resistant, so they survive. Each cell population is heterogeneous because it contains cells with different levels of resistance to the lethal agent.

Organisms also vary in their resistance to a given lethal agent. Culture A in Figure 10–2 is more resistant to the lethal agent than is culture B. Culture B dies at a faster rate, so that less time is required to

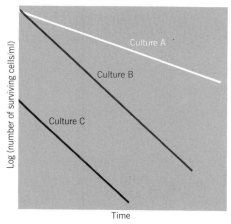

FIGURE 10–2

Death curves for three cultures exposed to a lethal agent. Culture B is more sensitive to the agent than is culture A. Culture C is killed at the same rate as culture B, but it reaches zero survivors more quickly because there are fewer organisms at zero time.

sterilize this culture. The time required to sterilize a culture is dependent on the number of organisms in the initial culture. Cultures B and C are both killed at the same rate (the slopes of the lines are equal), but culture C starts with fewer organisms, so it reaches a value of zero survivors/ml in a shorter time than does culture B.

PHYSICAL METHODS OF CONTROL

Microorganisms and viruses can be killed by heat or radiation; or they can be physically removed by filtration (Table 10–1). High temperatures inactivate proteins and nucleic acids by breaking their hydrogen bonds. This results in the unfolding of proteins and the separation of double-stranded nucleic acids. Radiation kills cells by causing chemical changes to the nitrogenous bases in their nucleic acids. Filtration does not kill, but it does remove cellular organisms from the solution that is filtered (Table 10–1).

Killing with heat

Organisms and viruses are susceptible to killing by heat. Heat is the most widely used method of sterilization; however its use is limited to heat-resistant materials. Plastics, clothing and gowns, liquids, and many organic substances (including vaccines and drugs) cannot be sterilized by heat because they decompose at high temperatures. The temperature, duration, and humidity are important parameters of

TABLE 10-1
Physical Methods of Control

Treatment	Conditions	Uses	Disadvantages
Heat			
Dry heat	160°C, 2 hr	Sterilization of laboratory glassware	High temperatures; charring organic materials
Moist heat	121°C, 15 min, 15 lb pressure	Sterilization of liquid organic compounds	Limited volume; expensive equipment
Incineration		Destruction of contaminated animals	Ash conversion
Pasteurization	62–66°C, 30 min	Destruction of pathogens in milk, beer, wine; increases shelf life	Sterilization not possible
Filtration		Decontamination of liquids and air	Viscosity; virus removal not possible
Radiation			
Ultraviolet		Decontamination of air, other gases, and surfaces	Penetration through glass not possible; danger to eyes
Gamma rays		Food preservation	Danger to humans

heat sterilization. A standard criterion for testing the ability of heat to sterilize a substance is the survivability of the endospores of *Clostridium* or *Bacillus*. These spores are among the most heat-resistant forms of life known.

Dry heat generated by an electric or a gas oven will kill spores if they are exposed for 2 hours at 160°C. The length of this procedure is necessary to kill all the spores, even though the vegetative cells of the same organism will die within the first few minutes. One disadvantage of dry heat sterilization is that organic compounds will char at this temperature. Moreover, liquid media cannot be heated to 121°C without undergoing excessive evaporation. These problems are solved by sterilizing liquids and organic compounds with moist heat in a pressurized autoclave.

Moist heat is more effective than dry heat in killing clostridial spores. Hydrated macromolecules are very sensitive to temperatures above 100°C (boiling water). These temperatures are generated with pressurized steam. An **autoclave** (Figure 10-3) is an industrial pressure cooker with a large pressure chamber for sterilizing. The steam (at 15 lb/in^2) in an autoclave chamber produces a temperature of 121°C, which is sufficient to kill clostridial spores in 2 minutes. The duration of heating must be increased if the spores are contained in a liquid, to allow time for the solution to reach 121°C. The normal sterilization time for an autoclave, fully loaded with test tubes, is 12 to 15 minutes at 121°C. This time is increased to sterilize flasks containing 500 ml or more of liquid.

Moist heat is widely used to sterilize microbiological media and glassware. Most autoclaves have an exhaust and dry cycle to dry glassware and pipets after sterilizing them. A normal autoclave cycle (pressure build-up, sterilization, exhaust) takes between 30 minutes and 1 hour.

Pasteurization. Food left in its natural state often spoils because of the actions of contaminating microorganisms. Before the widespread availability of refrigeration, food spoilage was a major problem. Milk often spoiled within a day or two and wines turned bad as often as not.

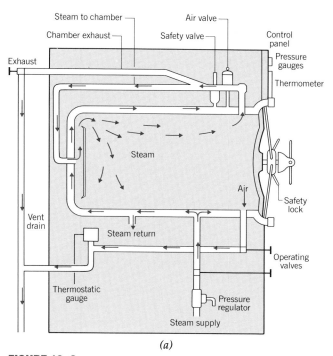

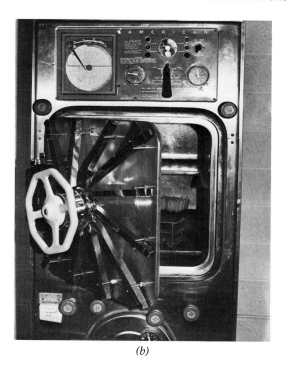

FIGURE 10–3

(a) Diagrammatic representation of a steam autoclave (side view) and (b) a photograph of a functional autoclave.

Louis Pasteur discovered the technique of heating a food just enough to preserve it without altering its composition. This is now known as **pasteurization** and is an ideal means of preserving milk. Milk contains butterfat and proteins that cannot stand excessive heat. When milk is heated at 62 to 66°C for 30 minutes and then quickly cooled, a great majority of the contaminating microbes are killed without precipitating the proteins. A newer technique, **flash pasteurization,** rapidly heats milk to 71.7°C, maintains it at this temperature for at least 15 seconds, and then rapidly cools it.

The U.S. Public Health Service establishes the conditions for pasteurizing milk based on the time and temperature required to kill *Coxiella burnetii.* This organism is the causative agent of Q fever and is the most heat-resistant pathogen found in milk. Pasteurization is designed to kill all the pathogens in milk and enough of the other milk microbes to ex-

tend its refrigeration shelf life. The shelf life of wine and beer can also be extended by pasteurization.

Incineration is the ultimate means of destroying life. Small laboratory animals used in the study of infectious disease are routinely destroyed by incineration. This is also an appropriate means of destroying burnable laboratory wastes.

Radiation

The emission and propagation of energy through space or through a substance in the form of waves is called **radiation.** The energy content of the different forms of radiation is dependent on the wave frequency (Figure 10–4). Each wave has electromagnetic properties and is composed either of particles or of light energy measured as a photon.

Cosmic rays, alpha rays, and beta rays are particulate forms of radiant energy. Alpha rays and beta rays are emitted from radioactive atoms that are in the act of decaying. These two electromagnetic waves have sufficient energy to penetrate solid substances, so they must be contained to prevent damage to humans. Gamma rays and X rays (Figure 10–4) are electromagnetic waves that are generated as a pulse of electromagnetic energy called a **photon**. The amount of energy in an electromagnetic wave is a product of its frequency (f) times Planck's constant (h). Gamma rays have higher frequencies than X rays and so possess more energy. Gamma rays are generated by the decay of radioactive compounds such as cobalt 60; X rays are generated by a combination of heat and electrical energy.

Ultraviolet radiation (Figure 10–4) is the spectrum of electromagnetic waves having longer wavelengths (shorter frequencies) than X rays, but having shorter wavelengths than visible light. Ultraviolet (UV) radiation can be generated by passing electrical current through vapors of mercury (black light). UV light is a low-energy, low-frequency radiation that is readily absorbed by glass and water. Even though ultraviolet light is produced naturally by the sun, most of it is absorbed by the ozone layers of the earth's atmosphere and does not reach the earth's surface.

Gamma radiation. Gamma radiation can be used to preserve foods and to sterilize specialized material. Its use requires special precautions because gamma radiation can seriously injure humans. Irradiation with gamma rays emitted from cobalt 60 is used in medicine to kill cancerous cells. Gamma radiation has applications in both experimental and therapeutic work. It ionizes chemicals to form free radicals and kills in the same manner that X rays do.

X rays. X rays penetrate tissue and are used in diagnostic medicine. An X-ray photograph is taken by placing a photographic emulsion behind a patient and then exposing the patient to a source of X rays. The X-ray photons penetrate the tissue and expose the photographic film.

FIGURE 10–4
The electromagnetic spectrum. The amount of energy in a given electromagnetic wave is directly proportional to its frequency. Visible light is only a small part of the electromagnetic spectrum.

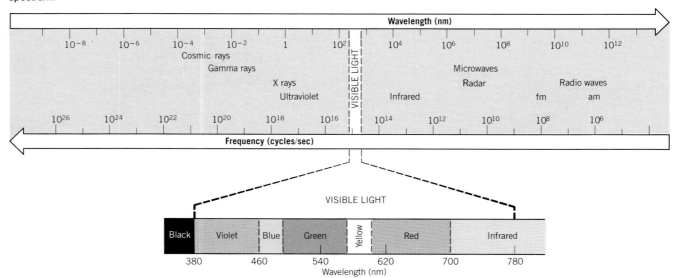

Not all the energy in the X-ray beam will pass through the body tissue. Some of the energy will be absorbed by atoms and will cause them to become ions through the gain or loss of electrons. Radiation that causes this to happen is called **ionizing radiation**. The process of ionization forms free radicals. Both X rays and gamma rays are forms of ionizing radiation. The hydroxyl radical (·OH) is the predominant radical formed when aqueous solutions are exposed to ionizing radiations. These free radicals react with many cellular proteins and nucleic acids and result in chemical alterations that can kill the cell. Ionizing radiation usually kills a cell when a free radical reacts with and chemically alters the cell's DNA.

Endospores are much more resistant to ionizing radiation than are their vegetative counterparts. This resistance may be a direct result of the low water content in endospores. Among the nonsporing bacteria, pseudomonads are very sensitive to radiation, whereas some *Micrococcus* and *Streptococcus* species are more resistant. Resistance in this instance may be due to the presence of free-radical scavengers such as sulfhydryl groups (R-SH).

Gamma radiation and X-ray radiation have limited use in generalized sterilization procedures because of the potential hazards they pose to humans. Cosmic rays are natural forms of ionizing radiation. The amount of cosmic radiation that reaches the earth is so small that it does not visibly affect the biological world.

Ultraviolet light. Light with wavelengths between 100 and 400 nm is termed ultraviolet (UV) light (Figure 10–4). Nucleic acids absorb ultraviolet light between the wavelengths of 250 and 270 nm. Ultraviolet light damages cells by disrupting hydrogen bonding and by causing chemical changes in nucleic acids. Structural changes in DNA lead to copying errors and thus increase the probability for the occurrence of a lethal mutation. By varying the dosage of UV irradiation, it can be used to produce nonlethal mutations in bacteria or to kill them.

UV light has limited application as a physical sterilizing agent because it is absorbed by glass and by water. It is used to sterilize exposed surfaces and air, particularly in microbial transfer rooms and in operating rooms. UV light is used cautiously because direct exposure can cause damage to the human eyes.

Filtration

Bacteria and eucaryotes can be removed from liquids and gases by filtration. Filters are made from natural substances, such as cellulose and diatomaceous earth, or they are manufactured from chemical polymers. The filters (Figure 10–5) retain the bacteria that are adsorbed to the filter material or are sucked into blind passages. Membrane filters of polycarbonate and cellulose acetate can be made with specific pore sizes that range from 8.0 μm to less than 0.05 μm. Most bacteria are retained by filters with a pore size of 0.45 μm; however, some of the spirochetes, which are very thin bacteria, can pass through filters with a pore size as small as 0.22 μm. Viruses are not usually retained by membrane filters. Some viruses are so small that they pass through filters with the smallest pores made. The inability of filtration to remove all viruses limits its use in sterilization.

Filtration of liquids is performed with sterile filters (Figure 10–6), using vacuum pressure to pull the liq-

FIGURE 10–5

Scanning electron micrograph of raw sewage collected on a membrane filter (10,000×). (Courtesy of Dr. A. M. Crundell.)

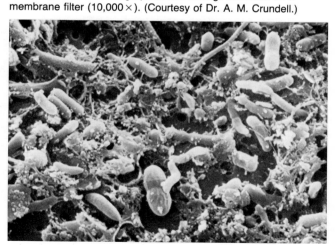

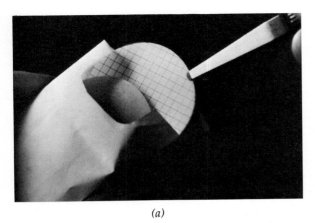

(a)

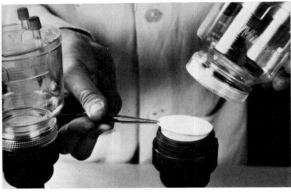

(b)

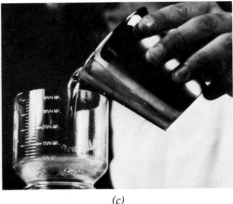

(c)

FIGURE 10–6
Membrane filtration can be used to remove microbes from liquids. (a) The sterile membrane is removed with sterile forceps and (b) is placed on the manifold. (c) The sample is then filtered under vacuum. (Courtesy of Millipore AV Services, Bedford, MA.)

uid through the filter. The filtrate is considered free of bacterial contaminants if a 0.22 μm filter is used and if the filtrate is collected in a sterile container. Filtration is used to remove microorganisms from solutions of heat-sensitive compounds and from gases. A practical problem of filtration is that the flow rate decreases with increasing viscosity of the solution and with decreasing pore size of the filter. Slow flow rates limit the volume of material that can be conveniently filtered.

Filtration techniques have been developed for use in determining the presence of bacteria in large volumes of air and water. Bacteria are collected on a filter that is placed on an appropriate growth medium (Figure 10–7). The number of colonies that grow is used to evaluate the environmental population of microbes.

CHEMICAL METHODS OF CONTROL

Various chemicals with diverse properties are used to control microorganisms. Chemicals that attack specific cells include the naturally produced antibiotics and the manufactured chemotherapeutic drugs. Chemicals that are nonselective for the cells they affect are termed disinfectants. A **disinfectant** is a

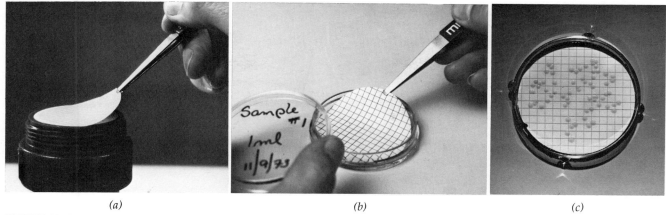

(a)   *(b)*   *(c)*

FIGURE 10–7
Bacteria retained on a membrane filter will grow into colonies when placed on a suitable
growth medium. (*a*) Removal of the filter membrane, (*b*) laying filter membrane on petri dish,
and (*c*) colonies growing on the membrane after incubation. (*a* and *b*, Courtesy of Millipore
AV Services, Bedford, MA., *c*, courtesy of Gelman Scientific, photo by Stanley Livingston.)

chemical that will inhibit the growth of or destroy an organism (but not necessarily their spores). The term disinfectant is usually restricted to those compounds or preparations that are caustic to humans. **Antiseptics** are a class of compounds that are able to destroy microorganisms capable of causing contamination or disease and are suitable for use on human beings.

Nonselective chemicals

Humans have many special needs for controlling microorganisms, and they have developed chemical disinfectants to meet special applications. The commercial criteria for selecting a chemical disinfectant are: (1) the compound must be an effective killer of microorganisms and, if possible, of viruses; (2) the compound should be soluble in water for ease of preparation and application; (3) the compound should have a low toxicity for humans; and (4) the compound should be available at a reasonable cost. Compounds that meet these criteria are listed by the chemical group to which they belong (Table 10–2).

Alcohols. Ethanol, isopropanol, and benzyl alcohol are organic alcohols (RCH_2OH) that are effective antiseptics when applied as 50- to 70-percent aqueous solutions. Alcohols precipitate proteins and solubilize lipids present in the cell walls and cell membranes of bacteria. They are used as antiseptics on human skin either individually or in combination with a halogen such as iodine. Alcohols effectively kill vegetative cells, but they are not effective against spores and some viruses.

Halogens. **Iodine** is a halogen that is an effective antiseptic, especially when solubilized in 70 percent ethanol. Iodine inactivates proteins and organic molecules by reacting with hydroxyl groups. This halogen is used extensively to treat cuts and abrasions of the human skin.

Chlorine gas is a halogen disinfectant that reacts with water to form hypochlorous acid (HClO).

$$Cl_2 + H_2O \rightarrow HCl + HClO$$

The hypochlorous acid formed reacts with water to form HCl and hydrogen peroxide (H_2O_2). Both hypochlorous acid and hydrogen peroxide are strong oxidants. Chlorine gas is used to decontaminate large amounts of water. Household bleach is another source of hypochlorous acid (contains 5.25% sodium hypochlorite) that can be used as a disinfectant on surfaces that will withstand bleaching.

TABLE 10–2
Antiseptics and Disinfectants

Class of Compounds	Action	Uses	Disadvantages
Alcohols Ethanol, isopropanol, benzyl alcohol (50–70% aqueous solutions)	Denature protein and solubilize lipids	Antiseptic used on skin	Not effective against spores and some viruses
Aldehydes Formaldehyde (8% solution), glutaraldehyde (2% solution)	Alkylates, reacts with —NH_2, —SH, and —COOH	Effective disinfectants, sporicides	Toxic to humans
Halogens Iodine (I_2) as tincture of iodine (2% in 70% alcohol)	Inactivates proteins (reacts with tyrosine)	Antiseptic used on skin, iodophores are nonstaining	
Chlorine (Cl_2) gas in neutral or acidic aqueous solutions	Reacts with water to make hypochlorous acid (HClO), strong oxidizing agent	Used to purify water, disinfectant in food industry	May react with water impurities to form toxic compounds
Heavy Metals Copper sulfate ($CuSO_4$)	Prevents growth of algae and fungi	Algaicide and fungicide	
Silver nitrate ($AgNO_3$)	Precipitates proteins	Antiseptic used in the eyes of newborns	Neutralized by organic compounds
Mercuric chloride ($HgCl_2$)	Inactivates proteins (reacts with —SH)	Disinfectant	Poisonous in high concentrations, inactivates organic compounds
Gases Sulfur dioxide (SO_2)	Reacts with many cell components	Food additive, especially to fruit juices	
Ethylene oxide (H_2C——CH_2) with O bridge	Alkylates	Used to sterilize heat-sensitive objects (i.e., plastics), sporicidal	
Propylene oxide (H_2C——CH_2——CH_3) with O bridge	Alkylates	Substitute for ethylene oxide, sporicidal	
Cationic Detergents Quaternary ammonium compounds with a long chain alkyl group	Disruption of the cell membrane	Skin antiseptics and disinfectants	Inactivated by metal ions, low pH, organic material, and phospholipids
Phenols Phenol, carbolic acid and derivatives, lysol, hexylresorcinol, hexachlorophene	Denature proteins and disrupt cell membranes	Disinfectant at high concentrations, used in soaps at low concentrations	Very toxic to human tissue

Aldehydes. Formaldehyde and glutaraldehyde are alkylating agents that kill microbes by reacting with the replaceable hydrogen atoms on organic compounds. Cellular targets include amines ($-NH_2$), sulfhydryl ($-SH$), and carboxyl ($-COOH$) groups of proteins and small organic molecules. **Formaldehyde** is an effective disinfectant when used as an 8 percent solution, and **glutaraldehyde** is a useful disinfectant when present in a 2-percent solution. Both of these aldehydes have limited application because they give off noxious vapors.

Heavy metals. Copper, mercury, and silver are heavy metals that are effective in killing microbes. **Silver nitrate** ($AgNO_3$) was used as eye drops for newborn infants to prevent infections by *Neisseria gonorrhoeae*. **Copper sulfate** ($CuSO_4$) is widely used as an algaecide, and mercuric compounds are used as disinfectants. Copper sulfate is toxic to the photosynthetic systems of algae and is used in marine bottom paints to prevent the attachment of fouling organisms (mussels and barnacles). The toxicity of heavy metals is due to their ability to precipitate proteins and organic molecules.

Lead, arsenic, and mercury are not widely used as disinfectants because they are concentrated by the human body and can cause long-term disorders. Mercury is added to ointments and solutions used in the topical treatment of skin infections. Mercurochrome is an organic mercury bromide compound that is widely used as an antiseptic.

Gases. **Sulfur dioxide** (SO_2) was the first gas to be used as a disinfectant. Sulfur was burned to disinfect houses and wine casks in ancient Greece. Sulfur dioxide is still used today as a food preservative.

The extensive use of plastics in microbiology and in hospitals has expanded the application of gases as sterilizing agents. **Ethylene oxide** (Table 10–2) is a gas that is effectively used as a sterilizing agent. Plastic petri dishes, tubes, pipets, and syringes are sterilized with ethylene oxide in a pressurized chamber that has controls for temperature and humidity. Ethylene oxide is a sporicide that readily penetrates packaged material. **Propylene oxide** is another sporicidal gas that can be used as a substitute for ethylene oxide.

Cationic detergents. Quaternary ammonium compounds have a low toxicity for mammalian tissue and are bacteriocidal. These compounds are cationic detergents that kill cells by disrupting their cytoplasmic membranes. They are used for preparing the vagina and other sensitive mucous membrane structures for surgery. Each cationic detergent has four groups (Figure 10–8) attached to a nitrogen atom. One of these groups is a long chain alkyl group that interacts with the membrane lipids. Cationic detergents are inactivated by low pH, phospholipids, organic compounds, and metal ions.

Phenols. Phenolic compounds and their substituted derivatives are extremely effective disinfectants. Low concentrations of phenol derivatives are used as antiseptics. Phenols function by denaturing proteins and by disrupting cell membranes. Although phenol itself is no longer used as a disinfectant, phenol derivatives such as carbolic acid and lysol are. **Hexachlorophene** is another phenol derivative that effectively kills staphylococci at concentrations as low as one part per million. Hexachlorophene was once widely used as an antiseptic, but now it is available only with a prescription because it is quickly absorbed through the skin and has been known to cause brain damage in infants.

Many disinfectants and antiseptics are sold commercially in the consumers' market. Hydrogen peroxide, mouthwashes, soaps, creams, and face wash pads contain antiseptic substances and are sold directly to the public. Disinfectants are also sold for the kitchen, bathroom, garbage cans, and other potentially infested areas. These commercial disinfectants and antiseptics are pleasant to use, are conveniently packaged, and have become a part of the contemporary way of life.

Selective chemicals

Antibiotics and some chemical drugs are selective in their ability to kill or inhibit the growth of a specific

(a) Quaternary ammonium compounds

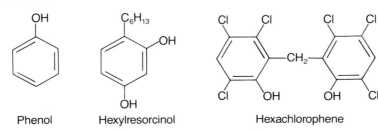

General formula   Ceepryn®

Roccal®

R represents a mixture
of alkyls from
C_8H_{17} to $C_{18}H_{37}$

(b) Phenols

Phenol   Hexylresorcinol   Hexachlorophene

FIGURE 10–8
Quaternary ammonium compounds and phenols are used as disinfectants at
high concentrations and as antiseptics at low concentrations.

cell type. Many of these substances are used to treat infectious diseases in humans because they have a low toxicity for human cells but a high toxicity for the infectious agent. **Chemotherapeutic drugs** are chemicals that are used to treat infectious disease. **Antibiotics** are substances synthesized by one organism that kill or inhibit the growth of another organism. Some antibiotics are extremely effective chemotherapeutic drugs, whereas other antibiotics are too toxic for humans and animals.

To be an effective drug, an antimicrobial chemotherapeutic agent must have properties in addition to its killing ability. The **efficacy** of a drug is the combination of qualities a compound possesses that contribute to its value as a chemotherapeutic agent. These qualities include stability in vivo, rate of absorption, rate of elimination, and penetration to the infected site. A low rating in one area can sometimes be bypassed. For example, streptomycin is inactivated by the low pH of the stomach, but this can be bypassed by injecting this antibiotic. Other drugs have been chemically modified to bypass problem areas. Penicillin G is sensitive to the pH of the stomach, so chemists have modified it by producing the acid-stable antibiotic ampicillin.

The **therapeutic index** is the ratio of the minimum dose of the drug that is toxic to the host divided by the minimum dose required for antimicrobial activity. The higher the ratio, the greater is the efficacy of the drug. Part of this index depends on the ability of the drug to be absorbed by the host animal. The level of a drug in the blood (Figure 10–9) depends on the dose of the drug, the host's body weight, the route of administration, the schedule of medications, and the rate of elimination of the drug by the host. The efficacy of a drug depends on the complex interaction between the host, the drug, and the invading microbe.

Discovery of antibiotics

Alexander Fleming described his accidental discovery of the first antibiotic in his initial (1929) report on penicillin. Fleming was a Scottish physician interested in staphylococcal variants. To select for these variants (mutants), he kept his culture plates for an extended period of time. One plate became contaminated with a mold. The staphylococcal colonies that were growing around this mold colony gradually became transparent because of cell lysis. He identified the mold as *Pencillium* and named the bacteriolytic substance produced by the mold *penicillin*.

Penicillin was first produced in large quantities and used to treat infectious diseases of humans in the early 1940s. Howard Florey headed a group of investigators at Oxford University (England) who developed the techniques for producing penicillin in commercial quantities and for testing the antimicrobial activity of penicillin. Penicillin was found to be extremely effective against Gram-positive bacteria. By the end of World War II, it was used extensively for treating infectious diseases in both the military and the civilian populations.

Production of antibiotics by microorganisms. Most of the effective antibiotics were discovered between 1940 and 1959 and are produced by a limited number of organisms. Bacteria that produce antibiotics are members of either the genus *Bacillus* or *Streptomyces* (Table 10–3). In addition, certain fungi belonging to the genera *Aspergillus*, *Cephalosporium*, and *Penicillium* also produce antibiotics. Some of

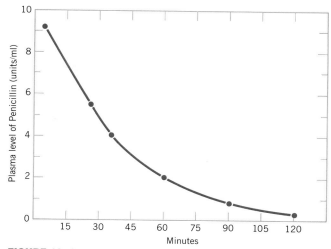

FIGURE 10–9

Blood concentration of penicillin G in an 18-kilogram dog following the intravenous administration of 50,000 units. (Courtesy of the American Physiology Society. Adapted from *American J. Physiol.*, 166:625–640, 1951.)

these antibiotics are effective against bacteria, some against fungi, and some against protozoa.

Antibiotics function by being bactericidal or bacteriostatic. Bacteriostatic antibiotics, which prevent the growth of the organism, include antibiotics that prevent protein synthesis. Bactericidal antibiotics actually kill the bacteria. Penicillin kills growing cells by preventing the synthesis of the cell wall, which in turn results in the loss of cellular integrity that leads to cell lysis. A given antibiotic may be most effective against a single group of organisms, or it

TABLE 10–3

Microorganisms that Produce Antibiotics

Group	Microorganism	Characteristics
Bacteria	*Bacillus* sp.	Aerobic, spore-forming
	Streptomyces sp.	Filamentous, found in soil
Fungi	*Penicillium* sp.	Aerobic
	Cephalosporium sp.	Marine
	Aspergillus sp.	Aerobic

TABLE 10–4
Antibiotics and Their Antibiotic Activities

Gram-positive Bacteria	Gram-negative Bacteria
Bacitracin	Neomycin
Cephalosporin	Penicillin (some)
Erythromycin	Polymyxin
Lincomycin	Streptomycin
Neomycin	Vanomycin
Novobiocin	
Penicillin	
Streptomycin	
Vancomycin	
Mycobacterium	**Many Bacteria (Broad Spectrum)**
Cycloserine	Chloramphenicol
Neomycin	Kanamycin
Streptomycin	Streptomycin
	Tetracycline
Protozoa	**Fungi**
Fumagillin	Amphotericin B
Quinine	Cycloheximide
	Griseofulvin
	Nystatin

can be effective against many different organisms (Table 10–4). **Broad-spectrum antibiotics** are active against both Gram-negative and Gram-positive bacteria and include kanamycin, chloroamphenicol, and tetracycline. The mode of action of the major antibiotics is listed in Table 10–5.

Inhibitors of cell-wall synthesis

Penicillins. The first antibiotic to be used effectively to treat systemic bacterial diseases was penicillin G. This antibiotic is produced by species of *Penicillium* and is primarily effective against Gram-positive bacteria. Penicillins are also effective against a limited number of Gram-negative organisms, such as *Neisseria*.

Penicillins either are synthesized naturally or are produced by chemically modified penicillanic acid

(Figure 10–10). The naturally produced penicillin G has the disadvantages of being inactivated by penicillinase (β-lactamase) and by the acid pH of the human stomach. Penicillin-resistant bacteria produce penicillinase, which breaks the β-lactam ring. Chemical modifications of penicillanic acid have resulted in penicillins that are resistant to both acid pHs and penicillinase. The modified penicillins include penicillin V, oxacillin, and ampicillin, which are acid resistant; and methicillin and oxacillin, which are resistant to penicillinase (Figure 10–10).

Penicillins inhibit the transpeptidase that synthesizes the peptide bridges of the peptidoglycan component of bacterial cell walls. Penicillins kill only growing cells. Inhibition of cell-wall formation in growing cells causes the cell to lose its cell-wall rigidity, making it vulnerable to osmotic pressure. Penicillin is a bacteriolytic agent that destroys the integrity of the cell wall, causing the cell to burst from osmotic pressure.

Penicillins have a high therapeutic index and can be taken orally as capsules or in liquid preparations. The liquid preparations are convenient for infants, but they should not be kept for long periods since penicillins are relatively unstable in aqueous solutions. Penicillins have a low toxicity for humans except for a small number of individuals who are allergic to them. Erythromycin can often be given to patients as a substitute for penicillin.

Cephalosporins. Marine fungi belonging to the genus *Cephalosporium* produce cephalosporins, which are similar to penicillins in that they have a β-lactam ring, can be chemically modified to produce special antibiotics (Figure 10–11), and can inhibit bacterial cell-wall synthesis. Cephalosporins are effective against both Gram-positive and Gram-negative bacteria. The β-lactam ring of cephalosporins can be cleaved by the enzyme cephalosporinase, which is produced by resistant bacteria. These antibiotics can be administered to penicillin-sensitive patients.

TABLE 10–5
Antibiotics: Their Source and Mode of Action

Antibiotic	Source	Mode of Action
Antibacterial Antibiotics		
Bacitracin	*Bacillus subtilis*	Cell-wall synthesis
Cephalosporin	*Cephalosporium* sp.	Cell-wall synthesis
Chloramphenicol	*Streptomyces venezuelae*	Protein synthesis
Cycloserine	*Streptomyces orchidaceous*	Cell-wall synthesis
	Streptomyces lavendulae	
Erythromycin	*Streptomyces erythraeus*	Protein synthesis
Kanamycin	*Streptomyces kanomyceticus*	Protein synthesis
Lincomycin	*Streptomyces lincolnensis*	Protein synthesis
Neomycin	*Streptomyces fradiae*	Protein synthesis
Novobiocin	*Streptomyces* sp.	DNA synthesis
Penicillin	*Penicillium* sp.	Cell-wall synthesis
Polymyxin	*Bacillus polymyxa*	Cell membrane
Streptomycin	*Streptomyces griseus*	Protein synthesis
Tetracycline	*Streptomyces aureofaciens*	Protein synthesis
Vancomycin	*Streptomyces orientalis*	Cell-wall synthesis
Antifungal Antibiotics		
Amphotericin B	*Streptomyces nodosus*	Membrane function
Cycloheximide	*Streptomyces griseus*	Protein synthesis
Griseofulvin	*Penicillium griseofulvum*	Cell wall, microtubules
Nystatin	*Streptomyces noursei*	Damages cell membranes
Antiprotozoan Antibiotics		
Fumagillin	*Aspergillus fumigatus*	Protein synthesis
Quinine	Cinchona bark	Unknown

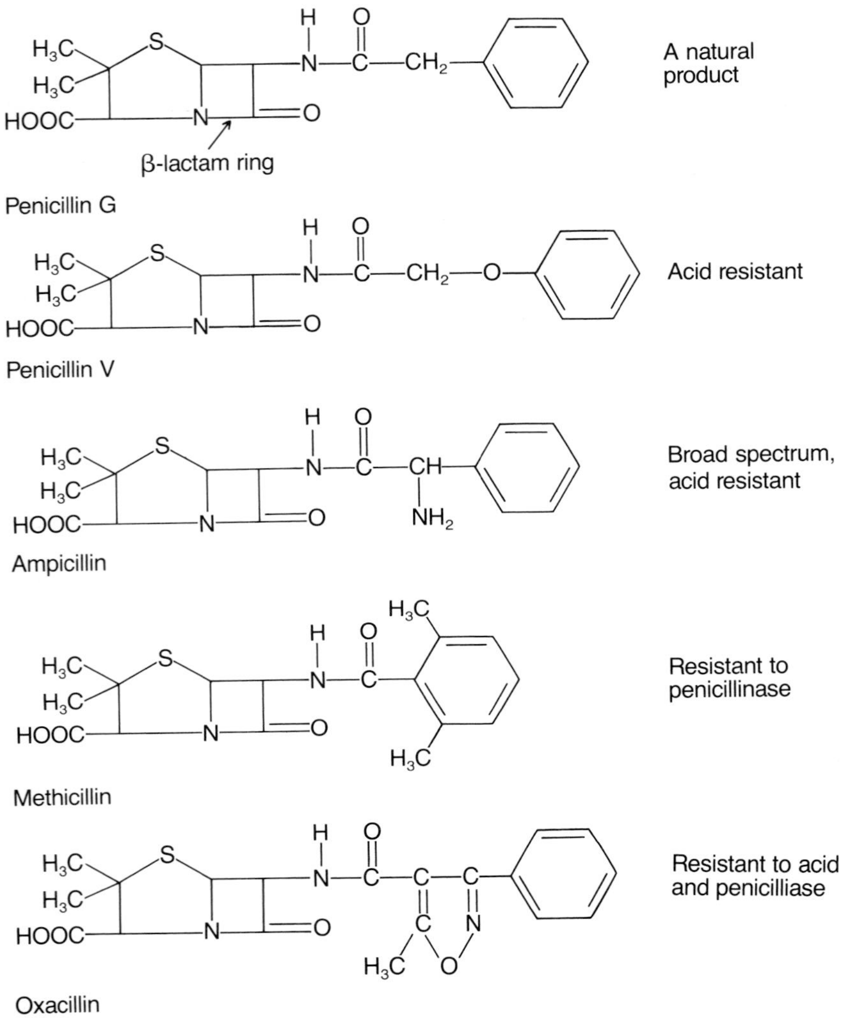

FIGURE 10-10
Structure of the penicillins that act by inhibiting cell-wall synthesis.

Other antibiotics that inhibit cell-wall synthesis.
Cycloserine and vancomycin are antibiotics produced by species of *Streptomyces* that inhibit cell-wall synthesis (Table 10–5). **Cycloserine** interferes with the production of D-alanine and its incorporation into the interpeptide bridges of the peptidoglycan molecule. **Vancomycin** is also produced by *Streptomyces* sp. and inhibits the formation of the peptide

of the peptidoglycan molecule. These antibiotics are effective against Gram-positive bacteria.

Bacitracin is a peptide antibiotic produced by *Bacillus subtilis*. The antibiotic-producing strain was isolated from the dirt in a wound suffered by a girl named Tracy and was thus named bacitracin. This antibiotic prevents peptidoglycan synthesis. It has a relatively high toxicity for humans and is poorly ab-

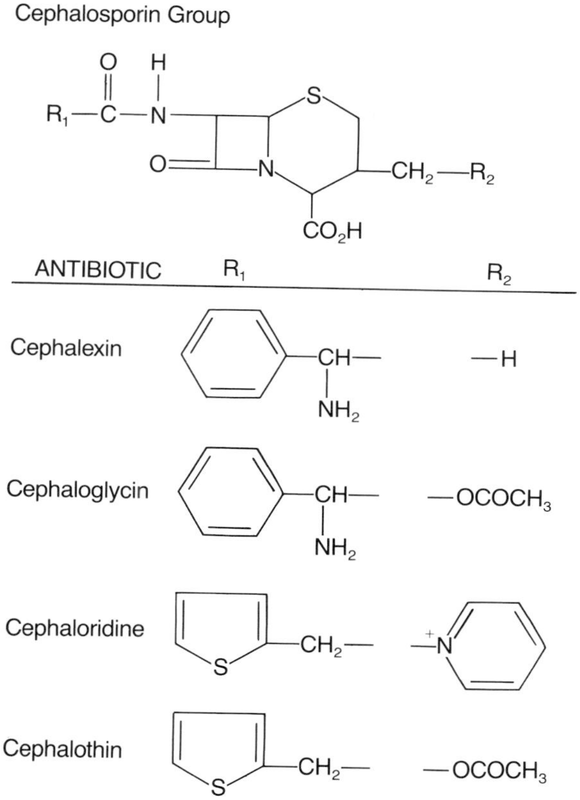

Cephalosporin Group

ANTIBIOTIC	R_1	R_2
Cephalexin	phenyl–CH(NH$_2$)–	–H
Cephaloglycin	phenyl–CH(NH$_2$)–	–OCOCH$_3$
Cephaloridine	thiophene–CH$_2$–	pyridinium
Cephalothin	thiophene–CH$_2$–	–OCOCH$_3$

FIGURE 10–11
Structure of the cephalosporins that act by inhibiting cell-wall synthesis.

sorbed. Bacitracin is mostly used in topical ointments to treat infections of the epidermis.

Inhibitors of protein synthesis in procaryotes

Procaryotic ribosomes are composed of 50S and 30S subunits, which join with messenger RNA to form a 70S ribosome mRNA complex. Protein synthesis (translation) begins with the binding of tRNA to this complex. At the termination of translation, the ribosomes revert to their subunit state and remain as 50S and 30S subunits until they form another complex with mRNA (see Chapter 5). Some antibiotics inhibit translation on the procaryotic 70S ribosomes. These same antibiotics also inhibit the functioning of the 70S ribosomes found in mitochondria and chloroplasts, but this inhibition is not lethal to eucaryotic cells.

Chloramphenicol, erythromycin, and lincomycin. These three antibiotics are produced by some *Streptomyces* (Table 10–5). They are structurally quite diverse (Figure 10–12), yet they all inhibit protein synthesis by binding to the 50S procaryotic ribosomal subunit. Their probable mechanism of inhibition is to prevent peptide bond formation by binding to the peptidyl transferase center on the ribosome.

Chloramphenicol is a structurally simple molecule that is now produced by chemical synthesis. The advantages of chloramphenicol are (1) it is a broad-spectrum antibiotic; (2) it is readily absorbed by the circulatory system; and (3) it quickly penetrates into body tissue and the spinal fluid. The contraindications of chloramphenicol are that it interferes with the normal development of red blood cells. About one individual out of every 40,000 taking chloramphenicol develops **aplastic anemia.** Individuals with this disorder do not form a normal complement of white and red blood cells, which can lead to premature death. Aplastic anemia also occurs in individuals who are not taking chloramphenicol, so it is clear that other factors are involved in causing this disorder. Chloramphenicol is still used to treat patients when no alternative antibiotic is appropriate.

Erythromycin is produced by *Streptomyces erythraeus* and is effective against Gram-positive organisms. This antibiotic is often given to patients who are allergic to penicillin. Erythromycin is administered orally, is readily absorbed, and has a high therapeutic index. **Lincomycin** is produced by *Streptomyces lincolnensis* and is active primarily against Gram-positive bacteria. This drug has a high therapeutic index and is readily absorbed. Note that the names of these antibiotics are derived from the species names of the producing organisms.

Kanamycin, neomycin, and streptomycin. These three antibiotics are aminoglycosides (Figure 10–13)

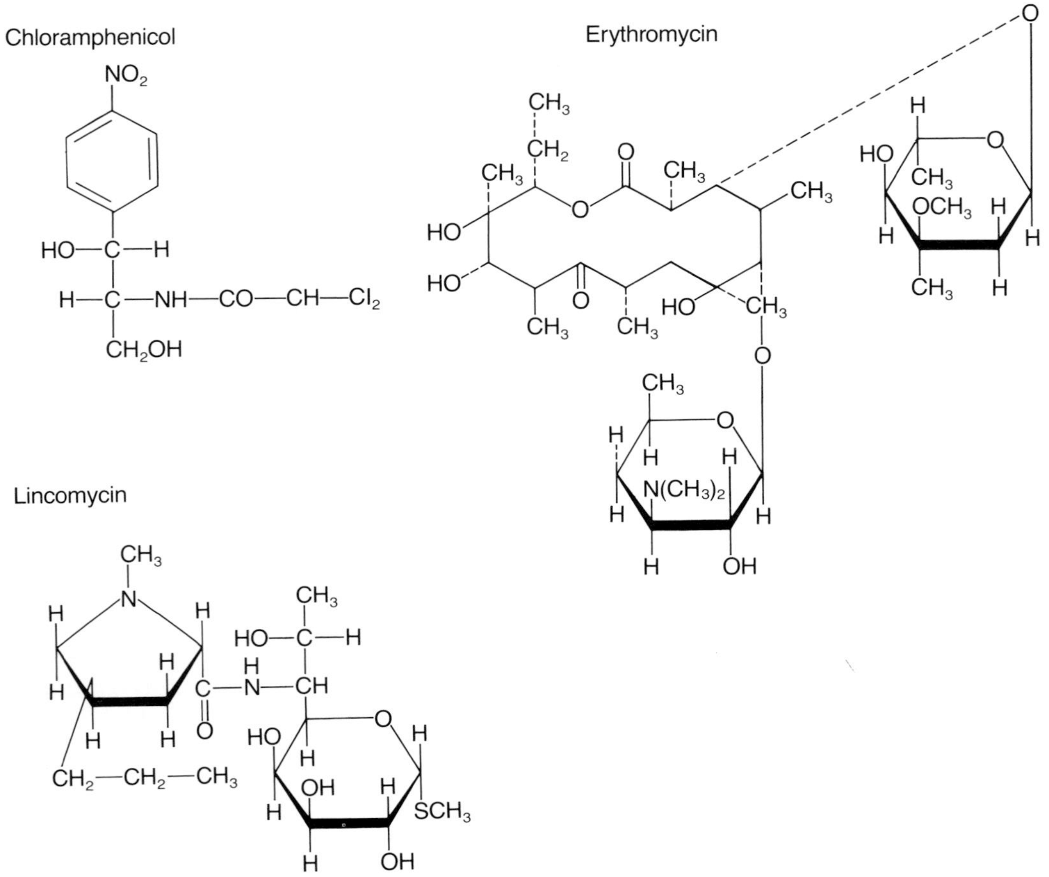

Chloramphenicol

Erythromycin

Lincomycin

FIGURE 10–12
Chloramphenicol, erythromycin, and lincomycin are antibiotics that inhibit procaryotic protein synthesis.

that bind to and prevent the dissociation of 70S ribosomes. **Streptomycin** binds to a specific protein on the 30S ribosomal subunit. This observation has helped to elucidate the mechanism of one form of streptomycin resistance. All three antibiotics are produced by soil isolates belonging to the genus *Streptomyces*. **Kanamycin** and streptomycin are broad-spectrum antibiotics; **neomycin** and streptomycin are especially effective against *Mycobacterium* sp.

Streptomycin was the first effective aminoglycoside discovered. Many bacteria are inhibited by streptomycin, but a considerable number of these develop a resistance to this antibiotic. The primary use of streptomycin has been in treating infections of *Mycobacterium tuberculosis*. Streptomycin together with isoniazid is credited with the significant reduction in the incidence of tuberculosis. The disadvantages of streptomycin are that it cannot be taken orally because of its acid sensitivity and its toxicity to the eighth cranial nerve, which can cause irreversible deafness.

FIGURE 10–13
Neomycin, kanamycin, and streptomycin are aminoglycoside antibiotics that prevent protein synthesis on 70S ribosomes.

Neomycin

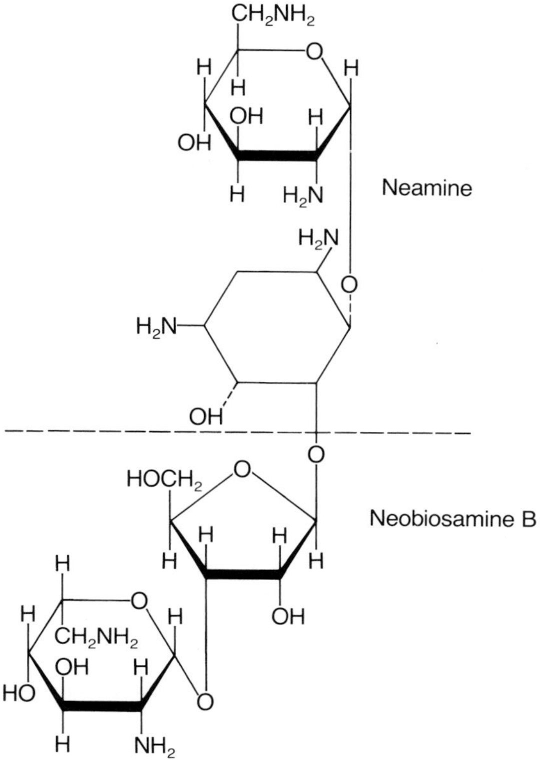

CH₂NH₂

Neamine

H₂N

Neobiosamine B

HOCH₂

Kanamycin

CH₂OH

Kanosamine

CH₂NH₂

Deoxystreptamine

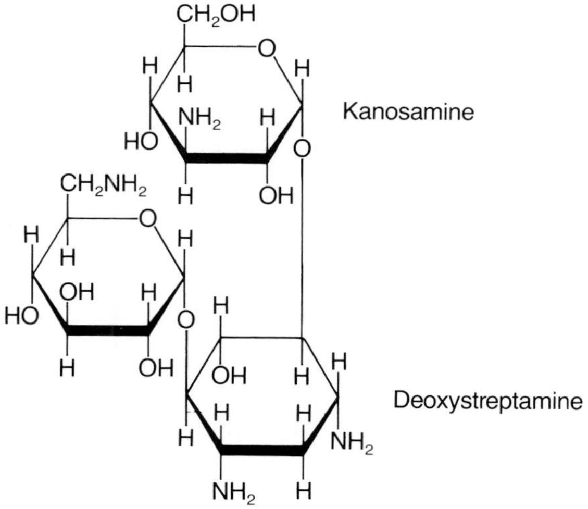

Streptomycin

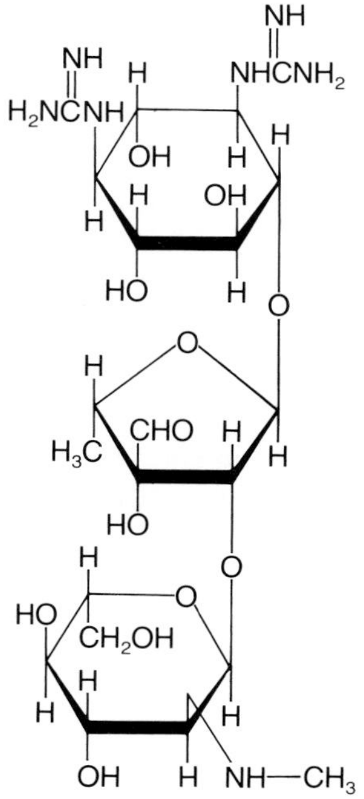

Tetracycline

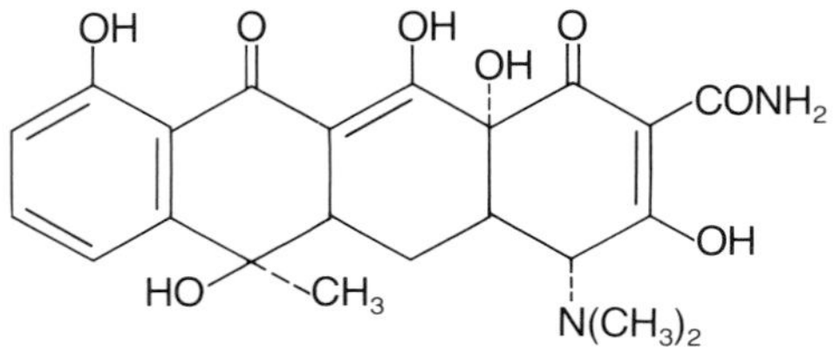

FIGURE 10–14
Tetracycline is a broad-spectrum antibiotic that prevents protein synthesis in procaryotes.

Tetracycline. Tetracycline is a broad-spectrum antibiotic (Table 10–5) that prevents the initiation of protein synthesis by preventing the binding of tRNA to the mRNA ribosome complex. Tetracycline (Figure 10–14) has a low therapeutic index in large part because it binds to proteins in food and to serum proteins in the blood. To be effective, high doses of tetracycline must be given. The side effects of tetracycline are diarrhea and the discoloration of teeth. The drug also breaks down on prolonged storage, and the products of decomposition can cause kidney damage. The advantages of this broad-spectrum antibiotic are that it can be administered to patients with multiple infections.

Antibiotics acting on cell membranes

Bacillus polymyxa produces the antibiotic **polymyxin,** which inhibits the normal function of the cell membrane. Polymyxin is a polypeptide antibiotic that is too toxic for humans to take internally, so its use is restricted to topical applications. Its effectiveness as a drug is further limited by inactivating agents that are present in pus.

Fungal antibiotics

Many antibiotics that interfere with cellular processes in fungi have been isolated. Some of these antibiotics also interfere with eucaryotic cell functions and are to some degree toxic to humans. A few have unusual characteristics that make them useful for treating fungal diseases.

Nystatin and **amphotericin B** are polyene antibiotics (Figure 10–15) produced by *Streptomyces*. These antibiotics bind membrane components, making the membrane leaky to small molecules. They are used to treat systemic mycoses but are ineffective in treating cutaneous mycoses. Long-term treatment can lead to intoxication from of the antibiotic's side effects on animal cells.

Cycloheximide (Figure 10–16) inhibits protein synthesis by interacting directly with the 60S subunit of the eucaryotic ribosomes. This antibiotic is toxic to fungi and protozoans as well as to humans. Cycloheximide is not used as a drug for humans. It is mentioned here because of its experimental use as an inhibitor of protein synthesis in eucaryotes.

Griseofulvin is produced by the mold *Penicillium griseofulvin*. This antibiotic inhibits fungal growth by preventing cell-wall and nucleic acid synthesis. It accumulates in the hair, nails, and other keratinous structures of the body when administered orally. Long-term treatment builds up sufficient concentrations in these structures to effectively treat subcutaneous mycoses.

Protozoan antibiotics

Quinine (Figure 10–17) is found in cinchona bark, which was used for centuries by the natives of Peru to treat malaria. It interferes with the life cycle of *Plasmodium falciparum* during its development in the mammalian circulatory system. **Fumagillin** inhibits protein synthesis in protozoa and is produced by the fungus *Aspergillus fumigatus*. This antibiotic has been used to treat amoebic dysentery, which is caused by *Entamoeba*.

Resistance to antibiotics

From the beginnings of antibiotic therapy, scientists have realized that susceptible bacteria can develop resistance to antibiotics. There are two broad types of antibiotic resistance: (1) bacterial structures can be altered to prevent the action of the antibiotic at its target site, and (2) enzymes can be produced that inactivate the antibiotic by chemically modifying it. Resistance of type 1 can be produced in the labora-

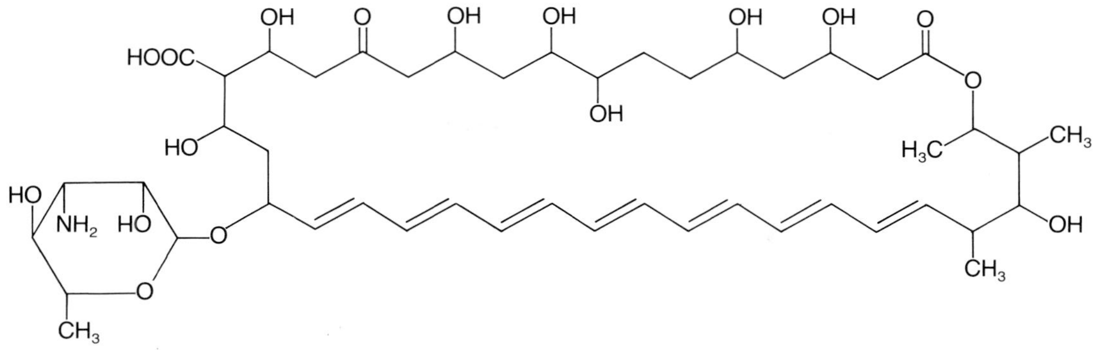

Amphotericin B

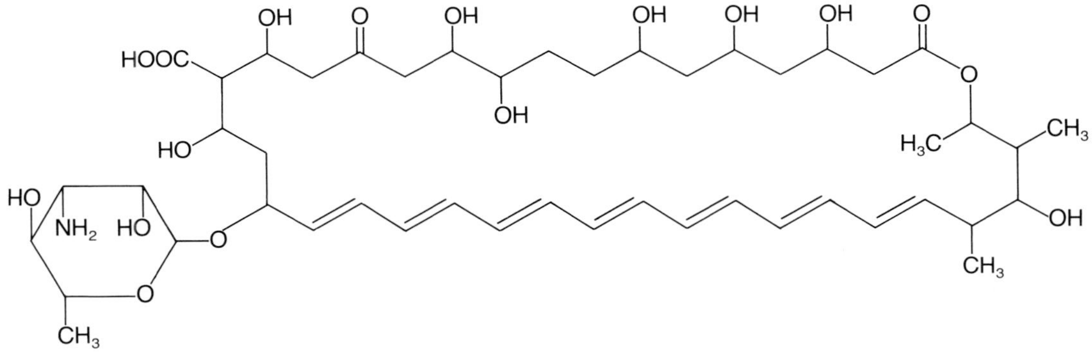

Nystatin

FIGURE 10–15
Amphotericin B and nystatin are antifungal polyene antibiotics.

FIGURE 10–16
Cycloheximide prevents protein synthesis in eucaryotes and is used in experimental biology.

Cycloheximide

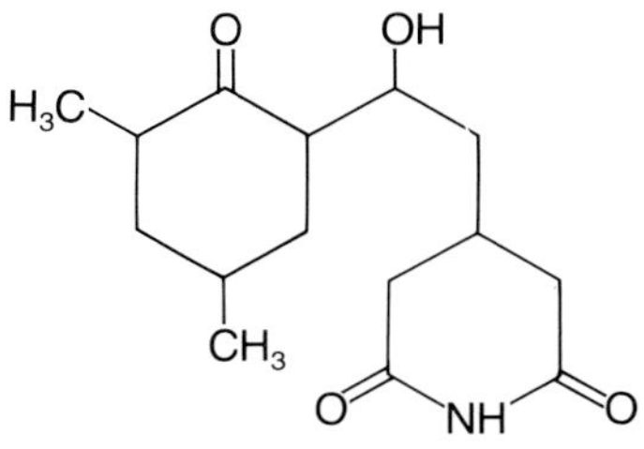

FIGURE 10–17
Quinine is isolated from cinchona bark and is used to treat malaria.

Quinine

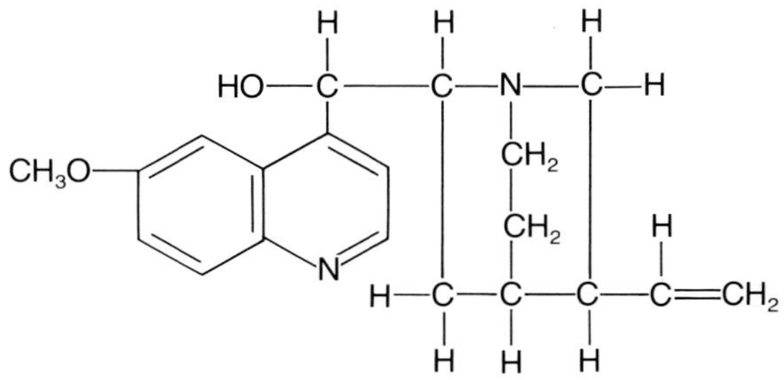

tory by mutations and is sometimes found in clinical isolates. These resistant strains contain an alteration in their chromosomal genes. Resistance of type 2 is found primarily in clinical isolates and is mediated by proteins coded for by extrachromosomal DNA.

Resistance to penicillin is due to the presence of penicillinase. This enzyme cleaves the β-lactam ring of penicillin (Figure 10–10) and thus inactivates its antibiotic activity. Penicillinase is coded for by a plasmid gene and, as such, can be transferred from one cell to another.

Another mechanism for antibiotic inactivation is the addition of an acetyl group, an adenyl group, or a phosphate group to the antibiotic. Gentamycin and kanamycin can be inactivated by **acetyl transferases.** Gentamycin and streptomycin can be inactivated by **adenyl transferases,** and all these aminoglycosides can be inactivated by **phosphotransferases.** The known aminoglycoside-inactivating enzymes are coded for by extrachromosomal genes. Resistance to chloramphenicol is mediated by an R-factor determined acetyl transferase. The plasmid location of these genes make them available for transfer between strains and between related species by conjugation. Tetracycline resistance is also located on the R factor, but its mode of action is unknown.

Resistance to streptomycin and erythromycin can be caused by alterations to the proteins of the procaryotic ribosomes. Mutations that bring about these changes occur in the chromosomal DNA and are not readily transferred between organisms. Streptomycin resistance has been traced to alterations in a protein in the 30S ribosomal subunit. Resistance to erythromycin is believed to be caused by an alteration in a protein of the 50S ribosomal subunit. This type 1 mechanism of resistance is the only way for cells to become erythromycin resistant.

Heavy use of any antibiotic will select for mutants that are resistant to it. Some authorities suggest that antibiotics have been indiscriminately used in veterinary medicine, in animal feeds, and in the less-developed countries where antibiotics can be obtained as over-the-counter drugs. Widespread and constant use of antibiotics as preventive drugs increases the chance of selecting resistant strains. This indeed did happen in the Philippines, where a penicillin-resistant strain of *Neisseria gonorrhoeae* developed and was later transferred to the United States.

Extensive use of antibiotics, such as tetracyclines, as additives to animal feeds has increased the incidence of R factors in the normal bacterial flora of animals. This practice has now been discontinued in England, but it is still used in the United States. In England this practice did select for tetracycline-resistant microbes that could negate the benefits to humans of this antibiotic. Many scientists feel that antibiotics should be discreetly used only to treat infectious diseases.

Chemotherapeutic agents

Paul Ehrlich (1854–1915) was the first scientist to try to develop chemicals that would selectively destroy infectious microorganisms. He began experimenting with aniline dyes because these compounds visibly reacted with microbes. His most successful discovery was called **salvarsan.** This drug is an arsenic-containing organic compound that inhibits *Treponema pallidum* and was used to treat syphilis. Ehrlich coined the word *chemotherapy* to describe the use of selective chemicals to cure patients of infectious diseases.

For years little research was done in chemotherapy. In 1939, however, the first sulfa drug (**sulfanilamide**) was discovered. Chemotherapy developed theoretically when D. D. Wood reasoned that the inhibitory action of sulfanilamide was a result of its structural similarity to *p*-aminobenzoic acid (Figure 10–18). Bacteria require *p*-aminobenzoic acid to synthesize folic acid, which they require for growth. When they grow in the presence of sulfanilamide, they are unable to make folic acid because sulfanilamide acts as a competitive inhibitor for an enzyme of folic acid synthesis. Since bacteria are unable to make their own folic acid, they cease to grow. Animal cells assimilate dietary folic acid, so they are not affected by sulfanilamide. Wood's theoretical approach to chemotherapy stimulated investigators to synthesize and test other metabolic analogues.

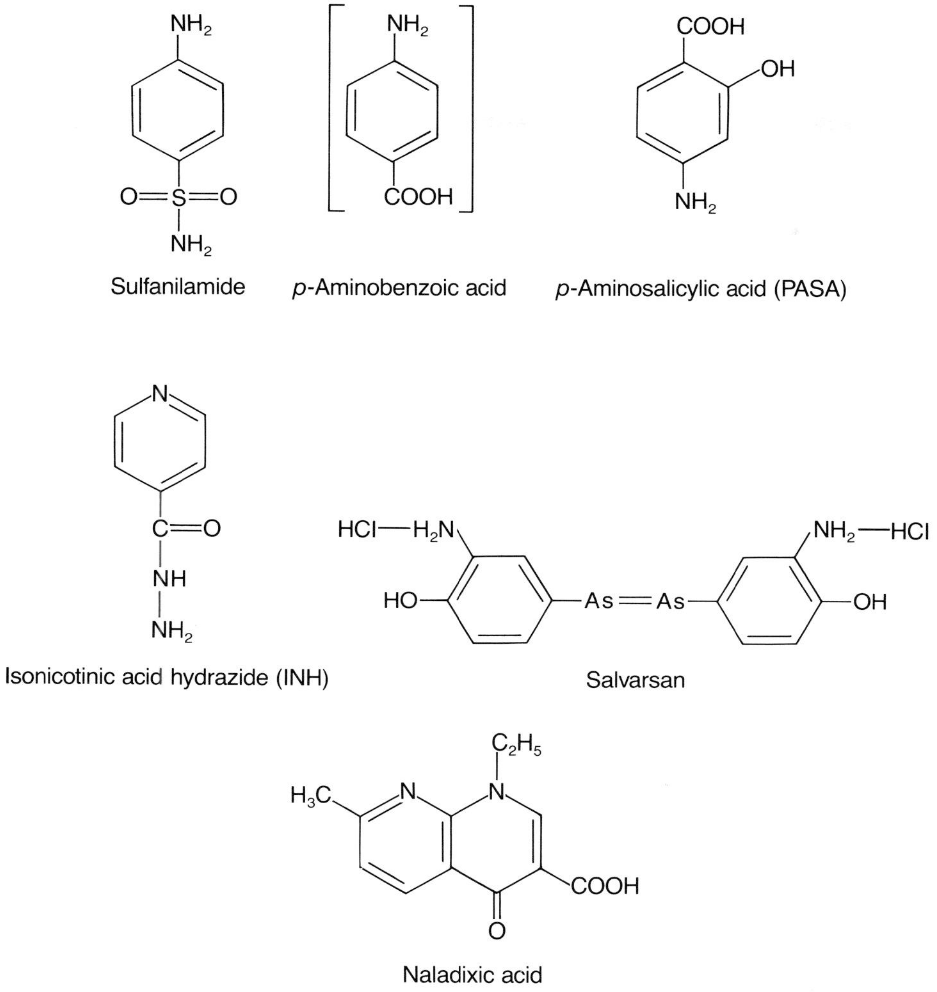

FIGURE 10–18
Synthetic chemotherapeutic agents used to treat human diseases. Sulfanilamide is an analogue of *p*-aminobenzoic acid (pABA is not a drug). PASA and INH are used to treat tuberculosis. Paul Ehrlich discovered salvarsan, which was the first chemotherapeutic agent effectively used to treat syphilis. Naladixic acid prevents DNA synthesis by inhibiting bacterial gyrase.

Synthetic drugs. Sulfanilamide has a high therapeutic index and is readily absorbed by humans. This small molecule penetrates infected tissue and crosses into the spinal fluid. The chemically manufactured drugs containing sulfur are collectively called the sulfa drugs. They have been widely and effectively used, but now there are many pathogens that are resistant to them.

Naladixic acid is a synthetic chemotherapeutic drug used to treat urinary tract infections. This compound (Figure 10–18) prevents the activity of gyrase, an enzyme necessary for the synthesis of DNA in procaryotes. Gyrase makes supercoils in DNA by breaking and then rejoining the double-stranded DNA. Naladixic acid prevents DNA synthesis in microbes by specifically inhibiting the function of gyrase.

The **imidazoles** are the newest class of antifungal drugs: some are truly broad-spectrum agents. **Ketoconazole** (NIZORAL®) is a substituted imidazole that shows a great deal of promise. It is the first orally administered, broad-spectrum, antifungal agent to have proven activity against some of the systemic mycoses affecting humans.

Certain basic dyes react with microorganisms and prevent their growth. **Crystal violet,** used to treat vaginal yeast infections when it is applied in a saturated tampon, is one such dye.

Antiviral drugs

Our main defenses against viral infections are our humoral immunity and our production of interferon. A few antibiotics have antiviral activities, but they are also toxic to human cells. **Actinomycin D** prevents RNA synthesis from DNA by binding to the DNA double helix. **Rifampin** inhibits the DNA-directed RNA polymerase of bacterial cells and some viruses. Both these antibiotics can interfere with viral replication.

Amantadine hydrochloride is an antiviral drug licensed to treat systemic viral infections. It prevents the replication of influenza A and C, but it does not inhibit influenza B. Purine and pyrimidine analogues, such as **idoxuridine** (IDU), **adenine arabinoside** (ara-A), and **trifluorothymidine** can prevent viral nucleic acid replication. IDU and ara-A are currently used to treat herpes keratoconjunctivitis.

Sensitivity to antimicrobial agents

Clinical microbiologists are responsible for advising physicians of the drug susceptibility of the microorganism(s) affecting their patients. Microbes develop resistance to antibiotics, so it is essential to know the antibiotic sensitivity of each isolated pathogen. The two techniques used to determine antibiotic susceptibility are: (1) the tube dilution technique, and (2) the use of standard disks.

Tube dilution method. The susceptibility to a given antimicrobial agent is tested using a pure culture of the infectious agent. Mueller-Hinton broth is widely used for antibiotic sensitivity testing because most bacterial pathogens grow in it and it has a low level of substances that inactivate antibiotics. The antimicrobial agent is added in decreasing concentrations to the tubes of the broth medium, which is then inoculated. Growth will occur only in tubes having an insufficient amount of the antimicrobial agent to inhibit growth. The tube with no growth and the lowest concentration of antibiotic contains the **minimum inhibitory concentration** (MIC) of the antimicrobial agent.

Sensitivity disk method. Filter paper disks containing standard concentrations of an antibiotic are used to determine antibiotic sensitivities. Eight or more different antimicrobial agents can be tested at one time (Figure 10–19) when this technique is used. The procedure is to spread a pure culture of the test organism on a suitable solidified growth medium, such as Mueller-Hinton agar. Antibiotic disks are available in a dispenser that is used to position the disks on the petri dish in a symmetrical order (Figure 10–19). Each disk is marked to indicate the antimicrobial agent and its concentration. After the plate is incubated for 16 to 18 hours at 35°C, sensitivity is read by measuring the size of the zone of no growth around each disk. This value (measured in mm) is compared to numbers on a chart (supplied by the disk manufacturer) and indicates whether the organism is resistant, intermediate, or sensitive to the antimicrobial agent.

Disk sensitivity is not a standardized procedure because there are too many variables involved. The inoculum used, the medium used, selection and concentration of the antimicrobial disks to be used, storage and handling of the disks, and the criteria for interpreting the results can all vary greatly. Nevertheless, sensitivity-disk testing is convenient, fast,

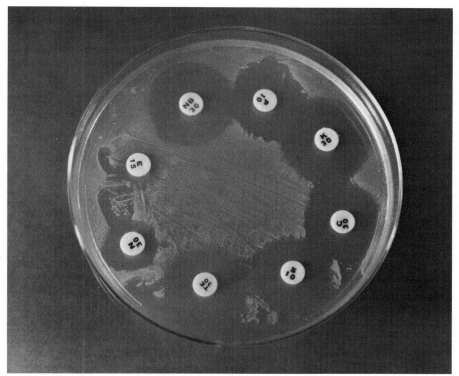

FIGURE 10–19
Antibiotic sensitivity disk testing. Each filter-paper disk contains a set concentration of
antibiotic. The zone of growth inhibition indicates the culture's sensitivity to that antibiotic.

and economical. Today it is the most widely used
form of antimicrobial testing.

SUMMARY

Microorganisms are controlled by preventing their
growth or by killing them. Sterilization is the process
of killing all life in an area or a contained space.
Cells die exponentially during sterilization. Endospores are the most resistant forms of life known,
yet sterilization procedures must ensure that no
spore survives. Both physical and chemical techniques are used in these procedures.

Physical methods of controlling microorganisms
include heat, radiation, and filtration. Moist heat is
more effective in killing bacterial spores than is dry
heat. Liquids are routinely sterilized under pressure
in an autoclave, whereas glassware is easily sterilized with dry heat in an oven. Pasteurization is a
milder form of heat treatment that eliminates common pathogens from milk and increases its shelf life.
Wine and beer can also be pasteurized. Gamma rays
and X rays are penetrating forms of ionizing radiation that can kill cells by producing free radicals. Ultraviolet light does not penetrate glass or water but
can be used to decontaminate air and the surfaces of
objects. Filtration is used to remove microorganisms,
but not necessarily viruses, from heat-sensitive solutions and from air or other gases.

Both selective and nonselective chemicals are used to control microbes. The nonselective chemicals are the disinfectants and include chlorine gas, formaldehyde, glutaraldehyde, ethylene oxide, sulfur dioxide, propylene oxide, and the higher concentrations of phenolic compounds. Antiseptics are mild disinfectants that can be used on humans. These include alcohol, iodine, iodine-alcohol mixtures, silver nitrate, mercuric compounds, cationic detergents, and low concentrations of phenolic compounds.

Compounds that selectively kill include the antibiotics and the chemically synthesized drugs. Antibiotics are produced by bacteria of the genera *Bacillus* and *Streptomyces* and by molds of the genera *Aspergillus*, *Cephalosporium*, and *Penicillium*. Antibiotics either inhibit the growth of or kill microorganisms by interfering with protein synthesis, nucleic acid synthesis, cell-wall synthesis, or cell membrane function. Cells develop resistance to these antibiotics either by altering the structure affected or by producing enzymes that modify or destroy the antibiotic. Sulfa drugs are examples of chemotherapeutic drugs. They act as analogues of essential metabolites. Antibiotic-susceptibility testing is done on clinical isolates to determine their sensitivity to antibiotics and chemotherapeutic drugs.

QUESTIONS AND TOPICS FOR STUDY AND DISCUSSION

Questions

1. What are the advantages and disadvantages of using dry heat versus moist heat in sterilization procedures?
2. What types of radiation can be used to inhibit or control microbial growth? Describe a practical application of each type.
3. Define or explain the following terms.

sterile	disinfectant
aseptic	antiseptic
bactericidal	antibiotic
bacteriostatic	therapeutic index
pasteurization	

4. Name five nonselective chemicals used to control microbial growth and describe a practical use for each one.
5. What groups of organisms produce antibiotics? What is the function of antibiotics in nature?
6. Name and describe the inhibition caused by two antibiotics that inhibit cell-wall formation and two that inhibit protein synthesis.
7. What are broad-spectrum antibiotics?
8. Describe two mechanisms of antibiotic resistance observed in bacteria.
9. What are sulfa drugs and how do they work?
10. Describe a practical method for determining antibiotic sensitivity.

Discussion

1. Why are there fewer antibiotics available for use against eucaryotic cells than against procaryotic cells?
2. What are the long-range implications of a cell developing resistance to an antibiotic by (a) altering a cellular structure, and (b) acquiring an enzyme capable of inactivating that antibiotic?
3. Are there biological reasons for science's inability to develop effective broad-spectrum antiviral drugs?

FURTHER READINGS

Books

Borick, P. M., *Chemical Sterilization*, Dowden, Hutchinson & Ross, Stroudsburg, Penn., 1973. A collection of selected papers on the use of chemicals in sterilization.

Finegold, S. M., and W. J. Martin, *Baily and Scott's Diagnostic Microbiology*, 6th ed., Mosby, St. Louis, 1982. A detailed reference source or advanced textbook that covers the techniques used in diagnostic microbiology. The first few chapters deal with general laboratory methods and the collection of clinical specimens.

Garrod, L. P., H. P. Lambert, and F. O'Grady, *Antibiotic and Chemotherapy*, Churchill Livingston, New York, 1981. An authoritative reference work on the biology, biochemistry, and pharmacology of chemotherapeutic agents.

Articles and Reviews

Benveniste, R., and J. Davis, "Mechanism of Antibiotic Resistance in Bacteria," *Ann. Rev. Biochem.*, 42:471–506 (1973). A review of the genetic and biochemical mechanisms through which bacteria develop antibiotic resistance.

Blumberg, P. M., and J. L. Strominger, "Interaction of Penicillin with the Bacterial Cell: Penicillin-binding Proteins and Penicillin-sensitive Enzymes," *Bacteriol. Rev.*, 38:291–335 (1974). A biochemical review dealing with the interaction of penicillin with the components of bacterial cells.

Kobayashi, G. S., and G. Medoff, "Antifungal Agents: Recent Developments," *Ann. Rev. Microbiol.*, 31:291–308 (1977). A review that covers the structure and function of antifungal agents.

Whitley, R. J., and C. A. Alford, "Developmental Aspects of Selected Antiviral Chemotherapeutic Agents," *Ann. Rev. Microbiol.*, 32:285–300 (1978). A review of the use of chemicals to prevent or decrease the effects of viral infections.

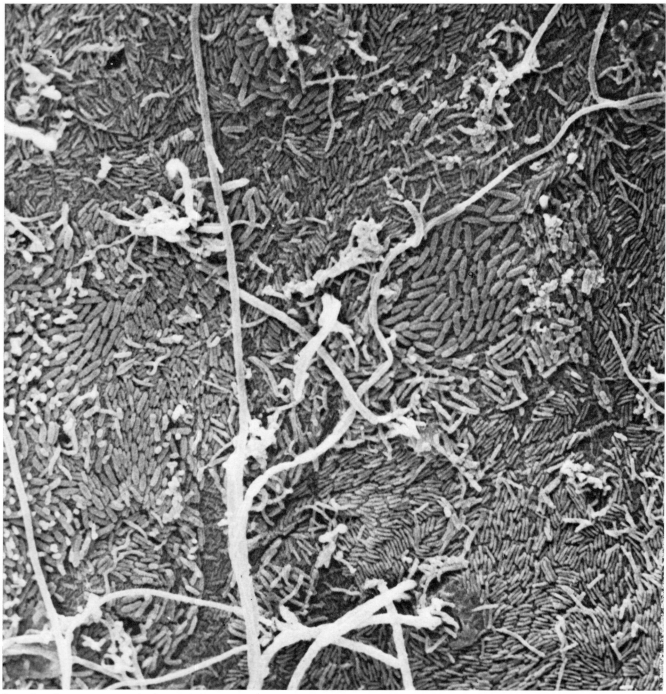

Scanning electron micrograph of bacteria in the termite gut. (Courtesy of Dr. J. A. Breznak.
From J. A. Breznak and H. S. Prankratz, *Applied Environ. Microbiol.*, 33:406–426, 1977,
with permission of the American Society for Microbiology.)

PART TWO

HOST-PARASITE RELATIONSHIPS

Healthy humans live in a state of dynamic symbiosis with numerous microorganisms. Bacteria are found on the skin, in the nasopharynx, and in the intestine, while other parts of the healthy human body are free of microbes. When illness does occur it is usually caused by an organic disorder or by an infectious agent.

A **disease** is any departure from the normal state of health. **Organic diseases** occur when a basic body function ceases to operate properly, as during a heart attack. **Infectious diseases** are caused by viruses, bacteria, fungi, or protozoa that can cause illness in more than one individual. The **etiological** (causative) agents of most infectious diseases are now known, and many infectious diseases can be treated with chemotherapy or prevented by immunizations. Also, only a few of the bacteria associated with healthy humans actually cause disease. This concept is brought out in Chapter 11, which discusses the normal microbial flora of the human.

When infectious agents do cause disease in a hosts, they have won the dynamic battle against the host's resistance. Humans have the ability to resist disease through a combination of physical, chemical, and cellular barriers. The physical and cellular aspects of host resistance are discussed in Chapter 12. Immunological principles and their impact on host resistance and on diagnostic microbiology are covered in Chapter 13.

Infectious agents cause epidemics when they infect a large proportion of a population. Epidemiology (Chapter 14) is the study of the factors that determine the occurrence of infectious disease in a population. All together, these four Chapters (11–14) comprise a coherent discussion of host-parasite relationships.

11

MICROBIOLOGY OF THE HUMAN

Many microorganisms live in a state of cohabitation with the human body. This relationship will continue as a stable, balanced relationship until a state of disease develops. Certain viruses, bacteria, fungi (including yeasts), and protozoa are capable of causing infectious diseases. Microorganisms that have the potential to cause disease are called **pathogens.** Some pathogens consistently cause disease, whereas others, called **opportunistic pathogens,** only cause disease when opportune conditions exist. Obtaining a general knowledge of the indigenous human microbial flora is the first step to understanding the dynamic interactions between microbes and humans.

MICROBIAL FLORA OF THE HEALTHY HUMAN

Indigenous populations of microorganisms inhabit specific parts of the human body. Many of these microbes are nonpathogenic and coexist with humans. Other microorganisms cause disease in humans either when the host is compromised by illness or when microorganisms colonize parts of the human body in which they are not normally found. Areas of the human body that are normally colonized by microbes include the skin, mouth, nasopharynx, eyes, ears, respiratory tract, gastrointestinal tract, anterior urethra, and vagina. The majority of these inhabitants are bacteria.

Respiratory tract

The respiratory tract includes the mouth, tonsils, nasopharynx, throat, trachea, bronchi, and lungs (Figure 11–1). The microbial flora in the mouth of an infant at birth corresponds to the organisms in the mother's vagina, whereas the nasopharynx of the newborn is sterile. These areas are soon colonized by many different microbes (Table 11–1). In adults, microorganisms are normal inhabitants of the mouth, nasopharynx, teeth, tonsils, and throat, whereas the trachea, bronchi, and lungs in both infants and adults are normally sterile. If bacteria and/or viruses do infect the human lungs, the disease is called **pneumonia.**

The growth of microorganisms on the surfaces of human teeth can contribute to the formation of dental caries (tooth decay). Filamentous bacteria belonging to the genera *Leptotrichia* and *Fusobacterium* can form colonies on the surfaces of human teeth. These

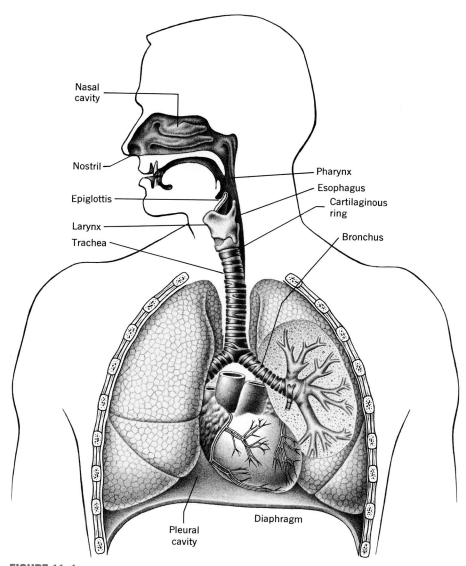

FIGURE 11—1
The upper torso of a human showing the respiratory tract. (From A. Nason, *Modern Biology*, copyright © 1965, Wiley.)

bacteria, together with streptococci and diphtheroids, are often associated with the dental plaque formed on tooth surfaces. **Dental plaque** is composed of bacteria enmeshed in a polysaccharide (dextran) film. The production of organic acids from the fermentation of sugars and the production of polysaccharides by the bacteria in dental plaque significantly contribute to the formation of dental caries.

TABLE 11-1
Normal Flora of the Human Respiratory Tract

Organism	Anatomical Locale	Potential Disease Processes[a]
Acinetobacter sp.	Nasopharynx	Meningitis, bacteremia, pneumonia
Actinobacillus sp.	Teeth	Periodontal disease
Actinomyces sp.	Mouth, tonsils	Actinomycosis
Bacteriodes sp.	Mouth	Lung abscesses, bacteremia
Candida albicans (yeast)	Mouth, throat	Thrush
Capnocytophaga sp.	Teeth	Periodontal disease
Corynebacterium sp.	Mouth, nose	Bacterial endocarditis, lung abscesses
Eikenelle sp.	Teeth	Periodontal disease
Enterobacter sp.	Nasal passages	No specific disease
Fusobacterium sp.	Mouth, tonsils	Lung abscesses
Hemophilus sp.	Mouth, nasopharynx, throat	Meningitis, conjunctivitis, pneumonia, bacteremia
Klebsiella sp.	Nasal passages	Pneumonia
Lactobacillus sp.	Mouth, saliva	No specific disease
Leptotrichia buccalis	Mouth, tooth surfaces	No known disease
Micrococcus sp.	Mouth, tonsils	No known disease
Mycoplasma sp.	Mouth	Atypical (mycoplasmal) pneumonia
Neisseria sp.	Mouth, nasopharynx, nose	Meningitis
Staphylococcus aureus	Mouth, nose, tonsils, nasopharynx	Pneumonia, otitis, pharyngitis
Staphylococcus epidermidis	Mouth, nose, tonsils, nasopharynx	Bacterial endocarditis
Streptococcus pneumoniae	Mouth, nose, tonsils, throat	Pneumonia, conjunctivitis, meningitis
Streptococcus (pyogenes)	Nasopharynx	Streptococcal pharyngitis
Streptococcus (viridans)	Mouth, throat	Subacute bacterial endocarditis
Treponema denticola	Mouth	No known disease
Veillonella sp.	Mouth, tonsils	Bacterial endocarditis
Vibrio sputorum	Mouth	No known disease

Source: Adapted from H. D. Isenberg and B. G. Painter, "Indigenous and Pathogenic Microorganisms of Humans," in E. H. Lennett (ed.), *Manual of Clinical Microbiology*, pp. 25–39, American Society for Microbiology, Washington, D.C., 1980.
[a]Potential for disease if shifted to another locale or if normal flora is disturbed.

Periodontal diseases affect the gums and the bones that support the teeth. Microorganisms that get trapped in pockets between the gums and the teeth are involved in these complex diseases.

Most organisms in the respiratory tract live in symbiosis with the adult human. Some of these organisms (Table 11–1) do not cause disease in humans, whereas others are pathogens. This latter group will cause disease if the host becomes compromised or if the organisms are transferred (1) to other parts of the body or (2) to humans who are susceptible to the infectious agent. Certain individuals actually carry pathogenic bacteria without showing clinical symptoms of a disease. These individuals are called **carriers.** A large number of people in the United States are carriers of *Hemophilus* sp., *Streptococcus pneumoniae,* and *Neisseria* sp. These organisms are carried in the human mouth and nasopharynx (Table 11–1), and under certain circumstances they pose a disease threat to the host.

Gastrointestinal tract

The stomach, gallbladder, duodenum, upper ileum, lower ileum, and the large intestine compose the human gastrointestinal tract (Figure 11–2). The stomach and duodenum contain a few microbes (between 10^3 and 10^6 bacteria/g of solids) that are usually derived from ingested food. The bacteria in the human stomach are normally just passing through and do not grow there because of the low pH. One exception is *Sarcina ventriculi,* which grows at pHs below 2.0 and has been isolated from patients with stomach ulcers.

Bacteria are prevalent in the lower ileum and the large intestine, where populations of between 10^8 and 10^{11} bacteria/g of contents are normal. Obligate anaerobes make up 95 percent of the microbes in the large intestine.

At birth, infants lack an intestinal microbial flora, but very soon thereafter their intestine is colonized by microorganisms. The predominant organisms in the gastrointestinal tract of breast-fed infants are *Lactobacillus acidophilus, Bacillus* sp., *Clostridium* sp., coliforms,* and enterococci. Children develop the normal intestinal flora found in adult humans after their diet is switched to solid foods.

Microorganisms in the intestine (Table 11–2) contribute to the bulk of feces. Their presence usually does not cause a diseased state. Some intestinal microbes can cause disease following surgery, a ruptured appendix, malfunction of the gallbladder, or other abnormal state of the host. Diseases of the gastrointestinal tract include peritonitis, cholecystitis, and gastroenteritis. **Peritonitis** is an inflammation of the serous membrane that lines the human abdominal cavity. This disease can be caused by microbes originating in the bowel following surgery or following the rupture of the patient's appendix. **Cholecystitis** is an inflammation of the gallbladder that can be caused by intestinal microbes. **Gastroenteritis** is an inflammation of the mucous membranes of the stomach and the small intestine. Specific bacteria produce toxins that cause the symptoms of gastroen-

*"Coliforms" are those fermenting Gram-negative rods that inhabit the intestinal tract of animals without causing disease.

TABLE 11–2
Normal Flora of the Human Gastrointestinal Tract

Organism	Potential Disease Processes
Lower Ileum and Large Intestine	
Bacteroides sp.	Peritonitis, abscesses, cholecystitis
Clostridium sp.	Food poisoning, cholecystitis
Corynebacterium sp.	Not known
Enterobacter sp.	Not known
Enterococcus	Peritonitis, cholecystitis
Escherichia coli	Peritonitis, gastroenteritis
Fusobacterium sp.	Abscesses, bacteremia
Klebsiella sp.	Not known
Lactobacillus sp.	Not known
Pseudomonas aeruginosa	Gastroenteritis, meningitis, bacteremia
Staphylococcus aureus	Food poisoning, gastroenteritis
Streptococcus (viridans)	No known disease
Vibrio sp.	Not by indigenous organisms

Source: Adapted from H. D. Isenberg and B. G. Painter, "Indigenous and Pathogenic Microorganisms of Humans," in E. H. Lennett (ed.), *Manual of Clinical Microbiology,* pp. 25–39, American Society for Microbiology, Washington, D.C., 1980.

teritis. Toxin production can be localized in the patient's intestine or the patient can ingest the bacterial toxins by eating contaminated food.

Escherichia coli is an inhabitant of the lower ileum and the large intestine. It is found in the lower bowel of warm-blooded animals and is prevalent in almost all humans. The presence of *E. coli* in water and food is often measured as an indicator of contamination by human feces. *Streptococcus faecalis* and *S. faecium* are also present in the human intestine and are collectively referred to as the **enterococcus group.** The presence of enterococci in food and water is also used as an indicator of fecal contamina-

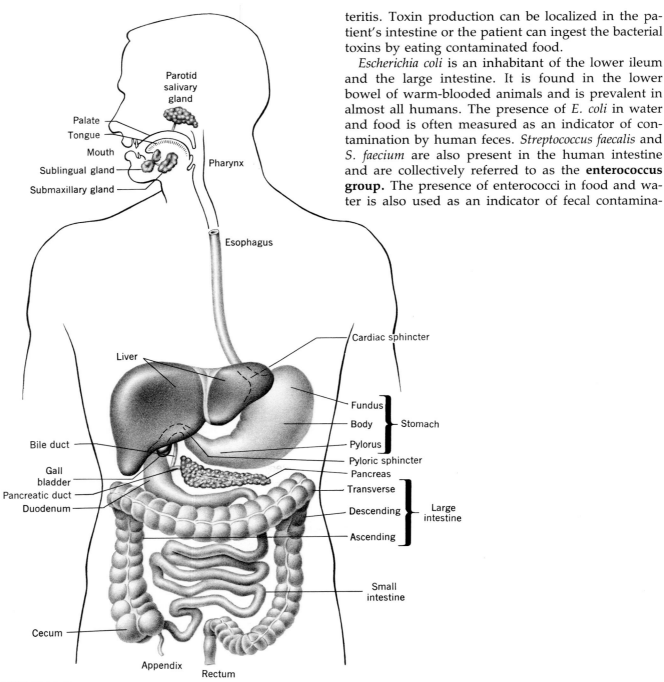

FIGURE 11–2
The upper body of a human showing the organs of digestion. (From A. Nason, *Modern Biology,* copyright © 1965, Wiley.)

tion. Since streptococci are also found in vegetable matter, they are not necessarily an indicator of human fecal contamination. Measuring these organisms is referred to as **fecal coliform,** or **fecal streptococci, counting.**

Normal flora of the genitourinary tract

The male and female genitourinary tract are diagramed in Figure 11–3. The human kidneys, bladder, and urethra (except for the anterior urethra) are normally free of microorganisms; however, these or-

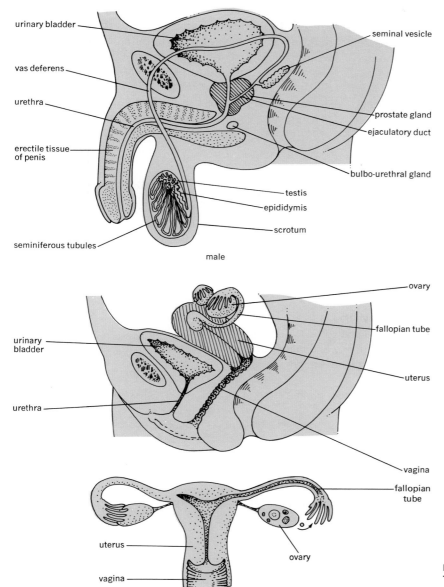

male

female

FIGURE 11–3
The male and female reproductive systems.
(From J. R. McClintic, *Physiology of the Human Body,* copyright © 1978, Wiley.)

gans can become infected. **Urethritis** is an infection of the urethra, **cystitis** is an infection of the bladder, and **pyelonephritis** is an inflammation of the kidney. These infections can develop during surgical procedures or catheterization, and they can be caused by organisms normally associated with the external genitalia. Males are less susceptible to these infections. The normal microbial flora of the male genitourinary tract is restricted to the anterior urethra. The genitalia of the female are more prone to microbial colonization, and females have an indigenous microbial flora in the anterior urethra, the external genitalia, and the vagina (Table 11–3). For this reason, females are more susceptible to urinary tract infections than are males.

The normal flora of the vagina changes during sexual maturation. *Staphylococcus epidermidis* and *Lactobacillus acidophilus* are predominant in the adult vagina, and these organisms are even more predominant during pregnancy. Micrococci, streptococci, coliforms, and diphtheroids are the predominant microorganisms in the vagina of prepubertal and postmenopausal women. Low numbers of yeasts are also present in the human vagina. **Vaginitis** is an inflammation of the vagina. Vaginitis is observed in women being treated with broad-spectrum antibiotics or other drugs that upset the microbial ecology of the vagina. *Candida albicans* is a yeast that is both a normal inhabitant of the human vagina and a cause of vaginitis. Vaginitis can also be caused by the pro-

TABLE 11–3
Normal Flora of the Human Genitourinary Tract

Organism	Anatomical Locale	Potential Disease Processes
Acinetobacter sp.	Anterior urethra, vagina	Urethritis
Bacteroides sp.	External genitalia	Infections following surgery
Clostridium sp.	Vagina	Infections following surgery
Corynebacterium sp.	External genitalia, anterior urethra, vagina	Not known
Enterobacteriaceae (*Escherichia, Proteus*)	External genitalia, anterior urethra, vagina	Pyelonephritis, cystitis, bacteremia
Fusobacterium sp.	External genitalia, vagina	Not known
Hemophilus vaginalis	Anterior urethra, vagina	Vaginitis
Lactobacillus sp.	Vagina (between puberty and menses)	None
Mycobacterium sp.	External genitalia, anterior urethra, vagina	None
Mycoplasma sp.	External genitalia, anterior urethra, vagina	Nonspecific urethritis
Neisseria sp.	External genitalia, anterior urethra, vagina	Specific species cause disease
Peptostreptococcus	External genitalia, vagina	Puerperal fever
Staphylococcus aureus	External genitalia, anterior urethra, vagina	Urethritis, furunculosis
Streptococcus (viridans)	External genitalia, anterior urethra, vagina	None
Yeasts (*Candida*) and Protozoa (*Trichomonas*)	External genitalia, anterior urethra, vagina	Vaginitis

Source: Adapted from H. D. Isenberg and B. G. Painter, "Indigenous and Pathogenic Microorganisms of Humans," in E. H. Lennett (ed.), *Manual of Clinical Microbiology*, pp. 25–39, American Society for Microbiology, Washington, D.C., 1980.

TABLE 11–4
Normal Flora of Human Skin, Ears, and Eyes

Organisms	Anatomical Locale	Potential Disease Processes
Corynebacterium sp.	Skin, ear, eye	Complication of cardiac surgery
Hemophilus aegypticus	Eye	Eye diseases
Hemophilus influenzae	Eye	Eye diseases
Micrococcus sp.	Skin	Not determined unequivocally
Neisseria sp.	Skin, eye	No diseases known for indigenous species
Propionibacterium acnes	Skin	Pimples, acne, endocarditis
Staphylococcus aureus	Skin, ear	Boils, impetigo, mastitis
Staphylococcus epidermidis	Skin, ear, eye	Pimples, acne, endocarditis
Streptococcus (viridans)	Skin, eye	No known disease
Trychophyton sp. (mold)	Skin	Skin diseases

Source: Adapted from H. D. Isenberg and B. G. Painter, "Indigenous and Pathogenic Microorganisms of Humans," in E. H. Lennett (ed.), *Manual of Clinical Microbiology*, pp. 25–39, American Society for Microbiology, Washington, D.C., 1980.

tozoan *Trichomonas vaginalis,* which is also a common inhabitant of the vagina.

Urine is presumed to be sterile, although voided urine normally contains up to 1000 bacteria/ml. These contaminating microorganisms usually originate from the normal flora of the anterior urethra or adjacent areas. Contamination of voided urine is more prevalent in the human female than in the human male because of external anatomical differences.

Normal flora of the human skin, ears, and eyes.

Human integument is the outermost barrier to infectious agents. The skin harbors a normal flora of microorganisms (Table 11–4), some of which are also present in the external auditory canal of the ear and in the healthy conjunctiva of the eye. *Staphylococcus aureus* is the major skin organism that has a potential to cause disease in humans. This organism can cause boils, impetigo, or mastitis. **Boils** are quite common infections of hair follicles or sebaceous glands and are characterized by the accumulation of pus. **Mastitis** is an inflammation of the female breast. **Impetigo** is an infection of the skin that is usually caused by *Staphylococcus aureus* or *Streptococcus pyogenes.* **Acne** is another disease of human skin and is characterized by the development of pimples primarily in adolescents. *Staphylococcus epidermidis* and *Propionibacterium acnes* are indigenous microflora of the skin that are often associated with acne.

The healthy human conjunctiva often contains microorganisms derived from the skin. Likewise, the external canal of the human ear contains a microbial flora derived from resident skin organisms. The middle and inner ear are usually sterile. When infections of the inner ear do occur **(otitis media),** they are often caused by the normal microbial flora of the nasopharynx and not by the normal skin flora.

Anatomical locations lacking microbial flora

The blood and the cerebrospinal fluid (CSF) of healthy humans are devoid of infectious agents. When microorganisms are found in human blood or in human CSF, it is an indication of a disease state. **Meningitis** is an inflammation of the membranes surrounding the brain and the spinal column. These membranes are called the **meninges.** Meningitis is diagnosed by demonstrating the presence of microorganisms in the spinal fluid. When bacteria are present in the blood, the condition is termed a **bacteremia.** This term implies that the organisms present in the blood are unable to multiply. When there are microorganisms present and multiplying in the blood, the condition is referred to as **septicemia.**

PLATE 1.

Morphology of blood elements. (Courtesy of L. W. Diggs, M.D. From L. W. Diggs, L. W. Strum, and A. Bell, "The Morphology of Human Blood Elements," 3rd ed., Abbott Laboratories, 1954.)

Legend Key. Cell Types Found in Smears of Peripheral Blood from Normal Humans. The arrangement is arbitrary and the number of leukocytes in relation to erythrocytes and thrombocytes is greater than would occur in an actual microscopic field.

- A Erythrocytes
- B Large lymphocyte with azurophilic granules
- C Neutrophil
- D Eosinophil
- E Neutrophil segmented
- F Monocyte with blue-gray cytoplasm, coarse linear chromatin, and blunt pseudopods
- G Thrombocytes
- H Lymphocytes
- I Neutrophilic band
- J Basophil

PLATE 2.

Gram-positive diplococci in sputum of a patient with pneumococcal pneumonia.

PLATE 3.

Capsulated diplococci in the sputum of a patient with pneumococcal pneumonia as demonstrated with the Quellung reaction.

PLATE 4.

Typical clumps of Gram-positive cocci in the sputum of a patient with staphylococcal pneumonia.

PLATE 5.

Gram-negative diplococci inside leukocytes from the urethral exudate of a man with gonorrhea.

Plates 2, 3, 4 and 5: From G. L. Mandell, R. G. Douglas, Jr. and J. E. Bennett, *Principles and Practices of Infectious Diseases,* Volume 1. John Wiley & Sons, 1979.

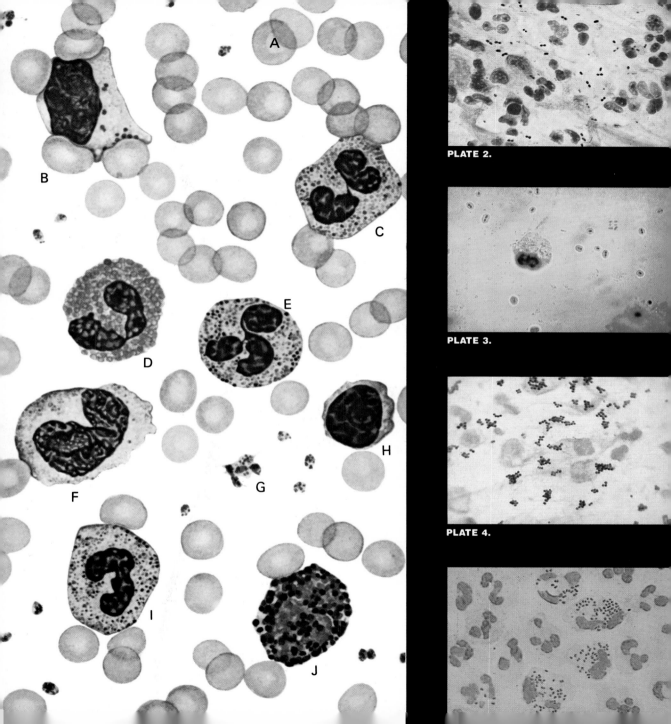

PLATE 2.

PLATE 3.

PLATE 4.

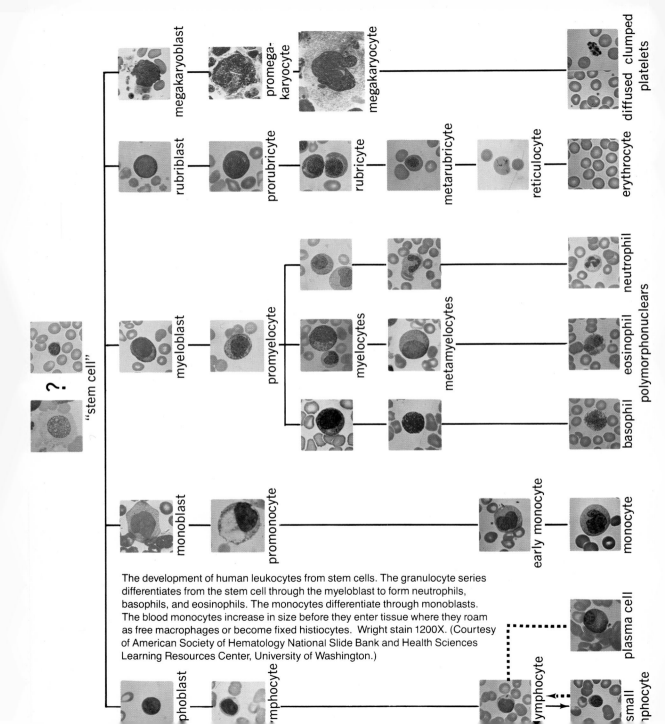

megakaryoblast — promega-karyocyte — megakaryocyte — diffused clumped platelets

rubriblast — prorubricyte — rubricyte — metarubricyte — reticulocyte — erythrocyte

"stem cell"

myeloblast — promyelocyte — myelocytes — metamyelocytes — neutrophil

eosinophil
polymorphonuclears

basophil

monoblast — promonocyte — early monocyte — monocyte

The development of human leukocytes from stem cells. The granulocyte series differentiates from the stem cell through the myeloblast to form neutrophils, basophils, and eosinophils. The monocytes differentiate through monoblasts. The blood monocytes increase in size before they enter tissue where they roam as free macrophages or become fixed histiocytes. Wright stain 1200X. (Courtesy of American Society of Hematology National Slide Bank and Health Sciences Learning Resources Center, University of Washington.)

plasma cell

lymphocyte

lymphoblast — lymphocyte — small lymphocyte

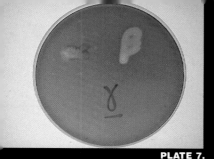

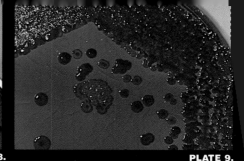

PLATE 7.

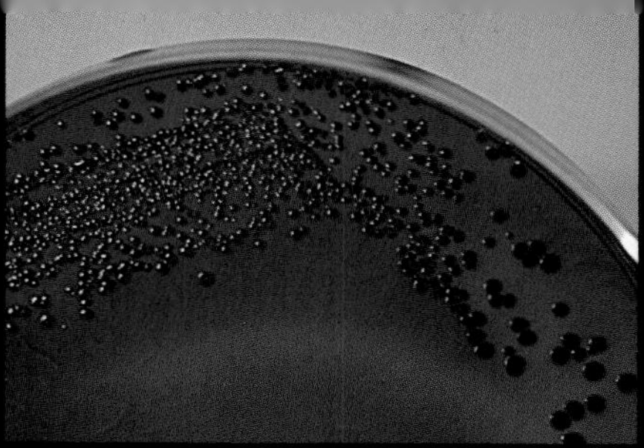

PLATE 8.

PLATE 9.

PLATE 7.
Alpha, beta, and gamma hemolysis caused by different streptococci when they grew on sheep red blood cells.

PLATE 8.
Escherichia coli produces colonies with a green sheen when it grows on EMB agar.

PLATE 9.
Enterobacter aerogenes produces pink mucoid colonies when it grows on EMB agar.

PLATE 10.
Lactose fermenters growing on McConkey agar.

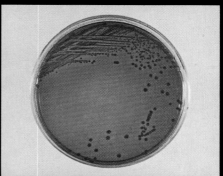

PLATE 10.

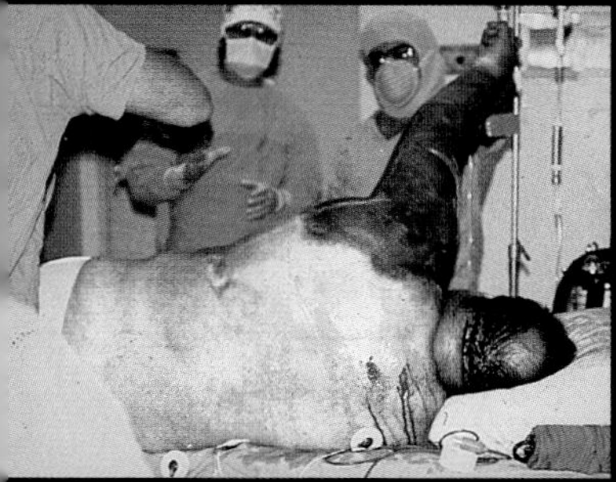

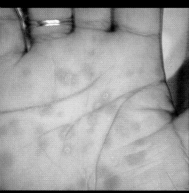

PLATE 11.
Clostridial gas gangrene of left upper extremity.

PLATE 12.
Lesions of secondary syphilis on the palm.

PLATE 13.
The gray membranelike growth of *Corynebacterium diphtheriae* in the pharynx of a diphtheria patient four days after the onset of symptoms.

PLATE 14.
The maculopapular skin rash on the trunk of a patient with endemic (murine) typhus; also characteristic of epidemic typhus.

PLATE 11.

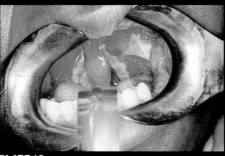

PLATE 13.

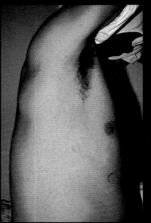

PLATE 12.

Plates 7, 11, 12, 13 and 14: From G. L. Mandell, R. G. Douglas, Jr. and J. E. Bennett, *Principles and Practice of Infectious Diseases*, Volume 1, John Wiley & Sons, 1979.

PLATE 14.

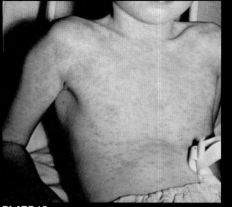

PLATE 15.

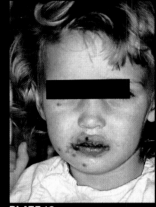

PLATE 16.

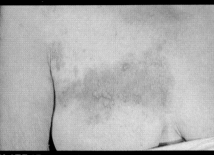

PLATE 17.

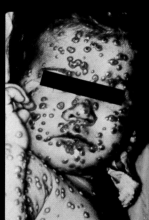

PLATE 18.

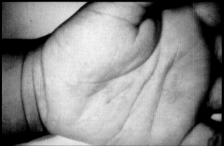

PLATE 19.

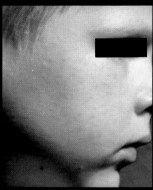

PLATE 20.

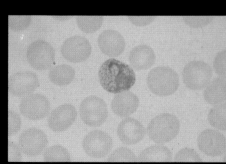

PLATE 21.

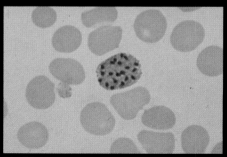

PLATE 22.

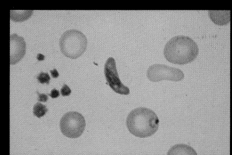

PLATE 23.

PLATE 15.

Typical measles rash on patient's trunk.

PLATE 16.

Herpes labialis lesions on the face of a child infected with HSV-1.

PLATE 17.

Typical rash of zoster on the chest of a 67-year-old woman.

PLATE 18.

Smallpox caused by variola major.

PLATE 19.

Papulovesicular lesions on a patient with hand-foot-and-mouth disease caused by coxsackievirus A16. (Courtesy A. Nahmias.)

PLATE 20.

Rubelliform rash caused by echovirus 16. (Courtesy F. Neva.)

PLATE 21.

Curved trophozoite of *Plasmodium vivax* inside an infected erythrocyte.

PLATE 22.

Schizont of *Plasmodium vivax*.

PLATE 23.

Gamont of *Plasmodium falciparum*.

From G. L. Mandell, R. G. Douglas, Jr. and J. E. Bennett, *Principles and Practice of Infectious Diseases,* Volume 1, John Wiley & Sons, 1979.

Bacteremia and septicemia are usually observed in diseased patients. Conditions that can lead to the presence of bacteria in the blood and/or the spinal fluid include surgery, trauma, burns, injury to bones and joints, brain abscesses, abortions, and many diseases of the viscera.

Infectious diseases are characterized by the dynamic interaction between the invading microorganism and the host. When physical or organic damage occurs to the host, some of the indigenous flora can change from living in peaceful coexistence to being a disease-causing microbe. When this occurs or when infectious agents from nonhuman sources establish a disease state in a human, it becomes the responsibility of the clinical microbiologist to participate in the characterization of the **etiological agent** (the organism or virus causing the disease).

CLINICAL LABORATORIES

Clinical microbiology laboratories are established to isolate and identify the etiological agents from diseased patients and to provide data on the drug susceptibility of the isolate. This information is used by physicians to make a diagnosis and to prescribe a therapeutic regimen. For these reasons, clinical microbiologists serve a central role in the treatment of infectious diseases. Microbiologists receive the samples collected by the attending medical staff, do the necessary laboratory experiments, and transmit the results to the attending physician.

Disease reporting and statistics

There are more than 8000 accredited hospital laboratories and at least another 25,000 private clinical laboratories in the United States. Both hospital clinical laboratories and private clinical laboratories perform microbiological analyses (Figure 11–4). The state and federal governments also operate clinical laboratories that perform specialized tests and serve a regulatory role. Each state department of health runs its own laboratories, which perform tests and compile and analyze data on morbidity and mortality. The United States Department of Health and Human Services operates the Center for Disease Control (CDC) in Atlanta, Georgia. This center will perform specialized tests such as phage and immunological typing of cultures on specimens supplied by health organizations. In addition, the CDC conducts research into national health problems, compiles national health statistics on morbidity and mortality, and has a regulatory role in licensing clinical laboratories. The CDC also publishes *Morbidity and Mortality Weekly Report,* which summarizes data on a weekly and a yearly basis.

Laboratory regulations

Laboratories are regulated by the state in which they are operating. Those laboratories that accept samples from other states also must abide by the federal regulations issued by the United States Department of Health and Human Services, Public Health Service. Licenses can be issued by the federal government after a laboratory satisfies the following requirements.

1. Maintains an adequate quality-control program.
2. Maintains records, equipment, and facilities according to specifications.
3. Is staffed by qualified personnel.
4. Participates in proficiency testing programs established by the CDC.

Federal licenses are issued under the auspices of the Clinical Improvement Act of 1967. An "accredited laboratory" is one approved by the Joint Commission on Accreditation of Hospitals, by the American Osteopathic Association, or by the Commission on Inspection and Accreditation of the College of American Pathologists. Accredited laboratories do not require a federal license.

Licenses are issued to a laboratory to perform tests in one or all of six different areas.

1. Microbiology and serology.
2. Clinical chemistry.
3. Immunohematology.
4. Hematology.
5. Pathology.
6. Radiobioassay.

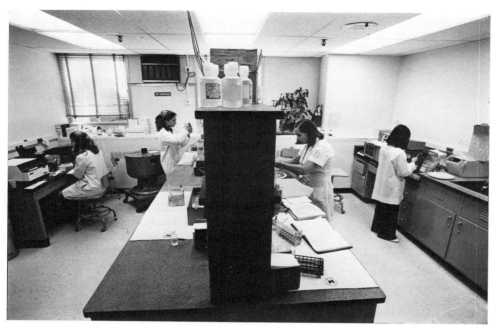

FIGURE 11—4
Wide-angle view of a hospital's clinical laboratory. (Joel Gordon)

The licensing and accreditation procedures in effect are designed to assure quality analyses in all diagnostic procedures performed.

Personnel

Federal regulations specify that the responsibility for the quality of a laboratory's work rests with the director who administers the technical and scientific operation of the laboratory. The director of a clinical microbiology laboratory is an individual who has earned a Ph.D. degree in an appropriate scientific discipline or the M.D. degree. He or she is then certified by a professional organization such as the American Board of Medical Microbiology. Federal personnel regulations apply to any individual who assumed the position of laboratory director after July 1, 1968. Each laboratory must also have one or more supervisors present in the laboratory during all hours in which tests are being performed. This person is held responsible for the proper performance of all laboratory operations in the absence of the di-

rector. Supervisors direct the work of technologists who are trained in the specific techniques performed in the laboratory.

A licensed clinical microbiology laboratory is capable of performing diagnostic tests in bacteriology, parasitology, virology, and serology. Those who actually do the tests are either clinical microbiologists or medical technologists. Medical technologists are qualified to perform tests in all areas of the clinical laboratory, whereas clinical microbiologists are restricted to microbiological testing. Medical technologists are registered by the state after an internship and after passing a qualifying examination. These laboratory personnel analyze specimens that are usually collected by physicians or other health care professionals.

COLLECTION OF SPECIMENS

Specimen collection and handling is an essential prelude to diagnostic microbiology. Some microbes are easily cultured and identified by their growth capabilities; other microbes are difficult or impossible to grow, but they can be detected by direct observation of stained smears or by serological techniques. The success and accuracy of any diagnostic technique will depend in part on the quality of the specimen being investigated. Clean and appropriate sampling techniques must be used to collect the specimen for the clinical microbiology laboratory.

Wounds and excised material

Specimens from wounds and from diseased organs must be procured with aseptic techniques to avoid contamination by the indigenous microbial flora. Specimens from an abscess should include pus in addition to the diseased tissue. Enough material should be collected for both microscopic observation and for culturing. Surgical specimens can be aseptically bisected by the surgeon to provide an appropriate sample for the clinical microbiology laboratory. Surgical samples are finely minced with sterile scissors and then ground into a suspension that is used for culturing. Samples should be cultured immediately, and anaerobic collection techniques should be used.

Blood specimens

Septicemia is a serious condition that requires the prompt characterization of the etiological agent. Blood must be collected aseptically by first cleansing the skin with 70 percent alcohol followed by applying a solution of 2 percent iodine. Between 10 and 20 ml of adult blood (less for children) should be collected by venipuncture for each culture required. Both aerobic and anaerobic culture media should be inoculated immediately after drawing the blood. If this is not possible, the blood can be transported to a laboratory by transferring it to a sterile evacuated tube containing the anticoagulant sodium polyanetholsulfonate. Multiple sample collection during the fever peaks is usually necessary to isolate an etiological agent from blood. It is better to draw blood from patients before they are placed on an antibiotic regimen, because the presence of antibiotics in the blood decreases the chances of culturing the causative pathogen.

Ear and eye specimens

Samples are rarely taken from the inner ear because of the surgical procedures required. Infections of the inner ear are treated with antibiotics that inhibit *Streptococcus pneumoniae*, *Streptococcus pyogenes*, and *Hemophilus influenzae*: these bacteria are the most common etiological agents of inner ear infections. Swabs of the eye are taken to establish the causative agent of conjunctivitis and keratitis. To prevent the sample on the swab from drying out, the swab should be stored and transported in a moist container. Because only small samples can be obtained from the eye, laboratory personnel commonly spot-inoculate agar plates with the material instead of streaking the agar plate.

Feces

Stool specimens that cannot be cultured immediately are placed in a buffered (0.033 M phosphate) glycerol medium following collection. This medium prevents the normal drop in pH in excreted feces that leads to the death of many of the indigenous microorganisms. In this medium, the specimen can be transported safely to the clinical laboratory. Stool specimens of 0.3 to 2.0 g of material are sufficient. Each stool sample should be accompanied by a clinical history of the patient. This history is important because many pathogens can be excreted in stools and because the microbiologist needs to narrow down the number of possible pathogens in order to quickly and efficiently identify the etiological agent.

Cerebrospinal fluids

Untreated bacterial meningitis is a rapidly progressing fatal disease. Cerebrospinal fluid (CSF) examinations are usually performed under emergency conditions and take priority in the clinical microbiology laboratory. Samples are taken by lumbar puncture after disinfecting the skin. The smears of the CSF should be made and observed, and CSF should be inoculated into appropriate media. Confirmation of bacterial contamination is obtained by culturing the organism(s) involved.

Specimens from the respiratory tract

Specimens from the nasopharynx and the throat are taken with sterile swabs attached either to a flexible wire or to a straight applicator stick. The results from these cultures are interpreted with due thought given to the indigenous flora of the anatomical locale. Carriers of *Neisseria meningitidis*, *Corynebacterium diphtheriae*, and *Streptococcus pyogenes* are detected by culturing samples from the nasopharynx. Specimens from the throat are taken to diagnose streptococcal pharyngitis and whooping cough. Throat swabs should be placed in a fluid transport medium to maintain the viability of the specimen.

Sputum from the tracheae is difficult to obtain in a form that is not contaminated by the normal flora of the upper respiratory tract. Patients who are able to cough deeply can expectorate a specimen that can be sent to the laboratory. These samples are often contaminated by the flora of the upper respiratory tract. Sputum samples from seriously ill or comatose patients are more difficult to obtain, but they can be collected by percutaneous transtracheal aspiration using a local anesthesia. This is a cumbersome technique at best. Actually, there is no convenient, reliable, satisfactory technique available to obtain sample material for the isolation and identification of the etiological agents of pneumonia. Often lung infections are treated with broad-spectrum antibiotics without isolating the causative agent.

Urine samples

Urine specimens are often contaminated by the indigenous microbial flora. Cleanly voided urine from human females can be obtained by collection of two or three samples. Human males are able to produce cleanly voided urine more easily, and usually only one sample is necessary. Urine samples should be cultured either within an hour or refrigerated immediately. Urine is an excellent culture medium, and the number of microorganisms present in urine will increase rapidly if the sample is not refrigerated.

Bacteriurea exists if a patient has 100,000 or more bacteria/ml of urine. Patients who have between 1000 and 100,000 bacteria of a single species/ml of clean voided urine are possibly infected and should be retested.

Bacterial causes of venereal diseases can be diagnosed by detection of the causative agent in vaginal exudate, in urethra discharge, or in lesions. Gonorrhea is detected by observing the bacteria in smears of a urethral discharge from the male patient. This disease in female patients is characterized by gonococcus in the cervical discharge. *Neisseria gonorrhoeae* does not survive well outside the human body, so samples should be cultured immediately. The causative agent of syphilis, *Treponema pallidum*, cannot be cultured in the laboratory, so it is detected by dark-field microscopy in samples taken from syphilitic lesions. Fluorescent antibody and other immunological techniques are also used to detect *T. pallidum* (see Chapter 13).

RESPONSIBILITIES OF THE CLINICAL MICROBIOLOGIST

Clinical microbiologists are involved in the collection and processing of specimens and in analyzing and reporting the laboratory results of microbiological tests. The rapid and accurate analysis of the microbiological content of a specimen is important to the successful recovery of the patient. Sometimes it is more important for the attending physician to know that a microorganism is present in a normally sterile anatomical locale than to wait a few days or a week for the isolation and classification of the etiological agent. The clinical microbiologist has the responsibility of obtaining and reporting as much information as is possible to the physician as soon as it is feasible.

SUMMARY

Many microorganisms coexist with humans. They reside in the mouth, nasopharynx, eyes, external ears, respiratory tract, gastrointestinal tract, anterior urethra, and the vagina. Some of these organisms are opportunistic pathogens that are capable of causing disease in compromised hosts, whereas others are not known to cause disease in humans. Not all parts of the human body contain an indigenous microbial flora. Blood, cerebrospinal fluid, the kidneys, the urinary bladder, and the urethra (except the anterior urethra) are free of microbial contaminants in the healthy human.

The clinical microbiology laboratory is charged with the responsibility of isolating and identifying the causative agents of infectious diseases. All accredited hospitals have a clinical laboratory for this purpose. Private laboratories, state laboratories, and federal laboratories are also involved in diagnostic microbiology. These laboratories process specimens and are responsible for analyzing and reporting the results of their laboratory tests. The success and accuracy of all diagnostic techniques depend on the proper collection of specimens from human patients. Samples are routinely collected with due regard for the indigenous microbial flora. The successful isolation and identification of the etiological agent(s) depend on the use of proper procedures for the transportation and handling of specimens.

QUESTIONS AND TOPICS FOR STUDY AND DISCUSSION

Questions

1. What changes occur in the intestinal flora of a breast-fed infant as the infant grows into childhood?
2. How does the normal flora of the vagina change during sexual maturation? Which microorganisms in the vagina are potential pathogens?
3. Define and explain the following.

   peritonitis   urethritis
   cholecystitis   cystitis
   gastroenteritis   pyelonephritis
   bacteremia   septicemia
   otitis media

4. What anatomical parts of a healthy human are free of microorganisms? Can these organs become infected, and, if so, under what conditions?

5. Describe one important public health function of your county, state, and federal public health agencies.
6. What problems are involved in collecting urine specimens? Are these problems different in males versus females? How are the problems surmounted?

Discussion

1. Under what conditions does an opportunistic bacterium become a pathogen?
2. *Staphylococcus* is implicated in most cases of toxic shock syndrome. The incidence of this disease has been correlated with the use of superabsorbent tampons. What are the possible relationships between these facts and the normal flora of the vagina?

FURTHER READINGS

Books

Finegold, S. M., and W. J. Martin, *Baily and Scott's Diagnostic Microbiology*, 6th ed., Mosby, St. Louis, 1982. The first few chapters deal with general laboratory methods and the collection of clinical specimens.

Lennette, E. H., A. Balows, W. J. Hausler, and J. P. Truant, *Manual of Clinical Microbiology*, 3rd ed., American Society for Microbiology, Washington, D.C., 1980. Section 10 is devoted to "infection prevention and quality control" in both the hospital and the clinical laboratory.

Articles and Reviews

Moss, M. L., C. A. Horton, and J. C. White, "Clinical Biochemistry," *Ann. Rev. Biochem.*, 40:573–604 (1971). A summary of analytical methods used in analyzing chemicals of clinical importance.

Pamphlets

Mikat, D. M., and K. W. Mikat, "A Clinician's Dictionary Guide to Bacteria and Fungi," 3rd ed., 1976, Eli Lilly and Company, Indianapolis. A convenient guide to the clinically important bacteria and fungi, distributed as a service to the medical profession.

12

HOST-PARASITE RELATIONSHIPS

Many microorganisms live in close association with animals. When both organisms benefit from the relationship, the organisms live in **symbiosis.** For example, the N_2-fixing bacteria and the cellulytic protozoa found in the termite gut have a symbiotic relationship with the termite. Another symbiotic relationship exists between humans and bacteria in their large intestine. These bacteria break down the fibrous material consumed in the human diet into products that appear to be absorbed and utilized by the human. Organisms that cause damage to their hosts are referred to as **parasites,** and the relationship is known as **parasitism.** A small group of helminths (worms), bacteria, fungi, and protozoa are human parasites.

Infectious diseases develop when the relationship between a host and a microbe results in damage to that host. A disease is infectious when it is caused by an etiological agent that can be transmitted from one individual to another. Infectious disease-causing agents are either viruses or microorganisms (bacteria, fungi, or protozoa). Some etiological agents of infectious diseases are **obligate parasites** because they are unable to reproduce outside of their host.

Other microbes are **opportunistic parasites** because they cause disease only under specific conditions. They normally exist in a symbiotic relationship with their host; however, they are capable of causing disease following a significant change in the resistance of the host and/or following a change in the parasite. Infectious diseases are characterized by the dynamic interaction between the microbe's ability to persist and the host's battle to resist. The following discussion provides the groundwork for understanding the dynamic nature of infectious disease.

ABILITY TO CAUSE DISEASE

The ability to cause infectious disease in humans is observed among certain species of bacteria, fungi, protozoa, helminths, and viruses. The diversity among these organisms is paralleled by the variety of human diseases they cause. The present discussion of the general properties of infectious agents will ignore the viruses. Animal viruses are distinctly different from the other infectious agents, so they are discussed separately in Chapter 22.

TABLE 12–1
Properties of Exotoxins and Endotoxins

Exotoxins	Endotoxins
Protein in composition	Complexes containing lipopolysaccharide
Heat labile	Heat stabile
Soluble products of bacterial metabolism	Low solubility, components of cell-wall structures
Usually very high toxicity, specific in effect	Low toxicity, nonspecific
Produced by Gram-positive and Gram-negative bacteria	Produced by Gram-negative bacteria
Detected by biological effect and laboratory methods	Detected by *Limulus* amebocyte lysate assay and other methods
Toxoids formed by chemical alteration	Toxoids usually not formed (polysaccharide is antigenic)

Pathogens* are organisms that are capable of causing disease. This term is used to describe species that have caused disease in the past and therefore are likely to cause disease in the future. Not all isolates of a given pathogenic species will be equal in their ability to cause disease. The measure of the degree to which a given isolate or culture is able to cause disease is termed **virulence.** For example, it would require only a few cells of a highly virulent strain to cause disease in a susceptible host, whereas many cells of a strain with low virulence would be required to cause a similar disease state.

Intoxication versus invasive diseases

Bacteria cause disease by invading tissue, destroying tissue through chemical means, and/or by stimulating the body's inflammatory response. Organisms that invade tissue usually cause localized tissue damage and stimulate the body's inflammatory response. During this process, they often produce chemicals, known as **toxins,** that cause damage to cells or tissues. Diseases attributable to the effects of toxins are described as **intoxications.**

Some intoxications can occur when the toxin-producing organism is not present in the host. An ex-

Pathology is the branch of medicine that studies the nature of diseases and their causes.

ample is botulism food poisoning. *Clostridium botulinum* can produce a neurotoxin during growth in improperly prepared canned food. Persons who consume the neurotoxin in the food will exhibit the clinical symptoms of botulism. This is an intoxication that is caused by the toxin alone: the presence of the producing organism is not necessary to cause the disease.

In contrast, **invasive** diseases are caused by the growth of the microorganism in the host animal. Syphilis is an invasive disease caused by *Treponema pallidum.* This bacterium penetrates the mucous membranes of the genitourinary tract, enters the circulatory system, and then invades numerous tissues of the human body. *T. pallidum* causes syphilis in humans through its ability to invade and grow in human tissue.

Many pathogens cause disease through a combination of toxigenic and invasive mechanisms. An example is *Streptococcus pyogenes*, which can cause both strep throat (pharyngitis) and the red rash of scarlet fever. Growth of *S. pyogenes* in the throat causes pharyngitis. While growing in the throat, certain strains of *S. pyogenes* will produce erythrogenic toxin. This toxin causes the red scarlet-fever rash on the patient's extremities. Most bacterial diseases are a result of both the toxigenic and the invasive characteristics of the infectious agent.

Toxins

Toxins are natural substances that chemically damage cells or tissues to cause disease. Many snakes, jellyfish, plants, fungi, and bacteria are able to produce toxins. Bacterial toxins are grouped into two major types: exotoxins and endotoxins (Table 12–1). **Exotoxins** are usually highly toxic, heat-labile proteins produced during the growth of either Gram-negative or Gram-positive bacteria. The effects of these toxins on human tissues are usually very specific. In contrast, **endotoxins** are heat-stable components of the outer membrane of Gram-negative bacteria, are of lower toxicity, and are composed of lipopolysaccharide.

Exotoxins. Bacterial exotoxins are produced by a variety of Gram-negative and Gram-positive bacteria (Table 12–2). Exotoxin-producing bacteria are often named after the disease they cause; for example, *Clostridium botulinum, C. tetani, Corynebacterium diphtheriae,* and *Vibrio cholerae.* Exotoxins are proteins that are released to the surrounding environment following their synthesis in the cell's cytoplasm. They often react with a single target tissue in which they cause specific damage. The toxins of botulism and tetanus are nerve toxins; diphtheria toxin is an inhibitor of protein synthesis; and certain enterotoxins alter the retention of fluid by the small intestine. Because exotoxins are proteins, most are destroyed by heating at cooking temperatures. Staphylococcal enterotoxin is an example.

TABLE 12–2
Properties of Selected Bacterial Toxins

Toxin (Organism)	Properties	Action
Exotoxins		
Botulism toxins (*Clostridium botulinum*)	Heat-labile protein, 6 antigenic types	Neurotoxin, muscle paralysis
Tetanus toxin (*Clostridium tetani*)	Heat-labile protein	Neurotoxin, spasmodic muscle contraction
Diphtheria toxin (*Cory. diphtheriae*	Heat-labile protein	Inhibition of protein synthesis in eucaryotes
Enterotoxins (*Staphylococcus*) (Enterotoxic *E. coli*) (*Shigella*) (*V. cholerae*)	Proteins, sometimes heat-stabile	Emetic (causes vomiting), net loss of fluid from small intestine
Erythrogenic toxins (*Streptococcus*)	Protein types A, B, and C	Scarlet-fever rash
Whooping cough toxin (*Bordetella pertussis*)	Heat-labile protein	Dermal necrosis (slows ciliary action)
Plague toxin (*Yersinia pestis*)	Protein types A and B	Necrosis, hemorrhage
Shigella neurotoxin (*Shigella dysenteriae*)	Heat-labile protein	Paralysis (mice), hemorrhage
Endotoxins		
Pyrogen (Gram-negative bacteria)	Toxic lipid A, heat-stabile protein antigen	Diarrhea, fever shock, intestinal hemorrhage, necrosis

Toxoids are chemically inactivated toxins that are still immunogenic. Normal individuals who are immunized with a toxoid will develop antitoxins against the toxin. Antitoxins will react with their specific toxin and will neutralize the toxin's effects on its target tissue. Toxoids are used to immunize individuals against toxigenic diseases. In the United States, infants are immunized with tetanus toxoid and diphtheria toxoid to prevent the clinical symptoms of tetanus and diphtheria.

Botulism toxin is the most toxic naturally produced substance known. This toxin causes paralysis in humans and can lead to death from respiratory failure. Humans are not immunized against botulism because the incidence of the disease is low (average of 25 cases in the United States per year—1950 to 1977). When cases are diagnosed, the patients are treated with antitoxin preparations.

Enterotoxins are a group of bacterial exotoxins that act on the intestine (Gr. *enteron,* intestine). Enterotoxic *Escherichia coli* and *Vibrio cholerae* infect the human intestine and produce enterotoxins that cause diarrhea. These enterotoxins appear to be similar because they both stimulate the secretion of chlorine ion (Cl^-) and inhibit the uptake of potassium ion (K^+) by the human intestine. This physiological change results in a great outpouring of fluid into the intestine.

Many strains of *Staphylococcus aureus* produce **staphylococcal enterotoxins,** which, unlike other exotoxins, are relatively heat stabile. These toxins are produced when *S. aureus* grows in unrefrigerated food. They cause staphylococcal food poisoning in persons who consume the contaminated food. In humans, this illness is characterized by diarrhea, nausea, vomiting, and cramps.

Another group of exotoxins causes necrosis (tissue destruction) or hemorrhage. *Bordetella pertussis* produces **whooping cough toxin,** which specifically destroys the cilliary epithelial cells in the human trachea. The **plague toxin** (murine toxin) produced by *Yersinia pestis* causes necrosis. It also affects the vascular system, resulting in subcutaneous hemorrhages. The exact role of the plague toxin in causing the human disease is unknown. *Shigella dysenteriae* produces an exotoxin that inhibits protein synthesis in mammalian cells. This toxin is called the **shigella neurotoxin** because in mice and rabbits it causes peripheral paralysis (not seen in humans) and death. *Shigella dysenteriae* causes bacillary dysentery (Gr. *dys,* bad, *enteron,* intestine) in humans; however, the role of shigella neurotoxin in this human disease is unknown.

Bacterial endotoxins. **Endotoxins** are heat-stabile, poisonous substances that are structural components of bacterial cells. They are an integral part of the bacterial outer cell wall and, as such, can be released as subcomponents of the cells only after the cell lyses. Endotoxins are effective poisons both in the bound state and as soluble products of cell lysates. Endotoxins are large lipopolysaccharides that are usually associated with the outer envelope of Gram-negative bacteria (Table 12–2). Their toxicity resides in the lipid A portion of the molecule.

Endotoxins have been isolated from many Gram-negative bacteria. Injection of the isolated endotoxins into animals results in diarrhea, shock, and fever. These symptoms are thought to be mediated by the noradrenalin, histamine, and serotonin that are released from host cells in response to endotoxin irritation. Noradrenalin, histamine, and serotonin directly affect the vascular system of animals. The endotoxins of Gram-negative bacteria are also called **pyrogens** (Gr. *pyros,* fire) because they cause fever. In comparison to exotoxins, endotoxins are generally less potent and have less tissue specificity.

The *Limulus* amebocyte lysate assay is used to detect endotoxins in picogram quantities. The horseshoe crab *Limulus* (Figure 12–1) has a primitive resistance mechanism associated with the amebocytes in its circulatory system. Amebocyte proteins coagulate when they react with endotoxin molecules. This reaction is presumed to be beneficial to the horseshoe crab by localizing the infection in a walled-off area. The *Limulus* amebocyte lysate assay has been adapted to detect endotoxins in commercial biological preparations and to detect Gram-negative bacteria in natural environments. Unknown samples that contain endotoxin coagulate commercial preparations of lysed *Limulus* amebocytes. The assay is theoretically able to detect 10 bacteria/ml.

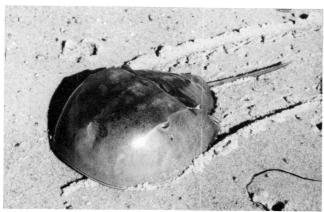

FIGURE 12–1
Limulus polyphemus is the Atlantic Coast horseshoe crab. Its primitive circulatory system contains amebocytes that react with the endotoxin of Gram-negative bacteria. (Courtesy of Dr. Thomas J. Novitsky and Associates of Cape Cod, Inc.)

Hydrolytic enzymes.   Bacteria produce a variety of enzymes that hydrolyze components found in animal tissues. When these enzymes cause cellular damage, they are considered to be toxins. **Hydrolysis** is the process of cleaving a covalent bond with the concomitant addition of water to the reactants (Figure 12–2). All cells produce hydrolytic enzymes to recycle essential components within their cells and to utilize storage products. These enzymes are found in the periplasmic space of Gram-negative bacteria: Gram-positive bacteria produce hydrolytic exoenzymes because they do not have a periplasmic space. Pathogenic bacteria produce a variety of hydrolytic enzymes that can cause damage to host tissue (Table 12–3).

Collagenase and **hyaluronidase** are bacterial enzymes that hydrolyze components of human connective tissue. Collagen is the most abundant pro-

FIGURE 12–2
Reactions of hydrolytic enzymes produced by pathogenic bacteria.

Enzyme	Substrate	Products	Reaction
Collagenase	Helical regions of collagen	Polypetides	Hydrolysis of peptide bonds
Fibrinolysin	Fibrin	Soluble products	Hydrolysis of peptide bonds (esp. arg and lys)
Hyaluronidase	Hyaluronic acid 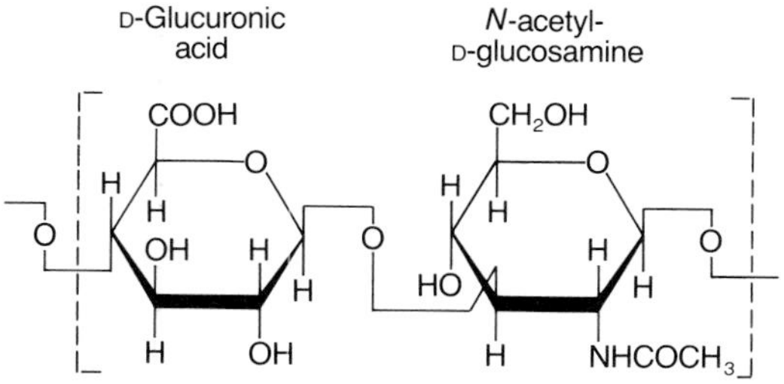	D-glucuronic acid N-acetyl-D-glucosamine	Hydrolysis B1-4 glycosidic bond
Lecithinase (phospholipase A)	Lecithin 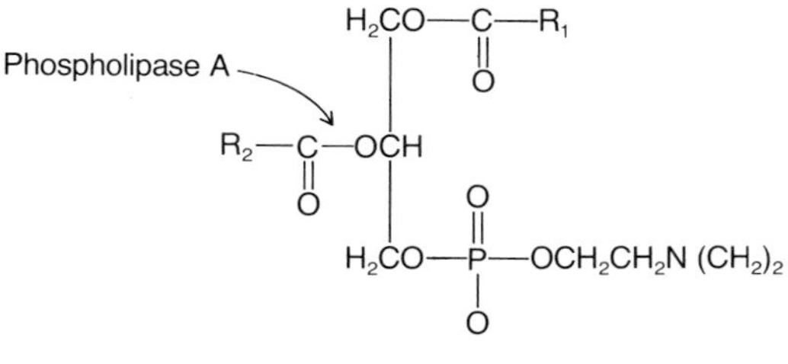	1-Acylglyceryl-phosphinicocholine + a fatty acid anion	Lipid hydrolysis

TABLE 12–3
Bacterial Enzymes Involved in Virulence

Enzyme	Action	Role in Disease
Coagulase	Activation of fibrin clot formation	Unclear function: may coat bacteria, useful in diagnosis
Collagenase	Hydrolysis of collagen	A factor in invasiveness
Hyaluronidase	Hydrolysis of hyaluronic acid in tissue	A factor in invasiveness
Lecithinase (alpha toxin)	Hydrolysis of membrane lipids	Lysis of cells, destroys cell membrane
Streptokinase (plasmin[a] or fibrinolysin)	Hydrolysis of fibrin clot to soluble products	A factor in invasiveness, used in diagnosis
Proteinases	Hydrolysis of proteins	A factor in invasiveness

[a]Plasmin is the recommended name for this enzyme.

tein in higher animals, where it is a structural component of connective tissue. Collagenase hydrolyzes collagen into polypeptides. Hyaluronic acid is the most abundant mucopolysaccharide in higher animals. It is a heteropolysaccharide (D-glucuronic acid and N-acetyl D-glucosamine) found in the connective tissue of vertebrates. Hyaluronidase hydrolyzes the glycosidic bond in hyaluronic acid. These enzymes contribute to the invasiveness of the pathogens that produce them.

Lecithinase hydrolyzes lecithin, which is a phospholipid found in animal cell membranes. Lecithin is the common name for choline phosphoglyceride. The activity of lecithinase can destroy the integrity of an animal cell's plasma membrane, which causes the cell to lyse.

Forming a fibrin clot is one way that animals localize an infection. Some bacteria negate this action by producing **fibrinolysin** (also called streptokinase), which hydrolyzes fibrin clots into soluble products. This enables bacteria to invade adjacent tissue.

The pathogenic role of coagulase produced by *Staphylococcus aureus* is still unclear. Most virulent strains of staphylococci produce coagulases, which are exoenzymes that clot plasma by hydrolyzing fibrinogen to produce fibrin. The presence of coagu-

lase has been used to identify virulent strains of staphylococci. However, the role of coagulase in pathogenesis is unclear because coagulase-nonproducing strains of staphylococci also cause human disease and healthy humans carry coagulase positive *Staphylococcus aureus* without ill effects.

Proteinases hydrolyze proteins to peptides. They are prevalent in invasive organisms that cause severe damage to animal tissue such as skin and muscle. Bacterial proteinases are diverse in their action: some proteinases hydrolyze many different peptide bonds, others hydrolyze only bonds formed between two specific amino acids.

The type of hydrolytic enzymes, their specificity, and the quantity produced by an infectious microorganism all contribute to the virulence of that organism. The hydrolytic enzymes produced will also influence the anatomical locale in which the organism can establish an infection.

Capsules

Some bacteria produce extracellular polymers of amino acids or carbohydrates that form capsules around the producing cell. Capsular material is deposited outward of the bacterial cell wall and confers a smooth viscous appearance on the producing colonies. Simple staining techniques are used to demonstrate the capsules that surround microorganisms (Figure 12–3).

Capsules often prevent or retard phagocytosis by animal leukocytes. This antiphagocytic property often makes capsulated strains more virulent than noncapsulated strains, as was elegantly shown by Griffith's transformation experiments. When injected intraperitoneally, the capsulated smooth colony strain of *Streptococcus pneumoniae* (Color Plate 3) caused death in mice, whereas the noncapsulated rough colony strain did not. It is now known that smooth colonies of *S. pneumoniae* type 3 produce an antiphagocytic polysaccharide capsule composed of glucose and glucuronic acid.

The virulence of *Bacillus anthracis* is also related to the presence of a capsule. Noncapsulated strains are avirulent, whereas the strains of *B. anthracis* that produce a *D*-glutamic acid polypeptide capsule can cause anthrax.

Adherence or colonization

Bacteria that colonize specific regions of the animal body appear to have surface antigens that facilitate adherence to that tissue. Colonization of tooth surfaces by species of streptococci is an important part of the process that leads to dental caries. The presence of pili on the surface of gonococci appears to facilitate the adherence of these bacteria to urethral epithelium. Once adherence has taken place, the bacteria are able to colonize that tissue.

Measuring virulence

Pathogens can possess one or many virulence factors. Some virulence factors can be measured by simple biochemical techniques, whereas others represent a combination of properties detectable only by a biological assay. The ability to multiply inside a phagocytic leukocyte is an example of the latter. A standard biological assay measures the amount of toxin, or the number of bacteria, that will cause death in 50 percent of a population of susceptible

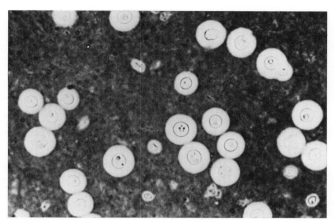

FIGURE 12–3
Microbial capsules can be observed in the light microscope with simple staining procedures. The capsule of *Cryptococcus neoformans* are clearly visible when the background is stained with india ink. (Courtesy of Dr. N. L. Goodman.)

animals. This is determined experimentally by measuring the **lethal dose 50 percent** or LD_{50}.

To determine an LD_{50}, one must first choose a susceptible experimental animal. Individual animals are exposed to different numbers of pathogenic organisms or to different amounts of toxin. The number of animals that survive is determined after a standard time period. These data are analyzed by statistical methods, and the number of organisms, or the amount of toxin needed, to kill 50 percent of the population of animals is determined.

Only a few organisms of a highly virulent strain are necessary to cause the death of a susceptible animal, whereas many organisms of a strain of low virulence would be required to cause the death of the same animal. The toxicity of purified toxins can also be measured with a biological assay. Botulism toxin has an LD_{50}/mg of 1,500,000 in guinea pigs. This means that 1 mg of botulism toxin is 1,500,000 times the amount needed to kill 50 percent of the guinea pigs injected. In comparison, 1 mg of *E. coli* endotoxin has only 10 lethal doses for the mouse. Obviously, the botulism toxin is much more toxic than the endotoxin, even though different animals were used.

HOST RESISTANCE TO DISEASE

Experiments with animals have shown that the establishment of an infectious disease is dependent on the route of infection, the dose received, and the health of the animal. The animal is an active participant in the disease process, and under normal circumstances it launches its own defense mechanisms to ward off infectious agents. Species of animals vary greatly in their susceptibility to infectious agents. Even among humans, differences in resistance to certain diseases are discernible between different races and even between regional populations of the same race. Animals also have anatomical, cellular, and humoral defense mechanisms against infecting parasites.

Species, genetics, and race

Some bacterial pathogens or viruses can cause disease in humans but not in other animals. *Yersinia pestis* causes human plague, which is usually fatal if untreated. At the same time, *Y. pestis* is carried by ground squirrels and apparently causes no ill effects to the infected squirrels and to the fleas that transmit this pathogen to humans. Another example is the poliovirus, which infects humans and monkeys but does not infect quadrapeds or other animals unrelated to humans. Animals that never succumb to an infectious disease are said to have **species resistance** to that disease.

Most pathogens exhibit species specificity and will cause disease only in a limited number of hosts. This is beneficial to humans since there are only a few infections that we can contract from domestic animals. On the other hand, species resistance is a major obstacle to pathologists because diseases that cannot be mimicked in laboratory animals are difficult to investigate. Syphilis and leprosy are two such diseases. Neither disease is mimicked in an experimental animal, and the etiological agent of leprosy, *Mycobacterium leprae*, is almost impossible to grow under any conditions.

There is some historical evidence that **gene pools** of a host population can confer either resistance or susceptibility to an infectious agent. During the European explorations of the world, infectious diseases caused many deaths among the aborigines. For ex-ample, the population of the Massachusetts Bay Indians prior to the European colonization was estimated to be about 30,000 individuals. By the middle of the 1600s, less than 1000 survivors remained following severe smallpox epidemics. A similar devastation occurred when the United States Plains Indians lost two-thirds of their population to smallpox and tuberculosis. The American Indians had a very low resistance to these diseases, whereas the European settlers, whose descendants had been exposed to these diseases, survived.

A group of human beings possessing a common set of genetically determined physical characteristics is designated a **race.** The American Indians are a race, as are the Caucasian and the Negro peoples. Racial resistance and susceptibility to a disease are perpetuated in the gene pool of that race. For example, members of the Negro race have a high resistance to erysipelas—a streptococcal skin infection. In addition, blacks respond more readily to treatments for gonorrhea. Subgroups of Caucasians also have differences in racial resistance and susceptibility to a disease. People of Irish descent have a low resistance to tuberculosis, whereas people of Jewish descent have a very low mortality rate from tuberculosis.

Resistance to malaria by individuals with sickle-cell anemia is a well-documented case of genetic resistance. Individuals with sickle-cell anemia produce abnormal hemoglobin, which in turn causes red blood cells to assume a sickle shape. Protozoa belonging to the genus *Plasmodium* cause malaria. Part of the replication cycle of *Plasmodium* occurs in the human red blood cell. Individuals with the inherited sickle-cell trait have a high resistance to malaria because the sickle-cells are unable to support the replicative needs of the parasite. Sickle-cell anemia is prevalent in members of the negroid race in the endemic malaria regions of the tropics. This is a clear-cut case of inherited resistance to a specific disease within a race of humans.

Sex

Human sexuality plays a role in resistance to disease. In the United States, more males are conceived (120/100) than females. However, more male fetuses are naturally aborted, which results in a ratio of males to females at birth of 105/100. After birth, the survival rate for female infants is higher than for male infants. Human females are also more resistant to infectious diseases than are their male counterparts. Males are more susceptible than females to respiratory infections, viral infections of the central nervous system, viral gastrointestinal diseases, and hepatitis.

Age

Except for the first few months of life, resistance to infectious disease increases during the lifetime of the human. This is largely attributed to the development of the immune response to various infectious agents (see Chapter 13). Infants acquire from their mother a short-lived immunity to infectious diseases. This immunity lasts for 6 to 12 months. Subsequently, individuals develop their own immune response to infectious agents either by receiving immunizations

or by surviving sublethal cases of infectious diseases.

Tuberculosis and pneumonia appear to be exceptions to the general rule of increased resistance with age. The incidence of tuberculosis increases with age (Figure 12–4) with the absolute number of cases being greatest among the 45 to 65 age group. When the cases per 100,000 population are plotted against age (Figure 12–4), the incidence of tuberculosis increases with age beginning with the 5 to 14 age group. The same pattern is observed for pneumonia. The decreased resistance to pneumonia and tuberculosis is attributed to the accumulation of degradative changes in elderly persons.

Physiological state of host

Resistance to infectious disease decreases directly with any decline in the physiological well-being of the host. Surgery, physical wounds, organic disease, nutritional deficiencies, exhaustion, and fatigue all

FIGURE 12–4
Cases of tuberculosis by age group in the United States during 1978: (a) plotted as the total number of cases, and (b) plotted as cases per 100,000 population. (Centers for Disease Control: "Reported Morbidity and Mortality in the United States," 1978. *Morbidity Mortality Weekly Report,* 27, 54: Annual Suppl., 1979.)

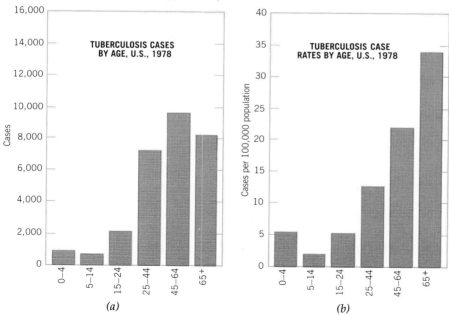

lead to a diminished host resistance. Whenever the human body is called on to repair diseased tissue, fewer resources are available to fight infectious diseases.

Poor nutrition and outright starvation make humans extremely susceptible to infectious diseases. Refugees in strife-torn countries are particularly vulnerable because they are more likely to suffer fatigue, nutritional deficiencies, and/or starvation. Fatigue and crowding increase a human's susceptibility to infectious disease. For example, outbreaks of meningococcal meningitis among military recruits have been attributed to the rigorous basic training (fatigue) and the crowded living conditions (barracks).

The composite of all these factors—species, genetics, race, sex, age, and the physiological state of the host—contributes to the susceptibility of humans to infectious disease. When an individual actually comes in contact with a virulent infectious agent, there are additional mechanisms of resistance that are important. These include anatomical structures together with the cellular and humoral defense mechanisms of the host.

Mechanical barriers to infectious agents

The human body poses anatomical barriers to pathogens. These barriers represent the **first line of defense** against infectious agents. Anatomical barriers include the human skin; the conjunctiva and tears, which protect the eyes; mucous membranes in the nasopharynx; ciliated epithelium of the trachea; and the mucous membranes of the genital and urinary tracts.

Human skin.   Healthy skin is an effective mechanical barrier to the invasiveness of most infectious agents. Many bacteria are normal inhabitants of the skin, where they live in symbiosis. In addition to serving as a mechanical barrier to penetration, the outer layer of skin is continually sloughed off, and skin contains sweat glands that produce bactericidal fatty acids (especially oleic acid). When bacteria do penetrate these barriers to infect hair follicles or se-

baceous glands, the infections are normally localized by the host deposition of a fibrin barrier.

Human eye.   The conjunctiva is the mucous membrane lining the eyelid. Underneath the eyelid is the fluid that bathes the cornea and the white of the eyeball. The tear ducts carry fluid from the lachrymal glands to the conjunctiva. Lachrymal fluid (tears) contains the enzyme lysozyme and immunoglobulins (principally IgA). Lysozyme hydrolyzes peptidoglycan in bacterial cell walls, whereas the immunoglobulins react specifically to inhibit the action of infectious agents. The human eye is well protected by the conjunctiva and the tears, which lubricate the eyeball's movement, wash away foreign matter from the eye surface and protect the eye from infectious agents.

Respiratory tract.   The respiratory tract is protected against infectious agents by hairs, by ciliary epithelium, and by a mucous membrane. Mucus is secreted by the membranes lining the nasopharynx and is moved to the oropharynx on a regular basis. The mucus in the back of the nasal cavity is replaced every 10 to 15 minutes. Foreign particles and infectious agents inhaled through the nose are either filtered out by hairs in the anterior nares or trapped in this flow of mucus. Mucus itself is not bactericidal, but its viscous composition traps bacteria and prevents their entrance into the lungs.

The trachea is also lined with mucous membranes interspersed with the ciliated epithelium. Mucus containing trapped foreign matter is propelled upward toward the oropharynx either by the ciliated epithelium or by coughing. This material is then expectorated or swallowed. These mechanisms normally protect the bronchioles in the lungs from infectious agents. As a matter of fact, expired air from healthy lungs is normally sterile. If microorganisms are present in expired air, they are exhaled in water droplets generated in the nasopharynx region by coughing or sneezing.

Digestive tract.   Many bacteria are normally found in the human mouth on the tongue, tooth surfaces, and gums. Saliva contains many bacteria that have been washed from these surfaces. When saliva is swallowed, these bacteria meet their demise in the strongly acidic gastric juices of the stomach. The bactericidal environment of the stomach usually prevents infectious agents from gaining entrance to the intestine. Viable bacteria and viruses enmeshed in food are protected from the acidity of the stomach and do reach the intestine.

Another protective mechanism of the stomach is the ability to vomit. Involuntary vomiting is a mechanism for voiding the contents of the stomach. Vomiting serves to protect the digestive system from excessive toxic material.

Urinary and genital tract. Voiding of urine by both males and females cleanses the urethra and normally maintains the urinary tract in a bacterial-free state. In contrast, bacteria inhabit the female vagina, which is colonized during childhood and remains colonized by bacteria, albeit by different species, thereafter. Vaginal mucus and the acidity of the vagina are to some degree bactericidal.

Cellular defense mechanisms

Anatomical barriers including the skin, tears, conjunctivae, mucous membranes, and ciliary epithelia serve as the first line of defense against invading microorganisms and viruses. The **secondary line of defense** is the body's complement of phagocytic cells. These cells are capable of destroying infectious agents that penetrate the anatomical barriers.

Leukocytes. Animals contain "white cells" in their blood, lymph, and tissues that are collectively called **leukocytes** (Table 12–4). This term formerly described the white cells of the blood. However, white cells are found both in the blood and in tissues, so we must expand the definition of leukocyte to include all the white cells of an animal. Leukocytes are identified by their function, anatomical location, morphology, and their staining reactions (Color Plate 1). Human leukocytes are derived from stem cells that reside primarily in the bone marrow. These

TABLE 12–4
Leukocytes in Normal Human Blood

Cell Type	Percentage Range
Granulocyte Series	
Neutrophils	40–80%
Eosinophils	1–7%
Basophils	0–1%
Monocyte Series	
Monocytes	2–11%
Lymphocytes[a]	15–50%

Source: Adapted from W. R. Clark, *The Experimental Foundations of Modern Immunology*, Wiley, New York (1980).
[a]About 70–80 percent of the lymphocytes are T lymphocytes; the remainder are B lymphocytes.

stem cells differentiate into functional white cells (Figure 12–5 and Color Plate 6), which are found in various parts of the body. The two major morphological groups of leukocytes are the granulocytes and the monocytes.

The **granulocyte series** contains white blood cells possessing a lobed or irregular-shaped nucleus and a granular cytoplasm. **Neutrophils** (also known as polymorphonuclear granulocytes or PMN) are identified by their lobed nucleus and by the pink to violet staining granules present in their cytoplasm. Neutrophils are the major phagocytic white cell in the circulatory system. **Eosinophils** comprise 1 to 7 percent of the blood's white blood cells. They are morphologically similar to neutrophils; however, they take up acid eosin, which stains their cytoplasmic granules red. Eosinophils are involved in allergic reactions and in resisting infections by helminths. **Basophils** have an irregular-shaped nucleus and possess large cytoplasmic granules. These granules contain substances such as histamine, serotonin, and heparin that are released when basophils participate in allergic reactions. Basophils are present in the blood, where they make up 0 to 1 percent of the leukocytes, and in tissues.

Leukocytes possessing a spherical nucleus include the monocytes and lymphocytes (Table 12–4). Lymphocytes, which are involved in the immune response, are described in Chapter 13. Monocytes are

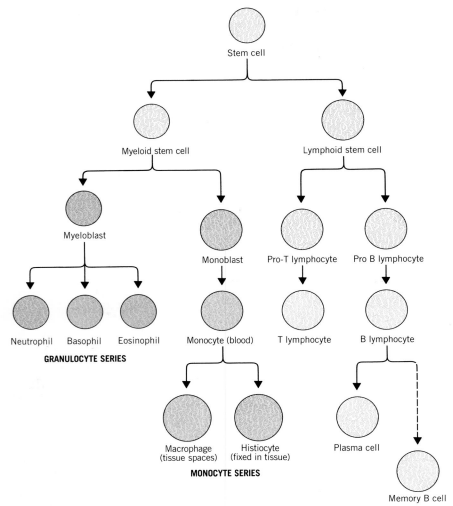

FIGURE 12–5
Leukocytes are all derived from stem cells through the process of differentiation. For a color interpretation, see Color Plate 6.

the circulating form of differentiated stem cells that eventually become macrophages (Figure 12–5). Monocytes have phagocytic activity in the circulation; however, blood monocytes probably represent a transition stage in the development of macrophages.

Phagocytosis by white blood cells. Neutrophils are the major phagocytic cells of the blood, where they comprise 40 to 80 percent of the normal white blood cell population. They are attracted to the site of bacterial infection, where they kill and phagocytize many of the invading microorganisms. Neutrophils represent a terminal stage in the differentiation of stem cells.

Monocytes are mononuclear phagocytic cells that make up to 2 to 11 percent of the circulating white blood cell population in humans. They remain in the blood for only a few days prior to migrating into tissue spaces. Here they increase in size (by as much as tenfold) and differentiate into **macrophages** (Figure 12–6). These cells are present in most human tissue and function as scavengers by removing and destroying foreign matter and breakdown products of human tissue. Macrophages are found free in tissue spaces. Other macrophages become fixed in the reticulum of the spleen, lymph nodes, and liver, where they are known as **histiocytes.**

The first step in phagocytosis is the formation of a bond between the particle and the phagocytic cell. The particle is then engulfed (Figure 12–7) by the plasma membrane, which invaginates and pinches off to form a phagocytic vacuole. When the phagocytic vacuole collides with a lysosome, an explosive rupture of the lysosome occurs. This releases the contents of the lysosome into the phagocytic vacuole. Substances within the lysosome usually kill bacteria within 10 to 30 minutes. Digestion of the material within the phagocytic vacuole follows. Unwanted microorganisms, viruses, and cell debris can be scavenged by neutrophils and macrophages and eliminated from the host through the mechanism of phagocytosis.

Inflammation. Infectious agents can cause damage to tissue that results in redness, swelling, pain, heat, and tenderness. This animal response is known as **inflammation.** Under certain circumstances, inflammation is accompanied by the accumulation of pus. The swelling is due to the local dilation of blood vessels and allows fluid and white blood cells to penetrate into the area. Redness is a result of the increased flow of blood to the area. Neutrophils gain entrance to the inflamed area through the dilated capillaries, whereas macrophages migrate to the inflammation site through tissue spaces.

Lymphokines are a large group of animal cell products that affect other animal cells. Many lympho-

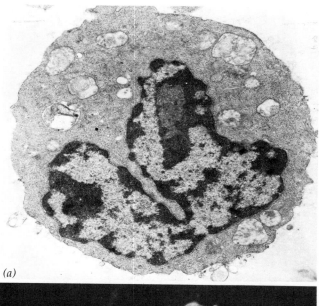

(a)

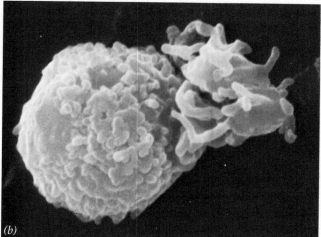

(b)

FIGURE 12–6

(a) Transmission electron micrograph of an activated macrophage containing numerous phagocytic vesicles (Courtesy of Dr. T. E. Mandel. From T. E. Mandel, "The Ultrastructure of Mammalian Lymphocytes and Their Progeny," pp 11–42, in J. J. Marchalonis, ed., *The Lymphocyte: Structure and Function,* copyright © 1977 Marcel Dekker.) (b) A scanning electron micrograph of a lymphocyte associated with platelets and red blood cells. (Courtesy of Dr. R. Chao.)

kines are involved in the inflammatory reaction at the infection site. Lymphokines are named and described by their effects on other cells. Among the

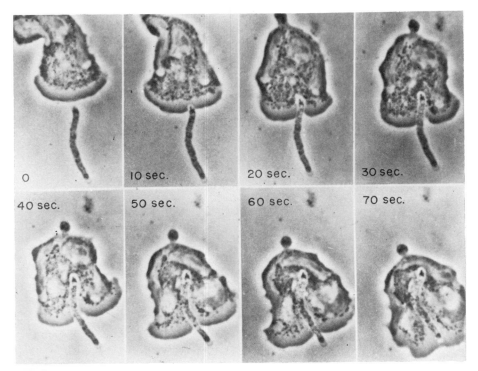

FIGURE 12–7
Sequence of light micrographs that show the phagocytosis of a bacterium by a macrophage.
(Courtesy of Dr. J. G. Hirsch, The Rockefeller University, N.Y.)

known lymphokines are the migration-inhibiting factor, macrophage chemotactic factor, macrophage-activating factor, pyrogen-releasing substance, and lymphocyte chemotactic factor. Most lymphokines are produced by activated T lymphocytes; however, researchers have recently shown that some lymphokines are produced by B lymphocytes, macrophages, and virus-infected fibroblasts. Most of the characterized lymphokines are glycoproteins, so they are chemically different from immunoglobulins.

The human defense mechanisms just described provide the first and second line of defense against infectious agents. Many bacteria and viruses are able to evade these mechanisms to establish infections in humans. To protect against these persistent infectious agents, animals have a third line of defense, which is the immunological response. This defense mechanism is discussed in detail in the next chapter.

SUMMARY

Infectious diseases can be characterized as a dynamic interaction between the microorganism's ability to persist and the host's battle to resist the infectious process. Infectious, disease-causing agents are either viruses, helminths, or microorganisms (bacteria, fungi, or protozoa). Pathogens are organisms that are capable of causing a disease. Virulence is a measure of the degree to which a given strain or culture is able to cause disease. Virulence factors include exotoxins, endotoxins, hydrolytic enzymes, capsules, and the property of adherence. Bacterial exotoxins are usually heat-labile proteins of high toxicity that cause specific damage to animal tissue. Humans are immunized with toxoids against some diseases manifested by exotoxins. Endotoxins are less toxic than exotoxins and are structural components of the bacterial cell. They are heat-stable lipopolysaccharides that are released from the cells only after lysis. Invasive pathogens gain entrance to the host and then cause disease by disrupting the normal functions of the host and/or by producing toxins. Invasive factors include hydrolytic enzymes capable of breaking down host tissue and capsules that are antiphagocytic. Bacterial capsules often protect the organism against phagocytosis, and other surface structures enable bacteria to adhere to specific animal tissues. The virulence of a pathogen or the potency of a toxin can be determined by measuring the LD_{50}.

Animals are not all subject to the same infectious agents. The resistance and susceptibility of an animal to an infectious agent depend on the species, gene pools within the population, race, sex, age, and the general physiological state of the animal.

Many animals possess species resistance to specific infectious agents. The first line of defense against infectious agents includes the human skin; the conjunctiva and tears, which protect the eyes; mucous membranes in the nasopharynx; ciliated epithelium of the trachea; and the mucous membranes of the genital and urinary tracts. A second line of defense becomes operative when organisms penetrate the body. Invading microorganisms are phagocytized by specialized leukocytes. Neutrophils are the major phagocytic cells in the circulation, whereas macrophages and histiocytes are the major phagocytic cells in tissue and tissue spaces. These white blood cells are attracted to the infection site by lymphokines. Lymphokines also participate in the inflammatory response. Long-term resistance against infectious agents is provided by the immunological response.

QUESTIONS AND TOPICS FOR STUDY AND DISCUSSION

Questions

1. Compare the characteristics of an invasive pathogen with those of a pathogen that causes a toxigenic disease.
2. Describe the mode of action of four exotoxins that affect human tissue. Which organisms produce these toxins?
3. What enzymes contribute to bacterial virulence? Do they contribute to the virulence of invasive or toxigenic pathogens? Explain.
4. How does a capsule contribute to the virulence of a bacterium?
5. Use the accumulated totals in the following experiment to determine the LD_{50} of the bacterial culture. Each animal was injected with bacteria and then maintained at 23°C. The number of animals still alive were counted after 24 hours. Can this animal assay be used to determine the toxicity of a toxin and/or the virulence of a virus? Explain.
6. Are all human races equally susceptible to all infectious diseases? Provide specific examples to support your answer.
7. How do age and sex influence a person's susceptibility to disease?
8. What anatomical barriers do humans possess that protect them against infectious agents?
9. Describe the human white blood cells that participate in the defense of the human body. Where are these cells found in the human body?

Bacteria Cells Injected	No. of Animals	Animals Dead	Animals Alive	Accumulated Dead	Total Alive	% Total
10^3	5	0	5	0	13	?
10^4	5	0	5	0	8	?
10^5	5	3	2	3	3	?
10^6	5	4	1	7	1	?
10^7	5	5	0	12	0	?

Discussion

1. Should the human race be concerned about introducing infectious agents into extraterrestrial environments? Discuss the historical evidence that supports your answer.

FURTHER READINGS

Books

Ajl, S. J., S. Kadis, and T. C. Montie (eds.), *Microbial Toxins*, vols. 1–5, Academic Press, New York, 1970. A six-volume series on bacterial toxins composed of articles written by experts in this specialized field. A good source for reactions and molecular data on specific toxins.

Bellanti, J. A., and D. H. Dayton (eds.), *The Phagocytic Cell in Host Resistance*, Raven, New York, 1975.

Articles and Reviews

Hirsch, J. G., "The Digestive Tract of Phagocytic Cells," in R. C. Williams and H. H. Fudenberg (eds.), *Phagocytic Mechanisms in Health and Disease*, pp. 23–38. Intercontinental Medical Book, New York, 1972.

Spector, W. C., and D. A. Willoughby, "The Inflammatory Response," *Bacteriol. Revs.*, 27:117–154 (1963). An early review of the physiology of inflammation.

13

IMMUNOLOGY

Many epidemics raged throughout Western Europe during the eighteenth and nineteenth centuries, just as science was raising its head above religious control. Smallpox, diphtheria, plague, tuberculosis, and cholera were diseases that incapacitated, disfigured, and killed large segments of the European population.

The first major scientific contribution to the control of infectious diseases was the development of a vaccine against smallpox. An English country physician, Edward Jenner (1749–1823), believed in the folklore that milkmaids resisted the devastating effects of smallpox because of their occupational exposure to cowpox. Jenner experimented with this folk belief by injecting individuals with material taken from cowpox lesions. These individuals experienced mild cases of cowpox but rarely contracted smallpox. The process became known as vaccination (*vacca* in Latin means "cow"), and the injected material was called a vaccine. Many cases of smallpox were averted by vaccination. However, it wasn't until Louis Pasteur's time that the general public accepted vaccination as an effective means of preventing disease.

Louis Pasteur (1822–1895) made the accidental observation that chickens inoculated with an old culture of fowl cholera were resistant to subsequent injection of disease-causing cholera cultures. In 1881, Pasteur used this basic knowledge to develop vaccines against anthrax and against rabies. The rabies vaccine was widely publicized and brought worldwide attention to the significance of vaccination.

Our understanding of human disease developed very rapidly between 1880 and 1900 (see Table 1–1). During this time, antitoxins against diphtheria and tetanus toxin were developed. Paul Ehrlich developed procedures to measure toxins and antitoxins. In addition, Elie Metchnikoff discovered phagocytosis through his observations of the devouring capabilities of invertebrate amoeboid cells. Metchnikoff (1883) maintained that phagocytosis was a major mechanism by which animals defended themselves against invading microorganisms. The processes of phagocytosis and vaccination became important areas of investigation by twentieth-century scientists.

Most major microbial diseases have now been brought under control, and one disease, smallpox, has been eliminated completely. Immunology has played a major role in accomplishing this feat. We now have a basic understanding of the mechanism of immunity, including an understanding of the genetics, biochemistry, and physiology of immunity. An indeterminable amount of pain, suffering, and death have been avoided through the practical application of immunology. This chapter explains the basic principles of immunology and their use in our modern medical society.

IMMUNITY

Immunity to a disease indicates that a given individual or population has an increased resistance to an infectious agent. No individual is "impervious" to a disease, because if a large enough dose of an infectious agent is administered in an appropriate fashion, it can overcome the defenses of even the most resistant individual.

The human population possesses different kinds of immunity. **Innate immunity** is inborn resistance to disease possessed by a given population or race. For example, humans have innate immunity against dog distemper, a common disease of domestic dogs. Innate immunity is inborn, has no dependency on previous exposure to the infectious agent, and largely depends on the nonspecific resistance factors discussed in Chapter 12.

Acquired immunity occurs when the host is treated in a manner that establishes a specific immune state within the host's body. This type of immunity can be acquired in four different ways: naturally acquired by an active or a passive means or artificially acquired by an active or a passive means (Table 13–1).

Naturally acquired active immunity develops during a sublethal case of an infectious disease, for example, measles. The host makes specific antibodies against the virus following infection. **Naturally acquired passive** immunity is the resistance to disease passed from mothers to their newborns or infants. Passive means that the host did not form the antibodies. For several months after birth, newborns are protected by the immunoglobulin that they acquired

TABLE 13–1
Immunity, Acquired and Innate

Immunity	Means of Acquisition	Host Response
Naturally Acquired		
Active	Recovery from sublethal or transient infection	Antibodies formed against agent, long-lasting
Passive	Transfer of antibodies to fetus through the placenta, to infants through mother's colostrum	IgG, short duration
Artificially Acquired		
Active	Immunization	Antibodies against toxoids or attenuated infectious agents, long-lasting
Passive	Injection of antibodies (antibodies formed in another animal)	Host receives antibodies from another animal; temporary, specific resistance
Innate Immunity		
Innate immunity	Inborn	Natural resistance to infectious agents

when their mother's antibodies crossed the placental barrier into the fetal circulation. Breast-fed infants also acquire antibodies from their mother's colostrum.

Individuals can be artificially immunized in two distinct ways. To prevent an individual from contracting a specific disease, the person can be immunized with a vaccine or a toxoid. Individuals immunized with these commercial preparations develop **artificially acquired active** immunity. This is an active process because the patient is the animal that produces the antibodies. When a patient is diagnosed as having a disease to which he/she has no immunity, the physician can passively immunize the patient by administering antibodies formed in another animal or person. Injection of antibodies formed in another organism results in **artificially acquired passive** immunity. Artificially acquired passive immunity is always of short duration (a few months), whereas artificially acquired active immunity can last an individual's lifetime.

Antibodies, antigens, and immunogens

Antibodies are proteins produced by the animal body in response to a foreign substance (antigen) that will react specifically with that substance. Antibodies are found either attached to animal cells, in animal blood, or in secretions of the exocrine tissues. Humoral* antibodies are present in animal serum; the study of these antibodies is termed **serology. Antigens** are substances that specifically react with an antibody to form a stable complex. An antigen that elicits an immune response is more properly called an **immunogen;** however, since most antigens are immunogens, we will use the term antigen. Most antigens are large proteins or polysaccharides that are foreign to the animal. Small molecules that serve as antigenic determinants but are unable to elicit the formation of antibodies are called **haptens.** Antibody-antigen reactions are widely used in biology for diagnostic purposes.

*The fluid or fluidlike substances of the body including the blood and lymph.

Antibody structure. Antibodies were shown by E. A. Kabat and A. Tiselius (1939) to belong to a class of serum protein called gamma globulins. Later these proteins were named the **immunoglobulins.** It is now possible to isolate specific antibody molecules and to investigate their structures by biochemical techniques. The basic immunoglobulin molecule is composed of two light polypeptides and two heavy polypeptides joined by disulfide bridges (Figure 13–1). The amino-terminal ends of the light and heavy chains have regions where the amino acid sequence varies greatly from molecule to molecule. These variable regions contain different amino acid sequences, making each immunoglobulin able to react uniquely with its specific antigen. The remainder of the amino acid sequences in the light and heavy chains are relatively constant from antibody to antibody. Geneticists are beginning to understand the process of gene transcription that enables a protein to have both variable and constant regions.

Immunoglobulin molecules have been taken apart biochemically and analyzed. The results demonstrate that the N-terminal ends (Figure 13–1) of the immunoglobulin molecules are responsible for specifically interacting with the antigen molecules. Since there are two pairs of N-terminal groups on each immunoglobulin molecule (each pair composed of one light chain and one heavy chain N-terminal end), there are two antigenic combining sites on each immunoglobulin. This structural arrangement results in **bivalance,** which is the ability of an immunoglobulin molecule to react with two separate, but identical, antigenic determinants.

There are five classes of immunoglobulin (Ig) found in humans. These proteins are designated IgA, IgD, IgE, IgG, and IgM. Each class of immunoglobulins is functionally and structurally different. Table 13–2 is a list of the differences between the immunoglobulin's molecular weight, serum concentration, half-life in serum, and characteristic properties.

Immunoglobulins belonging to the IgG class make up the highest percentage of the antibody molecules in the blood. This class is composed of four subclasses (IgG_1, IgG_2, IgG_3, IgG_4) that vary in the struc-

297

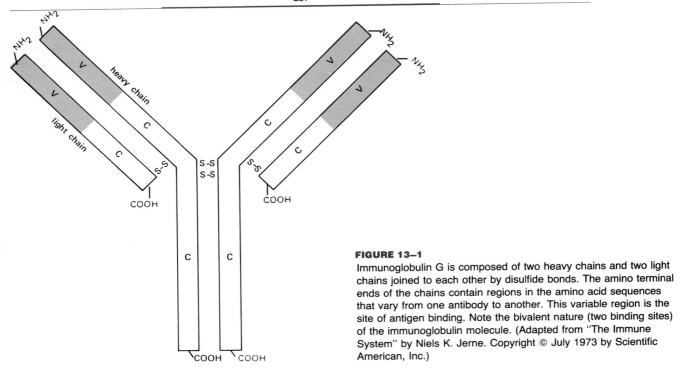

FIGURE 13–1

Immunoglobulin G is composed of two heavy chains and two light chains joined to each other by disulfide bonds. The amino terminal ends of the chains contain regions in the amino acid sequences that vary from one antibody to another. This variable region is the site of antigen binding. Note the bivalent nature (two binding sites) of the immunoglobulin molecule. (Adapted from "The Immune System" by Niels K. Jerne. Copyright © July 1973 by Scientific American, Inc.)

TABLE 13–2
Properties of Antibody Molecules

Immunoglobulin Class	Serum Concentration (mg/100 ml)	Molecular Weight	Half-Life (days)	Characteristic Properties
IgG (total)	range (900–1800)			Precipitins, antitoxins, complement
IgG$_1$	900	146,000	23	fixation (except IgG$_4$), late
IgG$_2$	300	146,000	23	antibody, placental transfer
IgG$_3$	100	165,000	8–9	(except IgG$_2$)
IgG$_4$	50	146,000	23	
IgA	156–294	160,000	6–8	Mucous membrane surface
(Secretory IgA)		400,000		protection
IgM	67–134	900,000	5	Agglutinins, opsonins, early antibody
IgD	0.3–4.0	184,000	2.8	On surface of B lymphocyte
IgE	0.0001–0.0007	190,000	2.5	Antibody to allergens

ture of their heavy chains (Table 13–2). IgG$_1$ is present in the greatest quantity and makes up 60 percent of the IgG in the serum. The different subclasses of IgG vary in their function. For example, all the IgGs bind complement except IgG$_4$, and all members of this class, except IgG$_2$, are able to cross the placenta. Immunoglobulins of the IgG class are responsible for protection against toxins and other protein antigens. The average serum half-life of human IgG is between 18 and 23 days, which makes IgGs the longest-lived immunoglobulin molecules.

Secretions of mucous membranes contain immunoglobulins of the A class. IgA molecules are similar in size to IgG; however, IgA molecules tend to polymerize into larger complexes. IgA is excreted by exocrine glands and is a component of breast milk, respiratory and intestinal mucin, saliva, tears, vaginal secretions, and prostatic fluid. This immunoglobulin protects these parts of the body from infectious agents. Humans normally produce equal amounts of IgA and IgG in a given time period. This is not apparent in the serum data because significant quantities of IgA are lost in secretions. The serum level of IgA is actually about one-fifth the level of serum IgG (Table 13–2).

IgM (M = macroglobulin) is synthesized in almost all immune responses as the early antibody. This immunoglobulin is a large complex that is basically a pentamer of the IgG structure. It is composed of five monomeric units held together by disulfide bonds and a polypeptide J chain that connects the heavy chains (Figure 13–2). IgM is synthesized early in the immune response; however, it has a short half-life. It binds complement and is very active in agglutination and opsoninization (renders bacteria susceptible to phagocytosis) reactions. These reactions protect the animal against invading microorganisms. IgM does not cross the placenta.

The remaining two classes of immunoglobulins are present in the serum in low concentrations. Although IgD can be isolated from serum, its function is at present unknown. IgE is found in serum in extremely low concentrations. This antibody is cytophilic, which means that it readily binds to cells (especially basophils and mast cells). Immunoglobulin

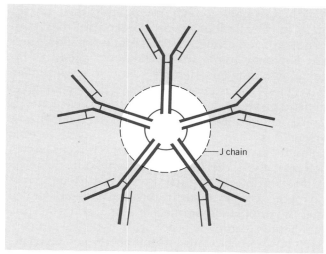

FIGURE 13–2
Immunoglobulin M is a pentamer of five monomeric subunits that individually are the size of an IgG molecule attached by a J chain and disulfide bonds. Immunoglobulin M is formed early during an animal's immunological response to an antigen.

E is responsible for allergic reactions that are discussed in more detail later in this chapter.

Structure of antigens. Antigens are substances foreign to the animal body, usually proteins or polysaccharides that provoke an immune response. Antigens react specifically with an immunoglobulin molecule. Lipids and nucleic acids act as antigens, but they have little or no ability to stimulate antibody formation in animals. Antigens must be large molecules and as such are usually multivalent. Multivalent antigens have numerous determinants, each of which is able to elicit the formation of a specific antibody. Bacterial cells are large multivalent antigens that will stimulate an animal to form many different antibodies. Since antibodies are specific in their reaction with their antigen, the specificity of the antibody reaction can be used to demonstrate differences between complex antigens such as bacteria.

An antigenic determinant is the smallest chemical unit that will react with an antibody. **Haptens** are low-molecular-weight foreign compounds that are too small to elicit antibody formation and yet they function as antigenic determinants. Many common drugs are haptens. Some drug breakdown products become immunogenic after they bind to large protein molecules. The experiment depicted in Figure 13–3 demonstrates this characteristic of haptens. Proteins can be chemically conjugated with *p*-aminobenzene arsenate (pABA). pABA by itself is unable to elicit an antibody response. However, the protein-hapten complex elicits the formation of antibodies when it is injected into an animal. By using various immunological assays, investigators have demonstrated that the antibodies, formed in response to the protein-hapten complex, react with both the protein-hapten complex and *p*-aminobenzene arsenate. These experiments demonstrate that small molecules such as pABA serve as antigenic determinants even though they do not elicit antibody formation.

Anamnestic response

Up to this point, we have viewed antibodies as biochemical entities that can be studied by chemical techniques. Another aspect of immunology is the mechanism by which animals form antibodies. Animals form antibodies following exposure to an antigen. They have a built-in memory system that recognizes an antigen to which they have been previously exposed. The ability to remember antigens is called the anamnestic (memory) response.

Immunologically competent animals make antibodies on exposure to an antigen in a very specific manner. On first exposure, there is a delay or latent period (usually 3 to 4 days in humans) during which no circulating antibody can be detected. Following the latent period, antibody concentration increases in the serum, reaches a peak level, and then decreases (Figure 13–4). This is called the **primary response.** There is a gradual decrease in the level of circulating antibody if and when the antigen is removed. This is caused in part by the short half-life of circulating antibodies (see Table 13–2).

On subsequent exposure to the same antigen, the animal dramatically increases the level of circulating antibody with a much shorter latent period. The animal behaves as if it remembers the previous experience with the antigen. This secondary response is referred to as the **anamnestic response.** It is extremely important in establishing resistance to infectious disease.

A secondary exposure stimulates the animal to produce an antibody at an accelerated rate. The level

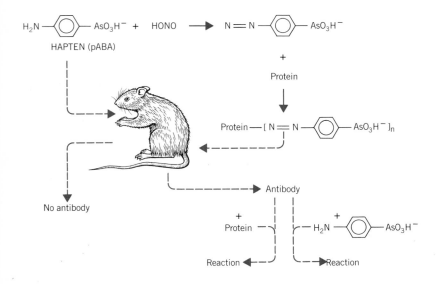

FIGURE 13–3
Hapten molecules are too small to elicit an immunological response. *p*-Aminobenzene arsenate (pABA) is a hapten that is easily attached to a large protein. In this state, pABA can stimulate an animal to produce specific antibodies against both the protein and pABA.

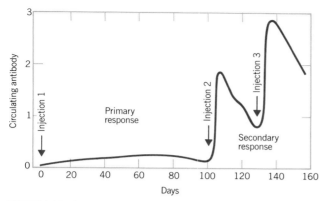

FIGURE 13–4
Animals form higher levels of circulating antibody more quickly on the second and subsequent exposure to an antigen. This is termed the anamnestic or memory response.

of the circulating antibody continues to rise as long as the antigen is present in the system. When the antigen is removed, the level of circulating antibody decreases because of the short half-life of serum immunoglobulins. The secondary response can be repeated many times to increase the level of circulating antibody. **Booster shots** are injections that stimulate the secondary response.

The absolute amount of antibody formed by an individual will depend on (1) the nature of the anti-gen, (2) the route of exposure, and (3) the dosage and sequence of exposure. The best procedures for routine immunizations have been established through clinical trials. For maximal protection, children should be immunized against bacterial and viral diseases (Table 13–3) at the recommended intervals.

These immunizations are administered through the oral route or by injecting the antigen intramuscularly. Polio vaccine is taken orally (TOPV = trivalent oral poliovirus vaccine), whereas the DTP (diphtheria, tetanus, pertussis) shots are given intramuscularly. The nature of the antigens also vary. Immunization against polio is accomplished by ingesting an attenuated strain of poliovirus. A formaldehyde-inactivated preparation of diphtheria toxin is used to immunize people against diphtheria, whereas killed cultures of *Bordetella pertussis* are used to immunize people against whooping cough. Clinical trials have established the best antigens to use and the best route and sequence of administration to protect people against the common childhood diseases.

Cells involved in immunity

An explanation of the immune response must take into account the foreign nature of antigens, the specificity of antibodies, and the anamnestic response. In

TABLE 13–3
Active Immunization Schedule for Normal Children and Infants

| Immunization | Vaccine | Schedule of Immunizations | | | | | Route |
		1st	2nd	3rd	4th	5th	
Diphtheria	DTP	2 mo	4 mo	6 mo	1.5 yr	4–6 yr	Intramuscular
Pertussis	DTP	2 mo	4 mo	6 mo	1.5 yr	4–6 yr	Intramuscular
Tetanus	DTP	2 mo	4 mo	6 mo	1.5 yr	4–6 yr	Intramuscular
Poliovirus	TOPV	2 mo	4 mo	1.5 yr	4–6 yr		Oral
Measles Mumps Rubella	Combined vaccine	15 mo					Intramuscular

DTP = diphtheria and tetanus toxoids combined with pertussis vaccine.
TOPV = trivalent oral poliovirus vaccine.
Combined vaccine = measles, mumps, and rubella vaccine.

TABLE 13–4
Properties of Leukocytes

Leukocyte	Cell Type	Morphology	Body Location	Functions
Granulocyte	Neutrophil (PMN)	Lobed nucleus	Circulation, few in tissue	Phagocytosis
	Basophil	Lobed nucleus granules in cytoplasms	Circulation	Release of histamine, serotonin
	Eosinophil	Lobed nucleus red-yellow staining granules	Circulation	Control of inflammatory response
Monocytes	Monocytes	Single nucleus, abundant cytoplasm	Circulation	Phagocytosis, precursors of macrophages
	Macrophages (free) Histiocytes (fixed in tissue)	Single nucleus, abundant cytoplasm	All tissues	Phagocytosis and destruction of cell debris
Lymphocytes	Lymphocytes	Single nucleus, little cytoplasm	Lymphoid tissue and circulation	Participation in immunological response
	Plasma cells	Single nucleus, ovoid cell	Lymphoid tissue	Antibody synthesis

part, the immunological response can be explained through the role of the "white cells" known as **leukocytes.** Leukocytes differentiate from the embryonic stem cells, which in adult animals are found primarily in the bone marrow and in lymph. Differentiated leukocytes are subdivided into major groups based on the distribution of their nuclear material, size, staining properties, and location in the body (Table 13–4).

Leukocytes can be conveniently divided into the granulocyte series and the monocyte series based on cell morphology. The phagocytic leukocytes are found in both series. **Neutrophils** are the major phagocytic cell type in the blood. The blood also contains monocytes that are precursors of macrophages. **Monocytes** (Figure 13–5) only stay in the circulatory system for a few days before they grow in size and move into tissue spaces where they are known as **macrophages.** Here they roam freely and phagocytize unwanted material and cells. Macrophages that become fixed in tissue are known as **histiocytes.**

Basophils are leukocytes of the granulocyte series that contain numerous cytoplasmic granules. They are often found in tissue as well as in blood where they represent 0 to 1 percent of the leukocyte population. Basophils possess surface receptors for IgE and are involved in immediate hypersensitivity reactions. When the IgE on a basophil reacts with its antigen (also called an allergen), the cell degranulates whereby it releases histamine and serotonin into the environment. These compounds are directly responsible for immediate hypersensitivity reactions. **Mast cells** are morphologically and functionally similar to basophils; however, mast cells are derived from peripheral mesenchyme late in embryogenesis and are found in connective tissue. The granules of mast cells contain histamine and serotonin, which they release on degranulation.

Lymphocytes belong to the monocyte series of leukocytes. They arise through the differentiation of stem cells (see Color Plate 1) and are involved in antibody production or in cell-mediated immunity. Lymphocytes are subdivided into two types of cells

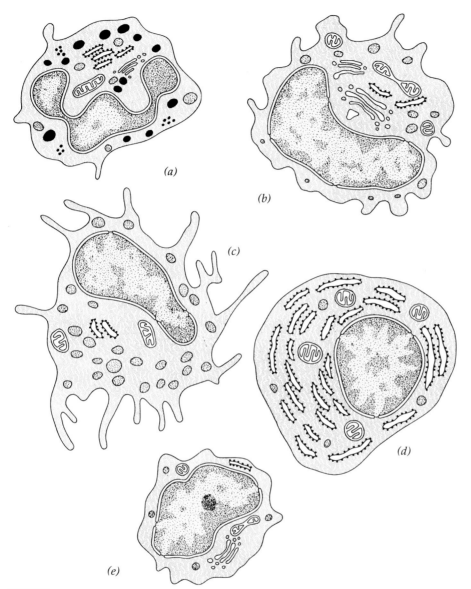

FIGURE 13–5
Leukocytes are the white blood cells of animals. Cross sections of (a) polymorphonuclear neutrophil, (b) monocyte, (c) mast cell, (d) plasma cell, and (e) lymphocyte. If an eosinophile were drawn to scale, it would be twice as large as the mast cell.

that are involved in antibody formation; the T lymphocytes and the B lymphocytes. Embryonic stem cells give rise to the bone marrow during develop-

ment. Some bone marrow stem cells are influenced by the thymus gland and differentiate into T lymphocytes (T for thymus). Other bone marrow stem cells develop into B lymphocytes. *B* stands for bursa of Fabricius, which is the structure in the chicken that produces B lymphocytes. Mammals have no analogous structure; however, the "chicken" terminology is retained for convenience.

The B lymphocytes and T lymphocytes are structurally and functionally distinct cell types that can be differentiated by immunological techniques. For example, mouse T lymphocytes contain the antigen *Thy-1* on their surface. T lymphocytes are involved

in **cell-mediated immunity** as well as other immunological reactions. B lymphocytes contain immunoglobulin molecules (IgD and IgM) on their surface. After reacting with their antigen, B lymphocytes are transformed into **plasma cells** that actively produce a specific immunoglobulin (Figure 13–6). Plasma cells possess an extensive rough endoplasmic reticulum for synthesizing protein (Figure 13–5). A given plasma cell can synthesize and secrete about 2000 identical antibody molecules a sec-

FIGURE 13–6
The clonal selection theory suggests that lymphocytes form clones of antibody-producing cells following reaction with their antigen. B lymphocytes are thought to be involved in the production of clones of plasma cells (antibody producing) and memory B lymphocytes. T lymphocytes are involved in cell-mediated immunity, delayed hypersensitivity, and allograph rejection. Activated T lymphocytes produce lymphokines and may also be involved in positive cooperation with B lymphocytes in initiating certain immunological responses.

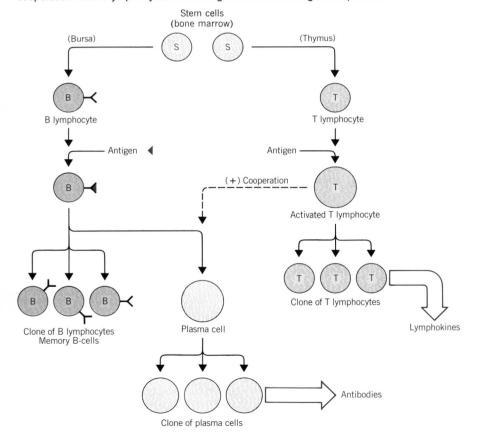

ond and usually lives only a few days after it is formed from a B lymphocyte. Other B lymphocytes become memory cells (Figure 13–6). Both B and T lymphocytes are involved in the process of antibody production.

Antibody formation. Sir MacFarlane Burnet proposed the **clonal selection theory** of antibody formation in 1957. This theory is widely held today since it explains the major phenomena of the immune response (Figure 13–6). The clonal selection theory proposes that antigens in an animal react with a specific cell carrying an antibody on its surface. Animals contain millions of these cells, each with a different and specific antibody on its surface. Combination of the antigen with a particular cell-bound antibody stimulates that cell to divide and to synthesize more antibody molecules. Each new cell of this **clone** is stimulated to produce antibodies and to divide as long as the antigen is present. When the antigen disappears from the body, descendants of this cell line remain in the body as a clone of memory cells. The animal responds to subsequent exposure to the antigen by stimulating the memory cells to again divide and to synthesize antibody molecules. This mechanism explains the anamnestic response in animals.

B lymphocytes are now known to be the cells making up the clone. Some B lymphocytes are transformed into antibody-synthesizing plasma cells after they react with their specific antigen, whereas others become memory cells (Figure 13–6). It now appears that certain clones of B lymphocytes can be triggered to develop into plasma cells that produce immunoglobulins independently of T lymphocytes, whereas other B lymphocyte clones require T lymphocyte cooperation (T lymphocytes, however, do not make antibodies). Each clone produces only one specific antibody. Since animals have many different antibodies, each animal has many different clones of B lymphocytes.

Most of the reactions between antibodies and antigens protect the host by neutralizing the effects of the antigen or by rendering the antigen susceptible to phagocytosis. Other immunological responses are deleterious to humans. The harmful effects of the immunological system include allergies, asthma, and graft rejection.

HYPERSENSITIVITY

Immunity is a double-edged sword because there are immune reactions that are detrimental to the host. One class of immunological reactions that cause deleterious effects in the host are called **hypersensitivities.** The key characteristics of hypersensitivities are prior exposure of the animal to the antigen and the ability to transfer the sensitivity from one patient to another by transferring either serum or leukocytes. Classically, hypersensitivities were divided into two groups based on the time required to elicit a response in a suitable host. **Immediate hypersensitivities** are manifested minutes after the second and subsequent exposure to the antigen and are mediated by antibodies. Classic delayed hypersensitivity reactions in sensitized animals do not appear until hours or even days after exposure to the antigen. **Delayed hypersensitivity reactions** are initiated by T lymphocytes and, for this reason, are classified with other cell-mediated immune reactions. Cell-mediated immune reactions include delayed hypersensitivity, allograph rejection, and resistance to certain infectious agents.

Immediate hypersensitivity

Common types of immediate hypersensitivities are asthma, hay fever, and anaphylactic shock. The symptoms of these diseases occur immediately on exposure to the antigen or allergen,* are passively transferred with serum, and require prior sensitization. These reactions are significantly different from the protective reactions of the immune response (Table 13–5) and involve a specific class of immunoglobulins.

Recent technical advances have enabled researchers to detect a new class (IgE) of immunoglobulins. Immunoglobulin E is chemically different from the other immunoglobulins and is present in very low concentrations in serum (usually 1 μg/ml or less).

---

*Allergens** are substances capable of inducing an allergic reaction.

TABLE 13–5
Immediate Hypersensitivity and Cell-mediated Immunity

Type	Time Course	Characteristics	Key Mediators	Reactions
Immediate				
IgE-mediated	Immediate	Transferred by serum	IgE antibodies attached to mast cells, basophils	Asthma, hives, hay fever, anaphylactic shock
Cytotoxicity	Immediate	Transferred by serum	Humoral antibodies and complement	Blood transfusions, mismatched blood
Delayed Hypersensitivity				
Cell-mediated	Peak reaction in 24–48 hours after contact	Transferred by lymphocytes	Sensitized T lymphocytes	Positive tuberculin test, poison ivy, graft rejection

IgE is an antibody that readily binds to basophils and mast cells and is called a cytophilic antibody. This immunoglobulin is responsible for some of the immediate hypersensitivities observed in humans. People who have allergies usually contain higher than normal concentrations of IgE in their serum.

Anaphylactic shock. The most severe form of immediate hypersensitivity is **anaphylactic shock** (anaphylaxis means "reverse protection"). Anaphylactic shock results when a sufficient dosage of an antigen is directly injected into the blood of a sensitized individual. This situation (very rare in humans) occurs when sensitized individuals are stung by a bee or wasp or when drug-sensitive patients are given injections of that drug. The antigens react with the cytophilic antibodies (IgE) bound to basophils and mast cells. These cells contain histamines and serotonin in their cytoplasmic granules. Reaction of the antigen with the cytophilic antibody on the surface of these cells causes them to release the histamines and serotonin into the environment. The physiological effect of histamine and serotonin is to increase capillary permeability and to cause constriction of smooth muscles. The first sign of anaphylactic shock is labored breathing. This is followed by contraction of the smooth muscles controlling the bladder and the intestine, resulting in involuntary urination and defecation. These symptoms are often followed

within a few minutes by death. Anaphylaxis can be mimicked with injections of histamine, and it can be prevented or lessened by injections of antihistamines and epinephrine.

Asthma. Allergic reactions that cause wheezing, coughing, and difficulty in breathing are referred to as asthma. This affliction is a hypersensitivity that varies in severity from individual to individual, depending on a genetic predisposition to the allergic state and the nature of the allergens. Individuals who are sensitized to an allergen can become asthmatic by inhaling the allergen. Common allergens include dust; animal dander (scales from hair and skin); pollens of trees, flowers, and weeds; and mold spores. As in anaphylaxis, the symptoms of asthma are mediated by the release of histamine and serotonin by mast cells; however, these mast cells are localized in the lungs. Bronchial constriction can be alleviated by administering antihistamines or epinephrine; in severe cases, patients are treated with oxygen. Hay fever allergens interact with the mucous membranes in the eyes and the nasal passages to cause the symptoms of hay fever. Certain people are also allergic to some foods or to the metabolic products of foods. Food allergies are manifested as hives or gastrointestinal upset.

Desensitization to certain allergens is successful with some patients. To determine one's allergies, small quantities of known allergens are injected into a patient's arm or back. If the patient is sensitive to the allergen, the skin swells and becomes red in the typical wheal and flare reaction. This reaction is immediate. The degree of sensitivity to the allergen can be determined by the amount of swelling and redness. Allergists use this information to prepare a sterile allergen solution that is injected into the patient's muscle. Under these circumstances, the allergens serve as immunogens and elicit the formation of IgG antibodies. These are called **blocking antibodies,** since theoretically they react with allergens before the allergens combine with the IgE cytophilic antibodies attached to mast cells. Increasing concentrations of the allergens are given to the patient over a period of years to build up the circulating levels of IgG antiallergens. Desensitization is more of a preventive measure than a cure.

Sodium cromolyn and steroids are among the drugs currently available to treat asthma. Asthma attacks can be lessened by taking sodium cromolyn, which prevents the degranulation of mast cells in the lungs. Severe cases of asthma can be treated with steroids that suppress the immunological response. The symptoms of asthma can be treated by injecting epinephrine and/or by taking antihistamines.

Serum sickness. IgG (not IgE) is the class of antibodies involved in the hypersensitivity reactions of serum sickness. **Serum sickness** occurs when immune complexes react with complement and other serum factors to cause fever, joint pain, and a skin rash. This can occur when a patient is passively immunized with an antibody produced in another animal, such as a horse. The foreign proteins in the transferred serum act as immunogens and stimulate the animal to form antibodies. The persistent foreign serum proteins are then available to react with their antibodies to form soluble immune complexes. Spontaneous recovery from serum sickness usually occurs in a few days. The antibodies involved in the immune complex syndromes, such as serum sickness, are generally IgG.

Cell-mediated immune reactions

In addition to the humoral antibodies produced by B lymphocytes, animals possess another immune system that involves cells. Cell-mediated immunity has been recognized since Robert Koch first observed the tuberculin reaction in 1891. When an extract of *Mycobacterium tuberculosis*, called *tuberculin,* is injected under the skin of a tubercular animal, an area of inflammation develops at the site of injection within 24 to 48 hours. The reaction is not present in humans who have never been exposed to *M. tuberculosis,* nor is the reaction evident in those who received transfusions of serum from an infected human. The response to tuberculin can be passively transferred by injecting viable, washed white blood cells from an exposed person to a nonexposed individual. This phenomenon is a delayed form of hypersensitivity, because white blood cells are involved and prior sensitization to the tuberculin antigen is necessary for the reaction to occur.

Cell-mediated immunity is an important mechanism by which animals resist infectious diseases such as tuberculosis. This resistance is mediated through the T lymphocytes. When sensitized T lymphocytes react with their specific antigens, they release cell products called lymphokines. **Lymphokines** are a large group of animal cell products, primarily glycoproteins, that affect other animal cells. The function of lymphokines include attracting macrophages to an infection site, immobilization of macrophages at the site, and stimulating macrophages to form degradative enzymes. Certain lymphokines, produced by sensitized T lymphocytes, actually kill other cells nonspecifically. T lymphocytes respond to their specific antigen by dividing and producing a clone of like cells within the body.

Cell-mediated immunity can be used as a diagnostic tool. Sensitized individuals develop delayed hypersensitivity reactions on exposure to certain microbial agents. Delayed hypersensitivity reactions are widely used to screen people for exposure to tuberculosis by using the tuberculin test. Individuals who are hypersensitive to tuberculin will show an induration (hard swelling) of 10 mm or greater at the site

TABLE 13-6
Hypersensitivity Reactions Used in Diagnosis

Disease	Type of Infectious Agent	Antigenic Preparation
Tuberculosis	Bacteria	Tuberculin
Leprosy	Bacteria	Lepromin
Mumps	Virus	Noninfectious virus
Coccidioidomycosis	Fungus	Concentrated culture filtrate
Histoplasmosis	Fungus	Concentrated culture filtrate
Blastomycosis	Fungus	Concentrated culture filtrate
Leishmaniasis	Protozoan	Extract of culture

of injection 24 to 48 hours after exposure. Hypersensitivity to tuberculin means that the patient either has an active case of tuberculosis or has had tuberculosis in the past. Delayed hypersensitivity reactions are also used to diagnose certain fungal diseases (Table 13–6).

Contact dermatitis results from skin contact with an allergen. It is a cell-mediated, delayed hypersensitivity reaction. Sensitization usually occurs by skin contact with small molecules such as the catechols of poison ivy. Subsequent contact with the plant will elicit a response with a delayed time course similar to that observed in the tuberculin reaction. The erythema (abnormal redness of the skin) and swelling are maximal in 24 and 48 hours. In severe cases of contact dermatitis, large blisters filled with leukocytes and serous fluid are formed.

Other deleterious forms of cell-mediated immunity are the rejection of allographs (tissue transferred from one individual to another individual of the same species), certain drug allergies, and certain autoimmune diseases.

ANTIBODY-ANTIGEN REACTIONS

Antibodies are immunoglobulin molecules that react specifically with their antigens. Since antibodies are extremely specific and since almost any natural product is immunogenic in some animal, biologists have used antigen-antibody reactions as a sensitive and accurate means of measuring biological material.

Practical methods for detecting either antigens or antibodies are available for use in diagnostic medicine.

Serology is the branch of immunology that analyzes blood sera to determine the presence and concentrations of antigens and antibodies. Human blood is composed of cells and a straw-colored liquid called **plasma.** Plasma contains nutrients, ions, fibrinogen, and a variety of proteins including immunoglobulins. Blood drawn from a patient will naturally clot. Removal of the clot by centrifugation separates the cells and fibrinogen (the pellet fraction) from the liquid phase. The remaining solution, also straw-colored, is called the **serum** and is defined as the plasma minus fibrinogen. Immunoglobulins are present in the serum. Numerous techniques have been developed for detecting antigens and antibodies.

Precipitin reactions. A multivalent antibody and its soluble multivalent antigen (for example, a protein such as albumin) will react to form a complex. If this complex is large enough, it will form a large aggregate called a **precipitate.** The antibody in this reaction is called a **precipitin.** A precipitin reaction is performed in a series of tubes that contain an identical amount of serum (Figure 13–7). When increasing amounts of antigen are added to the tubes, a precipitate forms in those tubes containing the correct ratio between antigen and antibody. The results depicted in Figure 13–7 show a visible precipitate in tubes 4, 5, and 6. Tubes 1 and 2 contained excess antibody, so there was not enough antigen to form

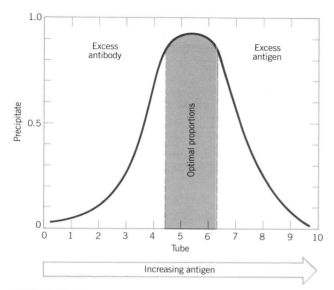

FIGURE 13–7
Precipitin reaction. A visible precipitate is formed when the concentration of antigen and antibody are optimal. If either the antibody or the antigen is in excess, a precipitate will not be formed.

large, visible complexes. Tubes 8 through 10 contained excess antigen, so only small, nonprecipitating complexes were formed. The **optimal proportion** between antigens and antibody molecules occurred in tubes 5 and 6. These antibody-antigen complexes

are large because of the multivalent nature of both the antigen and the antibody molecules (Figure 13–8). This is unlike chemical reactions, where the proportion of reactants to each other and to their products are constants for a given reaction.

Modifications of the precipitin reaction have been devised to allow the visualization of the precipitate formed. In the single-diffusion technique, the antibody is suspended in an agar matrix contained in a small tube. Antigen preparations are layered on top of the agar and allowed to diffuse into the antibody-containing gel (Figure 13–9). Precipitin bands will form at positions representing the optimal proportions of antigen to antibody.

O. Ouchterlony devised a similar technique in which both the antigens and the antibodies were allowed to diffuse. A typical Ouchterlony double-diffusion plate is shown in Figure 13–10. Symmetrical holes are cut in an agar matrix in a petri dish, and each well is filled with either an antigen or an antibody. The assay is called a double-diffusion test since both antigen and antibody diffuse out from their respective locations in the plate. A precipitate forms at the position in the agar where optimal proportions between the antigen and the antibody occur. The structure of the precipitate band indicates whether the antigens are identical, partially identical, or nonidentical. Identity is demonstrated when the precipitin bands join smoothly at the apex and

FIGURE 13–8
Schematic representation of the zone of (*a*) excess antibody, the zone of (*b*) excess antigen, and the (*c*) optimal proportions for a precipitin reaction.

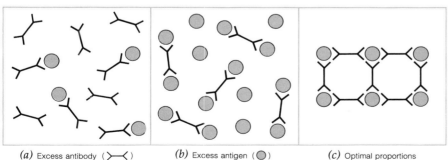

(*a*) Excess antibody (⟩—⟨)   (*b*) Excess antigen (⬤)   (*c*) Optimal proportions

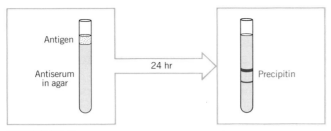

FIGURE 13–9
Single-diffusion precipitin reaction, also called an Oudin reaction. Immune serum is mixed in agar, and then antigen is layered on top of the tube. Diffusion of the antigen molecules into the agar gel creates a concentration gradient. Precipitin bands form at the position of optimal proportions.

show no spurs. Partial identity is indicated by the presence of a single spur at the apex, and nonidentity is indicated by the presence of two spurs at the apex (Figure 13–10). The Ouchterlony precipitin reaction is used to demonstrate the degree of similarity between antigens or antisera.

Agglutination reactions. Antigens that are particulate (particle or cell) clump together, or agglutinate, on reaction with antibodies specific for them. Bacterial cells and red blood cells are examples of large

FIGURE 13–10
Ouchterlony precipitin reaction. Wells in the agar are filled with immune serum or antigen. Precipitin bands form where the reactant concentrations are at optimal proportions. The wells contain different antigens (an$_1$, an$_2$, an$_3$) or immune sera (ab) prepared against all three antigens. A single spur (b) represents partial identity, a double spur (c) represents nonidentity, and a smooth continuous precipitin band (a) represents identity.

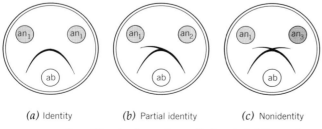

(a) Identity (b) Partial identity (c) Nonidentity

an$_1$, an$_2$, an$_3$ = three different antigens; ab = antibody against all three antigens

antigens. Agglutination reactions are done by diluting out the serum and adding aliquots of these dilutions to a constant concentration of the antigen. Typical results of this procedure are diagramed in Figure 13–11. The serum containing the antibody is said to have a specific titer. The **titer** is the reciprocal of the highest dilution that causes clumping of the antigen. Therefore, if clumping occurs in the tube with a dilution of $\frac{1}{32}$, but not in the tube with a dilution of $\frac{1}{64}$, the titer would be the reciprocal of $\frac{1}{32}$ or 32. The titer of a patient's serum is used to indicate the patient's relative resistance to an antigen. Agglutination tests can also indicate if the patient has been exposed to a specific antigen and are used in the diagnosis of certain diseases, for example, mycoplasmal pneumonia.

Certain antigen-antibody reactions do not result in agglutination, even though the antigen is large. Often the antibody's combining sites are all bound to the same large, multivalent antigen and no visible precipitate is formed. The **Coombs' antiglobulin assay** circumvents this problem (Figure 13–12). The antibody in question combines with a red blood cell (RBC) to form an activated, but nonagglutinating, RBC. Only when the activated RBC is treated with antihuman IgG does the agglutination of the RBC occur. The antihuman immunoglobulin is usually prepared in rabbits or goats and is known as the **Coombs' reagent.** This process was first developed by Coombs to detect anti-Rh antibodies in human sera: now the technique has wide applications in systems that form nonagglutinating complexes.

Radioimmunoassay. Very small quantities of antigenic substances can be detected by radioimmunoassay (RIA). This technique has been used for the accurate measurement of human hormones following its development by Solomon Berson and Rosalyn Yalow in the early 1960s. To be detected by RIA, a compound must be immunogenic. Haptens can be conjugated to proteins to make them antigenic. The compound must also be amenable to labeling with a radioactive element. Radioactive labeling of organic compounds is done by utilizing radioactive atoms during chemical synthesis. Isolated proteins can be

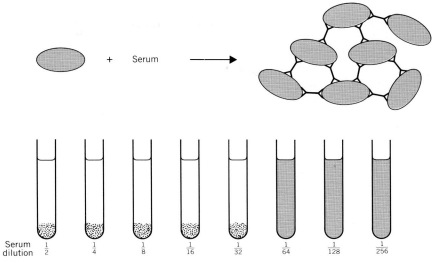

FIGURE 13–11

Agglutination reactions occur when antibodies react with large antigens causing them to clump. The serum is diluted out in tubes, and then a constant amount of antigen is added. The titer of this serum is the reciprical of the dilution in the last tube in which agglutination occurred (the titer is 32 in the example shown).

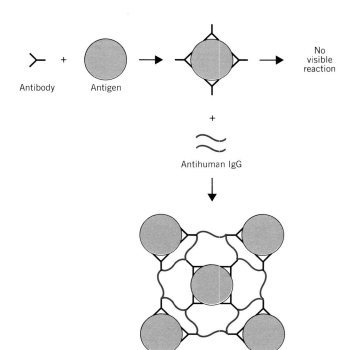

labeled by reacting their tyrosine residues with radioactive iodine (^{125}I).

RIA is a technique for measuring competitive binding. The antibody is bound to an immobile support in a tubular column. The specific radioactive *antigen is added until complete binding between the antibody and the *antigen has occurred. The unknown sample is then placed in contact with the *antigen-antibody complex, and the unlabeled antigen in the sample competes with the labeled *antigen for the antibody binding sites. A quantity of labeled antigen is released in this competitive process. The amount of released *antigen can be detected by radioactive counting techniques and is proportional to the amount of antigen in the unknown sample. Concentrations of compounds in the picogram

FIGURE 13–12

The Coombs' antiglobulin test uses antihuman immunoglobulin to precipitate antigen-antibody complexes that otherwise fail to react. Since the antibody being assayed is from human serum, it will react with the Coombs' antihuman globulin.

(10^{-12}gm) range have been measured with an RIA. The importance of RIA was recognized by the Nobel committee when they awarded Dr. Rosalyn Yalow the Nobel Prize in Medicine in 1977.

Complement-mediated cell lysis. The serum of all normal animals contains the nonspecific serological reagent called complement. **Complement** is a heat-labile (56°C for 30 minutes) group of at least 14 serum proteins that act in concert with one another, with antibody, and with membranes to cause cell lysis. These proteins bind to antigen-antibody complexes when the antibody is of the IgM or IgG immunoglobulin (except IgG_4) class. Complement functions by bringing about the cytolysis of cellular antigen-antibody complexes. It is most active against white blood cells, erythrocytes, and Gram-negative bacteria. When complement binds to an antigen-antibody complex, complement is said to be fixed. Complement-fixation reactions are a very sensitive way to measure antigen-antibody reactions and have been used extensively in diagnostic serology.

Special serological tests

It is not always possible to obtain large quantities of the antigen one wishes to work with. This is true of the venereal disease syphilis. Syphilis is caused by *Treponema pallidum*, a spirochete that has never been grown in vitro in pure culture. Investigators who wish to work with *T. pallidum* grow it in the testicles of rabbits.

Treponema pallidum immobilization test. In the *Treponema pallidum* immobilization test (TPI), motile *T. pallidum* cells from rabbit testes are combined with the patient's serum. If the serum contains antibodies against *T. pallidum*, it will inhibit the motility of the bacteria. This inhibition is readily detected in the dark-field microscope.

Fluorescent treponemal antibody test. Fluorescent compounds can be used to detect antibodies that have reacted with microscopically visible antigens. Antibodies against human IgG are prepared in a rab-

bit or goat, purified, and made visible by attaching fluorescent compounds to them. The resulting fluorescent antihuman antibody is used to detect reactions between a known organism, such as *T. pallidum*, and antibody in a patient's serum (Figure 13–13). If the patient's serum contains anti-*T. pallidum* antibodies, they will react with *T. pallidum*. The patient's excess serum is washed off before the antihuman fluorescent antibody is added. If the patient's serum contains treponemal antibodies, the cells of *T. pallidum* will be highlighted by a fluorescent outline when viewed under the fluorescent microscope.

Complement fixation—the Wasserman test. Complement fixation is a very sensitive test for detecting either antigen or antibody. Although the Wasserman test has been superceded by cheaper and more accurate tests, it is a good illustrative example of a complement-fixation assay. The Wasserman antibody can be detected with an indirect complement-fixation test (Figure 13–14) that uses purified mammalian cardiolipin as the antigen. A complement-fixation system is used to detect the complex formed between the Wasserman antibody and the cardiolipin.

Guinea pig serum is a standard source of complement for this type of test because it is available and it cross reacts nicely with human immunoglobulins. No visible reaction occurs when complement is bound to the antibody-antigen complex, so a test system must be employed. In the Wasserman test, the test system consists of sensitized sheep red blood cells (RBC) that are prepared by reacting sheep RBC with antisheep RBC antibodies. Unbound complement lyses sensitized RBC, whereas complement bound to another antigen-antibody complex (complement fixation) will not (Figure 13–14).

The Wasserman test measures the amount of complement fixed when a known amount of cardiolipin is mixed with a patient's serum. The amount of complement added and the amount of antigen added must be known. To control the amount of complement, the patient's serum is first heated to 56°C for

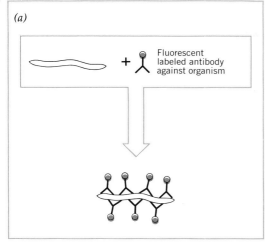

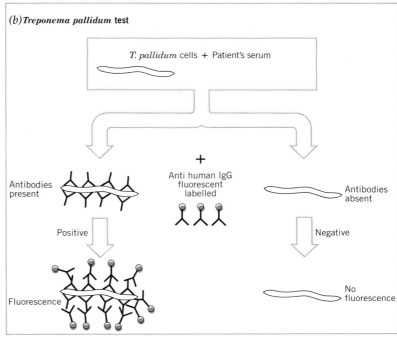

FIGURE 13–13
The fluorescent antibody test is used to (a) identify specific microorganisms or (b) detect the presence of antibodies in human serum that specifically react with a given microorganism.

30 minutes to destroy human complement. Next, a known amount of guinea pig complement is added. If the Wasserman antibody is present in the serum, it will react with the cardiolipin (Figure 13–14). This complex will then fix complement; no lysis will occur when the test system (sensitized sheep RBC) is added. When the Wasserman antibody is absent from the patient's serum, complement will not be fixed. The free complement is then free to lyse the sensitized sheep RBC.

Toxin neutralization. Antigens that cause a biologically demonstrable effect can be assayed by the ability of antibodies to negate that effect. Certain toxins kill mice. Mixing the toxin (antigen) with immune serum will neutralize the killing effect of the toxin. The degree of neutralization depends on the concen-

tration of the antitoxin in the serum. By varying the serum concentration, one can measure the amount of antitoxin present. Such an assay is called a **toxin neutralization test.**

Hemagglutination and hemagglutination inhibition tests. Certain viruses agglutinate red blood cells when a surface antigen (called a **hemagglutinin**) on the viral surface reacts with a receptor on the red blood cell. This reaction results in clumping of the RBC and is known as **hemagglutination.** Antibodies against the viral hemagglutinin will prevent the agglutination of red blood cells. This is called a **hemagglutination inhibition test** (Figure 13–15). Hemagglutination is used to assay for the presence of a virus, whereas hemagglutination inhibition is used to assay for the presence of antiviral antibody.

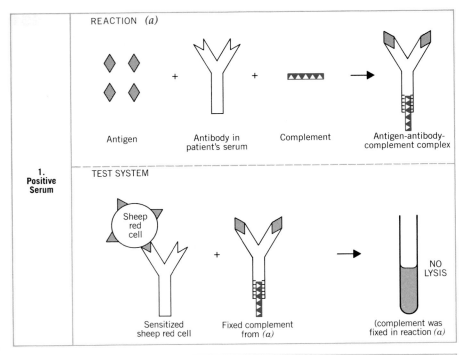

REACTION (a)

Antigen + Antibody in patient's serum + Complement → Antigen-antibody-complement complex

TEST SYSTEM

Sensitized sheep red cell + Fixed complement from (a) → NO LYSIS (complement was fixed in reaction (a))

1. Positive Serum

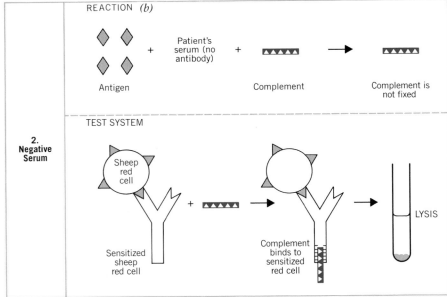

REACTION (b)

Antigen + Patient's serum (no antibody) + Complement → Complement is not fixed

TEST SYSTEM

Sensitized sheep red cell + Complement binds to sensitized red cell → LYSIS

2. Negative Serum

FIGURE 13–14
The Wasserman test is a classic complement-fixation test. When the patient's serum contains antibody against cardiolipin, there is an antibody-antigen complex formed that fixes complement. When complement is fixed, there is no lysis in the test system. In the absence of antibody against cardiolipin, complement is not fixed and is therefore available to react with the test system to cause lysis of the sheep red blood cells. (Reprinted with permission of Macmillan Publishing Co., Inc. From *Serology and Immunology: A Clinical Approach* by William D. Stansfield, copyright © 1981, William D. Stansfield.)

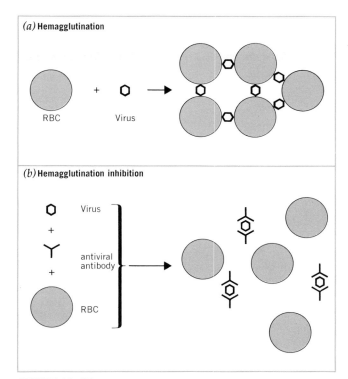

(a) Hemagglutination

RBC   +   Virus   →

(b) Hemagglutination inhibition

Virus

+

antiviral
antibody

+

RBC

FIGURE 13–15
Certain viruses are able to agglutinate red blood cells (RBC). *(a)*
Hemagglutination is used to detect viruses. *(b)* Hemagglutination
inhibition is used to detect antibodies against hemagglutinating
viruses.

Immunity against cancerous cells

Cancer is an unrestricted growth of eucaryotic cells.
Animals appear to have an immune surveillance system that removes potential cancerous cells by participating in their destruction. The evidence supporting this contention is: (1) procedures that reduce the immunological response increase the incidence of tumor formation; and (2) animals are more likely to form cancers during the stages of life where the immune response is minimal, namely, neonatal and elderly animals. Animal cells are continuously being turned over and replaced by normal body processes. Although we do not know the cause of human cancers, there are experimental animal cancers that are caused by viruses and/or chemicals. In these cancers, the cancerous cells contain new antigens that are immunogenic. In some cases, it is a viral protein that alters the cell surface to make the cell immunogenic. The animal responds by making antibodies against the new antigen on the cancer cell, and, with the help of macrophages and leukocytes known as **natural killer cells,** the animal destroys the cancer cell.

Animals containing tumors have both humoral antibodies and cell-mediated immune responses directed against the cancer cells. One theory of cancer proposes that tumors develop in animals when the cancerous cells outgrow the ability of the immune system to remove these cells from the body.

Blood groups

Human erythrocytes can be classified according to the antigenic determinants on their surface. These antigens are used to type human blood into one of four major blood groups and into numerous minor blood groups. The major human blood groups are designated by a letter, A, B, AB, and O, representing the presence of antigen A and/or B or the absence of these antigens, type O. These antigens are glycolipid complexes, of known structures, that are integral parts of the red blood cell surface. Individuals have either the antigen or the antibody to that antigen in their blood (Table 13–7).

The blood group antibodies are called **isohemagglutinins** since they agglutinate red blood cells from other individuals of the same species that contain the complementary antigen. Individuals with type O blood have anti-A and anti-B isohemagglutinins, whereas individuals with type AB blood have no isohemagglutinins against A or B in their blood. Humans with type B blood contain anti-A, and those with type A blood contain anti-B isohemagglutinins. The origin of the isohemagglutinins in human blood and their purpose for being there are unknown.

Often during surgery, or following severe accidents, patients need transfusions of blood. Transfusions of the wrong type of blood can result in massive hemagglutination. During transfusions, the

TABLE 13–7
Human Blood Groups

Patient's Blood Group	Isohemagglutinins in Blood	Antigens on RBC	Donor Blood Can Be
A	Anti-B	A	O, A
B	Anti-A	B	O, B
AB	Neither anti-A nor anti-B	AB	Universal recipient
O	Anti-A; anti-B	Neither A nor B	Universal donor

Major cross-match: Donor's RBC × recipient's serum.
Minor cross-match: Donor's serum × recipient's RBC.

donor's blood (0.5 liters) is diluted when it is transferred into the recipient's circulatory system (volume of 4.7 to 5.7 liters). Because of this dilution, the antibodies in the donor's blood do not react with the recipient red blood cells to cause hemagglutination. The recipient's isohemagglutinins and the donor's antigens are the key considerations in transfusion reactions. Type O individuals can be considered as universal donors since their red blood cells contain no A or B antigens; AB individuals can be considered as universal recipients since their serum contains no isohemagglutinins (Table 13–7). A person's blood type can be determined by a slide agglutination test that is performed before a transfusion. A major cross-match is performed by mixing the recipient's serum with the donor's red blood cells. The minor cross-match is performed by mixing the patient's red blood cells with the donor's serum. If hemagglutination occurs in a major cross-match, the blood types are incompatible and the transfusion is not done.

Rh factor is another important immunological component of blood. Individuals who are Rh positive contain D antigens on their red blood cells. Rh-negative individuals lack the D antigen and harbor no anti-D immunoglobulins. Problems occur if an Rh-negative woman and an Rh-positive man produce an Rh-positive child. The child produces the D antigen, which gains access to the mother's circulation when the placenta ruptures during childbirth or in certain instances during an abortion. The Rh-negative mother responds by manufacturing anti-D antibodies. These antibodies belong to the subclass of IgG that are able to cross the placenta. During the second or subsequent pregnancy, the Rh-negative mother can have enough anti-D antibodies in her blood to cause the death of her Rh-positive fetus. This disease in the fetus is called **erythroblastosis fetalis.** Modern medicine treats Rh-negative mothers with anti-D antibody within 72 hours postpartum. This procedure of passively immunizing the mother against the fetal Rh+ red blood cells prevents the mother's body from developing antibodies against D antigen. Since passive immunization is of short duration, subsequent pregnancies are similar to the first pregnancy in that no anti-D antibody is present in the mother's circulation.

SUMMARY

Animals develop immune resistance to infectious agents by forming antibodies that react specifically with the infectious agent. Immunity can be formed by the protected animal (active immunity), or it can be formed in another animal and transferred (passive immunity). Either type can be acquired in a natural or an artificial manner. Antibodies are immunoglobulins that are formed by animal cells in response to a foreign antigen. Antigens are molecules that interact specifically with their immunoglobulin molecules to form a stable complex.

Lymphocytes are involved in the immune response and originate from stem cells in bone marrow. They differentiate to B lymphocytes under the influence of the "bursa" or its equivalent and to T lymphocytes under the influence of the thymus. B lymphocytes contain surface immunoglobulins that interact with their specific antigens. The antigens stimulate B lymphocytes to form antibody-producing plasma cells and a clone of memory B lymphocytes. This is the cellular basis for the anamnestic response. T lymphocytes are involved in allograph rejection, delayed hypersensitivity, and in cell-mediated immunity. On reaction with their specific antigen, T lymphocytes are stimulated to divide and/or to release lymphokines. Cell-mediated immunity is involved in tumor surveillance and in resistance to certain microbial diseases. American children are actively immunized against the bacterial diseases of diphtheria, tetanus, and whooping cough and against the viral disease of rubella, mumps, polio, and measles.

One class of immunological reactions that cause damage to animals are called hypersensitivities. Immediate types of hypersensitivity include asthma, hay fever, and anaphylactic shock. Allergies are manifested through sensitized basophils and mast cells. On reaction with their specific allergen, these sensitized cells release histamines and serotonin: substances that cause the symptoms of allergies. Anaphylactic shock results from a direct injection of the allergen into the circulatory system, as is the case in bee stings. Anaphylactic shock can result in death if it is not treated immediately. Delayed hypersensitivity reactions, including contact dermatitis, allograft rejection, and certain drug allergies, require 12 to 24 hours to develop and are transferred with T lymphocytes. T lymphocytes are also involved in the inflammatory response. Cell-mediated immune reactions protect animals against certain microbial infections, such as tuberculosis.

Humoral antibodies can be detected by studying human sera. Precipitin reactions occur when soluble multivalent antigens react with their multivalent antibody. Precipitins can be detected by the precipitin test, Ouchterlony double-diffusion assay, or toxin neutralization tests. Cells are multivalent antigens that normally agglutinate on reaction with antibody formed against them. Specialized tests include hemagglutination inhibition and fluorescent antibody tests that use the Coombs' antiglobulin reagent. The study of the specific immunological reaction of a patient's serum is called serology.

QUESTIONS AND TOPICS FOR STUDY AND DISCUSSION

Questions

1. Describe the four types of acquired immunity. What is innate immunity?
2. Describe the physical properties and functions of the different classes of immunoglobulins. Which ones can cross the placental barrier?
3. Define or explain the following.

plasma	anamnestic response
serum	booster shots
titer	hemagglutination
hapten	cell-mediated immunity
serology	lymphokines
antigen	optimal proportions
immunogen	complement

4. What is the basic structure of an antibody? How does this structure explain the ability of an antibody molecule to react with two separate antigenic determinants (bivalence)?
5. Describe the role of B and T lymphocytes in the immune response.
6. Describe two forms of immediate hypersensitivity. What steps can be taken to prevent these diseases? How are they treated?
7. What is delayed hypersensitivity? How is this phenomenon used to screen patients for tuberculosis?
8. What are the differences between a precipitation reaction and an agglutination reaction?
9. What is the Coombs' antiglobulin assay, and how is it used?
10. Describe how isotopes (for example ^{125}I) can be used to assay for antibodies.
11. Describe a direct test for syphilis. Why can't you measure a simple antigen-antibody reaction when testing for syphilis?
12. What happens when type A blood is transferred into a type B patient? What tests are used to prevent this from happening?
13. Under what circumstances does the D antigen function as an immunogen in a mother? What are the consequences of this?

Discussion

1. Immunity has been described as a two-edged sword. Is this a valid characterization and, if so, why?
2. Smallpox has been eliminated from the human population. Can other infectious agents be eliminated from nature using immunology? Explain.

FURTHER READINGS

Books

Barrett, J. T., *Basic Immunology and Its Medical Application*, 2nd ed., Mosby, St. Louis, 1980. An introduction to the fundamentals of immunology for allied health students. The clinical applications of immunology are nicely brought out in the patients' case histories presented at the end of the chapters.

(Sir) Burnet, F. M., *The Clonal Selection Theory of Acquired Immunity*, University Press, Cambridge, England, 1959. An historically important book on this widely held theory of antibody formation.

Hyde, R. M., and R. A. Patnode, *Immunology*, Reston, Reston, Va., 1978. The fundamentals of immunology are presented in lecture-note form. The extensive questions (answers in the back of the book) at the end of each chapter help the student to use this paperback as a self-study textbook.

Roitt, I., *Essential Immunology*, 4th ed., Blackwell, Oxford, Eng., 1980. An introductory textbook in immunology for the college undergraduate.

Articles and Reviews

Buisseret, P. D., "Allergy," *Sci. Am.*, 247:86–95 (August 1982). The author presents recent advances that have led to a greater understanding of allergy.

Cooper, M. D., and A. R. Lawton, III, "The Development of the Immune System," *Sci. Am.*, 231:58–72 (November 1974). An introduction to the development of B and T lymphocytes and their role in the immune response.

Edelman, G., "Antibody Structure and Molecular Immunology," *Science*, 180:830–840 (1973). The Nobel lecture of Gerald Edelman delivered when he accepted the Nobel Prize in Physiology and Medicine.

Jerne, N. K., "The Immune System," *Sci. Am.*, 229:52–60 (July 1973). An introduction to the human immune system.

Milstein, C., "Monoclonal Antibodies," *Sci. Am.*, 243:66–74 (August 1980). The technique for creating hybrid cell lines that produce a single, highly specific antibody.

14

EPIDEMIOLOGY

During these times there was a pestilence, by which the whole human race came near to being annihilated . . .
Procopius of Caesarea, written about 550 A.D.

Epidemiology is the study of the occurrence of disease within a population. We are concerned with infectious diseases that are unique in that they can spread from one susceptible host to another. Infectious disease can occur as an **epidemic,** which is a sudden outbreak of illness that affects a large number of individuals. In contrast, an infectious **endemic** disease is an illness that persists in a restricted geographical location. Epidemiologists work to prevent human disease through their understanding of the forces that cause them.

Even though twentieth-century science has made great advances in the treatment and prevention of disease, infectious diseases still cause major human illness. Major epidemics of childhood and other diseases occur yearly throughout the world, and many geographical areas have persistent endemic diseases. The potential threat posed by infectious diseases is still very real; however, they will never again cause the devastation suffered by past civilization.

HISTORICAL PERSPECTIVE

Infectious diseases have altered the course of civilization by causing the depopulation of entire nations. Early reports of pestilence were recorded in both China and Egypt between 1500 and 1000 B.C. History has recorded these diseases because of the human suffering, death, and the subsequent disruption to the political and social structure of the societies they affected. Centuries later, the Roman Empire suffered a major epidemic (probably caused by smallpox) that occurred toward the end of the Parthean War, 161–166 A.D. So many Romans died during this epidemic that Marcus Aurelius was forced to recruit conquered peoples to serve in his armies and to settle his lands. The Roman Empire was again decimated by an epidemic (probably plague) that began in 251 A.D. and lasted until 266 A.D. As an indication of this extensive devastation, the major Roman city of Alexandria lost two-thirds of its population.

The 52-year plague that almost annihilated the human race was documented by Procopius of Caesarea, the historian for Justinian (Byzantine emperor who ruled from 527 to 565 A.D.). In his writings, Procopius accurately described the clinical symptoms of plague. Individuals who contracted the disease usually died within the week. There were no cures, and only rarely did an individual survive. The plague so devastated the population of the Byzantine Empire that the social structure never recovered. Leaders became powerless as they lost the work force required to run their empires. There were no farmers to cultivate the land, no produce to tax, and no armies to defend the outlying territories. The devastation of the Byzantine Empire marked the beginning of the Middle Ages and the end of the glory and magnificence that was the Graeco-Roman culture.

The Black Death was a devastating plague epidemic that began in Central Asia and spread to Italy by the 1340s. One account of this period tells of the siege of the fortified cathedral town of Kaffa (now Feodosiya in the Ukraine) by a rival army. When the plague struck, the attacking army quickly became sick and began to die in great numbers. So many soldiers died that the disposal of bodies became a problem. The commanding officer of the attacking army ordered that the bodies be catapulted into the city as projectiles propelled by their hurling machines. The plague made Kaffa uninhabitable and caused the survivors to flee in their galleys into the Mediterranean Sea. In their search for refuge, they carried the plague to many port cities, and soon the disease spread throughout Europe.

Colonial America battled epidemics during much of its history. By some accounts, fewer than 40 percent of the early settlers survived the Atlantic passage and the hardships of colonialism. The population of the Colonies grew very slowly in large part because of infectious diseases. The American Indians suffered and died along with the colonists. The populations of many American Indian tribes were decimated by the infectious diseases introduced by the Europeans.

Diphtheria and yellow fever seriously affected the colonists. Diphtheria caused many deaths during the middle of the 1700s, especially among children under 10 years of age (Table 14–1). Since no cure was known, it was not unusual for a large family to lose four or five children to diphtheria in a single year. Epidemics of yellow fever occurred in colonial port cities, especially in those located from Philadelphia south. Yellow fever was carried from the tropics to the northern port cities by the ships involved in the West Indies trade. The spread of yellow fever was curtailed when the colonial authorities began to quarantine all ships arriving from the West Indies.

Epidemiology developed out of this tragic history of suffering, death, and social upheaval. John Snow (1813–1858) published the first logical approach to controlling epidemics in his classic report on cholera. Snow was an English physician who studied cholera in a section of London that was serviced by two separate water companies (Table 14–2). Both companies obtained water from the Thames River. The Lambeth Company took water from the river upstream of London; the Southwark and Vauxhall Company took water from the populated London portion of the river. Snow discovered that the incidence of deaths from cholera in houses supplied with water from the Southwark and Vauxhall Company was significantly higher than in houses supplied by the Lambeth Company. From these results, he concluded that cholera was carried in the water supply that originated in the sewage-polluted basin of the

TABLE 14–1

Diphtheria in Colonial New Hampshire

Age Group	Deaths	Percentage of Total
Under 10	802	81.5
10–20	139	14.1
20–30	35	3.6
30–40	4	0.4
40–90	3	0.3
Above 90	1	0.1
Total	984	100

Source: Adapted from the pamphlet "An account of the Numbers that have died of distemper in the Throat . . . In New Hampshire," Jabez Fitch, July 1736.

TABLE 14–2

Cholera Deaths in London During 1853 in Houses Supplied by Different Water Companies

Water Company	Number of Houses	Deaths from Cholera	Deaths per 10,000 Houses
Southwark and Vauxhall Company	40,046	1263	315
Lambeth Company	26,107	98	37
The rest of London	256,423	1422	59

Source: Adapted from "Snow on Cholera," a reprint of two papers by John Snow, M.D., The Commonwealth Fund, New York, 1936.

Thames River. He also proposed that cholera was caused by a microorganism.

Snow used this same reasoning to solve the mystery of the Broadstreet cholera epidemic of 1854. People living within walking distance of a water pump on Broadstreet had a very high incidence of cholera. Snow surmised that the well was the source of the cholera epidemic. After he removed the pump handle from the well to prevent the use of the well water, the epidemic stopped. These early studies led to the science of **epidemiology,** which today is broadly defined as the study of the factors that determine the occurrence of disease in a population.

EPIDEMIOLOGY OF INFECTIOUS DISEASES

Our current comprehension of the etiological basis of infectious diseases, the progressive effects of diseases, and their mode of transmission have led to the development of a scientific approach to epidemiology. The control of infectious diseases is exercised in hospitals and health care facilities, in community schools, at the county level through the local and state health departments, and nationally through the Centers for Disease Control (CDC). The efforts of these professional organizations have greatly reduced the morbidity and mortality from infectious diseases in the United States.

Mortality from infectious diseases is largely preventable through the widespread use of immunization procedures and chemotherapy. Currently in the United States the mortality from organic diseases such as cancer and heart disease is significantly

higher than mortality from infectious diseases. **Morbidity** is a measure of the incidence of disease, both fatal and nonfatal, in a population. Nonfatal diseases greatly affect a population through lost workdays, discomfort, and, in some diseases, through permanent physical handicaps. Prevention of both morbidity and mortality in a population is a constant concern of the health care profession.

Nature of epidemics

An epidemic occurs when a significant proportion of a given population contracts a specific infectious disease. The baseline for determining an epidemic state varies with each disease. For example, death from pneumonia associated with influenza occurs at an annual mortality rate of between 400 and 650 deaths in 121 large U.S. cities (Figure 14–1). Only when the mortality exceeds these expected levels is the disease considered to be an epidemic.

Each epidemic must have an origin and a mode of transmission. Diseases transmitted by person-to-person contact often begin in the cold months, when people are indoors, and are characteristic of a **propagated epidemic.** The incidence of such a disease (Figure 14–2) increases gradually and then drops as the infected patients recover or die. **Common-source epidemics** originate from a single contaminated source, have a rapid onset, quickly reach a maximum incidence of new cases, and then decline (Figure 14–2). This type of epidemic can be caused by infectious agents found in contaminated swimming water or in food and water that is consumed by a

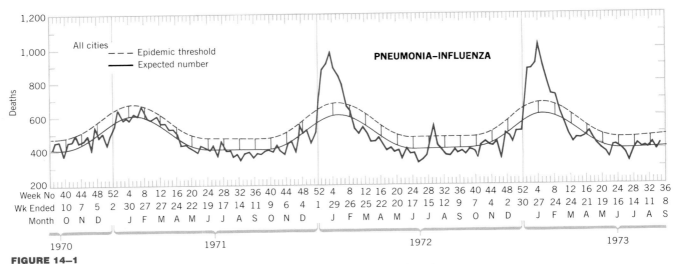

FIGURE 14–1

Reported deaths in 121 U.S. cities from pneumonia-influenza. There is an expected number (—) of deaths at any given time of the year in the U.S. population. Epidemiologists know that there is an influenza epidemic when the number of deaths from pneumonia-influenza exceed the epidemic threshold (---). (Centers for Disease Control. "Annual Summary 1979: Reported Morbidity and Mortality in the United States," *Morbidity Mortality Weekly Report*, 28, no. 54:1980)

large number of people. The occurrence of common-source epidemics can be prevented by eliminating the source of contamination.

Endemic diseases occur at a constant (usually low) frequency in a population. An example is endemic typhus (Figure 14–3), which is caused by a bacterium whose natural reservoir is wild rats and field mice. This rickettsial disease is transmitted sporadically to humans by fleas. Its natural reservoir provides a constant source of the infectious agent. There is a low, constant level of endemic typhus within the susceptible population of humans who have not had the opportunity to develop a natural immunity. Endemic typhus is geographically restricted because of the distribution of its natural reservoir (Figure 14–3).

A **pandemic disease** is one that spreads around the world, causing extensive morbidity. Influenza is able to cause pandemics because it is easily transmitted between humans and because the influenza virus has the propensity to alter its antigenic makeup (see Chapter 23). New antigenic types of influenza vi-

ruses arise that are able to bypass immunological resistance formed by most humans during previous epidemics. Influenza is still a serious viral disease that causes high morbidity throughout the world.

Factors influencing epidemics

Climate, seasons, geography, and social practices are major factors that affect the occurrence of infectious diseases. Certain infectious agents are restricted to geographical regions of the world because they require a reservoir and/or a vector to survive. Climate and seasonal variations affect the survival of the infectious agents, reservoirs, and vectors. Social practices often dictate human behavior that in turn can increase the transmission of, or the susceptibility to, infectious diseases.

Vectors.   A living agent that is capable of transferring a pathogen from one animal to another is referred to as a **vector**. Ticks, lice, fleas, and mosquitoes are arthropod vectors (Table 14–3) that are

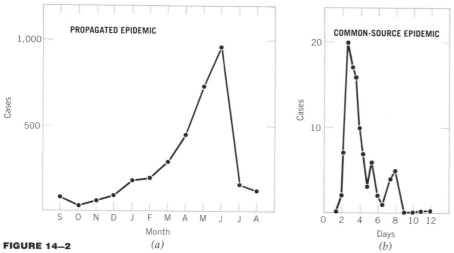

FIGURE 14–2

(a) A propagated epidemic of German measles (rubella) in Michigan (1978). Very few cases occurred in the summer months while children were out of school. The gradual increase in the number of cases during the winter and then the abrupt decline as the summer recess began are characteristics of a person-to-person mode of transmission. (b) A common-source epidemic caused by *Vibrio parahaemolyticus* aboard a cruise ship. Ninety-one of the 1059 persons on board were afflicted by a gastroenteritis illness that was traced to a seafood salad. This type of epidemic is characterized by a rapid increase in the number of cases. (Centers for Disease Control. "Annual Summary 1979: Reported Morbidity and Mortality in the United States," *Morbidity Mortality Weekly Report,* 28, no. 54:1980.)

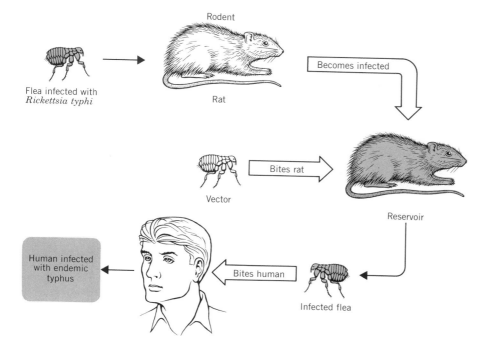

FIGURE 14–3

Rickettsia typhi causes endemic typhus fever in humans. This bacterium lives in a rodent (such as the rat) reservoir until it is transferred to other rodents or to humans by fleas.

involved in the transfer of specific viral and bacterial diseases.

Mosquitoes are necessary vectors for the transfer of the viruses that cause human encephalitis. Mosquitoes pick up the infectious agent as they take a blood meal from an infected reservoir (Table 14–3). These agents are then transferred to other reservoirs and/or humans. Rickettsia are obligate intracellular parasitic bacteria. They are unable to live outside of animal tissue and must be transferred between animals by vectors. Rat fleas, body lice, and wood ticks are arthropod vectors that are involved in the transfer of rickettsial diseases.

Death of the vector, prior to passage of the pathogen to a human or a reservoir, usually results in the death of the pathogen. In some vector-parasite relationships, however, the pathogen can be passed to the progeny of the insect by egg infection. *Rickettsia rickettsii* is the bacterial cause of Rocky Mountain spotted fever; it survives by this mechanism. *R. rickettsii* is naturally transmitted from one generation of ticks to the next by **transovarian passage.**

Reservoirs. Animals that harbor pathogens without themselves being affected are known as **reservoirs.** The reservoirs for the arthropod-borne diseases (Table 14–3) are animals in which the pathogen can coexist. Perching birds, rodents, and horses are reservoirs for the encephalitis viruses.

Rickettsial disease and bubonic plague (nonpulmonary) are major arthropod-borne bacterial diseases that are maintained in natural reservoirs. Rats, ground squirrels, dogs, foxes, and humans are reservoirs for these arthropod-borne bacterial diseases. In most cases, the pathogen replicates in the vector or reservoir without causing damage to this intermediate host. If a specific disease is not passed between humans, the human becomes a dead-end host.

Geographical considerations. Survival of many infectious agents depends on the climate (temperature, humidity, rainfall) and the local fauna of a geographical region. Because arthropod vectors live in distinct geographical areas, the incidence of the arthropod-borne diseases are directly related to the geographical boundaries of their reservoirs and vectors. For example, Rocky Mountain spotted fever is a bacterial disease that has a restricted geographical distribution. This disease is transmitted during the bite of an infected tick. *Rickettsia rickettsii* is carried by the wood tick in the Rocky Mountain states and by the dog tick in the eastern United States. The disease occurs most frequently in the east-central United States, where it is transferred by the dog tick (Figure 14–4). Very few cases are reported in the northern, western, or Rocky Mountain states.

Seasonal variations in climate also restrict the dis-

TABLE 14–3
Selected Arthropod-borne Diseases of Humans

Viral Diseases	Animals Affected	Reservoir	Vector
St. Louis encephalitis	Humans	Perching birds	Mosquito (*Culex* sp.)
Western equine encephalitis	Horses and humans	Wild birds	Mosquito (*Culex* and *Culiseta* sp.)
Venezuelan equine encephalitis	Horses (rare in humans)	Rodents and horses	Mosquito (*Culex* sp.)
Bacterial Diseases	**Etiological Agent**	**Reservoir**	**Vector**
Rocky Mt. spotted fever	*Rickettsia rickettsii*	Rodents, dogs, and foxes	Wood tick (*Dermacentor* sp.)
Epidemic typhus	*Rickettsia prowazekii*	Humans	Body louse (*Pediculus vestimenti*)
Endemic (murine) typhus fever	*Rickettsia typhi*	Rats and field mice	Rat flea (*Xenopsylla cheopis*) Rat louse (*Polyplax spinulosa*)
Bubonic plague	*Yersinia pestis*	Rats and ground squirrels	Flea (*Xenopsylla cheopis*)

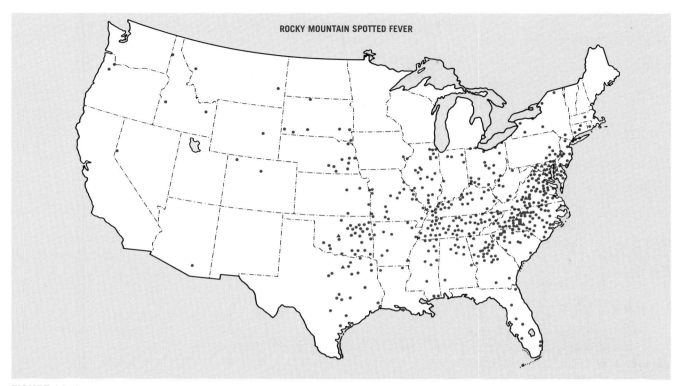

ROCKY MOUNTAIN SPOTTED FEVER

FIGURE 14—4
Incidence and distribution of Rocky Mountain spotted fever in the United States reported by
county in 1978. No cases were reported outside of the contiguous continental United States.
● 1–5 cases, ▲ 6–10 cases, ■ > 10 cases. (Centers for Disease Control. "Annual
Summary 1979: Reported Morbidity and Mortality in the United States," *Morbidity Mortality
Weekly Report*, 28, no. 54:1980.)

tribution of arthropod-borne diseases. For example,
viral encephalitis is transmitted by mosquitoes that
hatch during the summer months, so major outbreaks occur between July and September (Figure
14–5). A major epidemic of St. Louis equine encephalitis occurred in Illinois (429 cases), Ohio (416
cases), and Indiana (290 cases) during August 1975.
The epidemic reached its peak in September and
then dropped rapidly during October and November. The normal decline in the incidence of encephalitis coincides with the first mosquito-killing frost.

Some fungal diseases are prevalent in distinct climatic regions. Coccidioidomycosis is a fungal dis-

ease caused by *Coccidioides immitis,* which is found
in the soil of arid regions of the southwestern United
States and Mexico. This disease is transmitted by the
inhalation of the fungal spores that become airborne
in dry desert regions. Climatic conditions play a major role in the geographical distribution of coccidioidomycosis.

Social practices. Certain forms of human interaction can augment the transmission of human diseases. Shaking hands is a Western convention of
greeting that is a major method of transferring bacteria and viruses. Sexual promiscuity among teen-

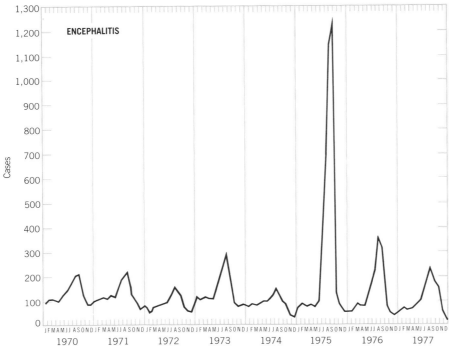

FIGURE 14—5

Incidence of all types of encephalitis in the United States (1970 –1977) reported by the month of onset. Epidemics occurred in the summer months when the mosquito population is at its peak. A major outbreak of St. Louis encephalitis occurred in 1975. (Centers for Disease Control. "Annual Summary 1979: Reported Morbidity and Mortality in the United States," *Morbidity Mortality Weekly Report*, 28, no. 54:1980.)

agers and young adults leads to a greater incidence of venereal disease. Finally, the congregation of young children in schools increases the incidence of infectious childhood diseases among this susceptible population. Chickenpox is one childhood disease that annually reaches epidemic proportions during the late winter and early spring (Figure 14–6), when children are in school.

Kuru is an example of a viral disease that was once perpetuated by an isolated social practice. Kuru is a degenerative disease of the human central nervous system that leads to death 4 to 5 years after infection. The disease was discovered among the young males and the women of a cannibalistic New Guinea tribe that followed the custom of consuming their dead tribesmen. The adult male members were always honored with the choicer portions of muscle,

whereas the women and the young males were left with the entrails and the brains. Kuru is caused by a virus that infects the brain, so it was prevalent in the women and young males of the tribe. When Westerners discovered the etiology of this disease, they convinced the tribal members to cease their cannibalistic customs and thus brought an end to the transmission of kuru.

Disease transmission

The etiological agent of an infectious disease is transferred to susceptible individuals during an epidemic. Epidemiologists recognize five major mechanisms involved in the transfer of infectious agents.

1. Person-to-person.
2. Airborne.

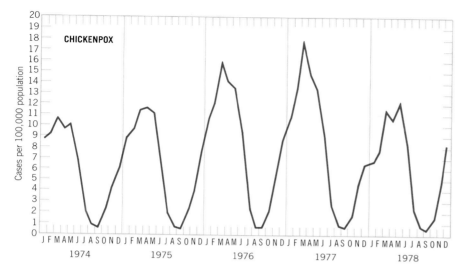

FIGURE 14–6
Reported case rates of chickenpox by month in the United States between 1974 and 1978. Chickenpox epidemics occur during the winter months primarily among school-age children. (Centers for Disease Control. "Annual Summary 1979: Reported Morbidity and Mortality in the United States," *Morbidity Mortality Weekly Report,* 28, no. 54:1980.)

3. Foodborne and waterborne.
4. Arthropod vectors.
5. Zoonoses.

Since most infectious agents are transferred by only one mechanism, epidemiologists can control the spread of infectious disease by interrupting the transfer mechanism.

Person-to-person. Venereal diseases infect the genital tract and are transferred by direct contact between individuals during sexual intercourse. The bacteria that cause gonorrhea and syphilis quickly lose their viability outside of the human body. Therefore, a person cannot contract these venereal diseases from inanimate objects such as toilet seats. Prevention of venereal diseases requires the education of individuals (1) to take certain precautions during intimate relationships and (2) to seek help if they become infected. Transfer of the nonviral venereal diseases can be physically prevented by the use of condoms; also, the bacterial diseases can be treated with chemotherapy (See Chapters 18 and 19). Common colds are viral respiratory diseases that are transmitted by direct contact. The custom of shaking hands and of kissing are involved in transfer of the common cold.

Inanimate objects such as water glasses, toothbrushes, combs, towels, and the myriad of objects that infants place in their mouths act as vehicles for the indirect person-to-person transmission of infectious agents. Interrupting this type of transfer is very difficult. Preventive measures include isolation or, in extreme cases, quarantine of the infected individual.

Airborne transmission. Respiratory diseases including diphtheria, influenza, and the common cold are readily transferred through the air. The air that is exhaled from the human lungs is normally free of bacterial and virus-sized particles. However, when a patient coughs or sneezes, the exhaled air picks up water droplets that may contain viruses and microorganisms from the mouth and the nasopharynx (Figure 14–7). Outside the body, the water quickly evaporates, leaving organic matter and infectious agents suspended in an aerosol. These suspensions move in the air currents and can be inhaled by healthy individuals.

Transmission of infectious agents through the air is most effective when people congregate in enclosed quarters. The high incidence of respiratory illness during the cold winter months corresponds with the large amount of time that people spend indoors. Wearing a face mask can prevent the transmission of airborne infections. This is done routinely in hospitals, but the practice is not widespread outside of health care facilities.

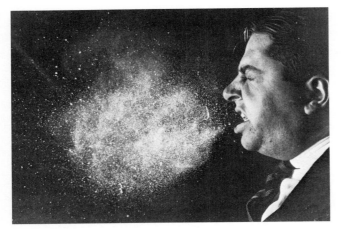

FIGURE 14—7
Violent, unstifled sneeze. (American Society for Microbiology.)

Foodborne and waterborne. Infectious agents that can establish an infection following ingestion are often transmitted by contaminated food and/or water. Certain bacteria, viruses, and protozoa cause waterborne diseases (Table 14–4). Many of these pathogens infect the gastrointestinal tract and are excreted in human feces.

Water becomes contaminated when untreated human sewage enters a water source. People are infected by contaminated water when it is consumed and/or when it is used for recreation. Waterborne outbreaks of infectious disease usually occur as common-source epidemics. During the years 1972–1977, *Shigella* was responsible for most outbreaks of waterborne bacterial diseases in the United States (Table 14–4). *Giardia lamblia* and hepatitis A were responsible for major outbreaks of waterborne protozoan and viral diseases, respectively.

Food can be contaminated with pathogens through improper handling, unhygienic practices, and contamination with human feces. *Clostridium botulinum*, *Salmonella*, and *Staphylococcus aureus* are the major causes of food poisoning (Table 14–5). *Cl. botulinum* grows in improperly prepared canned foods. *Salmonella* and *Shigella* are bacteria that normally enter the human food supply through the unhygienic handling of food by infected persons. Common-source outbreaks of food poisoning occur when infected food-handlers prepare meals for large numbers of people. *Staphylococcus aureus* causes staphylococcal food poisoning when food is improperly handled (unrefrigerated or improperly cooked) after preparation.

Trichinella spiralis is a nematode that infects pork and wild game and cause trichinosis in humans. Non-B hepatitis is the major waterborne viral disease. When this virus is present in sewage-contaminated saltwater, it can be taken in by filter-feeding shellfish. Oysters harvested from these waters are a major source of foodborne hepatitis. There are no known cures for trichinosis and hepatitis, which makes them serious foodborne diseases.

Arthropod vectors. Controlling the distribution of fleas, ticks, lice, and mosquitoes is the major approach used to control the spread of arthropod-borne diseases. These diseases usually occur on a seasonal basis and depend on the distribution of the vector. Some infectious agents are able to replicate in the vector, so the vector also serves as a reservoir. Other vectors function only to transfer the infectious agent from an infected reservoir to a susceptible host. Control can be exerted by reducing the vector population. If the reservoir is a domestic animal, control of the disease can be exerted by treatment of the diseased animals and/or by limiting their movement about the country.

TABLE 14—4
Etiology of Waterborne Disease Outbreaks Reported to the CDC, 1972–1977

Etiology	Number of Outbreaks	Percentage of Total
Giardia lamblia	20	27.0
Shigella	14	18.9
Hepatitis A	9	12.2
Nontyphoid *Salmonella*	5	6.8
Salmonella typhi	4	5.4
Enterotoxic *E. coli*	1	1.4
Miscellaneous chemicals	21	28.4
	74	100.1

TABLE 14—5
Major Foodborne Disease Outbreaks by Etiology

Etiology	1977	1978	1979
Bacterial			
Clostridium botulinum	20	12	7
Clostridium perfringens	6	9	20
Salmonella	41	45	44
Shigella	5	4	7
Staphylococcus aureus	25	23	34
Vibrio parahaemolyticus	2	2	2
Parasitic			
Trichinella spiralis	14	7	11
Viral			
Hepatitis non-B	4	5	5

Source: Centers for Disease Control, *Foodborne Disease Outbreaks Annual Summary,* 1979, issued April 1981.

Zoonoses. Infectious diseases that occur primarily in animals and only occasionally in humans are termed **zoonoses.** Diseases such as tularemia, rabies, and brucellosis are examples of zoonotic diseases. Tularemia is found in wild rabbits and is passed to humans through direct contact with the entrails of the rabbit during field dressing. Rabies is most prevalent in skunks, bats, raccoons, and foxes; but it is also found in domestic dogs, cats, and cattle. The rabies virus is present in the saliva of infected animals and is transmitted to humans when they are bitten by a rabid animal. Most domestic dogs in the United States are now immunized against rabies. This greatly reduces the chance that humans will come in contact with a rabid dog. Brucellosis is a disease of domestic cattle that can be passed to humans through milk. Modern procedures for pasteurizing milk have eliminated milk as a major source of this disease. The few widely scattered cases of brucellosis in the United States (179 in 1978) occur primarily among workers in the meat-packing and livestock industry.

Public health measures

Data collection. An effective method of accurately collecting data on morbidity and mortality is a pre-requisite for the effective control of infectious diseases. The attending physician is responsible for the diagnosis of the illness, and the clinical microbiologist is responsible for the identification of the infectious agent. In compliance with the federal law, this information is transmitted via each state's department of public health to the Centers for Disease Control (CDC) in Atlanta, where it is compiled and statistically analyzed. Special attention is given to new antibiotic-resistant strains of bacteria and to the increased virulence of infectious agents. The CDC compiles statistics on both morbidity and mortality and publishes these data in a weekly report that is available to health care professionals.

Controlling the spread of infectious diseases falls under the purview of the public health agencies, which include the federal Food and Drug Administration, the U.S. Department of Health and Human Resources, and the state health departments. These agencies make and enforce regulations governing the preparation and distribution of food, water quality, and immunization programs.

Water quality and sewage treatment. The amount of organic matter in and the hardness of the water we drink vary greatly depending on the region of the country and the type of water resource available. Human water supplies can come from springs, wells, reservoirs, or lakes. In addition to the aesthetic aspects of water quality, humans seek water sources that are free of pathogens.

Infectious agents can get into a water supply when they are excreted in the feces of infected hosts. *Salmonella, Shigella,* and *Vibrio cholerae* are prime examples of bacterial pathogens that are transmitted via water contaminated with human feces. Polio and infectious hepatitis are examples of viral diseases that are transmitted by water. A major means of preventing the spread of waterborne infections is to prevent sewage from entering the human water supply.

Humans naturally contain bacteria in their intestines. *Bacteroides fragilis* and *Escherichia coli* are found in the human intestine and are excreted in human feces. Since *E. coli* is easily grown in the laboratory, it is used as an indicator of human fecal contamination. Water that is free of *E. coli* is considered to be free of contamination by human sewage.

Modern sewage treatment is based on an aqueous system mainly because of the widespread use of the flush toilet. Sewage treatment facilities are designed for the individual home or an entire community (Figure 14–8). The goal of sewage treatment is to remove the undesirable material from sewage or to render that material harmless. Sewage treatment normally occurs in two distinct phases: the anaerobic digestion phase (not shown) and the aerobic oxidation phase.

Sewage is fed into an anaerobic digestion tank. Here microbial fermentation degrades the particulate matter in sewage, producing carbon dioxide, methane, and hydrogen sulfide gas; soluble organic matter; and insoluble particulate matter. The gases either escape into the atmosphere or are burned as a source of energy. The particulate matter (including dead microbial cells) is recovered as sludge, which can be burned or used as organic fertilizer.

Soluble organic matter and inorganic ions remain in the liquid phase. In the septic-field system, this liquid flows into the septic field, where aerobic mi-

FIGURE 14–8
(*a*) Sewage treatment plant showing a sprinkling filter in the forground and a sludge drying bed in the background. (*b*) Waste water treatment facility composed of an aerobic digester (foreground), a circular sludge thickener, and a clorination building. (Both Runk/ Schoenberger, Grant Heilman.)

(*a*)

(*b*)

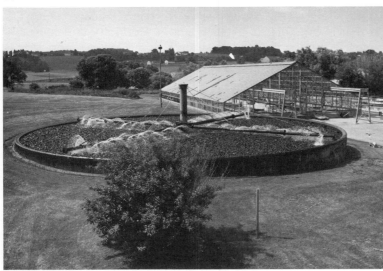
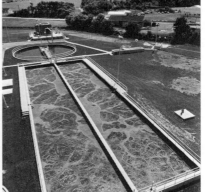

croorganisms oxidize the organic compounds as it trickles down through the soil into the water table. This process is optimized in sewage treatment plants by spraying the liquid effluent over a trickling filter (Figure 14–8a). Aerobic organisms colonize the surface area of the trickling filter and oxidize the organic matter to carbon dioxide and water. The aerobic microorganisms remain on the trickling filter, or they are filtered out by the soil in the septic field. Through this process, the microbial content of water that reenters the water supply is greatly reduced.

Even though pathogenic microorganisms do not survive an adequate sewage treatment facility, care must be exercised in positioning a septic tank and field to assure that direct seepage into the water supply does not occur. In many communities, the septic system must be approved by a certified civil engineer before a dwelling can be occupied.

Foodborne diseases. Contaminated food served to large groups of people in such places as restaurants, hospitals, and cruise ships is responsible for major outbreaks of foodborne diseases. Improper preparation of the food, infected food-handlers, and improper holding temperatures for prepared foods are the major causes of these epidemics. Foodborne outbreaks are monitored by the CDC in order to control current epidemics and to prevent future ones.

The case involving Mary Mallon and the spread of typhoid fever is a classic example of food being contaminated by an infected human. Mary Mallon (Typhoid Mary) was a cook who worked in the New York City area during the early part of the twentieth century. She recovered from typhoid fever only to become a chronic carrier of the causative agent, *Salmonella typhi*. Public health officials discovered her by tracing the source of a typhoid outbreak to a kitchen in which she was the cook. Microbiologists discovered that her intestine contained an essentially pure culture of *S. typhi*. Since she refused to give up her profession as a cook, health officials had her imprisoned to prevent her from spreading typhoid. If this case had occurred today, Mary Mallon would have been treated with antibiotics instead of being imprisoned.

Immunization programs. Large-scale immunization programs decrease the number of susceptible people, which in turn limits the spread of infectious agents. To maximize this approach, infants are immunized during their first 2 years of life. Children younger than 6 months old have some immunity, against infectious diseases, that they acquired from their mothers. This immunity is short-lived, so children should be actively immunized early in life. Infants in the United States are routinely immunized against tetanus, diphtheria, whooping cough, mumps, measles, rubella, and polio. Groups of adults, especially those who are vulnerable to influenza, are often immunized prior to expected epidemics of influenza.

The effect of a broad-based immunization program on the incidence of a disease can be dramatic. The incidence of polio dropped precipitously after the introduction of the inactivated (Salk) vaccine in 1955 (Figure 14–9) and continued to drop following the introduction of the oral (Sabin) vaccine in 1961. A similar dramatic decrease in the incidence of rubella (German measles) was observed following the introduction of the rubella vaccine in 1969. Rubella continues to occur at a fairly high rate in the United States mainly in high school students and in young adults who as a group were inadequately immunized.

International travel. Many infectious diseases are not indigenous to the United States but do occur in other parts of the world. Prevention of the spread of disease at the international level is governed by the International Health Regulations generated by the World Health Organization (WHO) in Geneva, Switzerland. This agency recommends the immunization certificates required of travelers who enter foreign countries, designates quarantinable diseases, and distributes a weekly "Blue Sheet" listing the areas infected with quarantinable diseases. When vaccinations are required for entry into a foreign country, the traveler must present an International Certificate of Vaccination. A complete listing of these requirements can be obtained from the Bureau of Epidemiology in the CDC.

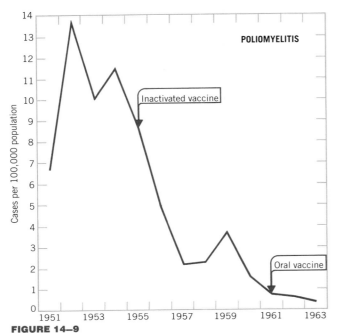

FIGURE 14–9

Poliomyelitis (paralytic) reported in the United States between 1951 and 1963. Since 1964, there have been fewer than 0.05 cases per 100,000 population in the United States per year. (Source: *Annual Summary, Morbidity and Mortality Weekly Report*, published by the Centers for Disease Control.)

Nosocomial infections

Hospitals represent a unique environment where both susceptible patients and infectious agents are concentrated. **Nosocomial infections** are diseases acquired during the course of a hospital stay. Current estimates are that between 3 and 4 percent of all patients admitted to general hospitals acquire nosocomial infections.

Incidence of nosocomial infections. Records of the number and types of infectious agents isolated in many hospitals are compiled on a routine basis. A 6-month summary report (January to June 1977) of nosocomial infections in 79 United States hospitals is shown in Table 14–6. This study involved 637,307 discharged hospital patients, of which 20,877 (3.3

percent) were identified as having acquired a nosocomial infection. The most frequent site of infection was the urinary tract. The second highest rate of infection involved surgical wounds. *Escherichia coli* was the most frequent pathogen found and was the predominant organism isolated from infections of surgical wounds and the urinary tract (Table 14–6). *Streptococcus* group D was the second most prominent pathogen isolated from the urinary tract. *Staphylococcus aureus* was a common pathogen that was isolated most often from surgical wounds.

Susceptible patients. More than 90 percent of the nosocomial infections reported in Table 14–6 occur in patients over 15 years of age. Infants less than 1 month old comprised only 4.2 percent of the affected patients. The highest percentage of infected patients by age were patients over 65 years: they represented 37.2 percent of the total.

Although modern medicine is able to prolong human life, it also has an impact on the incidence of nosocomial infections. Cancer patients, transplant patients, and individuals recovering from surgery are more susceptible to infectious diseases than is the average human. Moreover, transplant patients treated with immunosuppressant drugs and cancer patients treated with cytotoxic drugs have a suppressed immunological response. The insertion of mechanical devices or orthopedic prostheses and the exposure of internal structures to infection during extended surgery are hospital procedures that increase the patient's risk of infection.

Monitoring and control. Attending nurses serve as the first line of control against nosocomial infections. Nurses should constantly be alert to the signs of infection such as fever, chills, shock, pus, and diarrhea. This information should be recorded and acted on as soon as possible. The attending nurse also has the responsibility of following hygienic practices at all times and of protecting the patient from those who do not.

Monitoring of the hospital environment for potential sources of pathogens is another preventative practice. Hospital monitoring includes microbiological sampling of the operating and delivery rooms, biological testing of the effectiveness of the autoclaves and the ethylene oxide sterilizers, testing of the effectiveness of antiseptics and disinfectants, and monitoring for contamination of food including all in-house baby formulas. Hospitals establish standards for acceptable levels of microbial contamination in their monitored areas. Corrective measures are indicated when the measured levels exceed these standards. Special units of the hospital such as burn treatment facilities require even more frequent and more extensive bacteriological monitoring.

The antibiotic susceptibility profile of the isolates can contribute to the identification of potential nosocomial infectious agents. Hospitals are ideal environments for the development and transfer of bacterial resistance transfer factors (see Chapter 6). Since bacteria with multiple drug resistance are extremely difficult to control, special attention should

be paid to these pathogens. If an outbreak of an infectious disease does occur, appropriate steps should be taken by the epidemiologist to identify the source of the infectious agent and to prevent further spread of the disease.

SUMMARY

Epidemics of infectious diseases have caused extensive death, morbidity, and suffering and have even altered the course of ancient civilizations. Many outbreaks of infectious disease can now be controlled through immunization, public health measures, and through the use of chemotherapy. Epidemiology is the study of the factors that influence the occurrence of disease in a population. Among the biological factors involved in the spread of infectious disease are vectors, animal reservoirs, climate, and human social practices. Infectious agents can be airborne,

TABLE 14–6
Incidence[a] of Selected Pathogens Isolated from Hospital Patients, January–June 1977

Organism (isolate)	Primary Bacteremia	Surgical Wounds	Lower Respiratory	Urinary Tract	Cutaneous	Other	All Sites
Totals	15.9	109.2	67.1	157.5	23.3	41.5	414.5
Escherichia coli	2.6	16.6	4.8	50.9	1.7	3.7	80.3
Streptococcus Group A	0.1	0.8	0.2	0.2	0.3	0.5	2.1
Streptococcus Group B	0.4	2.0	0.3	1.5	0.2	0.7	5.1
Streptococcus Group D	1.2	10.8	0.9	23.0	1.7	2.4	40.0
Staphylococcus aureus	2.4	15.9	7.2	3.2	6.9	6.3	41.9
Staphylococcus epidermidis	1.3	5.3	0.5	6.0	1.3	1.4	15.8
Proteus-Providencia sp.	0.5	7.5	4.1	15.2	1.4	1.8	30.5
Klebsiella sp.	1.6	5.3	7.0	13.2	1.1	2.0	30.2
Pseudomonas aeruginosa	1.0	4.4	4.8	13.7	1.1	1.8	26.9
Enterobacter sp.	0.7	3.8	3.7	5.6	0.5	0.8	15.0
Candida sp.	0.5	1.1	2.3	6.9	0.7	3.5	15.0
Pseudomonas other sp.	0.3	1.3	1.3	3.6	0.2	0.8	7.5
Bacteroides fragilis	0.6	3.9	—[b]	—[b]	0.3	0.6	5.4
Serratia sp.	0.4	0.9	1.8	3.0	0.2	0.4	6.7
All others	2.4	29.7	28.0	11.7	5.8	14.9	92.5

Source: *National Nosocomial Infection Study Report 1977* (6-month summary), Centers for Disease Control, November 1979.
[a]Number of isolates per 10,000 patients discharged.
[b]Less than 0.1 per 10,000 patients discharged.

foodborne, waterborne, or transferred by person-to-person contact, by indirect contact, by arthropod vectors, or by animals. Preventing an epidemic can be accomplished by interrupting the mode of disease transmission. Public health measures that have been established to prevent disease transmission include sewage treatment, surveillance of and investigation of epidemics and outbreaks of diseases, surveillance of the proper handling of food, and immunization programs. Prevention of infectious diseases at the international level is under the auspices of the World Health Organization. This organization establishes the quarantinable diseases and advises travelers of the necessary immunizations for entry into foreign countries. Nosocomial infections are an important source of morbidity. Hospital patients are often more susceptible to infectious diseases, and hospitals are environments conducive to the development of antibiotic-resistant strains of bacteria. Epidemiologists attempt to control the spread of infectious agents at all levels of our society.

QUESTIONS AND TOPICS FOR STUDY AND DISCUSSION

Questions

1. What are the characteristics of an endemic, an epidemic, an enzootic, and a pandemic disease?
2. What role do vectors and reservoirs play in infectious diseases? What reservoirs and vectors of infectious diseases exist in your geographical area?
3. What social practices in your culture contribute to the spread of infectious disease? Should these practices be stopped or curtailed?
4. Name five modes of disease transmission and describe an infectious disease that belongs to each. What are some practical means of preventing the transmission of these diseases?
5. What are nosocomial infections and how serious a problem are they? What procedures and practices contribute to nosocomial infections?

Discussion

1. What effect has mankind's ability to control infectious diseases had on life expectancy and culture in your society? Has there been a differential effect on the countries of the world caused by the availability of modern medical technology?
2. How important is it to control the spread of infectious agents within your society? Are there still problems with the worldwide spread of infectious agents?

FURTHER READINGS

Books

Benenson, A. S. (ed.), *Control of Communicable Disease in Man*, 12th ed., American Public Health Association, Washington, D.C., 1975. A handbook of essential facts on infectious diseases of humans including symptoms, occurrence, infectious agents, reservoirs, transmission, incubation period, susceptibility, and methods of control.

Burnet, M., and D. O. White, *Natural History of Infectious Disease*, 4th ed., Cambridge, New York, 1972.

Burnett-Conners, E. B., H. J. Simon, and D. C. Dechairo (eds.), *Epidemiology for the Infection Control Nurse*, Mosby, St. Louis, 1978. A collection of essays on topics pertaining to the control of nosocomial infections.

Articles and Reviews

Henderson, D. A., "The Eradication of Smallpox," *Sci. Am.*, 235:25–33 (October 1976). An epidemiological report on the successful elimination of this serious human viral disease.

Kaplan, M. M., and R. G. Webster, "The Epidemiology of Influenza," *Sci. Am.*, 237:88–106 (December 1977). A review of influenza that covers its history, epidemiology, and virology.

Merson, M. H., et. al, "Traveler's Diarrhea in Mexico," *N. Engl. J. Med.*, 294:1299–1305 (1976). A case study of diarrhea among 73 physicians and 48 family members who visited Mexico City to attend a medical conference.

Salk, J., and D. Salk, "Control of Influenza and Poliomyelitis with Killed Virus Vaccines," *Science*, 195:834–847 (1977). A review article that presents scientific data in support of the use of the Salk vaccine in preference to the use of the TOPV.

Wishnow, R. M., and J. L. Steinfeld, "The Conquest of the Major Infectious Diseases in the United States: A Bicentennial Retrospect," *Ann. Rev. Microbiol.*, 30:427–450 (1976). A review of the progress made in the United States to control many of the major infectious diseases of humans.

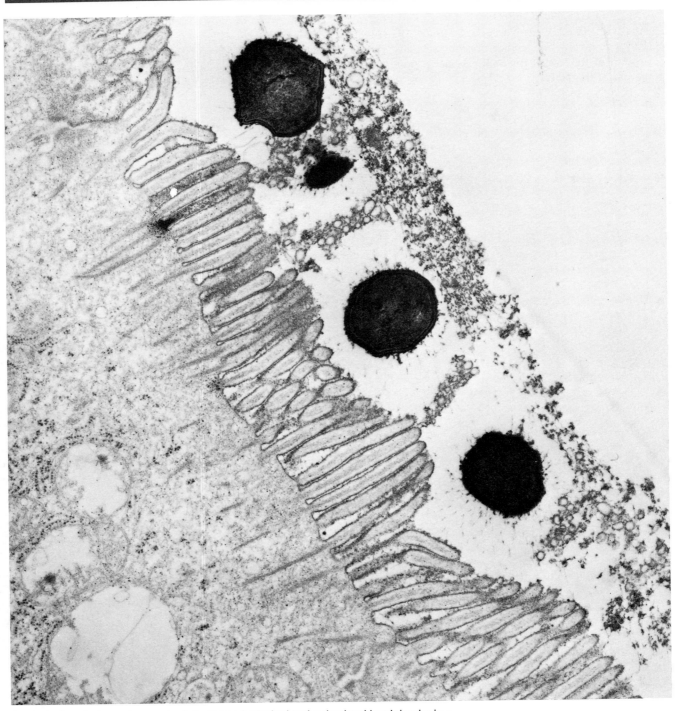

Transmission electron micrograph of streptococci attached to the duodenal brush border in a chicken infected with *Streptococcus faecium*. (Courtesy of R. Fuller. From R. Fuller, S. B. Houghton, and B. E. Brooker, *Applied Environ. Microbiol.*, 41:1433–1441, 1981.)

PART THREE

PROCARYOTIC PATHOGENS

The great variation in the nature of bacterial diseases is due in part to the biological diversity of the pathogenic bacteria. Within the 19 divisions of bacteria recognized by *Bergey's Manual,* 12 divisions contain genera of recognized pathogenic organisms. Within these 12 divisions, only a few genera, and usually only a few species, have the ability to cause human disease.

The organization of the chapters on procaryotic pathogens draws heavily on taxonomic groupings. The endospore-forming rods, spirochetes, rickettsias, Gram-positive cocci, and Gram-negative rods are natural groups containing pathogenic bacteria. A sixth group contains the closely related corynebacteria and the mycobacteria. Finally, there are a number of bacterial genera that taxonomists classify under the heading of "uncertain affiliation." The

pathogenic bacteria in this classification are grouped together in the final chapter entitled Other Pathogenic Bacteria.

Each bacterial pathogen has unique characteristics that enable it to cause disease in humans. The site of infection, the toxins or invasive factors produced, and the human body's response to the infectious agent all contribute to the clinical symptoms of a disease. Almost all bacterial diseases can be effectively treated with antibiotics and/or immunization procedures. These treatments depend on the accurate diagnosis of the clinical symptoms and in many instances on the identification of the bacterial agent responsible. The ability of the human race to control bacterial infections is one of the greatest accomplishments of the twentieth century.

15

ENDOSPORE-FORMING RODS

Endospore-forming rods and cocci are grouped together in the family Bacillaceae. Two of the five genera of this family contain bacterial species that cause human disease. The aerobic, pathogenic, endospore-forming rods belong to the genus *Bacillus,* whereas the anaerobic, pathogenic, spore-forming rods belong to the genus *Clostridium.* Three species of *Bacillus* cause human disease. *B. anthracis* causes anthrax, *B. cereus* is involved in food poisoning, and *B. subtilis* has been implicated in human eye infections. The major anaerobic spore-forming bacteria involved in human disease are *C. botulinum, C. tetani,* and *C. perfringens.* They cause botulism, tetanus, and gaseous gangrene, respectively.

Spores and vegetative cells of *Bacillus* sp. are widely distributed in air, soil, water, dust, some foods, and wool. These organisms are easily grown in the laboratory, and some produce antibiotics. Spores of the pathogenic clostridia are widely distributed in soil, rotting wood, and mud. They are sometimes found in the intestines of warm-blooded animals, including humans. The extreme heat- and chemical-resistance of bacterial endospores enable spore-formers to survive in many environments where other bacteria would perish.

BACILLUS

The genus *Bacillus* contains the Gram-positive, spore-forming, rod-shaped bacteria that grow aerobically or as facultative anaerobes on a wide variety of organic substrates. Almost all species of *Bacillus* are motile; however, the pathogen *B. anthracis* is nonmotile. The bacilli are differentiated on the basis of their size, metabolism, growth substrates, spore shape, and the position of the spore in the vegetative cell.

Anthrax

In 1877, Robert Koch demonstrated that anthrax was caused by the bacterium *B. anthracis.* Koch's work is acknowledged as the first scientific report to link a bacterium with an animal disease. Koch isolated bacilli from sheep that had died from anthrax and then watched these organisms grow in the aqueous humor of an ox's eye (see Chapter 1). When he inoculated these organisms into mice, the mice died of anthrax. Koch reisolated the bacteria from the spleens of these dead mice and then inoculated the isolates into healthy mice. These mice also died of anthrax.

Thus anthrax was the first disease to be conclusively demonstrated to be caused by a bacterium.

During Koch's lifetime, anthrax was a common disease that destroyed cattle and sheep. Once a pasture became contaminated, the spores of *B. anthracis* persisted in the soil for many years and contaminated the animals that used the pasture. Anthrax was and is transmitted to humans through animal products. People who work with sheep wool and goat hides are especially vulnerable.

The incidence of anthrax in the United States is very low; only 27 human cases were reported from 1969 to 1978. Sporadic outbreaks still occur among cattle and sheep, but the disease is usually controlled before it is transmitted to humans. Anthrax is more common in the Middle East, Africa, and Asia, where it infects sheep and goats. Most cases of human anthrax in the United States are contracted from imported wool and hides.

Bacillus anthracis. This bacterium is a relatively large (1.0 to 1.5 by 5 to 10 μm), nonmotile, spore-forming rod (Figure 15–1). Virulent strains of *B. anthracis* form capsules of glutamyl polypeptide when they grow in animals (in vivo). The major virulence factors of *B. anthracis* are the glutamyl polypeptide capsule and the anthrax toxin. These bacteria produce the capsule when they grow in tissue or in cultures with a CO_2-enriched atmosphere. The anthrax toxin is an exotoxin that plays a major role in the pathogenesis of this disease.

Anthrax in humans.   Humans are infected by *B. anthracis* when it is inhaled, ingested, or when it infects the epidermis through a scratch or an abrasion. **Cutaneous anthrax** is a localized infection that first develops as an abscess on the skin (Figure 15-2). *B. anthracis* enters the epidermis through a cut or an abrasion. This form of anthrax is often seen on the hands of persons who work with animal skins. A black eschar (scar tissue) develops on the cutaneous lesion when the lesion heals. At the other extreme, the infection can develop into a systemic infection.

Inhalation anthrax begins when spores of *B. an-*

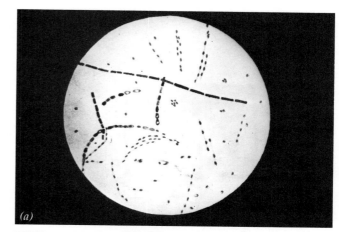

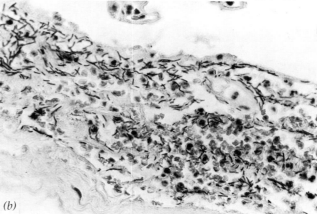

FIGURE 15–1

(a) Photomicrograph of *Bacillus anthracis* after it was stained with the fuchsin-methylene blue spore stain. (b) *Bacillus anthracis* in tissue taken from a patient with fatal inhalation anthrax. (Courtesy of the Centers for Disease Control.)

thracis are inspired into the lungs, where they are phagocytized by macrophages. The spores do not germinate in the lungs; instead they are transported in macrophages to the regional lymnph nodes. Here the spores germinate into vegetative cells: some are destroyed by phagocytosis, whereas others escape into the blood. The vegetative cells of *B. anthracis* multiply in the blood, causing a bacteremia, and readily infect the spleen. The infected spleen enlarges and turns black because of internal hemor-

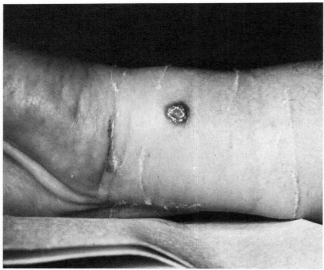

FIGURE 15–2
A cutaneous anthrax lesion on the arm of a 50 year-old female who had been a carder in a wool factory. (Courtesy of the Centers for Disease Control.)

rhaging. The patient usually dies during this stage of the disease. Chemotherapy is ineffective in treating anthrax once the bacteremia occurs even though the bacteria are susceptible to antibiotics. Inhalation anthrax is the most serious form of anthrax because it has a high mortality rate.

Ingestion of anthrax spores is a rare mode of human infection; however, it is the most common means of animal infection. The spores are ingested from an infected crop or they are consumed in contaminated grains. Among the few cases of human anthrax that are reported in the United States most are either cutaneous anthrax or inhalation anthrax.

Treatment and prevention. Both sulfanilamides and penicillins are effective against the anthrax bacillus. Humans are not immunized against anthrax because of the low incidence of the disease; however, cattle and sheep are immunized, especially when they are threatened by outbreaks of anthrax. Immunizations can be performed (1) with attenuated *B. anthracis* or (2) with a virulent spore suspension combined with immune serum. Controlling anthrax in domestic animals is the best method of preventing human infection.

Other bacillus

Two other *Bacillus* sp. have caused disease in humans. *B. subtilis* occasionally causes infections of the human eye, and *B. cereus* can cause food poisoning through the production of enterotoxin.

A vast amount of information concerning sporogenesis has been gained from the study of *Bacillus*. In addition, specific species of *Bacillus* are pathogenic to the larvae of moths. Commercial preparations of *B. thuringiensis* have been used as a biological insecticide for the control of certain insect pests. These bacteria produce a proteolytic protein that digests the intestinal wall of the insect larvae. Some species of *Bacillus* are also known to produce antibiotics. *B. polymyxa* and *B. subtilis* produce distinct polypeptide antibiotics that are used to treat bacterial infections. Members of the *Bacillus* genus are widely used as research tools because of the ease with which they are isolated, handled, and grown. This is in direct contrast with the clostridia, which are more difficult to grow.

CLOSTRIDIA

Clostridia (L. *clostridium*, spindle) are anaerobic, spore-forming, rod-shaped bacteria found in soils, mud, and animal intestines. Vegetative cells of clostridia are Gram-positive and are usually motile by peritrichous flagellation. These organisms are chemoorganotrophs that gain useful energy by fermenting organic compounds such as sugars, amino acids, purines, and/or polyalcohols. The classification of the clostridia is based in part on the substrates they ferment and their fermentation products. Clostridia do not produce cytochromes or catalase, which are heme-containing proteins. They are unable to perform aerobic respiration because they lack cytochromes. Moreover, the vegetative cells of clostridia are sensitive to oxygen in part because they lack catalase. Clostridial spores, on the other hand, are resistant to oxygen, heat, desiccation, and many toxic chemicals.

Clostridia cause diseases that are pure intoxications when the organism is absent or they cause limited invasive diseases. Pathogenic clostridia grow only in anaerobic environments such as deep puncture wounds, anaerobic portions of the lower intestine, or in anaerobic environments outside of the host. *C. botulinum* and *C. tetani* are the causative agents of **botulism food poisoning** and **tetanus**, respectively. The symptoms of these diseases are the direct result of potent neurotoxins. **Gaseous gangrene** is a degradative disease characterized by local muscle necrosis. *C. perfringens* is the major causative agent; however, *C. novyi* and *C. septicum* have also been isolated from gangrenous tissue.

Botulism

Human botulism was first described in 1785 as a disease associated with the consumption of sausage (L. *botulus*, sausage). The causative agent was first isolated by E. van Ermengem in 1896 and is now named *C. botulinum*. Three types of human botulism are now recognized: foodborne botulism, infant botulism, and wound botulism. All three types are caused by *C. botulinum*.

Clostridium botulinum. The cells of *C. botulinum* are large (0.8 to 1.3 by 4 to 8 μm) rods that are motile by peritrichous flagellation. The spores are oval and are located subterminally (Figure 15–3). Cultures of *C. botulinum* grow readily on laboratory media containing amino acids incubated under strict anaerobic conditions. In laboratory cultures, these bacteria can produce the potent botulism exotoxin, so all cultures must be handled with respect. *C. botulinum* is widely dispersed in mud and soil and causes toxicogenic disease in humans, cattle, chickens, and ducks. Although there are relatively few cases of human botulism in the United States, massive die-offs of ducks caused by botulism have been reported in Michigan and in California. The toxin is produced by *C. botulinum* growing in the mud in the bottom of shallow bodies of water. The ducks ingest the toxin when they feed on plant roots from the same body of water. The toxin kills the ducks by paralyzing them. The only way to prevent this natural disaster is to drain the water from these areas to prevent ducks from landing or to scare the ducks away from contaminated areas.

Botulism toxin. Botulism food poisoning of humans is a pure intoxication caused by a neurotoxin. In this disease, the clostridia do not infect the host. Instead, they produce the toxins while growing in canned foods. The toxins cause the disease when they are ingested. There are seven antigenically distinct types of botulism toxins (Table 15–1). Types A, B, E, and F are known to cause botulism in humans, whereas types C and D are the types most often isolated from fowl with botulism. The type of toxin responsible for a given illness is important because the treatment of the disease depends on the administration of the correct antitoxin. Each of the six antigenic types must be neutralized by a distinct antitoxin. Polyvalent equine antitoxin for types A, B, and E botulism toxins is now used to treat human botulism. Antitoxin will neutralize unbound toxin, but it will not reverse the symptoms caused by the bound toxin.

FIGURE 15–3

Photomicrograph of *Clostridium botulinum* stained with gentian violet. (Courtesy of the Centers for Disease Control.)

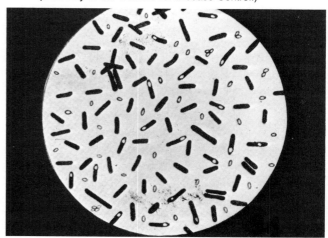

TABLE 15–1
Clostridium botulinum Types

Type	Disease	Source
A	Botulism of humans, chickens	Soil, Rocky Mountain states
B	Botulism of humans, chickens	Soil, Mississippi Valley and Great Lakes states
C	Paralytic disease of chickens; botulism in wild ducks	Fly larvae and mud
D	Disease in cattle	Soil, South Africa
E	Botulism of humans	Fish and fish producs
F	Botulism of humans	Salmon and crabs
G	Disease in laboratory animals	Soil

Toxoids can be produced from each type of botulism toxin. The toxoids are used to produce antitoxins in horses, and in rare cases they are used to immunize humans. Botulism toxins can also be inactivated by boiling them for 10 minutes or by heating them at 80°C for 30 minutes. One way to prevent botulism food poisoning is to heat food thoroughly to these temperatures prior to serving it.

Botulism toxins are neurotoxins that affect the peripheral nervous system by inhibiting transmitter release. They are among the most toxic biological substances known: 1 mg contains 2×10^8 minimum lethal doses (MLD) for the mouse. The toxin causes irreversible damage to the nerves. Type A toxin is a large protein molecule (900,000 daltons) of which the neurotoxin portion (120,000 to 150,000 daltons) is only a small part. The large nontoxic portion (measured by its hemagglutinating activity) appears to protect the neurotoxin from the acidity of the stomach's gastric juices during ingestion.

The reason for the production of a potent neurotoxin by a soil organism and the reason behind the variety of toxin types have long been a curiosity. Recently, researchers discovered that toxin types C and D result from lysogenic conversion of *C. botulinum* by a bacteriophage. Cultures that produce type C toxin can be cured by growing them in acridine orange. Cured vegetative cells can be reinfected with phage 1D and will then produce type D toxin. All the toxin-producing strains of *C. botulinum* carry temperate phage, but to date only the types C and D toxins have been shown conclusively to be produced by lysogenized bacteria.

Botulism in humans. Foodborne botulism is the most common form of the disease in the United States, with 65 cases reported in 1978. All the confirmed cases originated from home-processed vegetables, olives, fish, spaghetti sauce, tomatoes, or pork and beans. Spores of *C. botulinum* are commonly found on garden vegetables since soil is one of their normal habitats. Foods become poisonous when the spores survive the canning process, germinate in the anaerobic environment of canned food, and produce botulism toxin during growth. Outward signs of this growth include the swelling of a can, caused by the gas produced during fermentation, and the foul smell of putrefaction. These foods should not be eaten.

Symptoms of botulism appear usually within 12 to 48 hours and include a stiff neck, nausea, vomiting, double vision, difficulty in swallowing, and muscle paralysis. When death does occur, it is usually caused by the paralysis of the respiratory muscles. The death of untreated patients can occur between 24 hours and 1 week following the appearance of the symptoms. Patients with botulism poisoning should be treated with a polyvalent botulism antitoxin. The prognosis for survival is good if the disease is recognized early. The prognosis decreases progressively with the length of time between appearance of the symptoms and the initiation of treatment.

Botulism food poisoning can occur as an isolated case or as a point-source epidemic. The outbreak that occurred in Pontiac, Michigan, in 1977 was traced to home-canned peppers. The peppers were used to prepare an uncooked sauce that was served in a Mexican restaurant. Forty-five cases of botulism developed. Luckily, no deaths resulted, in large measure because of the rapid diagnosis and treatment of the patients at a nearby hospital. The local public health authorities quickly located the source of the infection and closed the restaurant to prevent further disease. In 1977, this single point-source outbreak accounted for 65 percent of the cases of foodborne botulism in the United States.

Since **infant botulism** was first recognized in 1976, more than 100 cases have been diagnosed in the United States, with single cases reported in Australia, Canada, and England. The disease affects infants between the ages of 3 and 26 weeks. Symptoms include unexplained weakness, difficulty in swallowing, respiratory arrest, and paralysis of the ocular muscle. Only botulism toxins type A and type B are reported in infant botulism. The disease is a toxico-infection in which toxin-producing *C. botulinum* grow and produce toxin in the infant's intestine. No common source of infection has been found. This has led epidemiologists to assume that the infants ingest viable spores of *C. botulinum* in food or by placing contaminated objects in their mouths. The spores germinate into vegetative cells that produce toxin in the patient's intestine. Patients do recover without the administration of antitoxin; however, some patients require respiratory assistance. These infants often excrete *C. botulinum* for several weeks following their recovery from the clinical symptoms.

Wound botulism is a rare disease that occurs when *C. botulinum* infects severe wounds. High-risk situations include car and farm accidents that are accompanied by major tissue damage and soil contamination of the wound. War-related wounds were once a major source of wound botulism; however, in a recent 8-year period, only seven cases of wound botulism were reported.

Tetanus

Tetanus is a toxigenic disease caused by the common soil bacterium *Clostridium tetani.* The disease in humans is characterized by spasms of the voluntary muscles, especially of the neck and jaw. Spasms of the jaw muscles prevent patients from opening their mouths, so the disease is also called ''lockjaw.'' Humans are in daily contact with the spores of *C. tetani,* yet few cases of tetanus occur. The disease develops from infections of deep wounds, deep lacerations, or puncture wounds. Protection is provided by immunizing individuals at an early age and by administering booster shots every 5 years.

Clostridium tetani. This anaerobic, spore-forming, Gram-positive rod is widely dispersed in soil. It grows under anaerobic conditions in complex media containing amino acids, vitamins, and purines. Most strains ferment amino acids but do not ferment sugars. The cells are smaller than *C. botulinum* (0.3 to 0.5 by 2 to 5 μm), and they move by peritrichous flagellation. The spherical spores are located at a terminal end of the cell (Figure 15–4). The spores are resistant to heating at 100°C and to many chemicals that are toxic to other bacteria.

Tetanus was one of the first diseases studied from an immunological point of view. S. Kitasato obtained pure cultures of *C. tetani* in 1889 and showed that tetanus was a toxicogenic disease. During the next year, he and E. von Behring discovered antitoxins to both tetanus toxin and diphtheria toxin. Today we known that tetanus toxin (tetanospasmin) is a neurotoxin that acts very much like botulism toxin.

Tetanus toxin is a protein with a monomeric molecular weight of between 140,000 and 160,000 daltons. One mg of tetanus toxin contains between 1 and 3 $\times$ 10^8 minimum lethal doses for the mouse. Tetanus toxin acts in the spinal cord, where it interferes with signal transmissions that stimulate muscle contraction. Death occurs from asphyxia fol-

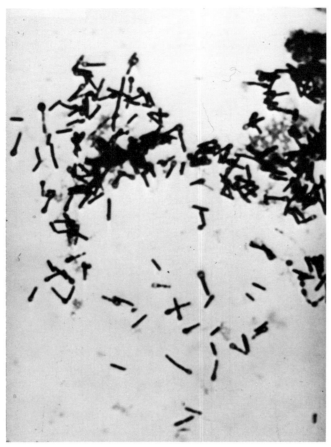

FIGURE 15–4
Clostridium tetani. Gram stain of cells from a 48-hour culture grown on chopped meat medium. 956X. (Centers for Disease Control, Atlanta.)

lowing the spasmodic contraction of the respiratory muscles.

Tetanus in humans. Infection begins when an anaerobic wound becomes contaminated with the spores of *C. tetani*. This can occur during farm accidents, severe auto accidents, or when a patient incurs a deep puncture wound from a rusty nail or wood splinter. Deep wounds having an impaired blood supply are likely sites of infection because *C.*

tetani only grows in anaerobic environments. The incubation time can vary from 2 to 50 days following the injury.

Vegetative cells of *C. tetani* grow in the wound. *C. tetani* is not invasive, but it is able to produce proteases that break down local tissue. The growing clostridia produce tetanus toxin at the wound site. The toxin molecules enter local nerve cells (motoneurons) and then move within the axons of these cells to the spinal cord. Immunized individuals do not display the symptoms of tetanus because the toxin is quickly neutralized by the antitoxin before it enters the motoneuron. If the tetanus toxin does enter the nerve axon, it is unavailable to the neutralizing effects of circulating antitoxin. The toxin then interferes with the normal functions of the interneuronal cells (Renshaw cells), causing muscle contraction to be exaggerated. About 50 percent of the patients with generalized tetanus who are treated with antitoxin are cured. Chemotherapy is of little use because it has no effect on the toxin already present in the system.

Neonatal tetanus occurs primarily in the less-developed countries of the world. *C. tetani* infects the umbilicus of newborns during delivery when insufficient care is taken to exclude soil and dust from the delivery area. The incidence of all types of tetanus is very low in the United States (less than 100 cases between 1976 and 1978) primarily because of our immunization programs.

Prophylactic treatment. In the United States, children 2 to 3 months old are given their first immunization shot of tetanus toxoid in combination with the diphtheria toxoid and the pertussis (DTP) vaccine. Five shots are recommended, the last being administered just prior to a child's entry into school (5 to 6 years of age). Booster shots are recommended for individuals who sustain serious wounds and who have not had a tetanus booster within the preceding 5 years.

Patients with tetanus should be given large doses of immune human globulin. This will neutralize the circulating toxin, even though it will not reverse the effects of bound toxin. The patient's symptoms can be treated with muscle relaxants combined with respiratory assistance. Patients who survive the first 4 days of tetanus will normally recover.

Histotoxic clostridial infections

Various clostridia that are normal inhabitants of soil, mud, and the intestines of warm-blooded animals (including humans) will opportunistically invade damaged tissue. When clostridia infect muscle tissue and cause local tissue necrosis, the disease is called **gaseous gangrene.** The causative agents grow in anoxic tissue and produce substances that destroy tissue. Bacteria capable of such infections are grouped together and referred to as the **histotoxic clostridia.** These bacteria can also cause infection of the uterus following abortions, low-level bacteremia, and food poisoning.

The histotoxic clostridia. *Clostridium perfringens* is the organism most commonly isolated from gaseous gangrene wounds. *C. novyi* and *C. septicum* can also be involved, but they are isolated from fewer cases. These bacteria are anaerobic, spore-forming rods that produce gas during the fermentation of carbohydrates. They are commonly found in the soil and in the human intestine. *C. perfringens* is found in more than 50 percent of the cases of gaseous gangrene. It also causes uterine infections, and it is the causative agent of clostridial food poisoning.

C. perfringens is not a highly invasive organism, but it does destroy local tissue. This bacterium produces a variety of toxins (Table 15–2) that are used to distinguish the five distinct types (A, B, C, D, and E) of this organism. Among the toxins are lecithinase (alpha toxin), lethal necrotizing toxin, lethal hemolytic toxin, collagenase, proteinase, hyaluronidase, and deoxyribonuclease. The alpha toxin kills cells and thereby causes tissue damage by breaking down lecithin in cell membranes. The production of some or all of these toxins enables *C. perfringens* to infect wounds and to cause progressive tissue destruction.

Gaseous gangrene. Severely damaged or anoxic tissue is susceptible to infections by clostridia in soil and animal feces. Gaseous gangrene (Color Plate 11) is a histotoxic clostridial infection characterized by progressive myonecrosis (muscle death) and by gas production. Local tissue death perpetuates the anoxic character of the infected area by cutting off the local blood supply. Gaseous gangrene is often a multiple infection that involves more than one species of clostridia.

The symptoms of gaseous gangrene include swell-

TABLE 15–2
Toxins Produced by *Clostridium perfringens*

Toxin	Designation	Activity
Lethal Toxins[a]		
Lecithinase	Alpha	Lethal to mice, hemolytic
Lethal, necrotizing	Beta	Lethal to mice, necrosis of skin, nonhemolytic
Lethal, hemolytic	Delta	Hemolytic
Lethal, necrotizing	Epsilon	Lethal to mice, necrosis of skin, nonhemolytic
Other Toxins		
Collagenase	Kappa	Protein hydrolysis
Proteinase	Lambda	Protein hydrolysis
Hyaluronidase	Mu	Hydrolysis of hyaluronic acid

[a]The five types (A through E) of *C. perfringens* are differentiated by the ability of antisera to neutralize their lethal toxins.

ing, a dark yellow appearance of the skin, and the presence of a thin, dark watery exudate. Hydrogen gas generated during fermentation is temporarily trapped in the tissue spaces. It escapes by bubbling up through the exudate of the wound. Symptoms can begin 6 to 72 hours after surgery or after the patient sustains an injury. Exploratory surgery of the affected tissue reveals necrotic muscle and a lack of a suitable blood supply.

The rapid progression of gaseous gangrene calls for excision or amputation of the infected tissue. Some success has been attained by treating the infected area in a hyperbaric oxygen chamber. This treatment forces oxygen into the infected tissue, where it kills the vegetative cells of the clostridia. Antibiotics are usually ineffective. They do not get to the site of infection because of the poor circulation at the infection site. Gaseous gangrene was a significant cause of disease during World War II because war wounds were severe and soil contamination was frequent. Today, gaseous gangrene develops in patients involved in serious automobile accidents and in elderly patients who have impaired circulation to their limbs.

Other clostridial infection

Clostridium perfringens is found in the uterus of adult human females (5 percent), where it has been known to cause disease following an abortion or procedures that might cause damage to the uterus. The organisms invade the uterine wall, where they cause tissue damage and a failure of the local circulation.

Clostridium perfringens type A is a major cause of food poisoning. Abdominal cramps and diarrhea develop within 9 to 15 hours after the ingestion of food contaminated with vegetative cells (several million per gram of food) of *C. perfringens*. Inadequate cooking and holding temperatures for boiled meats, gravy, and poultry are the major sources of these organisms in food poisoning. The diarrhea and cramps are caused by a heat-labile protein enterotoxin produced by growing vegetative cells. Patients recover rapidly from the disease following a bout of gastroenteritis.

SUMMARY

All the endospore-forming bacteria that cause disease in humans belong to the genus *Bacillus* or *Clostridium* (Table 15–3). When epidemics of these diseases do occur, they are point-source epidemics because these agents are rarely, if ever, transferred from person-to-person.

Anthrax is a disease primarily of animals that is caused by *B. anthracis*. Humans contract anthrax through the inhalation of spores or by the infection of an open sore on the skin. Pulmonary anthrax, the most serious form of the disease, occurs among workers who deal with animal products such as hides and wool. Anthrax is a rare human disease that can be treated with chemotherapy.

The anaerobic clostridia are widely distributed in soil, mud, and the intestines of animals. They are opportunistic pathogens that require special circumstances to cause disease in humans. *Clostridium tetani* can cause human tetanus as a result of a severe or deep puncture wound. The bacteria grow in the wound, producing the neurotoxin tetanospasmin. Muscle spasms, especially in the jaw (lockjaw), are caused by the toxin. Tetanus is prevented by immunizing individuals with tetanus toxoid. *C. botulinum* causes botulism food poisoning and infant botulism. There are seven antigenic types of botulism neurotoxin, each being produced by the vegetative cells of a specific strain. At least some toxins are coded for by prophage genes carried by lysogenized *C. botulinum*. The toxin is potent and lethal to humans. Contamination of food occurs from improper preparation of canned vegetables and meats. Polyvalent antitoxins are administered as the only successful method of treating botulism food poisoning. Infant botulism is caused by *C. botulinum* types A and B when they grow in the intestines of infants. The symptoms are similar but milder than botulism food poisoning; even untreated patients recover.

Clostridium perfringens is the major isolate from infections of gaseous gangrene. The organism is not invasive but locally infects and causes tissue damage to wound sites and unhealthy limbs. Histotoxic toxins produced by *C. perfringens* cause tissue necrosis,

TABLE 15—3
Summary: Endospore-forming Rods

Disease	Etiological Agent	Forms of the Disease or Common Name	Symptoms
Anthrax	*Bacillus anthracis*	Cutaneous anthrax	Lesion on skin covered by eschar
		Inhalation anthrax	Systemic infection, lymph nodes to blood to spleen
Botulism	*Clostridium botulinum*	Food poisoning	Stiff neck, nausea, vomiting, double vision, difficulty in swallowing, and muscle paralysis
		Infant botulism	Weakness, difficulty in swallowing, respiratory arrest, paralysis of the ocular muscles
Gaseous gangrene	*Clostridium perfringens* *Clostridium novyi* *Clostridium septicum*	Histotoxic disease	Progressive myonecrosis associated with gas production
Tetanus	*Clostridium tetani*	"Lockjaw"	Spasmodic contraction of muscles, especially in the jaw and neck, respiratory arrest
Food poisoning	*Bacillus cereus*	Gastroenteritis	Diarrhea, abdominal cramps, vomiting (sometimes)
	Clostridium perfringens	Gastroenteritis	Diarrhea, abdominal cramps

which leads to impaired circulation at the site of infection. Treatment requires removal of the infected area and/or hyperbaric oxygen treatment. Ingestion of large numbers of *C. perfringens* in improperly prepared and/or stored food can cause food poisoning. Recovery occurs spontaneously following a bout of abdominal cramps and diarrhea.

QUESTIONS AND TOPICS FOR STUDY AND DISCUSSION

Questions

1. The endospore-forming rods are primarily soil bacteria. Under what circumstances do they cause human disease?
2. Describe the discovery of the anthrax bacillus. Why is anthrax also called woolsorter's disease?
3. How does the presence of spores affect the epidemiology of the disease caused by species of *Bacillus* and *Clostridium?*
4. Describe the toxins responsible for botulism and tetanus.
5. What are the forms of human botulism, and how are they acquired?
6. Describe the clinical symptoms of tetanus. How is tetanus prevented and how is it treated?
7. Describe the symptoms and etiology of gaseous gangrene. Can this bacterial infection be effectively treated with antibiotics? Explain.
8. What organisms are involved in clostridial food poisoning? What is the seriousness of these infections?

Discussion

1. What special problems are caused by endospores in food preparation and preservation?
2. Devise selective enrichments for isolating members of the *Bacillus* and the *Clostridium* genera.

FURTHER READINGS

Books

Kadis, S., T. C. Montie, and S. J. Ajl (eds.), *Microbial Toxins*, vol. 2A, *Bacterial Protein Toxins*, Academic Press, New York, 1971. A collection of articles on toxins that includes papers on the clostridial toxins.

Smith, L. D. S., *Botulism, the Organism, its Toxins, the Disease*, Thomas, Springfield, Il., 1977.

Articles and Reviews

Albrink, W. S., "Pathogenesis of Inhalation Anthrax," *Bacteriol. Rev.*, 25:268–273 (1961). A brief review of anthrax in experimental animals and of the few reported human cases.

Duncan, C. L., "Role of Clostridial Toxins in Pathogenesis," *Microbiology-1975*, pp. 283–291. D. Schlessinger (ed.), American Society for Microbiology, Washington, D.C., 1975.

Gangarosa, E. J., et al., "Botulism in the United States 1899–1969," *Am. J. Epidemiology*, 93:93–101 (1971). An historic review of the incidence, morbidity, mortality, and the geographical distribution of botulism in the United States.

Nakamura, M., and J. A. Schulze, "*Clostridium perfringens* Food Poisoning," *Ann. Rev. Microbiol.*, 24:359–372 (1970). The authors discuss the pathogenicity of *C. perfringens* in cases of animal and human food poisoning.

Sugiyma, H., "*Clostridium botulinum* Neurotoxins," *Microbiol. Revs.* 44:419–448 (1980). An extensive review of the toxins responsible for botulism.

Van Ness, G. B., "Ecology of Anthrax," *Science*, 172:1303–1307 (1971). This article describes the soil ecology of *Bacillus anthracis* in relation to known outbreaks of anthrax in the United States.

16

ENTERIC BACTERIA AND RELATED GRAM-NEGATIVE RODS

Gram-negative, rod-shaped bacteria are found throughout the microbial world. These bacteria are morphologically very similar, but metabolically they are so diverse that each of the biological mechanisms for converting energy is represented. There are Gram-negative rods that are phototrophs, chemo-lithotrophs, or chemoorganotrophs. Their energy metabolism is used to classify them into families. Some of the chemoorganotrophic Gram-negative rods are human pathogens.

By far the most important group of pathogenic Gram-negative rods is the facultative anaerobes. They are widely distributed in nature. Some inhabit the human intestine and are referred to as the **enteric bacteria.** The enterics are present in two families: the Enterobacteriaceae contains the Gram-negative, facultative-anaerobic, oxidase-negative rods; and the Vibrionaceae contains the Gram-negative, facultative-anaerobic, oxidase-positive, curved or straight rods. Many of the enteric bacteria are normal inhabitants of the human intestine, whereas others are either obligate or opportunistic pathogens.

Escherichia coli is the major facultative enteric bacterium in the human intestine even though it comprises only 0.1 to 1.0 percent of the total bacterial population in human stools. Obligate anaerobes belonging to the Bacteroidaceae family make up the largest segment (95 to 99 percent) of the bacterial population in human feces. They are present to a lesser extent in the vagina, the external genitalia, and the mouth. Some members of this family cause infections of soft tissue.

The Pseudomonadaceae are Gram-negative, non-fermentative rods that are ubiquitous in soil and water. One species, *Pseudomonas aeruginosa*, causes human disease in compromised hosts. A classification scheme of the Gram-negative rods* is presented in Table 16–1.

ENTEROBACTERIACEAE

The Gram-negative, facultative-anaerobic, rod-shaped bacteria belong to the family Enterobacteriaceae or to the family Vibrionaceae. These families contain bacteria that are important human pathogens: *Salmonella typhi* (typhoid fever), *Shigella dysenteriae* (bacillary dysentery), *Vibrio cholerae* (cholera), and *Yersinia pestis* (plague). Other genera of the En-

*The other Gram-negative rods designated as being of uncertain affiliation are discussed in Chapter 21.

287

terobacteriaceae contain members that are opportunistic pathogens: *Serratia, Klebsiella, Enterobacter, Proteus,* and certain strains of *Escherichia.* Because these organisms are very similar in gross appearance, it is important to define them by biochemical and immunological techniques.

Classification and identification

Differentiation of the Gram-negative, facultative-anaerobic bacteria depends on morphological, biochemical, and, in some cases, immunological criteria. Most members of this group are straight, motile rods that are morphologically indistinguishable. The vibrios are distinct in that they are polarly flagellated, straight or curved rods; species of *Shigella* and *Klebsiella* are nonmotile. These bacteria range in size from 1 to 3 μm long and from 0.4 to 0.6 μm wide. Further subdivision among the Enterobacteriaceae depends largely on biochemical characteristics.

Metabolic characteristics. Many facultative bacteria lack cytochrome *c.* An **oxidase test** is a color reaction that is positive when cells contain cytochrome *c.* Cytochrome *c* participates in the oxidation of a *p*-phenylenediamine derivative that undergoes a color change. The Enterobacteriaceae are oxidase negative because they lack cytochrome *c,* whereas the Vibrionaceae and the Pseudomonadaceae are oxidase positive.

Because the Enterobacteriaceae are facultative anaerobes, the substrates they ferment and the products they produce are used in the identification of genera within this family. Table 16–2 is a simplified flowchart of the production of 2,3-butanediol, fermentation of lactose, motility, and the presence of urease. These are a few of the biochemical tests needed to identify the numerous bacteria in this family.

Most of the Enterobacteriaceae ferment glucose

TABLE 16–1

Principal Divisions of the Pathogenic Gram-Negative Rods

Principal Division	Genera	Disease Potential
I. Facultative Anaerobes A. RODS— Enterobacteriaceae	*Shigella*	Bacillary dysentery
	Escherichia	Opportunistic pathogen, travelers' diarrhea
	Salmonella	Typhoid, gastroenteritis septicemia, enteric fever
	Klebsiella	Respiratory tract infections
	Enterobacter *Serratia* *Proteus*	Opportunistic or secondary pathogens
	Yersinia	Plague
B. VIBRIOS— Vibrionaceae	*Vibrio*	Cholera
II. Anaerobes— Bacteroidaceae	*Bacteroides* *Fusobacterium*	Infections of soft tissue and wounds
III. Aerobes— Pseudomonadaceae	*Pseudomonas*	Opportunistic pathogen

TABLE 16—2

Properties of the Major Genera in the Enterobacteriaceae Family

Fermentation Products	Lactose	Motility	Urease	Genus
	Fermented	Motile (most strains)	Absent	*Escherichia*
		Motile	Absent	*Salmonella*
Do not produce 2,3-butanediol	Not fermented	Motile	Present	*Proteus*
		Nonmotile	Absent	*Shigella*
Produce 2,3-butanediol	Fermented (gas-produced)	Nonmotile	Present	*Klebsiella*
		Motile	Absent	*Enterobacter*
	Not fermented	Motile (most strains)	Absent	*Serratia*

FIGURE 16—1

(*a*) Lactose fermenters grow as brick-red colonies surrounded by zones of precipitated bile on MacConkey agar. (*b*) Lactose nonfermenters do not visibly alter the medium. (Photograph supplied by Oxoid Limited, Basingstoke, Hampshire, England.)

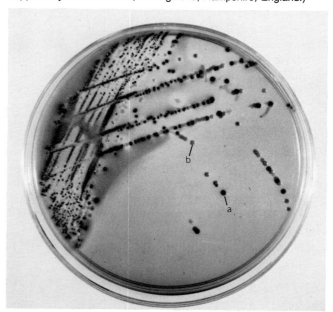

through the mixed-acid fermentation. The products of this fermentation include succinic acid, lactic acid, acetic acid, formic acid, H_2, CO_2, and ethanol. *Enterobacter, Klebsiella,* and *Serratia* also produce 2,3-butanediol; members of the other genera do not. Organisms that produce 2,3-butanediol as a product of the mixed-acid fermentation make fewer molecules of organic acids, so the final pH of their fermentation broth is relatively high. Because they cannot produce 2,3-butanediol, *Escherichia, Salmonella, Proteus,* and *Shigella* ferment sugars to organic acids, which lower the pH of their fermentation broths to 4.5 or less. The production of 2,3-butanediol is detected easily with a biochemical test, and a low pH (less than 4.5) of a fermentation broth is measured by adding a pH indicator dye to the medium.

The ability to ferment lactose is a key biochemical marker for this group (Table 16–1). *Salmonella, Shigella, Proteus,* and *Serratia marcescens* are unable to ferment lactose, whereas *Escherichia, Klebsiella,* and *Enterobacter* do. Lactose fermenters grow as red colonies on MacConkey agar (Figure 16–1 and Color Plate 10), whereas lactose nonfermenters grow as colorless or transparent colonies. In addition to lac-

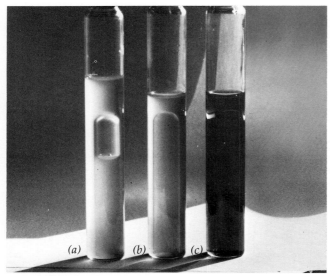

FIGURE 16–2
Durham tubes are used to detect gas production during bacterial fermentations. (a) *Escherichia coli* produces gas when it ferments lactose, whereas (b) *Enterobacter aerogenes* does not. The uninoculated tube (c) appears dark because of the presence of phenol red, a pH indicator.

tose and neutral red, MacConkey agar contains bile salts and crystal violet, which inhibit the growth of Gram-positive bacteria. Neutral red is a vital dye that is taken up by cells and turns red in response to acid production. The lactose fermenters produce acids that precipitate the bile salts and change the color of the neutral dye to red. The production of gas during lactose fermentation is detected by using a Durham tube (Figure 16–2). Durham tubes trap gas produced by those organisms that grow inside the inverted tube.

Motility can be observed with the light microscope or determined by observing an organism's growth pattern. Motile organisms produce a brushed-edge pattern (Figure 16–3) when grown in a motility medium.

Proteus and *Klebsiella* have urease (Table 16–2),

$$H_2N-\overset{\overset{\textstyle O}{\textstyle \|}}{C}-NH_2$$

which breaks down urea ($H_2N-C-NH_2$) to CO_2 and NH_3. Urease is detected when the pH indicator

in urea broth changes color in response to the alkaline products produced by urease.

The results of specialized tests that measure the presence of *Escherichia coli* in water are one indicator of water potability. Since *E. coli* is a human enteric organism, its presence in water is indicative of contamination by human feces. When *E. coli* is selectively grown on Levine eosine methylene blue (EMB) agar (Color Plate 8), it forms dark colonies possessing a green sheen (Figure 16–4). The number of *E. coli* colonies is termed a **fecal coliform count.** Because they form colonies with a characteristic green sheen, the number of *E. coli* colonies is easily determined even when colonies of other Gram-negative bacteria are present. For example, *Enterobacter* grow as pink-to-lavender colonies with dark centers (Color Plate 9); the lactose nonfermenters (Table 16–2) grow as white or transparent colonies.

Enterics can be further characterized by measuring their ability to metabolize different sugars and alcohols, their ability to grow on citrate, the presence of specific enzymes, and the production of hydrogen

FIGURE 16–3
Motility is detected by the brushlike growth in semisolid media. (a) The brushlike growth of a motile *Proteus* sp., and (b) the growth of the nonmotile *Streptococcus* sp. in the same medium.

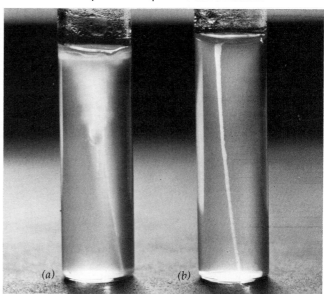

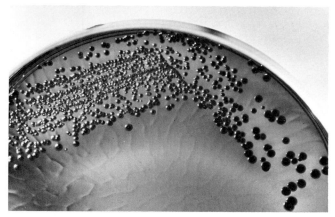

(a)

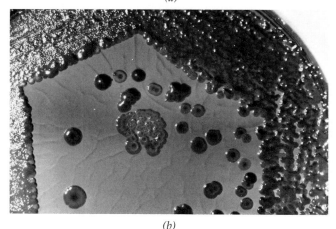

(b)

FIGURE 16—4
Levine EMB (eosin methylene blue) agar is used to select for Gram-negative bacteria and to differentiate *Escherichia coli* from *Enterobacter aerogenes*. Colonies of *E. coli* (a) are relatively small and have a greenish metallic sheen. Colonies of *E. aerogenes* (b) are lighter in color, possess dark centers, are larger than those of *E. coli,* and tend to grow together. For color presentation see Color Plate 11.

sulfide (H_2S). These tests can be performed in individual growth tubes or they can be done in commercial multitest systems (Figure 16–5) used to identify Gram-negative rods.

Antigenic structure. Gram-negative bacteria possess surface antigens that can be used in their identification. These surface antigens (Figure 16–6) are designated as the **O, H,** and **K antigens.** The H antigens are associated with flagella; nonmotile strains lack these antigens. The O antigens are the lipopolysaccharide component of the outer cell-wall found in Gram-negative bacteria. The polysaccharide portion (15 to 20 sugar residues) of the lipidpolysaccharide is the antigenic determinant of the O antigen. The great diversity of the O antigens depends on the nature and sequence of the sugar molecules in these polysaccharides. External to the O antigens are the K antigens (K is taken from the German, *kapsel*). K

FIGURE 16—5 (below)
The Enterotube® II is a multitest system used to identify Gram-negative bacteria. The 12 compartments in the tube are inoculated by touching the central wire needle to a bacterial colony and then pulling the wire through the tube. Following incubation, the Enterotube® is read by observing growth or color changes in the 12 compartments (Photograph courtesy of Joe Peterson, Hoffmann-LaRoche Inc., Nutley, N.J.)

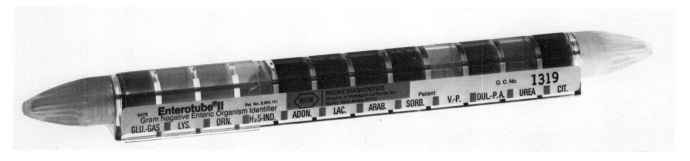

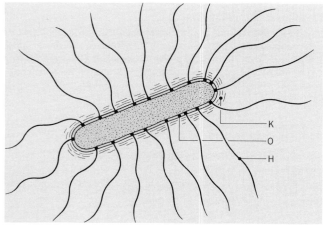

FIGURE 16–6
Antigenic structure of an enteric bacterium; K is the capsular antigen, O is the somatic antigen, and H is the flagellar antigen.

antigens are polymers of *N*-acetylgalactosamine and uronic acid, and they are removed by boiling. O antigens and H antigens are used as "fingerprints" for different isolates, and they have been used extensively to characterize species of *Salmonella*. The serological identification of specific species and/or strains of the enterics has been helpful in finding the origin of common-source epidemics.

Genetic relationships

Species of the Enterobacteriaceae share close genetic relationships, as is demonstrated by hybridization (Table 8–3) and other genetic experiments. Their genetic relatedness increases the frequency of plasmids and chromosomal gene transfer between species. R plasmids coding for multiple drug resistance together with plasmids coding for virulence factors (toxins and pili) are especially important to the pathogenesis of the enteric bacteria. Furthermore, the chance of such transfers occurring increases when the organisms live in the same ecological niche, the human intestine. The acquisition of drug resistance by plasmid transfer occurs among these bacteria and is a serious problem.

COLIFORMS

The facultative Gram-negative rods that normally inhabit the human intestinal tract without causing disease are referred to as the **coliforms.** *Escherichia, Enterobacter, Klebsiella,* and *Serratia* are important coliforms. Even though these organisms do not normally cause disease in humans, they must be considered as opportunistic pathogens that are capable of causing human diseases under special circumstances.

Escherichia

The bacterium *Escherichia coli* is named after Theodor Escherich. It is the only member of this genus. It is one of the most extensively studied organisms, in part because it is easy to isolate and grow under controlled conditions. Studies using *E. coli* have contributed greatly to the fields of genetics, biochemistry, and virology. In addition, *E. coli* is the predominant facultative anaerobe in the human lower intestine, so it is used as an indicator of human fecal contamination of water.

Pathogenesis. Three strains of *E. coli* are recognized as being involved in human disease. **Enterotoxic** *E. coli* (ETEC) carries plasmids that code for two toxins and a pilus. **Enteroinvasive** *E. coli* (EIEC) is able to invade the large intestine to cause a shigella-like syndrome. The regular *E. coli* causes urinary tract infections and is the most frequent Gram-negative bacterium isolated from patients with septicemia.

Enterotoxic *E. coli* has a heat-labile toxin, a heat-stable toxin, and a surface factor now identified as fimbriae. The **heat-labile toxin** activates adenylate cyclase, which forms 3′,5′-cyclic adenylate (abbreviated cyclic AMP or cAMP) as follows

$$ATP \xrightarrow{\text{adenylate cyclase}} cAMP + PPi$$

cAMP is a messenger molecule that stimulates the human intestinal mucosa to excrete Cl^- and bicarbonate. The electrolyte balance across the intestinal mucosa becomes unbalanced, resulting in the outpouring of water into the bowel. The excretion of copious amounts of water is the immediate cause of diarrhea. Cholera toxin has the same mechanism of action and causes similar symptoms. The **heat-stabile toxin** activates guanylate cyclase, which in turn increases the concentration of cGMP. The third factor is the presence of surface fimbriae that enables enterotoxic *E. coli* to colonize the small intestine, where both the heat-labile and heat-stabile enterotoxins act. All three virulence factors are coded for by plasmids. Enterotoxic *E. coli* causes severe infantile diarrhea, a choleralike syndrome, and is one cause of travelers' diarrhea.

Enteroinvasive *E. coli* is another strain of this bacterium that can invade the epithelium of the large intestine. It causes a shigellalike syndrome characterized by diarrhea and the presence of blood and pus in the stools.

E. coli strains that lack the plasmids coding for these virulence factors are still opportunistic pathogens. As normal inhabitants of the intestine, they do not cause disease, but they can cause invasive diseases of the urinary tract and of surgical wounds. *Escherichia coli* is the major cause of nosocomial infections (see Table 14–6).

Disease prevention and treatment. Enterotoxic *E. coli* causes acute diarrhea in infants and adults. The disease is more serious in infants since they have a lower physical resistance to this type of disease. Acute diarrhea caused by *E. coli* is transmitted by ingesting contaminated food or water. Enterotoxic *E. coli* is prevalent in underdeveloped countries where

sewage treatment facilities are unavailable. Foreigners should be careful of the food and water they consume when traveling in these countries. It is advisable to drink beverages made with boiled water (tea and coffee), canned or bottled carbonated beverages, and/or beer or wine. Ice cubes made with contaminated water should be avoided, as should glassware washed in contaminated water. Uncooked foods such as unpasteurized milk and cheese should also be avoided.

Treatment of diarrheal disease is aimed at replenishing the fluids lost from the body. Rehydration and establishment of the normal electrolytic balance can be accomplished by consuming the concoctions described in Table 16–3. The disease is usually self-limiting, and recovery follows the purging diarrhea, which removes the noxious substances from the bowel. Because the disease is more serious in infants, they are treated with colistin or neomycin.

Escherichia coli is a common cause of urinary tract infections that occur more often in women and in infants wearing diapers. An infection is indicated when the patient's urine contains more than 100,000 bacteria/ml. Bacteria in the urethra can infect the urinary bladder to cause **cystitis;** sometimes the bacteria infect the kidneys. Nosocomial urinary tract infections can result from catheterization and other urethral instrumentation. These infections are difficult to treat because many antibiotics do not penetrate the urinary tract from the blood. Uncomplicated urinary tract infections can be treated with sulfonamide or ampicillin.

TABLE 16–3
Treatment of Diarrheal Disease[a]

Concoction	Substance	Key Ingredient
Glass 1	Fruit juice, 8 oz	Rich in K^+
	Honey or corn syrup, ½ tb	Glucose necessary for ion absorbtion
	Salt, 1 pinch	Na^+ and Cl^-
Glass 2	Water (carbonated or boiled), 8 oz	Water
	Baking soda or powder, ¼ ts	$NaHCO_3$

[a]Drink the two concoctions in alternating fashion.

TABLE 16–4
Differentiation of Select Species of *Enterobacter*, *Klebsiella*, and *Serratia*

Characteristic	*Enterobacter aerogenes*	*Klebsiella pneumoniae*	*Serratia marcescens*
Motility	+	–	+
Ornithine decarboxylase	+	–	+
Ferments arabinose	+	+	–
Red pigment	–	–	+[a]

[a]Limited to specific strains of *Serratia marcescens*; growth temperature is a factor in pigment production.

Most strains of *E. coli* are susceptible to a broad range of antibiotics including ampicillin, cephalosporin, tetracyclines, carbenicillin, and the sulfanilamide drugs. Because of R factors, *E. coli* strains readily pick up multiple drug resistances. Determining the antibiotic sensitivities of the causative agent is necessary for effective treatment.

Enterobacter, Klebsiella, and Serratia

Enterobacter, *Klebsiella*, and *Serratia* are closely related genera. They all grow on citrate and mannitol as sole sources of carbon, and their growth is not inhibited by cyanide. They are identified by biochemical tests that include fermentation of sugars and sugar alcohols, their ability to decarboxylate ornithine, pigment production, and the presence of motility (Table 16–4).

Enterobacter is found in soil, water, sewage, dairy products, and in the human intestine. It is an opportunistic pathogen in that it causes urinary tract and surgical wound infections. *Enterobacter* is usually a secondary pathogen when it is isolated from these infections.

Species of *Serratia* are common inhabitants of air, soil, and water. They have been isolated from both healthy and diseased insects, animals, and birds. Of the three known species, *Serratia marcescens* is the one most often encountered in human infections. For decades, microbiologists have discounted the ability of *Serratia* to cause disease, but now it is known to cause various nosocomial infections. Certain strains of *S. marcescens* (Figure 16–7) and *S. rub-*

idaea produce a brick-red pigment, prodigiosin, especially when they are grown at room temperature. The species of *Serratia* are identified by their biochemical characteristics.

Nonpigmented *S. marcescens* are the predominant strains isolated from hospital settings. Multiple resistance and R-plasmid-mediated resistance to antibiotics appear to be found exclusively with these nonpigmented strains. They have been associated with respiratory illness, infections of intensive care patients, urinary tract infections, infections of surgi-

FIGURE 16–7
Some *Serratia* grow as brick-red colonies (they appear black in this photo) due to the production of prodigiosin.

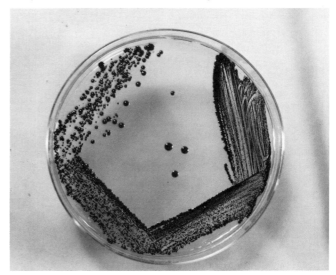

cal wounds, and septicemia of patients with intravenous catheters. *Serratia marcescens* is widely distributed in nature, so their presence in hospital wards is not unexpected. They are opportunistic pathogens that can cause disease in compromised patients.

Klebsiella are Gram-negative, encapsulated rods that can grow on citrate or glucose as a sole source of carbon. They are very similar to *Enterobacter*, and most strains produce 2,3-butanediol (Table 16–2). *Klebsiella* are differentiated from *Enterobacter* because they are nonmotile and are unable to decarboxylate ornithine. The most important human pathogen is *K. pneumoniae*. This organism is widely distributed in soil, water, and vegetable matter. Strains of *K. pneumoniae* can be subdivided serologically on the basis of their somatic (O) and capsular (K) antigens.

Between 5 and 10 percent of healthy Americans carry *K. pneumoniae* in their respiratory tract, whereas others carry this organism in their intestine. *K. pneumoniae* can infect the lungs of compromised patients and is responsible for approximately 3 percent of the cases of human pneumonia. The virulence of *K. pneumoniae* depends on the presence of an antiphagocytic capsule. This organism is also responsible for nosocomial infections of surgical wounds and the urinary tract (see Table 14–6). Patients with *K. pneumoniae* infections are treated with antibiotics: sulfonamides, ampicillin, and tetracyclines are used

to treat patients with uncomplicated urinary tract infections, whereas chloramphenicol, cephalosporins, and aminoglucosides are used to treat life-threatening infections.

Two other *Klebsiella* species have been implicated in inflammatory diseases of the nasopharyngeal region. *K. ozaenae* causes progressive atrophy of the nasal mucosa, and *K. rhinoscleromatis* causes hardening of the nasal tissue (Gr. *rhino*, nose).

SALMONELLA AND SHIGELLA

Salmonella

Typhoid fever, salmonella septicemia, and salmonella gastroenteritis (enteric fevers) are caused by species of *Salmonella*. The salmonella are motile, H_2S-producing, facultative, Gram-negative rods that do not ferment lactose. The classification of this genus is expansive because of the serological variations between isolates. The antigenic analysis of salmonella isolates has resulted in the designation of about 1500 serotypes. The Kaufmann-White scheme systematically assigns numbers and letters to the different O, H, and Vi (virulence) antigens (Table 16–5) to create groups of the salmonella.

Sal. typhimurium is the species most frequently isolated in the United States (Table 16–6). It is associated with salmonella gastroenteritis. *Sal. typhi*, found only in humans, causes **typhoid fever**. This

TABLE 16–5
Serotypes of Selected Species of *Salmonella*

Species	Group	O Antigen	H Antigen (Phase 1)
Sal. paratyphi-A	A	1, 2, 12	a
Sal. schottmulleri	B	1, 4, 5, 12	b
Sal. saint-paul	B	1, 4, 5, 12	e, n
Sal. typhimurium	B	1, 4, 5, 12	i
Sal. cholerae-suis	C	6, 7	c
Sal. infantis	C	6, 7	r
Sal. typhi	D	9, 12, Vi	d
Sal. enteritidis	D	1, 9, 12	g, m
Sal. anatum	E	3, 10	e, h

Source: From H. Chmel and D. Armstrong, *Am. J. Med.*, 60:203 (1976).

TABLE 16–6
Frequently Isolated Serotypes of *Salmonella*, United States, 1978

Serotype	Number	Percent
Sal. typhimurium	10,015	34.8
Sal. heidelberg	2,078	7.2
Sal. enteritidis	1,934	6.7
Sal. newport	1,879	6.5
Sal. infantis	1,225	4.3
Sal. agona	1,186	4.1
Sal. montevideo	703	2.4
Sal. typhi	604	2.1
Sal. saint-paul	602	2.1
Sal. javiana	528	1.8
Subtotal	20,754	72.2
Total (all serotypes)	28,748	100.0

Source: *Salmonella Surveillance Annual Summary*, 1978, USPHS, Centers for Disease Control, Atlanta, 1979.

organism is distinct from the other salmonella because it lacks ornithine decarboxylase and produces low amounts of H_2S from triple-sugar-iron (TSI) agar. Milder forms of enteric fever are caused by *Sal. schottmulleri* and *Sal. typhimurium*. *Sal. cholerae-suis* (cholera of a hog) is found primarily in domestic animals; however, it does cause salmonella septicemia and salmonella gastroenteritis in humans. *Sal. enteritidis* is the major cause of foodborne salmonella gastroenteritis (food poisoning).

Almost all salmonella infections are transmitted by the oral-fecal route. *Sal. typhimurium, Sal. cholerae-suis,* and *Sal. enteritidis* can be carried by turtles, domestic fowl (turkeys are prominent carriers), and other animals. Typhoid fever can be controlled by identifying and treating the human carriers of *Sal. typhi*. Carriers excrete *Sal. typhi* in their feces and often contaminate fomites, food, and water.

Typhoid fever. Typhoid fever is a bacterial infection of humans caused by *Sal. typhi*. Human volunteers have been used to study typhoid fever since this bacterium does not infect other animals. Humans must consume 10^5 to 10^7 bacteria to become infected within the average incubation period of 7.5

days. Incubation periods as long as 33 days have been observed when smaller doses were consumed. The clinical symptoms include malaise, headache, and loss of appetite followed by a prolonged fever. These symptoms are accompanied by abdominal pain and a rash that appears as "rose spots" on the trunk. Even though this bacterium infects its host via the intestine, diarrhea is an uncommon symptom of typhoid fever. The disease reaches its peak during the third week (Figure 16–8) and then subsides. The recovery stage can be accompanied by intestinal hemorrhages that can lead to peritonitis.

Sal. typhi infects the blood from the intestinal tract within the first week. As the concentration of serum agglutinins increases (Figure 16–8), the ability to detect *Sal. typhi* in the blood decreases. These organisms are next found in the feces and in the urine. *Sal. typhi* colonizes the biliary tract and from here infects the small intestine. Chronic carriers of typhoid have infected bile ducts and can be cured by cholecystectomy (removal of the gallbladder) if antibiotic therapy fails.

Typhoid fever should be suspected in patients with a fever persisting for 1 week or more. The demonstration of *Sal. typhi* in blood cultures is the most useful diagnostic tool. Chloramphenicol and ampicillin are used to treat typhoid fever; however, antibiotic sensitivity testing is important because resistant strains are known. The fever disappears in most patients after 3 to 5 days of treatment.

The incidence of typhoid fever is low in the United States (about 430 cases a year), but it remains a problem in other parts of the world. The cases in the United States are usually diagnosed in travelers returning from foreign countries where the climate is warm and the sewage treatment facilities are inadequate. Typhoid fever can be controlled in a society by (1) proper sewage disposal, (2) pasteurization of milk, (3) maintenance of unpolluted water supplies, (4) identification and treatment of infected individuals, and (5) the monitoring of food-handlers to detect carriers.

Salmonella septicemia and gastroenteritis. Salmonella food poisoning is manifested as gastroenteritis

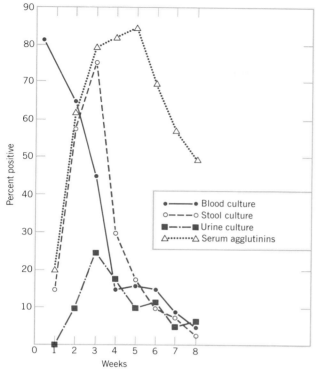

FIGURE 16–8
The kinetics of typhoid fever. The relative frequency of positive blood, urine, and stool cultures during the course of the disease. Notice that the serum agglutinin's peak corresponds to the decrease in the percentage of positive cultures. (From H. R. Morgan, "The Enteric Bacteria," in R. J. Dubos and J. G. Hirsch, eds., *Bacterial and Mycotic Infections of Man*, copyright © 1965, J. B. Lippincott Co.)

and is the most common cause of foodborne disease in the United States (see Table 14–5). A number of species are involved in these illnesses; however, *Sal. typhimurium* is the most common cause. The incubation period is between 6 and 48 hours after the person ingests contaminated food or water. The symptoms include sudden onset of headache, chills, and abdominal pain followed by nausea, vomiting, diarrhea, and a fever that lasts 1 to 4 days. The causative agent is excreted in the feces, but it rarely enters the circulatory system. Patients recover in due course; antibiotic treatment is not recommended,

except for the very young and for those patients over 60.

Occasionally patients develop **salmonella septicemia,** which does not involve the gastrointestinal tract. This disease is accompanied by a high fever and is most often caused by *Sal. cholerae-suis*. Salmonella septicemia is a serious infection that should be treated with appropriate antibiotics such as chloramphenicol and ampicillin.

Shigella

Bacillary dysentery (shigellosis) is caused by bacteria in the genus *Shigella*. Their distribution in nature is limited to the intestine of humans and primates. The disease is a problem to confined groups, such as the military, institutions for the mentally retarded, and Indian reservations. Historically, the disease has altered the outcome of military conflicts by rendering the soldiers temporarily unfit for battle.

Shigella are nonmotile, Gram-negative rods that do not ferment lactose. Kiyoshi Shiga isolated the first species, now named *S. dysenteriae*. The three other known species of *Shigella* are distinguished by fermentation of mannitol, by the presence of ornithine decarboxylase, and by serological typing. All four species cause dysentery in humans, with the most severe symptoms caused by *S. dysenteriae*.

Shigella infect the colon and the terminal ileum of the gastrointestinal tract. Here they produce lesions in the intestinal mucosa caused in part by the release of endotoxin from lysed cells. Shigella also produce an exotoxin known as the **shiga neurotoxin.** This toxin is a protein (mol. wt. ca. 75,000 daltons) that causes paralysis and death when injected into guinea pigs or rabbits. It is believed to have enterotoxin activity and may be responsible for the early diarrhea seen in bacillary dysentery.

The clinical symptoms of shigella dysentery include the rapid onset of abdominal cramps, diarrhea, and fever with the presence of both blood and mucus in the feces. This disease is clinically differentiated from amebic dysentery, because white blood cells are not usually observed in fecal specimens of amebic dysentery. Depending on the species of *Shigella*, infection can be established by as few as 180 viable bacteria and normally occurs when approximately 5000 bacteria are ingested.* The incubation period is between 1 and 4 days. The symptoms progress from abdominal cramps to bloody stools over a period of 100 hours. Recovery usually follows without antibiotic treatment. Severe cases can be treated with ampicillin.

Humans are the only important source of bacillary dysentery. The "four Fs" are recognized as the means of transmission: "food, feces, fingers, and flies." Prevention of bacillary dysentery can be accomplished only by controlling the spread of the organisms.

THE PLAGUE BACILLUS

Historical documents, literary accounts, and paintings remind us of the devastation wrought by the plague. This disease has been called the bubonic plague because it infects and swells the lymph nodes (buboes) in the groin. During the Middle Ages, the plague was called the Black Death because it is characterized by black patches under the skin caused by hemorrhages. Modern medicine refers to this disease as plague.

Epidemiology of plague—*Yersinia pestis*

The causative agent of plague is named after its French discoverer, Alexandre Yersin, and is classified with the Enterobacteriaceae. It is a Gram-negative, nonmotile, facultative coccobacillus. *Y. pestis* is foremost a pathogen of rodents and is found in infected populations of rats and ground squirrels. *Y. pestis* grows in these animal reservoirs and is found in their blood, feces, and urine. Other animals become infected by eating diseased rodents or by being bitten by an infected flea that once lived on a diseased rodent.

Y. pestis is transmitted to humans when they are bitten by a contaminated flea. The flea leaves its dead rodent host to seek another viable home. Ground squirrels are the most common animal reservoirs in the United States, so most of the U.S. cases of plague occur in the western United States where these rodents live. *Y. pestis* also infects the black house rat, *Rattus rattus;* the gray sewer rat, *Rattus norvegicus;* and, less commonly, *Rattus alexandrinus.* The ancient peoples who were devastated by the plague never understood the relationship between these rodents and the plague.

Plague in humans. Bubonic plague and pneumonic plague are the two forms of the human disease. Bubonic plague begins with a sudden onset of a high fever after a 2- to 5-day incubation period. During the incubation period, *Y. pestis* infects the regional lymph nodes. The enlarged tender **buboes** that form in the groin are swollen, infected lymph nodes. The disease becomes a septicemia resulting in the infection of the liver, spleen, lungs, and sometimes the meninges. Black hemorrhagic areas may develop under the skin. Patients either recover within 10 days of the onset of the symptoms or they die. Between 60 and 90 percent of the untreated cases are fatal.

Pneumonic plague is an infection of the lungs that occurs during the later stages of bubonic plague. *Y. pestis* can be transmitted from a pneumonic plague patient directly to another human. High numbers of *Y. pestis* are contained in the sputum of these patients and are transmitted by droplets expelled by coughing. Pneumonic plague spreads through a population very rapidly, and untreated cases are almost always fatal.

Y. pestis causes an invasive disease in which the bacteria are able to survive and multiply in monocytes. They also produce toxins, but the role of these toxins in the actual disease is not clear. The few patients who do recover from plague have a high state of immunity to reinfection.

Treatment and control. Streptomycin, chloramphenicol, and tetracyclines are used to treat both forms of plague. Drug therapy must begin soon after the onset of the symptoms, especially in patients with pneumonic plague who, may die if treatment does not begin within 12 to 15 hours after the onset of the fever. Elimination of the rodent reservoirs and

*These data were obtained with human volunteers.

the use of insecticides to control fleas are the major approaches to preventing plague. All cases of plague should be isolated to prevent person-to-person transmission of the disease. Plague is a rare disease in the United States where less than 25 cases are reported each year.

VIBRIONACEAE

Cholera has been pandemic since the early 1800s, and it still is in modern times. This disease is transmitted by water contaminated by human fecal matter, as was aptly demonstrated by John Snow (see Chapter 14). The most recent epidemic began in Macao and Hong Kong in 1960–61 (Figure 16–9), spread to India, and reached the Near East during the late 1960s. Cholera spread to Africa and then to parts of Europe during the early 1970s. The disease is most prevalent in the spring and early summer and is more common in tropical climates. Fewer than 20 cases a year are reported in the United States, and they are usually restricted to foreign travelers.

Cholera—*Vibrio cholerae.* The cholera-causing bacteria—*Vibrio cholerae*—are Gram-negative, polar-flagellated, oxidase-positive, curved rods that are classified in the family Vibrionaceae. They are facultative anaerobes that grow readily in alkaline media (pH 9.0 to 9.6) and 3 percent NaCl. They grow better under aerobic conditions, but they will ferment a wide selection of carbohydrates.

FIGURE 16–9
Global spread of cholera during the 1961–1971 pandemic. (World Health Organization.)

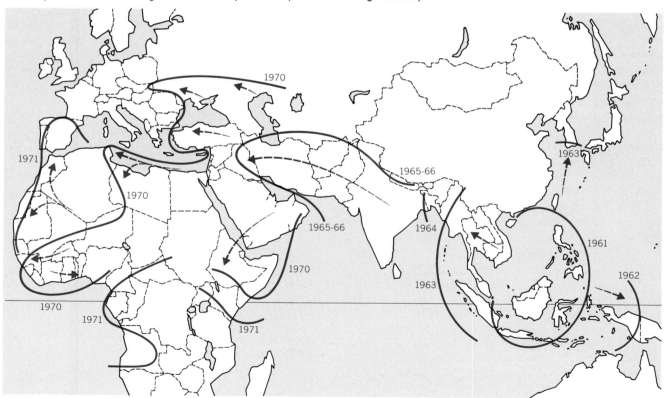

Cholera in humans. Humans ingest *V. cholerae* in contaminated food or water. The infection is established in the small intestine after a variable incubation time (between 24 hours and 5 days). Here *V. cholerae* grow and produce toxins that cause a purging diarrhea often accompanied by acidosis. The patient's stools are heavily contaminated with vibrios and also contain sloughed-off epithelial cells and mucus. The loss of water and electrolytes is so great that the patient becomes prostrate and eventually dies if not treated.

Vibrio cholerae produces a heat-labile enterotoxin that is responsible for the purging diarrhea of cholera. The toxin activates the membrane-bound adenylate cyclase in the intestinal epithelial cells. This enzyme increases the concentration of cAMP, which stimulates the intestinal mucosa to secrete Cl^- and bicarbonate. In turn, the cells lose copious amounts of water. The cholera enterotoxin has the same mechanism of action as the heat-labile enterotoxin of enterotoxic *E. coli*.

Treatment and control. Death from cholera results from severe dehydration. Treatment consists of replacing the lost fluids by oral and/or intravenous administration of fluids composed of an alkaline-saline solution containing bicarbonate and lactate. Up to 25 liters of this solution is required to treat a single patient. The case-fatality rate of untreated patients, which can be as high as 60 percent, can be reduced to 1 percent by restoring the fluids of cholera patients.

Chemotherapy is unable to affect the fatality rate directly, but it does decrease the duration of the diarrhea and the amount of fluid needed to restore the patient to health. Tetracyclines and chloramphenicol are the most effective antibiotics.

Vibrio cholerae survives poorly outside the human body. It is sensitive to drying, to heating (55°C for 10 minutes), and to many chemical disinfectants. Therefore, the occurrence of endemic cholera depends on human carriers of *V. cholerae*. Asymptomatic persons can be short-term carriers who excrete 10^2 to 10^3 vibrios per gram of feces, or they can be long-term carriers who probably have a persistent vibrio infection of their gallbladder. Because of these carriers, the only successful control of the disease is adequate sewage treatment combined with water purification systems.

BACTEROIDACEAE

The human body provides niches for strict anaerobes to grow even though we consider ourselves to be aerobic animals. The lower intestine provides a suitable environment for anaerobic bacteria, which comprise between 95 and 99 percent of the microbial population of the human lower intestine. The Gram-negative anaerobic rods are classified as a distinct group in the family Bacteroidaceae. Members of the genera *Bacteroides* and *Fusobacterium* are found in human feces and to a lesser extent in the vagina, external genitalia, and mouth.

The obligate anaerobes: *Bacteroides* and *Fusobacterium*

Bacteroides fragilis is an obligate anaerobe that is naturally found in the lower intestine of humans and warm-blooded animals (Figure 16–10). It is the most common species of anaerobic bacteria to be isolated from soft-tissue infections. As an opportunistic pathogen, it has been isolated from patients with appendicitis, peritonitis, heart valve infections, rectal abscesses, and surgical wounds. *B. fragilis* is often resistant to penicillin, but it is relatively sensitive to carbenicillin and chloramphenicol.

Fusobacterium sp. are obligate anaerobes that are isolated from the oral cavity and the upper respiratory tract of humans and warm-blooded animals. The pathogenic species cause infections of soft tissue and are secondary invaders of gangrenous tissue. The increased use of anaerobic culturing techniques in diagnostic laboratories continues to augment our knowledge of these obligate anaerobes.

PSEUDOMONADACEAE

The chemoorganotrophic, aerobic, oxidase-positive, Gram-negative rods are classified in the genus *Pseu-*

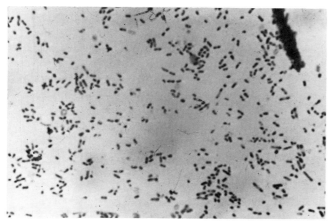

FIGURE 16—10
Bacteroides fragilis in a blood smear. (Courtesy of Dr. L. LeBeau.)

domonas. These bacteria are ubiquitous in aerobic environments and are recognized for their ability to metabolize an extensive variety of organic compounds. The classification of the pseudomonads is based on their biochemical reactions and their ability to produce water-soluble fluorescent pigments. A few pseudomonads are opportunistic pathogens that infect wounds and the urinary tract.

Pseudomonas aeruginosa. *P. aeruginosa* produces a blue-green fluorescent pigment that diffuses into its growth medium and gives a blue color to the pus produced during *P. aeruginosa* infections. The cells are polarly flagellated, motile, Gram-negative, non-spore-forming rods that oxidize a wide variety of organic compounds. *P. aeruginosa* is ubiquitous in nature and is found in sinks, on lab benches, and throughout most hospitals. For years it was thought to be a harmless saprophyte, but now it is known to cause human diseases, especially infections of burned tissue and of the urinary tract.

Burns on the epidermis provide an ideal growth environment for *P. aeruginosa*. This bacterium produces a heat-labile exotoxin that inhibits protein synthesis by a mechanism similar to the diphtheria toxin (see Chapter 17). It specifically inhibits protein synthesis, which in turn kills cells in eucaryotic tissue

by inactivating their elongation factor 2. *P. aeruginosa* infects burned tissue and prevents normal healing. Hospital burn centers are specially designed to control pseudomonad infections, which are difficult to treat because *P. aeruginosa* often carries drug-resistance plasmids. The topical application of polymyxin to burned tissue is one approach to controlling *P. aeruginosa* infections.

SUMMARY

The enteric pathogenic bacteria (Table 16–7) are classified in the families Enterobacteriaceae (oxidase-negative, facultative anaerobes) and Vibrionaceae (oxidase-positive, facultative anaerobes). The Enterobacteriaceae includes the genera *Escherichia, Enterobacter, Klebsiella, Serratia, Salmonella, Shigella,* and *Yersinia*. The first four genera are the coliforms that are normal inhabitants of the human intestine and normally do not cause human disease. Under special circumstances, they are opportunistic pathogens. Enterotoxic *E. coli* produces an enterotoxin and causes infantile diarrhea, choleralike syndrome, and/or travelers' diarrhea. Enteroinvasive *E. coli* causes a shigellalike syndrome. *K. pneumoniae* is capsulated and is responsible for about 3 percent of the cases of human bacterial pneumonia. *Enterobacter* and *Serratia* are opportunistic pathogens that can be found as secondary invaders. All these organisms infect the urinary tract or wounds under appropriate conditions.

Species of *Salmonella* are responsible for typhoid fever, salmonella gastroenteritis (enteric fever), and salmonella septicemia. These diseases are contracted by the fecal-oral route. *Sal. typhi* is found only in the human intestine, whereas other salmonella are found in the intestines of humans, birds, and animals. *Shigella* causes bacillary dysentery in humans and is transmitted by the fecal-oral route. This is a self-limiting disease of short duration that is characterized by bloody stools.

Yersinia pestis is primarily a pathogen of rodents, but it does cause plague in humans. Fleas living on diseased rodents transfer *Y. pestis* to humans. This

TABLE 16–7
Summary: Diseases of the Gram-negative Rods

Disease	Bacterium	Symptoms	Virulence and (Source)
Infantile diarrhea, travelers' diarrhea	Enterotoxic *E. coli*	Diarrhea, abdominal cramps	Enterotoxins LT and LS (food and water)
Shigellalike syndrome	Enteroinvasive *E. coli*	Blood, mucus in stools	Invasiveness (fecal-oral)
Cystitis	*Escherichia coli*	Urinary tract inflammation	Invasiveness, R factors
Pneumonia	*Klebsiella pneumoniae*	Lung congestion, cough	Capsules
Typhoid fever	*Salmonella typhi*	Malaise, headache, fever, septicemia	Endotoxins (food and water)
Sal. gastroenteritis *Sal.* septicemia	*Salmonella* sp.	Sudden onset, headache, chills, abdominal pain, vomiting, diarrhea	Endotoxins (humans, domestic fowl and wild animals)
Dysentery	*Shigella dysenteriae*	Abdominal cramps, diarrhea, blood and mucus in stool	Neurotoxin, enterotoxin (feces)
Plague	*Yersinia pestis*	High fever, infected lymph nodes, black skin patches	Invasiveness, toxins (fleas on rodents)
Cholera	*Vibrio cholerae*	Purging diarrhea	Enterotoxin (water)

Opportunistic Pathogens

Etiological Agent	Type of Infection
Bacteroides fragilis	Complications of bowel surgery, appendicitis
Enterobacter sp.	Urinary tract, surgical wounds
Pseudomonas aeruginosa	Burns
Serratia marcescens	Infections of compromised hosts

bacterium infects the lymph nodes, resulting in bubonic plague. Pneumonic plague is very contagious and can be passed to healthy humans by water droplets.

Vibrio cholerae causes a purging diarrheal disease in humans. The organism is ingested in contaminated water, multiplies in the intestine, and excretes an enterotoxin that is responsible for the disease symptoms. Treatment involves replenishing the fluid and electrolytes by oral and/or intravenous administration of a balanced saline solution.

The Gram-negative, anaerobic rods are classified as the Bacteroidaceae. *Bacteroides fragilis* is the major bacterium in the human intestine and can cause in-

fections of soft tissue. It has been isolated from patients with appendicitis, peritonitis, rectal abscesses, and surgical wounds. Another strict anaerobe, *Fusobacterium*, also causes infections of soft tissue. It is naturally found in the oral cavity and the upper respiratory tract.

The family Pseudomonales contains the Gram-negative, aerobic, oxidase-positive, rod-shaped bacteria. *P. aeruginosa* is an opportunistic human pathogen that is troublesome to burn patients. It produces a diphtherialike toxin that is cytotoxic. The ubiquitous nature of *P. aeruginosa* and its resistance to many antibiotics make prevention and control of these infections difficult.

QUESTIONS AND TOPICS FOR STUDY AND DISCUSSION

Questions

1. Create a chart of the genera of the Gram-negative rods that includes the characteristics of each, the disease(s) they cause, and the environment where they are naturally found.
2. Which Gram-negative bacteria are opportunistic pathogens? Under what conditions do they cause disease?
3. What specific criteria are used to classify the Enterobacteriaceae? How do these criteria distinguish between the genera in this family?
4. *Escherichia coli* is a normal inhabitant of the human intestine. Describe the diseases caused by enterotoxic *E. coli*, and explain how this strain differs from the normal *E. coli*.
5. Describe the disease caused by the following.
   Enterobacter aerogenes
   Klebsiella pneumoniae
   Serratia marcescens
   Bacteroides fragilis
   Fusobacterium sp.
6. Describe the diseases caused by *Salmonella* and their mode of transmission. What procedures are taken to limit the spread of these infections?
7. What were the problems faced by the public health authorities who had to deal with "Typhoid Mary" Mallon?
8. What are the signs of shigella dysentery that differentiate it from amebic dysentery and salmonella gastroenteritis?
9. What was the historic significance of *Yersinia pestis*? Does this bacterium still pose a serious threat to humans? If so, what, where, and why?
10. Describe the symptoms of and the treatment for cholera. How important is this disease (a) in your community and (b) in the world?
11. What is the mode of action of the cholera toxin? How does the cholera toxin relate to the toxin produced by enterotoxic *E. coli*?
12. Why is *Pseudomonas aeruginosa* a constant threat to burn patients? What steps are taken to prevent *Pseudomonas aeruginosa* infections of burn wounds?

Discussion

1. The Gram-negative rods are involved in a large proportion of the nosocomial infections reported in Table 14–6. Can you provide an explanation for this observation?
2. The acquisition of multiple drug resistance in bacteria was first observed in *Shigella dysenteriae*. How do bacteria acquire multiple drug resistance? Is the acquisition of drug resistance a special problem among the Gram-negative rods? Explain.

FURTHER READINGS

Books

Finegold, S. M., and W. J. Martin, *Baily and Scott's Diagnostic Microbiology*, 6th ed., Mosby, St. Louis, 1982. This book contains an extensive chapter on the classification and identification of the Enterobacteriaceae.

Articles and Reviews

Brenner, D. J., J. J. Farmer, F. W. Hickman, M. A. Asbury, and A. G. Steigerwalt, "Taxonomic and Nomenclature Changes in Enterobacteriaceae," Centers for Disease Control, Atlanta, 1977. The widely used Edward and Ewing classification scheme of the Enterobacteriaceae as modified by the CDC. There are a number of differences between this scheme and the classification scheme presented in *Bergey's Manual*.

Butler, T., A. A. F. Mahmoud, and K. S. Warren, "Algorithms in the Diagnosis and Management of Exotic Diseases XXIII. Typhoid fever," *J. Infect. Dis.*, 135:1017–1020 (1977). The diagnosis and management of typhoid fever.

Grimont, P. A. D., and F. Grimont, "The Genus *Serratia*," *Ann. Rev. Microbiol.*, 32:221–248 (1978). This review includes a discussion of the nosocomial infections cause by *Serratia*.

Hirschhorn, N., and W. B. Greenough III, "Cholera," *Sci. Am.*, 225:15–21 (August 1971). This article describes the physiological action of cholera toxin, the epidemiology, and the treatment of cholera.

Hornick, R. B., S. E. Greisman, T. E. Woodward, H. L. Dupont, A. T. Dawkins, and M. J. Snyder. "Typhoid Fever: Pathogenesis and Immunological Control," *N. Engl. J. Med.*, 283:686–690 (1970). A review of typhoid fever in humans that includes interesting dose response data obtained by infecting human volunteers.

17

CORYNEBACTERIA, MYCOBACTERIUM, NOCARDIAE, AND ACTINOMYCES

Four bacterial genera that have the potential to cause human disease, *Corynebacterium, Mycobacterium, Nocardia,* and *Actinomyces,* are grouped together as "The Actinomycetes and Related Organisms." This division includes a diversified group of organisms. Many are found in soil, some form branched filaments, and some have the ability to develop into mycelia.

Corynebacterium, Mycobacterium, and *Nocardia* share a number of characteristics. They possess a common cell-wall antigen, have arabinose and galactose in their cell walls, and produce mycolic acids. These acids are distinctive long chain α-branched, β-hydroxy acids (Table 17–1) and are present in a limited number of bacteria. Their similarities by no means make these genera a coherent group of organisms. They are morphologically diverse, and the types of human disease that they cause are even more distinctive. For these reasons, it is necessary to describe the pathogen(s) in each genus.

CORYNEBACTERIA

Diphtheria has been recognized as a human affliction (Table 17–2) since the time of Hippocrates, who first reported diphtherialike symptoms in humans. Much later, Pierre Bretonneau accurately described the formation of a veil in patients' throats as a symptom of diphtheria (Gr. *diphthera,* skin or membrane).

The causative agent of diphtheria, *Corynebacterium diphtheriae* (Gr. *coryne,* club), was first observed by Theodor Klebs in 1883. A year later, Friedrich Loeffler succeeded in growing this organism in an artificial medium. He was successful in using his isolates

TABLE 17–1
Mycolic Acids

Basic Structure

$$R_1 - \underset{\underset{OH}{|}}{\overset{\alpha}{CH}} - \underset{\underset{R_2}{|}}{\overset{\beta}{CH}} - COOH$$

	Range in Size	Formula
Mycobacterium	C_{79} to C_{85}	
M. tuberculosis		$(C_{78}H_{152}O_3)$
Nocardia	C_{48} to C_{58}	
Corynebacterium	C_{32} to C_{36}	
Corynemycolic acid		$(C_{32}H_{64}O_3)$
Corynemycolenic acid		$(C_{32}H_{62}O_3)$

304

TABLE 17–2
History of Diphtheria

Year	Scientists	Discovery
1821	Pierre Bretonneau	Recognized as specific disease
1883	Theodor Klebs	Described bacterial agent
1884	Friedrich Loeffler	Grew organism in artificial media
1888	E. Roux and A. Yersin	Discovered soluble toxin
1890	Emil von Behring and Shibasaburo Kitasato	Immunized animals with chemically inactivated toxin
1891	Berlin physicians	Used antitoxin to treat diphtheria
1909	Theobald Smith	Introduced active immunization with antitoxin-neutralized toxin
1913	Bela Schick	Developed assay to test for immunity
1920	G. Ramon	Produced formalin-inactivated toxin (toxoid) used today
1951	V. J. F. Freeman	Discovered that toxigenic *C. diphtheriae* is lysogenic

to cause diphtheria in guinea pigs. This bacterium caused tissue damage throughout the guinea pig's body even though the bacteria grew only in the nasopharangeal region. This tissue damage was attributed to the effects of diphtheria toxin, which was soon purified (in 1888) by Emil Roux and Alexandre Yersin.

Emil von Behring and Shibasaburo Kitasato performed studies on diphtheria and tetanus toxins that led to the development of the science of serology. The discovery of antitoxins was first reported in their 1890 paper.*

After many negative experiments, it was discovered that the blood of immune animals had the ability to neutralize the diphtheria toxin . . .

Von Behring used this discovery to develop an inactive diphtheria toxin that he used as an immunogen. Immunized animals developed an immunity strong enough to survive lethal injections of diphtheria toxin. Transfusions of blood from these immunized animals protected nonimmune animals against the effects of the active toxin. As a result of these experiments, German physicians began to use animal sera for passive immunization of diphtheria patients in 1891.

By the early 1900s, physicians used both active and passive forms of immunization to prevent diphtheria. Active immunization was the most appropriate means of controlling diphtheria; however, the production of an effective diphtheria toxoid remained a problem. Some of the early toxoids were ineffective and some were too toxic. To deal with this problem, Theobald Smith introduced antitoxin-neutralized diphtheria toxin as an immunizing agent. Later, G. Ramon found that formalin-inactivated diphtheria toxin (Table 17–2) was an effective antigen that was devoid of side effects. Formalin-inactivated diphtheria toxin is still used today for active immunization against diphtheria.

Diphtheria

The symptoms of diphtheria result from a systemic toxemia. *C. diphtheriae* grows in the nasopharynx, where it causes a typical sore throat. As the bacteria

*E. von Behring and S. Kitasato, "Ueber das Zustandekommen der Diphtherie-Immunitat und der Tetanus-Immunitat bei Thieren." *Deutsche Medizinische Wochenschrift*, 16:1113–1114 (1890).

grow, they form a whitish-gray membrane in the nasopharyngeal region (Color Plate 13). These bacteria produce diphtheria toxin, which is carried by the circulatory system to all parts of the body. The clinical symptoms of diphtheria include a slight fever, fatigue, and malaise. Many patients also experience a dramatic swelling of the neck. Death results from heart and kidney failure caused by the toxin. Diphtheria is an intoxication caused by a protein toxin produced by lysogenized bacteria.

Corynebacterium diphtheriae. The causative agent of diphtheria is a Gram-positive straight or slightly curved rod that is frequently swollen at one or both ends. Granules of polyphosphate are often observed in the cells. In stained smears, *C. diphtheriae* appears as "Chinese letters" that are formed by the sharp angles between dividing cells. *C. diphtheriae* is an aerobe that is selectively cultured on blood tellurite (K_2TeO_3) agar (Figure 17–1).

Virulence, toxin, production, and lysogeny. V. J. F. Freeman demonstrated that all toxin-producing (virulent) strains of *C. diphtheriae* are lysogenic for a β-prophage (see Chapter 9). The phage genome carries the *tox* gene responsible for diphtheria toxin. When virulent strains are cured of their prophage, they are no longer able to produce the toxin. In the reverse process, nonvirulent strains of *C. diphtheriae* become virulent following the establishment of a latent infection by β-phage (Figure 17–2).

Diphtheria toxin is commercially produced by the Park-Williams number 8 strain (PW8) first isolated in 1898. The greatest amount of toxin is produced by PW8 in media containing a low iron concentration (almost depleted, 0.14 μg/ml) that is aerated at a pH between 7.8 and 8.0. Up to 1.0 g of toxin per liter of culture fluid is produced under these conditions. The toxin used in the DTP vaccine is purified and then inactivated by being exposed to diluted formaldehyde at pH 8.0 at 37°C. This toxoid is antigenically identical to diphtheria toxin and is nontoxic to animals.

Diphtheria toxin. Purified diphtheria toxin is a protein composed of a single 62,000 dalton polypep-

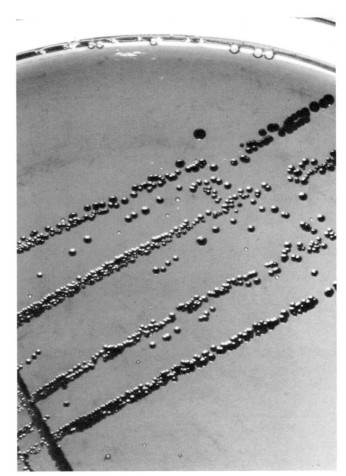

FIGURE 17–1
Corynebacterium diphtheriae growing on tellurite medium. (Courtesy of Dr. I. S. Snyder.)

tide. Diphtheria toxin acts by inhibiting protein synthesis in eucaryotic animal cells. Even at concentrations as low as 10^{-8}M, diphtheria toxin inhibits the uptake of ^{14}C-amino acids during protein synthesis in animal cells.

Diphtheria toxin specifically inactivates the eucaryotic cells' elongation factor (EF2). EF2 is necessary for the translocation of the tRNA polypeptide-ribosomal complex along the messenger RNA. Diphtheria toxin covalently modifies the EF2 by attaching an ADP-ribose complex (derived from NAD_{ox}) to it.

$$NAD_{ox} + EF2 \rightarrow nicotinamide + H^+ + ADP\text{-}ribose\text{-}EF2$$

Active	Inactive

When all the EF2 in a cell is converted to ADP-ribose-EF2, protein synthesis stops, which eventually kills the cell.

All the elongation factors thus far isolated from eucaryotic cells (including humans, plants, protozoa, and yeasts) are inactivated by diphtheria toxin. Diphtheria toxin enters only certain eucaryotic cells, so not all these organisms are affected.

Diphtheria toxin is inactive until it is enzymatically cleaved into two polypeptides (Figure 17–3). This process takes place on the surface of animal cells; the resulting polypeptides have distinct biological activities. The A polypeptide is a 21,150-dalton molecule that enzymatically inactivates EF2. The B polypeptide is a 39,000-dalton molecule that selectively binds to the surface of certain animal cells. In natural situations, the B polypeptide remains bound to the cell's surface, while the A polypeptide enters the cell after it is cleaved from the toxin molecule. Once inside the cell, it catalyzes the inactivation of EF2. One molecule of the A polypeptide is sufficient to inactivate all the EF2 in a cell.

Procaryotic cells also contain elongation factors (EF-G); however, these factors are not inactivated by diphtheria toxin. The enzymatic activity of diphtheria toxin uses NAD_{ox} (reduced forms and $NADP_{ox}$ do not work) and the EF2 found in eucaryotic cells as substrates.

Immunobiology and diphtheria. Successful control of diphtheria has been attained using active and passive immunizations. Passive immunization is used to

FIGURE 17–2

Nonvirulent *Corynebacterium diphtheriae* can be changed to a virulent, toxin-producing, lysogenized strain by β-phage. This bacteriophage can (a) reproduce phage by the lytic cycle or (b) mediate lysogenic conversion of *C. diphtheriae.*

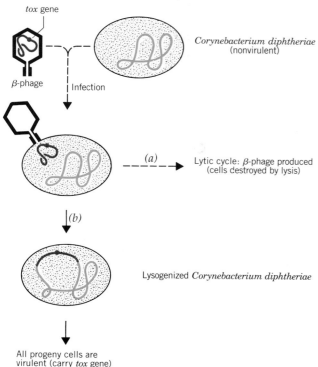

FIGURE 17–3

Diphtheria toxin can be cleaved into two polypeptides by trypsin. The B polypeptide binds to the cell's surface, but it has no toxic activity. The A polypeptide enters the animal cell and inhibits protein synthesis by inactivating the elongation factor (EF2) present in eucaryotic cells.

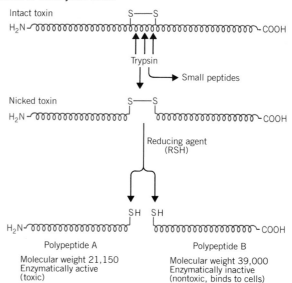

treat exposed nonimmune individuals, and active immunization is used to protect the general human population. A patient's resistance to diphtheria toxin can be determined with the toxin-neutralization test developed by Bela Schick.

Schick test. Since diphtheria is often fatal, the immune state of an exposed individual is an important medical consideration. A patient's immunity to diphtheria toxin can be tested by the injection of a small quantity of active toxin beneath the skin. In nonimmune individuals, the toxin will cause swelling, erythema, and tenderness at the site of injection, with a maximum response observed in 5 days. In immune persons, the toxin will be neutralized by circulating antibodies and no visible reaction occurs (Table 17–3). Because some patients are hypersensitive to components of the toxin preparation, an equal amount of heat-inactivated toxin is injected into the patient's other arm to check for hypersensitivity. Hypersensitive people develop a response within 36 hours. These responses quickly fade (short). Hypersensitive individuals who are also immune show reactions in both arms, but these reactions are of short duration. Nonimmune hypersensitive individuals show a reaction in both arms, but the reaction caused by the active toxin develops 120 hours after injection and persists (long). Through these reactions a physician can determine if an exposed patient is susceptible to diphtheria.

Passive immunization. Nonimmunized patients exposed to diphtheria should be passively immunized and treated with antibiotics. Antibiotic therapy alone is insufficient to cure the patient even though *C. diphtheriae* is susceptible to penicillins, tetracyclines, and erythromycin. Treatment with antibiotics hastens the elimination of the causative agent, but the diphtheria toxin is produced too rapidly for antibiotic treatment to prevent the patient's death.

Passive immunization with equine (horse) diphtheria antitoxin is the primary method of preventing the death of an infected patient. The antitoxin is injected intravenously as a single dose. This procedure will prevent the symptoms if neutralization of the diphtheria toxin occurs before the toxin enters the patient's tissues. A patient's sensitivity to horse serum should be determined prior to administering the antitoxin. Sensitive people can have a severe anaphylactic reaction following the injection of equine-diphtheria antitoxin.

Active immunization. Active immunization with the formalin-inactivated diphtheria toxoid is the primary means of controlling diphtheria in humans. Children are routinely immunized with diphtheria toxoid contained in the DTP shots. Countries that require active immunizations experience a low incidence of diphtheria. The United States has an extensive immunization program that contributes to the low incidence of diphtheria (from 1977 through 1980 there was a total of 222 cases).

Epidemiology of diphtheria. Diphtheria epidemics caused many deaths in colonial America and still oc-

TABLE 17–3
Response to Diphtheria Toxin[a]

	Hypersensitive		Normal	
	Immune	Nonimmune	Immune	Nonimmune
Diphtheria toxin (first arm)	+ (short)	+ (long)	−	+ (long)
Diphtheria toxoid (second arm)	+ (short)	+ (short)	−	−

[a]Each patient receives an injection of toxin in one arm and of toxoid in the other arm. If a reaction develops within 36 hours and then fades, it is labeled "+ (short)." Reactions that develop 120 hours after injection and persist are labeled "+ (long)."

cur in nonimmunized susceptible human populations. *C. diphtheriae* is spread by cough-produced droplets carried in the air. Both asymptomatic carriers and diseased patients can spread the infectious agent. Antibiotic therapy helps to eliminate the organisms from both groups of carriers, but the main control method is immunization of the population against the toxin.

MYCOBACTERIA

Tuberculosis and leprosy are two serious human diseases caused by mycobacteria. Even though leprosy was the first human disease reported to be caused by a bacterium (G. A. Hansen, 1880), this organism has not been grown outside of animals. In contrast, tuberculosis was one of the first human diseases to be proven, by Koch's postulates, to be caused by a bacterium. Koch isolated tubercle bacilli from diseased guinea pigs, grew them on serum agar, and then showed that they caused tuberculosis in healthy guinea pigs. Koch's work with anthrax and tuberculosis laid the foundation of medical bacteriology.

Tuberculosis

Tuberculosis was a devastating endemic disease that once killed one out of every seven humans. It is a progressive degenerative disease of the human lungs. Human resistance to tuberculosis develops through a cell-mediated immunity that further contributes to the unique nature of human tuberculosis.

Tuberculosis in humans. The major cause of human tuberculosis is *Mycobacterium tuberculosis*. Tuberculosis is acquired by person-to-person transmission of the causative agent present in droplet nuclei. The aveoli of the lungs are the foci of the initial infection. The host responds with a nonspecific inflammatory reaction at the infection site during which many of the tubercle bacilli are engulfed by phagocytic leukocytes. Some of the bacteria are killed by phagocytosis, whereas others multiply within the leukocytes. The infection spreads via these cells to the regional lymph nodes and from

there to other parts of the body. More foci of infection can be established at additional sites in the lungs.

After a period of 2 to 4 weeks, the patient develops a hypersensitivity to the *M. tuberculosis*. The host's immune response is necessary for the formation of tubercles (L., *tuberculum*, small lump) in the lungs. Macrophages that phagocytize the tubercle bacilli are attracted to the infection sites. After phagocytosis, the bacteria multiply within the macrophages. These infected macrophages undergo a dramatic change to form the cellular groundwork of the tubercle. Some of these cells fuse to form giant cells that are located in the center of the tubercle, and leukocytes converge on the periphery of the tubercle. Over a period of time, the animal cells in the center of the nodule die, and a cheesy residue forms in the nodule core. The lesion gradually heals accompanied by fibrosis and often by calcification, two processes that wall off the nodule from the rest of the lung. These tubercles are readily detected in chest radiographs. Healing is permanent in most patients; however, in a number of individuals the infection remains dormant for years or decades before it is reactivated.

M. tuberculosis infections can lead to the formation of semisolid, necrotic lesions in the lungs that can give rise to disseminated tuberculosis. In this form of the disease, the tubercle bacilli are spread through the lymph or via deteriorated pulmonary blood vessels. This condition can lead to the establishment of small tubercles throughout the body, which is characteristic of **miliary tuberculosis.**

Cell-mediated immunity in tuberculosis. Many of the host's responses to tuberculosis depend on cell-mediated immune reactions. Antigens of the tubercle bacilli react with activated T lymphocytes (Figure 17–4), causing them to multiply into a clone of cells and to secrete lymphokines. **Lymphokines** are a large group of glycoproteins (see Chapter 12) that function to (1) attract macrophages to the area, (2) activate macrophages, and (3) immobilize the activated macrophages at the infection site. Activated macrophages have numerous lysosomes and phagocytic vacuoles (Figure 17–5) that participate in en-

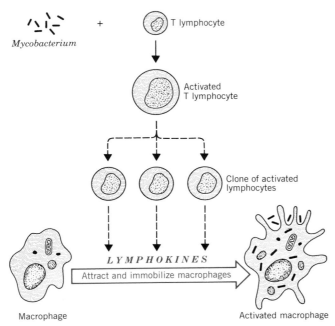

FIGURE 17–4
Cell-mediated immune response to *Mycobacterium tuberculosis.*
The tubercle bacilli that are engulfed by the activated
macrophages are not necessarily destroyed.

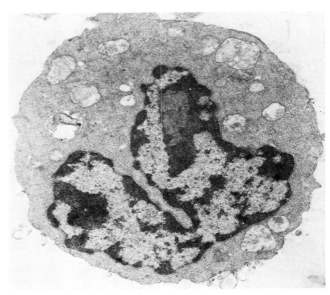

FIGURE 17–5
Electron micrograph of an activated T lymphocyte. (Courtesy of
Dr. T. E. Mandel. From T. E. Mandel, "The Ultrastructure of
Mammalian Lymphocytes and Their Progeny," pp 11–42, in J. J.
Marchalonis, ed., *The Lymphocyte: Structure and Function,*
copyright © 1977, Marcel Dekker.)

gulfing and destroying tubercle bacilli. However, not
all tubercle bacilli are destroyed. Some are able to
survive and to multiply within the macrophages, especially when they are phagocytized before the primary immune response. The cell-mediated immune
response plays a significant role in the host's defense against tuberculosis.

Mycobacterium tuberculosis. Active cases of tuberculosis can be diagnosed by demonstrating the presence of acid-fast, rod-shaped bacteria (Figure 17–6)
in a patient's sputum. The acid-fast stain is performed by steaming a specimen on a slide in the
presence of carbolfuchsin. Only acid-fast cells retain
this stain when the slide is washed with acidified
alcohol (Figure 17–6). Identification depends on the
acid-fast stain since mycobacteria stain poorly with
the Gram stain (they appear to stain as Gram-positive bacteria). Confirmation of the diagnosis and

measurements of drug sensitivity are determined by
growing the organism on laboratory media.

M. tuberculosis is a rod-shaped bacterium that
grows aerobically on ordinary laboratory medium
with a long generation time (14 to 15 hours). The
growing cells adhere to each other forming flowing
waves of aggregated cells (Figure 17–7). This growth
characteristic is often referred to as "serpentine
cords" and is directly related to the presence of the
lipid "cord factor" found in their cell wall.

Mycobacterial lipids and virulence. Between 20
and 40 percent of the mycobacterial cell's dry weight
is lipid. The lipids (1) contribute to the virulence of
the strain, (2) are necessary for the acid-fast reaction,
(3) contribute to the cell's resistance to acidic or alkali treatment, and (4) deter the bactericidal actions
of antibody and complement.

Mycobacterial cell walls are lipid rich (lipids make

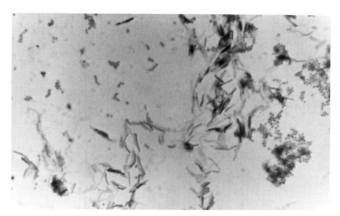

FIGURE 17–6
Acid-fast stain of *Mycobacterium smegmatis*. 1200X (Courtesy of Dr. L. LeBeau.)

up 60% of the cell wall dry weight) and contain unique complex lipids including glycolipids, peptidoglycolipids, and mycolic acids. **Mycolic acids** contain two long-chain, hydrophobic, aliphatic groups as shown in Table 17–1. The cord factor (Figure 17–8) is a complex mycolic acid that is directly related to the virulence and serpentine growth of *M. tuberculosis*. It is present in all virulent strains, it is lethal to mice, and it inhibits the migration of polymorphonuclear leukocytes. *M. tuberculosis* lso produces **wax D**, which plays a role in inducing delayed cell-mediated immune reactions. Wax D is not truly a wax; chemically it is composed of a mycolic acid and a glycopeptide. Even though these lipids play a role in virulence, the ultimate test of virulence is the ability of isolates to cause a progressive tubercular disease in guinea pigs.

Immunobiology of *Mycobacterium tuberculosis*. The diagnosis and treatment of *M. tuberculosis* depend on cell-mediated immune reactions. These reactions are transferred by the injection of leukocytes from an immune person into a nonimmune person.

Koch phenomenon. *M. tuberculosis* and its products will elicit a delayed cell-mediated hypersensitivity reaction in sensitized animals. This phenomenon, known as the **Koch phenomenon,** was first observed in guinea pigs. When sensitized animals are injected with killed tubercle bacilli (or their products), they develop a hardened red lesion at the site of injection. This reaction *cannot* be transferred to a nonsensitized animal in serum. Nonsensitized animals can, however, be artificially sensitized by an injection of washed viable lymphoid cells obtained from a sensitized animal. The Koch phenomenon is a delayed cell-mediated hypersensitivity reaction that takes 2 to 3 days to develop.

FIGURE 17–7
Serpentine cord growth of *Mycobacterium tuberculosis*.

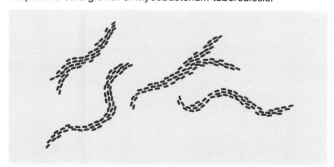

FIGURE 17–8
Cord factor present in virulent *Mycobacterium tuberculosis*.
6,6′ -Dimycolyltrehalose (cord factor)

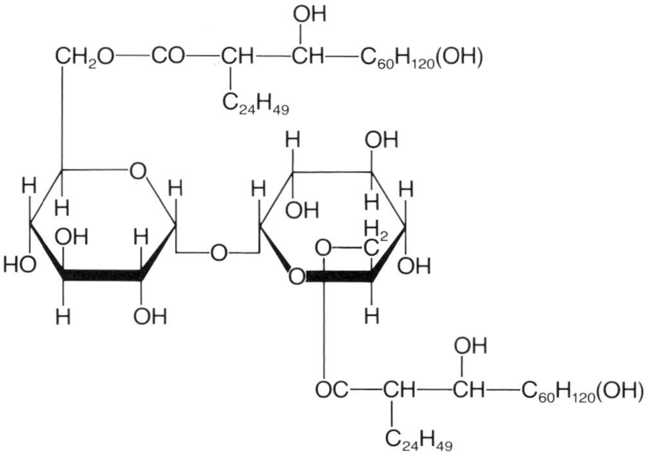

Tuberculin test. The Koch phenomenon is the basis for the tuberculin test that is used to detect hypersensitivity to *M. tuberculosis*. As early as 1 month after infection, a person develops a hypersensitivity to *M. tuberculosis* that can last for a lifetime. Screening for sensitized people is done by intradermally injecting a purified protein from *M. tuberculosis* known as **tuberculin.** Tuberculin-positive patients respond in 48 hours by forming a red, hardened area at the site of injection. A positive tuberculin reaction indicates that the patient either has an active case of tuberculosis or was previously infected.

Vaccines. The **bacille Calmette Guerin** (BCG) strain of *Mycobacterium* is an attenuated strain that is now used to immunize humans. Immunizations with the BCG strain have been used in Scandinavia and to a lesser extent elsewhere in Europe. BCG immunizations are effective in preventing childhood tuberculosis; however, their effectiveness in preventing adult tuberculosis is still in question. Most immunized individuals become tuberculin positive for about 4 years commencing 2 months after they are inoculated. Reversion to tuberculin negative is construed to require reimmunization.

Americans are not routinely immunized against tuberculosis. The United States controls tuberculosis by treating the active cases detected through routine tuberculin-screening procedures. The tuberculin-screening procedures are incompatible with a program of BCG immunization because immunized persons generally become tuberculin positive.

Human resistance. Cases of tuberculosis are unequally distributed between the sexes, different ages, and the human races (Figure 17–9). There is a higher incidence of tuberculosis among males of all races than among females. White males and females account for fewer cases than do the males and females of other races. American Indians, Eskimos, and blacks are particularly susceptible to this disease. The differential susceptibility to tuberculosis appears to be due in part to socioeconomic conditions and in part to genetic differences between races.

Age is another determining factor in susceptibility to tuberculosis. There is a higher incidence of tuber-

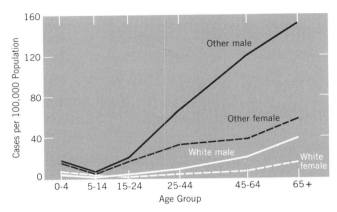

FIGURE 17–9
Incidence of tuberculosis in the U.S. population according to age, sex, and race. (Centers for Disease Control, "Annual Summary 1978: Reported Morbidity and Mortality in the United States," *Morbidity Mortality Weekly Report,* 27, No. 54, 1979.)

culosis in children less than 4 years old than among those between 5 and 14 years old. The highest incidence is among the 65-plus age group in all racial and both sex categories (Figure 17–9). Older people may have a higher incidence of tuberculosis because of the reactivation of dormant tubercles in their lungs. When tuberculosis does occur, it is exacerbated in elderly and malnourished patients and in those suffering from chronic alcoholism.

Epidemiology. Tuberculosis can be spread from active tubercular patients, or it can develop from the reactivation of dormant tubercles. Epidemiologists project that three-fourths of the cases of tuberculosis arise from the activation of dormant infections. Patients with active tubercles can spread *M. tuberculosis* in sputum and water droplets discharged by coughing. The tubercle bacilli can survive in moist or dried sputum for up to 6 weeks. Susceptible persons are infected by inhaling the organisms. Currently there are fewer than 30,000 cases of tuberculosis reported in the United States per year, of which approximately 10% result in death.

Prevention and treatment. Tuberculosis patients are treated with chemotherapeutic agents. Both streptomycin and isoniazid are effective against this disease. These two drugs have had a strong impact on the incidence of tuberculosis in the United States (Table 17–4).

Streptomycin, which was discovered in 1945 and was found to be bactericidal for *M. tuberculosis* has been widely used to treat tuberculosis in humans in spite of its numerous contraindications. It must be injected to avoid inactivation by gastric acid, prolonged treatment results in a loss of hearing as a result of its toxic effects on the eighth cranial nerve, and the development of resistant strains limits its effectiveness. These problems are compounded by the fact that the walled-off nature of the tubercle necessitates prolonged chemotherapy.

Isoniazid (INH) is a synthetic bactericidal drug that can be administered orally. INH is now widely used because of its low toxicity to humans, its effectiveness against *M. tuberculosis,* and its low cost. More recently, rifampin and ethanbutol have been found to be effective drugs for treating tuberculosis. Combinations of INH and ethanbutol or INH and rifampin are used to lessen the chance of selecting a mutant resistant to a single drug. Drug resistance is a serious problem during prolonged drug therapy.

INH is also used in chemoprophylaxis to prevent infection of family members or others living in close proximity to an active tubercular patient. Immuni-

TABLE 17–4
Reported Cases of Tuberculosis in the United States

Year	Total Cases	Cases/ 100,000 Population
1935	111,856	87.9
1940	102,984	78.0
1945	114,931	86.7
1950	121,742	80.5
1955	77,368	47.1
1960	55,494	30.8
1965	49,016	25.3
1970	37,137	18.2
1975	33,989	15.9
1980	27,749	12.3

Source: Centers for Disease Control, "Annual Summary, 1980: Reported Morbidity and Mortality in the United States." *Morbidity Mortality Weekly Report,* 27, no. 54, 1981.

zation with the BCG strain is used to protect high-risk individuals (persons working with tubercular patients) from tuberculosis.

Mycobacterium bovis. Cattle infected with *Mycobacterium bovis* can pass this organism to humans through air or through the consumption of milk. Ingested organisms infect the cervical lymph nodes and in later stages of the disease show a propensity to infect joints and bones. Infection of the vertebrae can lead to body disfigurement as is characterized by the hunchback posture. Inhalation of *M. bovis* can lead to pulmonary tuberculosis.

To eliminate the threat of *M. bovis* infections, the U.S. Department of Agriculture began to test the tuberculosis sensitivity of cattle in 1917. All the tuberculin-positive animals were destroyed. Now cattle are routinely checked for tuberculin sensitivity and less than 0.5 percent of the cattle in the U.S. are tuberculin positive.

LEPROSY

Leprosy, or Hansen's disease, is one of the oldest known human diseases. From biblical times through the colonial days in America, leprosy victims were ostracized to leper colonies. Leprosy is still a worldwide health problem affecting between 12 and 15 million people, primarily in Southeast Asia and Africa. In the United States, most of the estimated 3200 persons with leprosy are specially treated by the U.S. Public Health Service in their leprosy hospital in Carville, Louisiana.

Leprosy in humans

Mycobacterium leprae was shown by G. A. Hansen (1880) to cause leprosy. Early signs of leprosy appear as light, insensitive patches on the skin. *M. leprae* grows only in cool places in the body, which include the extremities (toes and fingers), the face, and the male testicles. These organisms prefer to grow in skin and nervous tissue. The organism grows so slowly that symptoms may not appear for 3 to 5 years and sometimes not until 40 years after infection.

Infection of the hands and feet gradually leads to

a loss of sensation caused by the progressive destruction of the nerve endings. Leprosy victims are unable to sense pain in their extremities. They continuously suffer physical injuries such as burned hands, crushed fingers, and swollen feet. Another form of physical injury is the progressive destruction of bone and nerve tissue of the extremities. Deterioration of these tissues results in the shortening and even the loss of fingers and toes. *M. leprae* also invade the facial tissue, causing severe disfigurement. These bacteria destroy the eyebrows and cause a thickening of the skin on the chin, nose, cheekbones, and forehead, resulting in the facial appearance likened to a lion.

Diagnosis of leprosy. *M. leprae* is an acid-fast rod that has not yet been grown in laboratory media. It has been grown in the foot pads of mice and in armadillos. *M. leprae* has a very slow growth rate and grows only in animals or tissues that have a low body temperature.

Leprosy is diagnosed by the demonstration of acid-fast bacilli in scrapings or exudates from surface lesions. Leprosy patients possess a delayed hypersensitivity to **lepromin,** which is an extract prepared from homogenized leprous tissue containing *M. leprae.* This reaction is similar to the positive-tuberculin test and is used in the diagnosis of leprosy.

Epidemiology and treatment. Humans are the only known natural host of *M. leprae.* Leprosy is spread at a very low rate, presumably by person-to-person contact. Yet in the last 25 years, only one staff member at the Carville Hospital has contracted leprosy. The epidemiology of leprosy is still poorly understood.

Early stages of leprosy can be effectively treated with dapsone (diaminodiphenylsulfone). This drug must be taken weekly for the life of the patient. Drug treatment does not reverse existing damage, but it prevents the progression of the disease. Thalidomide (a drug that causes severe birth defects) is used in nonchildbearing patients to control severe leprosy. Surgery is also used to treat existing deformities.

ACTINOMYCETES

Mycelia are long, continuous, protoplasmic cylinders characteristic of fungal morphology. Myceliated cells reproduce by fragmentation or by the production of aerial hyphae that differentiate into sporelike resting structures. The procaryotes that grow as branched cells or as extended mycelia were once considered to be fungi; however, now they are classified as bacteria.

Branching or myceliated bacteria are classified in the family Actinomycetes. They reproduce by fragmentation or by the production of aerial spores. The mycelium is usually small in circumference (1 μm or less) and is surrounded by a bacterial cell wall that contains diaminopimelic acid and/or muramic acid. Their growth is inhibited by the antibacterial antibiotics (penicillins, tetracyclines, and sulfonamides), not by the polyene antibiotics that inhibit fungal growth. *Nocardia* and *Actinomyces* are genera in this family that cause bacterial diseases in humans.

Nocardia

Nocardiae are similar to the mycobacteria and the corynebacteria in that they possess common cell-wall antigens, have arabinose and galactose in their cell walls, and produce mycolic acids. Nocardiae are Gram-positive, aerobic soil bacteria that grow in a simple medium (Sabauraud's glucose agar). Two closely related species cause disease in humans, *Nocardia asteroides* and *Nocardia brasiliensis*. These species are somewhat acid-fast, produce branched filaments in older cultures (Figure 17–10), and produce thin aerial mycelia. Fragmentation of the mycelia occurs after 4 to 5 days of growth and is the major form of reproduction.

Nocardiosis in humans. Pulmonary nocardiosis is the most common disease caused by nocardia. It primarily affects compromised patients and occurs at a low incidence. The major causative agent, *N. asteroides,* is inhaled into the lungs from its normal habitat in contaminated soil. These bacteria grow as a mass of intertwining mycelia in lesions that gradually become surrounded by fibrous tissue. *N. aster-*

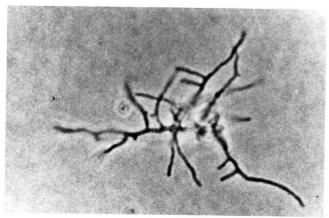

FIGURE 17–10
Photomicrograph of *Nocardia asteroides*. (Courtesy of Drs. R. J. Hawley and T. Imaeda.)

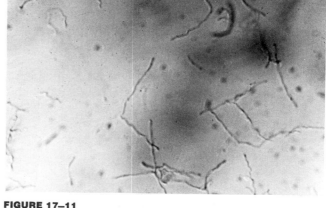

FIGURE 17–11
Photomicrograph of *Actinomyces israelii*. (Courtesy of Dr. L. LeBeau.)

oides can be transported in the blood from the pulmonary lesions to other parts of the body. They can form abscesses in subcutaneous tissue and in the central nervous system. Death usually results when abscesses are established in the brain or in the meninges.

Nocardiae cause **mycetomas** (chronic subcutaneous abscesses) when they infect skin wounds. Mycetomas are more common in tropical climates, where people are less likely to protect their feet with shoes. The abscesses originate when cuts and abrasions on the hands and feet become infected by *Nocardia* sp. The abscesses spread locally and destroy soft tissue and bones. In cattle, these infections result in the disease known as lumpy jaw.

Treatment. Nocardiosis is treated with antibiotics and/or sulfonamides. For chemotherapy to be successful, the disease must not be confused with similar clinical diseases caused by fungi, so identification of the etiological agent is essential. The surgical drainage of accessible abscesses is also employed as part of the treatment. Even with these procedures, the time delay between infection and diagnosis and the progressive invasive nature of these bacteria result in a 50% mortality for all forms of nocardiosis.

Actinomyces

Members of this genus are fermentative, Gram-positive, nonmotile, non-spore-forming bacteria that can form branching filaments (Figure 17–11). They never form extensive mycelia, and they are not acid-fast. *Actinomyces israelii* and *Actinomyces bovis* are found only in warm-blooded animals, where they are opportunistic pathogens. They require temperatures of 37°C for growth and are naturally found in the oral cavities of humans and warm-blooded animals.

Actinomycosis in humans. *A. israelii* is the primary human pathogen involved in actinomycosis. This bacterium causes chronic destructive abscesses in connective tissue. The disease can involve the abdomen, neck, face, lungs, and/or the chest wall. The organisms are invasive and form burrowing lesions that usually erupt at the skin surface. The lesions can be walled off through the deposition of connective tissue. Actinomycosis is not transmissible from person to person. Presumably, infections originate when a patient becomes compromised or experiences trauma. Since *A. israelii* can be cultured from almost all human tonsils and the majority of human gum scrapings, it is considered an opportunistic pathogen.

TABLE 17–5
Summary of Diphtheria, Tuberculosis, Leprosy, Nocardiosis, Actinomycosis

Disease	Etiological Agent	Symptoms	Epidemiology and (Treatment)
Diphtheria	*Corynebacterium diphtheriae*	Sore throat, membrane on tonsils, heart and kidney failure	Spread by cough (Immunize with diphtheria toxoid; treatment with antitoxin, antibiotics)
Tuberculosis	*Mycobacterium tuberculosis, M. bovis* (secondary)	Tubercles in lungs, malaise, excessive fatigue	Inhalation, reactivation of tubercles (Antibiotics, INH sulfonamides, BCG vaccine)
Miliary tuberculosis	*Mycobacterium tuberculosis, M. bovis* (secondary)	Tubercles throughout the body	Dissemination from lung tubercles (Antibiotics, sulfonamides)
Leprosy	*Mycobacterium leprae*	Deterioration of extremities, facial disfigurement	Unknown (Dapsone)
Nocardiosis	*Nocardia asteroides, Nocardia brasiliensis* (secondary)	Pulmonary lesions, abscesses in subcutaneous tissue	Inhalation of organism from soil (Antibiotics, surgical drainage, and sulfonamides)
Actinomycosis	*Actinomyces israelii, Actinomyces bovis*	Chronic destructive abscesses	Opportunistic pathogen (Antibiotics, surgical drainage)

Epidemiology and treatment. The occurrence of actinomycosis in humans is rare. The organism is sensitive to penicillin, tetracyclines, chloramphenicol, and streptomycin. Normal therapy combines penicillin treatment with surgical drainage of the abscesses. The cure rate for operable lesions is about 90 percent.

SUMMARY

Diphtheria is an intoxication caused by lysogenized strains of *Corynebacterium diphtheriae* (Table 17–5). This organism infects the human throat, where it produces a protein toxin that is circulated throughout the body. Diphtheria toxin inhibits protein synthesis by inactivating the elongation factor of eucaryotic cells. Untreated patients die from the necrotic effects of diphtheria toxin on the heart and kidneys. Exposed susceptible patients should be passively immunized with antitoxin and treated with antibiotics. Active immunization of people with diphtheria toxoid is the major means of controlling diphtheria.

Tuberculosis is caused by the acid-fast bacterium, *Mycobacterium tuberculosis*. Pulmonary tuberculosis develops in the human lung following the inhalation of *M. tuberculosis* or by the reactivation of dormant tubercles. The bacteria grow intracellularly and cause the formation of tubercles. Tubercle bacilli can be disseminated from the infected lung to other parts of the body, where they establish small tubercles characteristic of miliary tuberculosis. Humans respond to tuberculosis by developing a cell-mediated immunity. The tuberculin reaction is a measure of the delayed cell-mediated hypersensitive state found in persons who have a history of tuberculosis. Cell-mediated immunity is involved in localizing the infection and in removing and destroying tubercle bacilli. Tubercular patients can be cured by long-term treatment with a combination of antibiotics and chemotherapeutic drugs.

Leprosy is caused by *Mycobacterium leprae*, a bacterium that has never been cultured outside of an animal. *M. leprae* grows in the extremities and prefers to grow in nerves and skin. Growth of the bacterium causes a loss of sensation in the extremities, which in turn leads to the loss of fingers and toes. Invasion of facial tissue can cause severe disfigurement. Leprosy has a long incubation period (months to years) and is not very contagious. Early stages of leprosy can be treated with dapsone.

Nocardiosis occurs in compromised patients who inhale *Nocardia asteroides,* which is a normal bacterial inhabitant of soil. It forms abscesses in tissue throughout the body. These bacteria are disseminated from the primary pulmonary lesion to form abscesses in subcutaneous tissue and in the central nervous system. Nocardiosis can be treated with antibiotics and sulfonamides.

Actinomyces israelii is an opportunistic pathogen that is present as a normal inhabitant of the human mouth. Actinomycosis is characterized by the formation of chronic abscesses in connective tissue and occurs primarily in traumatized and/or compromised hosts. Actinomycosis is treated with antibiotics and surgical drainage of the abscesses.

QUESTIONS AND TOPICS FOR STUDY AND DISCUSSION

Questions

1. How is the β-bacteriophage involved in human diphtheria?
2. Describe the structure and the action of the diphtheria toxin? How does this toxin enter animal cells?
3. What are the clinical signs of diphtheria? How would you test for immunity against the diphtheria toxin?
4. How is diphtheria spread within a human population? What are the steps for preventing or, if necessary, treating human diphtheria?
5. What characteristics of a human *Mycobacterium tuberculosis* infection lead to a prolonged, insidious disease?
6. Describe the involvement of cell-mediated immunity in human resistance to tuberculosis and in the tuberculin reaction.
7. Describe the acid-fast stain and explain its use in microbiology.
8. What is the Koch phenomenon? Why is the Koch phenomenon not transferred with serum?
9. Describe and explain the key factors associated with

the incidence of tuberculosis in the human population?
10. What is the prescribed treatment for human tuberculosis? Explain the necessity for prolonged therapy.
11. In what ways is leprosy different from other bacterial diseases?
12. Why do leprosy patients often lose fingers and/or toes?
13. What is the treatment for leprosy?
14. What are the characteristics of the Actinomycetes that make them similar to fungi? Briefly describe the human diseases the Actinomycetes cause.

Discussion

1. Diphtheria is a disease of humans caused by a bacterial toxin that is coded for by a gene carried by a temperate bacteriophage. Can you think of why or how this complex situation evolved? Is there any selective pressure for this system?
2. What public health procedures should be taken to prevent the spread of tuberculosis? Should these procedures also be applied to leprosy? Why or why not?

FURTHER READINGS

Articles and Reviews

Barksdale, L., "*Corynebacterium diphtheriae* and Its Relatives," *Bacteriol. Revs.,* 34:378–422 (1970). An extensive, well-illustrated review of the bacteriology of *C. diphtheriae* that includes a section on the corynebacteriophages.

Barksdale, L., and K-S. Kim, "*Mycobacterium,*" *Bacteriol. Revs.,* 41:217–372 (1977). An extensive review of the Mycobacteria and the mycobacteriophages.

Beamann, B. L., J. Burnside, B. Edwards, and W. Caussey, "Nocardial Infections in the United States, 1972–1974," *J. Infect. Dis.,* 134:286–289 (1976). The distribution of species of *Nocardia* is correlated with the incidence of the diseases they caused.

Collier, J. B., "Diphtheria Toxin: Mode of Action and Structure," *Bacteriol. Revs.,* 39:54–85 (1975). A biochemical review of the action of diphtheria toxin on animal cells.

Pappenheimer, A. M., Jr., and D. M. Gill, "Diphtheria," *Science,* 182:353–358 (1973). A general review of diphtheria that emphasizes the production and action of the diphtheria toxin.

18

PATHOGENIC COCCI

The major pathogenic cocci belong to one of the three genera: *Streptococcus, Staphylococcus,* or *Neisseria.* The streptococci and the staphylococci are Gram-positive bacteria that grow in chains (streptococci) or in clusters (staphylococci). In contrast, the neisseria are Gram-negative bacteria that grow as pairs of bean-shaped cells. Most species of *Streptococcus* and *Staphylococcus* are widely dispersed in natural environments, whereas species of *Neisseria* are found associated exclusively with humans or other warm-blooded animals. Certain species of all three genera are normal symbionts of the human mouth, nasopharynx, intestine, and vagina.

Humans are natural carriers of pyogenic cocci. Members of all three genera cause suppurative (pus-forming) infections. The streptococci and the staphylococci cause diseases that range in severity from boils to generalized bacteremia and rheumatic fever. Neisseria are responsible for gonorrhea and meningococcal meningitis. The symptoms, the mode of infection, the organs affected, and the severity of the illnesses caused by these organisms vary greatly. Fortunately, these bacteria are easily grown in laboratory media, and they are susceptible to antibiotic chemotherapy.

THE STREPTOCOCCI

Streptococci are catalase-negative, Gram-positive, spherical, nonmotile cells that grow in pairs or chains (Figure 18–1). They ferment glucose through the glycolytic pathway to produce lactic acid as the major end product. Even though their metabolism is

FIGURE 18–1

Gram stain of *Streptococcus* in sputum. The cells stain blue and are arranged in chains, 1000X. (Courtesy of Dr. L. LeBeau.)

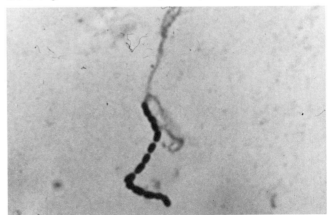

fermentative, they are able to grow slowly under aerobic or microaerophilic conditions. A distinguishing characteristic of the streptococci is their inability to make catalase. Streptococci cannot make the heme moiety of catalase; however, some streptococci can utilize the heme present in blood-containing media to produce a pseudocatalase. Catalase is an easily detectable enzyme, and its presence is used to differentiate between the catalase-negative streptococci and the catalase-positive staphylococci.

Classification of the streptococci

No simple system is available for classifying the streptococci. Instead, species of streptococci are recognized and defined by one or more of the following traits: Lancefield serotypes, hemolysins, growth in 6.5 percent NaCl, sensitivity to bacitracin or optochin, presence of capsules, and/or bile solubility (Table 18–1). Three artificial groups of streptococci can be constructed based on their hemolytic reactions

TABLE 18–1
Classification of Some Streptococci

Organism (Group Name)	Lancefield Group	Distinguishing Characteristics
I. The β-Hemolytic Streptococci Pyogenes		
S. pyogenes	A	β hemolysis, sensitive to bacitracin, does not grow in 6.5% NaCl or at 10° or 45°C
S. agalactiae	B	β hemolysis[a] (weak), bacitracin ±, CAMP +
Enterococci		
S. faecalis	D	β hemolysis, α hemolysis, or nonhemolytic, grows in 6.5% NaCl and at 10° and 45°C, survives heating at 60°C for 30 minutes
S. faecium	D	
II. The α-Hemolytic Streptococci Pneumococci		
S. pneumoniae		Sensitive to optochin, bile-soluble, positive Quellung reaction, oxygen-sensitive β hemolysis
Viridans		
S. mutans (nonhemolytic)		Optochin-resistant, grows at 45°C but not at 10°C or in 6.5% NaCl
S. mitior		
III. Nonhemolytic (γ-hemolytic) Streptococci Lactis		
S. lactis	N	Grows at 10°C but not at 45°C or in 6.5% NaCl

[a]Not present in all strains.

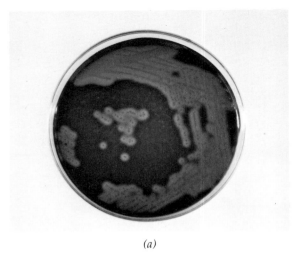

(a)

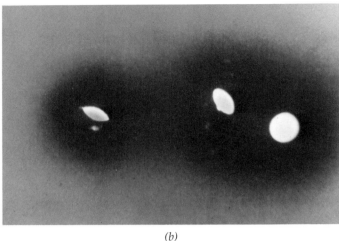

(b)

FIGURE 18–2

(a) β-hemolytic *Streptococcus pyogenes* growing on a blood agar plate. The clear zone of lysis is caused by β hemolysin produced by the bacteria. (Courtesy of J. R. Mcdonald, Oxoid Limited, Basingstoke, England.) *(b)* Colonies of an α-hemolytic *Streptococcus* growing on a blood agar plate. (Courtesy of Dr. L. LeBeau.)

(Color Plate 7). **β hemolysis** is recognized as a clear area surrounding a colony growing on a blood agar plate (Figure 18–2). β-hemolytic cells produce β hemolysin(s), which lyse red blood cells. β hemolysis can be caused by an oxygen-sensitive toxin (only seen when grown anaerobically) and/or by an oxygen-stabile toxin. **α hemolysis** is a partial lysis of red blood cells that results in a green area surrounding the producing colony (Figure 18–2). The green color is due to an unidentified reduced product of hemoglobin. **Nonhemolytic*** streptococci do not lyse red blood cells.

Serological identification of antigens, primarily of the β-hemolytic streptococci, has been used to classify these bacteria (Table 18–1) into the Lancefield groups (A to H and K to U). Groups A, B, and D contain human pathogens. All the group A β-hemolytic streptococci are classified as *S. pyogenes*. This species is the most important human pathogen of this genus. *S. pyogenes* is β-hemolytic and is sensitive to low concentrations of bacitracin. In group B,

S. agalactiae causes serious infections of newborns. It can be identified by the **CAMP test,** which measures the increased lysis of red blood cells in the presence of staphylococcal alpha toxin. The group D enterococci are common inhabitants of the human intestine. They are identified by their growth characteristics and by their ability to survive heating at 60°C for 30 minutes.

Streptococcus pneumoniae is the major human pathogen of the α-hemolytic streptococci. This organism produces a strong α hemolysis on aerobic blood agar plates. *S. pneumoniae* also causes β hemolysis when it produces pneumolysin, a toxin that is only active under anaerobic conditions. Virulent strains are encapsulated and can be identified and typed by the Quellung reaction (Color Plate 3). Cells of *S. pneumoniae* are sensitive to optochin and are solubilized by bile or bile salts that activate a cellular amidase that in turn lyses the bacteria. Other α-hemolytic streptococci include *S. mutans* and *S. mitior*, which inhabit the teeth and mouths of humans. These organisms are classically classified in the viridans (green) group (Table 18–1) because they are α hemolytic.

**These strains have also been designated as γ *hemolytic;* however, the term nonhemolytic is preferred.

The nonhemolytic (γ) streptococci are identified by their metabolic characteristics. *S. lactis* is representative of the Lactis group: it is found in milk and milk products. It is evident from Table 18–1 that there is no simple approach to the classification of the streptococci; however, this brief outline will be used as a guide to this genus.

Streptococcus pyogenes

Streptococcus pyogenes is an oval- to sphere-shaped organism (0.6 to 1.0 μm) that causes β hemolysis when grown on blood agar and is sensitive to low concentrations of bacitracin. *S. pyogenes* is widely distributed among the human population, where it is an opportunistic pathogen. It causes cutaneous and systemic human infections and is the major cause of acute bacterial pharyngitis.

Toxins and virulence factors. A variety of extracellular toxins and antiphagocytic substances contribute to the virulence of group A streptococci. These bacteria produce capsules of hyaluronic acid (Figure 18–3) that retard phagocytosis by polymorphonuclear leukocytes and macrophages. The capsule is not immunogenic in humans since hyaluronic acid is a component of human connective tissue. **M protein** (there are more than 60 serotypes) is another antiphagocytic virulence factor that is produced by group A streptococci. The M protein is found attached to fimbriaelike structures, which protrude from the cell surface.

Erythrogenic toxins are extracellular proteins that are responsible for the rash observed in scarlet fever patients. Lysogenized strains of *S. pyogenes* can produce one of the three antigenic types (A, B, and C) of erythrogenic toxin. Immunity to one of these toxins does not confer immunity to the other two.

The **Dick test** employs erythrogenic toxin to diagnose a patient's susceptibility to scarlet fever. When the toxin is injected into a susceptible patient, a swollen red area develops at the site of the injection. This reaction indicates that the patient has no antitoxin to erythrogenic toxin. Convalescent scarlet fever patients show a negative Dick test. These patients have circulating antitoxin that neutralizes the injected toxin before a cellular response occurs. In the **Shultz-Charlton test,** antitoxin is injected at the site of the red rash. If the antitoxin is specific for the toxin, it will neutralize it and the rash will blanch. Since there are three different antigenic types of erythrogenic toxin, a mixture of the three antitoxins is used in the Shultz-Charlton test. These tests are good examples of toxin neutralization reactions, but because of the multiple antigenic forms of erythrogenic toxins, they are not widely used as diagnostic tools.

β hemolysis of red blood cells is caused by two toxins called streptolysins. **Streptolysin S** is stable in air and lyses red blood cells on aerobic plates. Antibodies against the cell-bound streptolysin *S* have never been demonstrated. **Streptolysin O** is inactivated by oxygen, so it lyses red blood cells only under anaerobic conditions. Antibodies against strep-

FIGURE 18–3
Capsules of *Streptococcus pneumoniae* as demonstrated by the Quellung reaction. (Courtesy of Dr. G. Goodhart.)

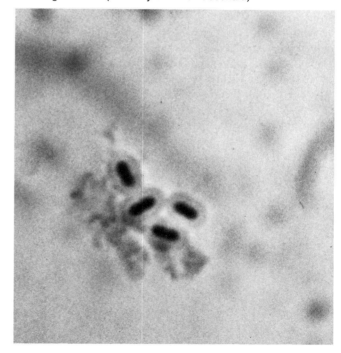

tolysin O are found in the serum of patients who have recovered from streptococcal infections. Both streptolysins S and O have the ability to lyse cells, and both take part in the destruction of phagocytic leukocytes.

Streptococci also produce a number of enzymes that contribute to their virulence. Streptokinase dissolves fibrin clots by breaking down plasminogen to plasmin. NADase breaks down NAD, and hyaluronidase breaks down hyaluronic acid in connective tissue. Since hyaluronidase can also attack the capsular material of streptococci, its role in pathogenicity is unclear. *S. pyogenes* also produce DNAase, which decreases the viscosity in tissue spaces and promotes bacterial invasiveness.

Human diseases caused by *Streptococcus pyogenes*. **Streptococcal pharyngitis,** also called strep throat, is the most common group A streptococcal infection. Streptococcal pharyngitis is caused by *Streptococcus pyogenes* that colonize the mucous membranes of both the pharyngeal region and the tonsils. The symptoms of this illness are fever, purulence (pus accumulation), and swelling and inflammation of the throat. The disease rarely leads to pneumonia or meningitis, but it can infect the middle ear (ostitis media) or the sinuses (sinusitis). Streptococcal pharyngitis is diagnosed by isolating from a patient's throat a β-hemolytic *Streptococcus* that is sensitive to low concentrations of bacitracin. Group A streptococci are sensitive to low concentrations (0.02 units) of bacitracin, whereas most other β-hemolytic streptococci are resistant to low concentrations of bacitracin. Streptococcal pharyngitis is one of the most common bacterial diseases of children between the ages of 5 and 15. This disease is treated with penicillin or erythromycin (in hypersensitive patients). Penicillin-resistant strains have not been demonstrated.

Scarlet fever is caused by lysogenic strains of group A *Streptococcus* that produce erythrogenic toxin. Established streptococcal infections in the throat, and occasionally wounds, release erythrogenic toxin into the circulation. The toxin causes a red rash that first appears on the chest and then spreads to the rest of the trunk and the extremities. Scarlet fever is now diagnosed by its clinical symptoms—the Schultz-Charlton test is rarely used. A patient can have scarlet fever more than once because of the multiple antigenic types of the toxin.

Puerperal sepsis (childbed fever) is a streptococcal infection of the mother's endometrium and surrounding structures that follows delivery or abortion. Ignaz Semmelweis in Vienna and Oliver Wendell Holmes in Boston simultaneously discovered the cause of this disease in the middle of the nineteenth century. Mothers were being infected with streptococci by the unsanitary practices of the attending medical staff. Many mothers died from the resulting streptococcal septicemia. Now the use of proper obstetrical techniques and antibiotics has essentially eliminated puerperal sepsis as a cause of death.

Group A streptococci can cause the human skin infections known as impetigo and erysipilas. **Streptococcal impetigo** (pyoderma) is a localized purulent dermatitis caused by group A streptococci. This disease commonly affects the face and hands and is very contagious. *S. pyogenes* causes 5 to 10 percent of the cases of impetigo, whereas between 30 and 80 percent of these skin infection cases are caused by *Staphylococcus aureus*. **Erysipilas** is an acute febrile disease of the skin caused by group A streptococci. Both impetigo and erysipilas can be treated with antibiotic ointments (aureomycin and bacitracin) or with ammoniated mercury ointments. Proper hygienic practices normally prevent the spread of these skin infections to susceptible patients.

Late sequelae of group A streptococcal infections are serious aftereffects of streptococcal pharyngitis. **Acute rheumatic fever** and **acute glomerulonephritis** are nonsuppurative sequelae to streptococcal infections. The symptoms of rheumatic fever occur 1 to 5 weeks (average of 19 days) following an acute, untreated streptococcal throat infection. Rheumatic fever is characterized by pains in the joints and long-term effects on the heart. The mechanism(s) by which streptococci cause acute rheumatic fever are unexplained. Possible mechanisms include the invasion of tissue by *S. pyogenes*, the effects of toxins, injury due to antibody-antigen complexes, and autoimmunity. This last theory suggests that group A streptococci and heart tissue share a common antigen. Antibodies against this antigen could react with human tissue to cause the symptoms of rheumatic fever. Rheumatic fever is prevented when streptococcal pharyngitis patients are treated with antibiotics. Glomerulonephritis is an inflammation of the kidneys that is sometimes observed following acute, untreated streptococcal pharyngitis or streptococcal skin infections. The mechanism by which streptococci cause glomerulonephritis is not known.

Streptococcus agalactiae

Streptococcus agalactiae is the major human pathogen belonging to the group B streptococci. It is becoming recognized as an important cause of meningitis, pneumonia, and bacteremia in newborns. The human female genital tract is the major reservoir for *S. agalactiae*, where it is present in as many as 25 to 35 percent of the female population. Newborns are presumably infected during birth or during their stay in the hospital nursery. Many infants are infected during the first 3 days of life, and some infections lead to pneumonia, meningitis, and bacteremia. These infections are responsive to treatment with the penicillin antibiotics.

Enterococci

Streptococcus faecalis and *S. faecium* are members of the Lancefield group D streptococci (Table 18–1). They are opportunistic pathogens that are normal inhabitants of the human intestine. Group D streptococci are a major cause of nosocomial infections (see Table 14–6). *S. faecalis* can infect the urinary tract, which in turn can lead to bacteremia. Other enterococci can cause bacterial endocarditis. Combinations of antibiotics (penicillin and aminoglycosides) are used to treat these infections because some enterococci are insensitive to penicillin.

Streptococcal pneumonia

Most human cases of bacterial pneumonia are caused by *Streptococcus pneumoniae* (Color Plate 2). This organism, which grows as an encapsulated diplococcus (Figure 18–3), was once called *Diplococcus pneumoniae*. Now it is classified in the genus *Streptococcus* since it is a Gram-positive coccus that produces lactic acid as a major product of glucose fermentation. *S. pneumoniae* is identified as an encapsulated, bile-soluble, optochin-sensitive α-hemolytic diplococcus. Encapsulated strains grow as smooth mucoid colonies on blood agar plates, whereas nonencapsulated strains form rough colonies (see Griffith's experiments, Chapter 6). The presence of the capsule and its specific type can be detected by the Quellung reaction using the appropriate antiserum.

Streptococcus pneumoniae is a normal inhabitant of the upper respiratory tract of 5 to 70 percent of human populations. It causes pneumonia in compromised hosts, especially elderly people, people who are ill or infirm, and people who are weakened by viral infections. *S. pneumoniae* establishes an infection in the lungs that results in edema and difficulty in breathing. Approximately 70 percent of the untreated patients spontaneously recover from pneumococcal pneumonia after 5 to 6 days. Recovery is accompanied by an increase in the anticapsular antibody in the serum and by a decrease in the severity of the symptoms. Other patients recover following treatment with either penicillin or erythromycin. A few pneumococcal-pneumonia patients—especially those over 70 years old—die even though they are being treated with antibiotics. Other bacteria that cause pneumonia include *Staphylococcus aureus*, *Klebsiella pneumoniae*, and *Mycoplasma pneumoniae*.

Viridans group streptococci

Streptococcus mutans, *S. mitior*, and *S. sanguis* are α-hemolytic streptococci belonging to the viridans group (Table 18–1). They are normal inhabitants of the human mouth and tooth surfaces, and both *S. mutans* and *S. mitior* are found in dental plaque. *S. mutans* produces dextran from sucrose, which is a major component of dental plaque. When these bacteria grow on the teeth, they produce acidic metabolic products (such as lactic acid), which contribute to the creation of dental caries. *S. mitior* and *S. san-*

guis are the most common bacteria of the viridans group to be involved in streptococcal endocarditis.

Epidemiology

Streptococci are transferred from person to person by direct contact or by coughing. Streptococci do not survive well on fomites. Outbreaks of streptococcal disease occur among children who have not built up a resistance to these bacteria. Outbreaks usually occur during the colder months and are more prevalent in dry areas of the country. The carrier rate for group A streptococci usually runs below 10 percent of the population, but it often increases just before an outbreak. Prevention of streptococcal infections depends on early detection of the causative agent followed by antibiotic chemotherapy.

THE STAPHYLOCOCCI

Staphylococci are Gram-positive, facultative-anaerobic bacteria that grow in clusters as shown in Figure 18–4. *Staphylococcus saprophyticus* is widely distributed in nature. It is considered to be nonpathogenic; however, in rare cases it causes urinary tract infections. *Staph. aureus* and *Staph. epidermidis* are common inhabitants of the human skin, respiratory tract, mucous membranes, and intestine. *Staph. aureus* is the major pathogen of this genus: it causes disease of the skin, food poisoning, and systemic diseases. *Staph. epidermidis* is an opportunistic pathogen that is a universal symbiont of human skin. The staphylococci are catalase-positive, so they can be differentiated from the catalase-negative streptococci. Staphylococci are very resistant to drying, they are viable after heating at 60°C for half an hour, and they grow in the presence of 6.5 percent NaCl.

Extracellular products

All *Staph. aureus* are coagulase positive. Coagulase production is used to differentiate *Staph. aureus* from *Staph. epidermidis*, which is coagulase negative. *Staph. aureus* also produces four hemolysins, leukocidin, and four distinct enterotoxins (Table 18–2).

Coagulase is an extracellular enzyme that causes citrated plasma to form a clot. Even though most pathogenic staphylococci produce this enzyme, the biochemical role of coagulase in virulence is unclear. Clots formed by coagulase may interfere with phagocytosis, or they may coat the bacteria to make them less susceptible to antibodies and phagocytosis. Coagulase-positive cultures produce other extracellular virulence products including hemolysins, lipase, hyaluronidase, DNAase, and fibrinolysin.

The four streptococcal hemolysins are differentiated by their ability to lyse red blood cells from different animals. α hemolysin lyses rabbit RBC and is a heat-labile protease. β hemolysin is the "hot-cold" hemolysin that lyses sheep RBC at cold temperatures after it is incubated at 37°C. γ hemolysin lyses human red blood cells and is heat-stabile. The δ hemolysin is toxic to leukocytes and many other cells. A single strain of *Staphylococcus* may produce up to three different hemolysins. Leukocidin lyses WBC, not RBC, so it is described as nonhemolytic. Cells that produce leukocidin have some protection against being phagocytized.

Enterotoxins are relatively heat-resistant polypeptides that are produced by about one-half of the coagulase-positive strains. The staphylococcal enterotoxins (six types) cause vomiting and diarrhea and are responsible for staphylococcal food poisoning.

FIGURE 18–4
Gram stain of *Staphylococcus aureus*. The cells stain blue and are arranged in clusters, 1000X. (Courtesy of Dr. L. LeBeau.)

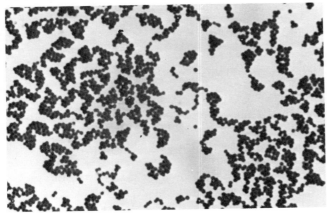

TABLE 18–2
Extracellular Products of Staphylococci

Extracelluar Product	Mode of Action	Properties
Hemolysins		
α hemolysin	Lysis of rabbit RBC	Heat-labile protein
β hemolysin	Lysis of sheep RBC	Inactive at 37°C
γ hemolysin	Lysis of human and rabbit RBC	Heat-stabile toxin
δ hemolysin	Toxic to leukocytes	
Leukocidins	Kill leukocytes	Three different types
Enterotoxin	Acute gastrointestinal upset (food poisoning)	Relatively heat-stabile toxin
Coagulase	Clots plasma	High correlation with virulence
Hyaluronidase	Breaks down hyaluronic acid in connective tissue	Invasive factor

Do not confuse the staphylococcal enterotoxin with the general term used to describe cell-bound toxins (endotoxins).

Staphylococcal diseases

Staphylococcus aureus is responsible for the majority of the staphylococcal infections in humans. This organism is carried in the nasal cavity and on the skin by a significant proportion of the human population. Staphylococci produce localized suppurative diseases involving the epidermis. These diseases include boils, carbuncles, and/or infected wounds. Staphylococci can also cause systemic infections that can lead to septicemia, pneumonia, or osteomyelitis (Color Plate 4).

Staph. aureus establishes an infection after invading the epidermis at a sebaceous gland opening, a hair follicle, or at a site of injury. White blood cells and plasma enter the area by passing through dilated capillaries to form a pimple. A fibrin clot forms around the infection site and prevents the spread of the organisms into the circulatory system. The swelling and redness of the pimple are due to an increase in the permeability of the local capillaries. The pimple becomes suppurative when leukocytes and bacteria accumulate at the site to form pus. A pus-filled blemish near the surface of the epidermis is called a **boil.** This can develop into a **furuncle** when the infection forms a lobed lesion that penetrates into the epidermis. Boils and furuncles are treated by surgical incision and drainage. These infections should be drained outwardly—they should never be ruptured so that the bacteria can gain entrance to the circulatory system. Chemotherapy is seldom effective against the localized staphylococcal infections because they are walled off from the normal circulation. In contrast, staphylococcal impetigo can be treated with topical antibiotics.

Staphylococcal infections of neonates is a major problem for nurseries. *Staph. aureus* is readily transmitted between carriers to newborns by direct contact. The umbilical cord and the eyes are two commonly infected sites. Staph infections in the nursery are especially problematical when antibiotic-resistant strains are encountered and when the infection rate is high. Hexachlorophene (hospital use only) and chlorhexidine are used as antiseptics to control infections of *Staph. aureus*.

More severe staphylococcal infections occur as complications of trauma following operations, accidents, burns, and/or debilitating diseases such as cancer or cirrhosis of the liver. Diseases caused by staphylococci under these conditions include pneumonia, osteomyelitis, deep tissue abscesses, endocarditis, meningitis, and purulent arthritis. These generalized bacterial diseases should be treated with prolonged intensive chemotherapy.

Staphylococcal food poisoning occurs most often in the warmer months when food is left unrefrigerated. The source of the disease is usually a foodhandler who unknowingly carried *Staph. aureus* and contaminates food during its preparation. Up to 30 percent of the adult human population carry *Staph. aureus* as part of the microbial flora of their nose, skin, and/or throat. In order to cause food poisoning, the bacteria must grow in the food and produce the toxin. Custards, stuffing, and creamed foods are favorable environments both for the growth of *Staphylococcus* and for the production of an enterotoxin. Since enterotoxin is relatively heat stabile, warming or even boiling the food does not inactivate it. Staphylococcal food poisoning is characterized by sudden nausea, vomiting, and diarrhea that occur within a few hours of ingesting the toxin. This is a classic example of toxemia. Recovery occurs within 24 to 48 hours.

Toxic shock syndrome. *Staph. aureus* and tampons are epidemiologically linked to the symptoms of toxic shock syndrome (TSS) in menstruating women. This syndrome was first reported in 1975 and was dramatically brought to the public's attention in 1980 when 299 TSS cases and 25 TSS deaths occurred between January and September. Ninety-five percent of these cases occurred in women during their menstrual period, and almost all the women used tampons. Analysis of the major tampon brands on the market (Table 18–3) showed that a new cellulose-based superabsorbent tampon was used in 71 percent of the cases. The increase in TSS paralleled the increased market share of this superabsorbent tampon. This brand was removed from the market in late 1980.

The symptoms of TSS include the sudden onset of high fever, vomiting, diarrhea, and muscle cramps (myalgia). A sunburnlike rash develops about 10 days after the symptoms first appear. Patients with severe cases go into shock. About 8 percent of the

reported cases resulted in death. Penicillin-resistant *Staph. aureus* was isolated from 43 (98 percent) of 44 TSS patients. It was not isolated from any of the unused tampons tested. TSS in men and in nonmenstruating women was also correlated with a penicillin-resistant *Staph. aureus* present in a focal lesion in the skin, bone, or lung. Both the symptoms and the preliminary bacteriological results implicate *Staph. aureus* as the cause of TSS.

The Centers for Disease Control recommend that women not use tampons continuously during a menstrual cycle. Presumably, the superabsorbent tampons traumatize the vaginal mucosa, which facilitates the growth of *Staph. aureus* and the uptake of toxin(s) from the vagina.

Epidemiology. Staphylococci are present among the normal bacterial flora of the human skin, the mucous membranes of the respiratory tract, and the gastrointestinal tract. Approximately 90 percent of infants become carriers of staphylococci within 10 days of birth. Adults carry *Staph. aureus* in their nose and spread these bacteria to their skin and clothing with their hands. The carrier rate is higher among medical personnel than among the general population. Infections are passed from person to person by direct contact. Staphylococcal infections should be

TABLE 18–3

Distribution of Tampon Brands Among Toxic Shock Syndrome Cases and Controls Using Only One Tampon Brand

Tampon Brand	Cases of TSS ($N = 42$)	Controls ($N = 114$)[a]
Brand 1 (superabsorbent)	71%	26%
Brand 2 (regular)	19%	25%
Brand 3 (regular)	5%	25%
Brand 4 (regular)	2%	12%
Brand 5 (regular)	2%	11%

Source: Centers for Disease Control, *Morbidity Mortality Weekly Report*, 29:441–445 (1980).
[a]Each patient was asked to provide the names of three female acquaintances within 3 years of their own age who lived within the same geographical region and who were not related to the patient. None of the controls had TSS; they used the brands indicated.

rapidly and effectively treated because these bacteria readily become resistant to antibiotics. Staphylococcal resistance to penicillin is carried on a plasmid that can be transferred between strains by bacteriophage. Staphylococci that are resistant to penicillin produce β lactamase, which enzymatically inactivates penicillin.

Diagnosis and prevention. *Staph. aureus* grows on blood agar plates as creamy colonies surrounded by zones of β hemolysis. In mixed infections they can be selectively isolated on culture media containing 7.5 percent NaCl, which inhibits the growth of many other bacteria. The isolated staphylococci are tested for coagulase and antibiotic sensitivity. Control of staphylococcal infections depends on the isolation of the causative agent, determination of its antibiotic sensitivity, and the administration of an appropriate chemotherapeutic regimen.

THE NEISSERIA

Humans are the only known reservoirs for two pathogenic species of *Neisseria*. *Neisseria gonorrhoeae* causes the venereal disease gonorrhea, and *Neisseria meningitidis* is a major cause of bacterial meningitis. These bacteria are commonly referred to as the gonococci and meningococci, respectively. Gonorrhea is the most frequently reported communicable disease in the United States with more than 1 million cases reported in recent years. Meningococcal meningitis is a serious illness that has a predilection for affecting children under 5 years old.

Descriptive characteristics. Neisseria are Gram-negative, nonmotile, nonspore-forming, bean-shaped diplococci (Figure 18–5). The six recognized species of *Neisseria* can be differentiated by the presence of capsules; growth at 22°C; fermentation of glucose, maltose, and/or sucrose; and growth on nutrient agar (Table 18–4). Only the nonpathogenic species grow at 22°C and on nutrient agar (without blood) incubated at 35°C. Pathogenic neisseria are difficult to grow because they are sensitive to fatty acids and metals. In addition, they contain an ami-

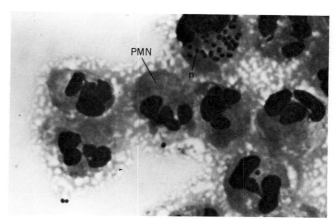

FIGURE 18–5
Typical Gram stain of a urethral smear from a male patient with gonorrhea. *Neisseria gonorrhoea* (n) appear as Gram-negative diplococci inside the polymorphonuclear neutrophiles (PMN). (Courtesy of E. J. Bottone and Abbott Laboratories. From *Schneierson's Atlas of Diagnostic Microbiology*, 7th ed., 1979.)

dase that causes their lysis outside of their human host. The laboratory cultivation of neisseria requires that they be quickly streaked on a suitable medium. They grow well on heated blood agar (called chocolate blood agar because of its brown color) that is incubated in an atmosphere of 5 to 10 percent CO_2. Chocolate blood agar is an appropriate medium because it binds heavy metals and fatty acids, which are growth inhibitors. Neisseria survive poorly outside of their animal hosts.

Most meningococci can be subdivided into serological groups based on their polysaccharide capsule. Meningococci in groups A, B, and C cause human diseases, with the majority of cases being caused by group A organisms. Many gonococci possess pili, which appear to enhance their ability to colonize mucous surfaces and are inhibitory to phagocytosis. The gonococci do not have a capsule, but they contain lipopolysaccharides in their cell walls that contribute to their virulence.

Meningitis. Meningococcal meningitis has a high incidence among children under 5 years of age and in physically compromised young adults. Military recruits who live in confined quarters belong to this

TABLE 18–4
Differential Characteristics of *Neisseria*

	Pigment	Capsules	Growth at 22°C	Fermentation Reactions			Growth (35°C) on Nutrient Agar
				Glucose	Sucrose	Maltose	
N. gonorrhoeae	−	−	−	+	−	−	−
N. meningitidis	−	v	−	+	−	+	−
N. mucosa	−	+	+	+	+	+	+
N. sicca	d	v	d	+	+	+	+
N. flavescens	+	−	+	−	−	−	+
N. subflava	+	+	d	+	v	+	d

(+) Most strains positive (>90%); (−) most strains negative (>90%); (d) some strains positive, some negative; (v) characteristic not constant.

latter group. *Neisseria meningitidis* commonly inhabits the human nasopharynx without causing disease. The adult carrier rate can be as high as 90%, especially before an epidemic. Physically fatigued individuals living in close contact appear to have a decreased resistance to meningococcal infections. This is also true of young children who have not built up their immunity against these bacteria.

The disease begins when the meningococci invade the host's circulatory system, causing a bacteremia. From the blood, the bacteria penetrate the meninges and infect the spinal fluid. Since the spinal fluid of normal humans is sterile, bacterial meningitis can be diagnosed by the presence of bacteria in the spinal fluid. Acute meningitis causes death in 85 percent of the untreated cases; however, these infections can be successfully treated with high doses of penicillin. The inflamed meninges are permeable to penicillin, even though penicillin does not penetrate the blood-brain barrier of healthy patients. Erythromycin and chloramphenicol are used to treat patients who are hypersensitive to penicillin.

The virulence of meningococci depends primarily on the antiphagocytic polysaccharide capsule. Most meningococcal illness is caused by encapsulated strains of the antigenic groups A, B, or C. The last major epidemic occurred during World War II (Figure 18–6) and was caused by meningococci of group A. Today, meningococcal meningitis occurs mostly in young children under the age of 5 years. Only 20 cases were reported among the military during 1980.

The current incidence of meningococcal meningitis in the United States is less than two cases per 100,000 population. Although two vaccines prepared from the group A and the group B polysaccharides are available, they are not widely used because of the low incidence of these infections. Prevention of meningococcal meningitis depends on the rapid diagnosis and antibiotic treatment of patients before the disease is transmitted to other susceptible patients.

Gonorrhea. Gonorrhea is caused by *Neisseria gonorrhoeae*, a bacterium that infects only humans. This venereal disease is transmitted by the sexual interaction of homosexual and heterosexual partners. The common symptoms of gonorrhea vary between men and women.

Men usually experience painful urination when they have gonorrhea. The gonococci penetrate the mucous membranes of the glans penis and the urethra, causing pain and a purulent discharge (Figure 18–5 and Color Plate 5). These symptoms usually develop within a few days after sexual contact with an infected partner. If untreated, the gonococci can infect the prostate and the epididymis. Sterility results if the sperm ducts are blocked when the host repairs the damage by the deposition of fibrous tissue. Humans develop no lasting immunity to gonorrhea, so they can be reinfected.

The symptoms of gonorrhea are less pronounced in women. Although the female urethra can be in-

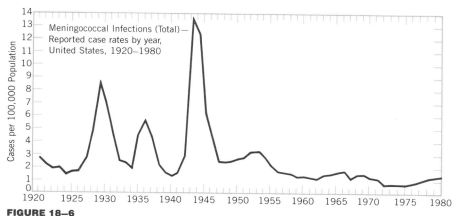

FIGURE 18–6

Meningococcal disease in the United States from 1920 to 1980. (Centers for Disease Control, "Annual Summary, 1980: Reported Morbidity and Mortality in the United States," *Morbidity Mortality Weekly Report*, 29, No. 54, 1981.)

fected, causing painful urination, the major infection occurs when gonococci enter the vagina and then move into the cervix of the uterus and the fallopian tubes. Women often become unknowing carriers of gonococci since there are few physiological symptoms associated with the infection. The only outward sign is a purulent vaginal discharge. Sterility, a long-term consequence of a gonococcal infection, occurs when fibrous tissue is deposited in a manner that blocks the patient's fallopian tubes. This is a normal body response to the damage caused by this infection. Another complication is the possibility of an ectopic pregnancy, which occurs when a fetus develops in the abdominal cavity or in a fallopian tube.

Pelvic inflammatory disease (PID) describes a general syndrome caused by ascending genital infections in women. Often it is difficult to identify the causative agent. When *N. gonorrhoeae* causes PID, significant female mortality can occur. This is a major reason for diagnosing and treating asymptomatic female carriers of *N. gonorrhoeae*.

The mouth and the rectum are other sites for gonococcal infections in both males and females. The rectum of female gonorrhea patients is a frequent site of infection. *N. gonorrhoeae* presumably is transmitted to the rectum in vaginal secretions. Rectal gonorrhea is also a disease of male homosexuals. Gonococci will infect the human pharynx when transmitted there by oral-genital contact.

The eyes of newborns can become infected with *Neisseria gonorrhoeae* as they pass through their mother's birth canal. Gonococcal infections of the newborn's eyes are known as **ophthalmia neonatorum,** and were once responsible for 15 percent of human blindness. Now this disease is prevented by placing drops of 1 percent silver nitrate ($AgNO_3$) solution or penicillin ointment in the eyes of newborns to inhibit the growth of gonococci.

Epidemiology. Gonorrhea is epidemic in the United States (Figure 18–7) with more than 1 million cases reported in each year between 1976 and 1980. This is the second major epidemic to occur since the early 1940s. The current epidemic gained momentum in the late 1960s and appears to have leveled off in 1975 at about 1 million cases. Sociologists and public health officials have attributed the latest epidemic to a loosening of sexual restrictions within the teenage and young adult segment of our society following the widespread availability and use of contraceptive pills.

Prevention of gonorrhea requires health professionals to develop educational programs and to in-

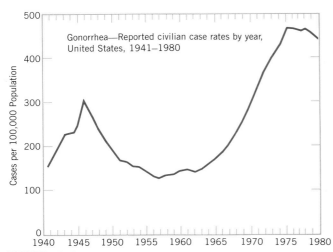

FIGURE 18–7
Civilian cases of gonorrhea in the United States from 1941 to 1980. (Centers for Disease Control, "Annual Summary, 1980: Reported Morbidity and Mortality in the United States," *Morbidity Mortality Weekly Report*, 29, No. 54, 1981.)

stitute public health measures. The use of condoms is one measure for preventing the spread of venereal diseases. The recent leveling off of the incidence of gonorrhea may be partially due to the screening of endocervical cultures for gonococci in asymptomatic young women. More than 200,000 cases of gonorrhea have been detected annually since 1971 by this screening program. Treatment of these patients decreases the number of asymptomatic carriers in the population.

Most gonococcal infections can be successfully treated with penicillin. Penicillin can also be used to prevent gonococcal infections when it is taken after a person makes contact with a potential carrier. Penicillin-resistant strains of *N. gonorrhoeae* have been isolated sporadically throughout the United States and England since 1976. These strains are designated as penicillinase-producing *N. gonorrhoeae* (PPNG). Infections by PPNG are treated with spectinomycin.

SUMMARY

The various species of pathogenic cocci are natural inhabitants of the human skin, mouth, intestine,

and/or vagina. They will cause suppurative infections (Table 18–5) under certain conditions. The three genera involved are the *Streptococcus, Staphylococcus* (both Gram-positive), and the Gram-negative *Neisseria*. Species of these genera cause diseases that vary in severity from mild skin infections to life-threatening systemic illnesses.

Streptococci are Gram-positive, catalase-negative, spherical cells that grow in chains. Many species do not cause disease; however, others produce streptolysins, hemolysins, and/or erythrogenic toxins that are major virulence factors. *Streptococcus pyogenes* (group A) is the major cause of streptococcal pharyngitis, scarlet fever, streptococcal impetigo, and puerperal sepsis. Untreated cases of streptococcal pharyngitis can lead to the late sequelae that include rheumatic fever and glomerulonephritis. *S. agalactiae* is a group B streptococcus that is a common cause of meningitis, pneumonia, and bacteremia in newborns. Encapsulated strains of *S. pneumoniae* are a major cause of human pneumonia. Streptococcal infections respond to treatment with penicillin or erythromycin.

Pathogenic staphylococci are coagulase-positive, Gram-positive cocci that grow in clusters. *Staph. aureus* can infect the human epidermis to cause impetigo, boils, and furuncles. Staphylococcal food poisoning occurs when people ingest food that has been contaminated by *Staph. aureus*. These organisms produce enterotoxin when they grow in improperly handled food. The symptoms have a rapid onset—spontaneous recovery usually follows in 24 to 48 hours. Toxic shock syndrome in menstruating women has been epidemiologically linked to *Staph. aureus* and certain brands of tampons.

Neisseria are obligate parasites of warm-blooded animals. Gonorrhea is a venereal disease caused by *Neisseria gonorrhoeae*. This bacterium can infect the genital tract, mouth, and rectum of both males and females. Both human sterility and pelvic inflammatory disease are serious consequences of gonococcal infections. Humans do not develop a lasting immunity against *N. gonorrhoeae*, so individuals can be reinfected. Gonococci can cause blindness in newborns whose eyes become infected during birth.

TABLE 18–5
Summary of Pathogenic Cocci

Organism	Virulence Factors	Organs Affected	Diseases	Transmission	Treatment
Streptococcus pyogenes	Capsules, M protein, erythrogenic toxin, streptolysins, β hemolysin, DNAase, NADase, hyaluronidase	Throat, skin, heart, kidneys	Strep throat (pharyngitis), scarlet fever, impetigo, rheumatic fever, glomerulonephritis	Person to person Late sequelae of strep infection	Penicillin, erythromycin
Streptococcus pneumoniae	Capsule, α hemolysin	Lungs	Pneumonia	Person to person	Penicillin, erythromycin
Staphylococcus aureus	Hemolysins, fibrinolysin, leukocydin, enterotoxin, DNAase, hyaluronidase	Epidermis Intestine	Boils, furuncles, osteomyelitis, impetigo, Staphylococcal food poisoning	Direct contact Ingestion of contaminated food	Chemotherapy (resistant strains)
Neisseria gonorrhoeae	Invasiveness, pili	Genitalia, eyes	Gonorrhea, PID, ophthalmia neonatorum	Sexual contact, during birth	Penicillin, 1% AgNO$_3$, or penicillin in eyes
Neisseria meningitidis	Invasiveness, polysaccharide capsules	Spinal fluid, meninges	Meningitis	Close contact	Penicillin, erythromycin, chloramphenicol

Neisseria meningitidis is a major cause of bacterial meningitis. This disease is most prevalent in children less than 5 years old and was once an important disease among military recruits living in confined quarters. Neisserial diseases can be treated by antibiotic chemotherapy.

QUESTIONS AND TOPICS FOR STUDY AND DISCUSSION

Questions

1. Construct a table of the pathogenic cocci that shows their characteristics and the human diseases they cause.
2. What are the virulence factors of the pathogenic strep-tococci? Which of these factors play a role in classifying these bacteria? Explain.
3. Describe the relationship between a strep throat and scarlet fever. What is the procedure that is used to diagnose a scarlet-fever rash?
4. Describe the late sequelae that can develop following a *Streptococcus pyogenes* infection? How are these diseases treated and/or prevented?
5. Describe the cocci involved in and the symptoms of impetigo and pneumonia.
6. What are the two pathogenic species of *Staphylococcus*? How are the staphylococci differentiated from the streptococci?
7. Describe the virulence of *Staphylococcus aureus*. How do these characteristics relate to this bacterium's ability to cause skin infections?

8. Compare staphylococcal food poisoning to botulism and clostridial food poisoning. What steps should be taken to prevent each type of food poisoning?

9. What evidence is there to support the contention that *Staphylococcus aureus* is responsible for toxic shock syndrome?

10. Why is *Nisseria gonorrhoeae* responsible for the most widespread bacterial epidemic in the United States?

11. How is gonorrhea diagnosed, treated, and prevented?

12. What are the signs of bacterial meningitis? How is this disease diagnosed, treated, and prevented?

Discussion

1. Should the manufacturers of the superabsorbent tampons be held liable for the effects of toxic shock syndrome?

2. How can a modern society prevent the long-term biological consequences of gonorrhea and herpes?

FURTHER READING
Books

Brooks, G. F., E. C. Gotschlich, K. K. Holmes, W. D. Sawyer, and F. E. Young, *Immunobiology of Neisseria gonorrhoeae*, American Society for Microbiology, Washington, D.C., 1978.

Cohen, J. O. (ed.), *The Staphylococci*, Wiley, New York, 1970.

Davis, D. B., R. Dulbecco, H. N. Eisen, H. S. Ginsberg, W. B. Wood, and M. McCarty, *Microbiology*, 3rd ed., Harper & Row, New York, 1980. Advanced, medicine-oriented textbook that contains a comprehensive chapter on each genera of the pathogenic cocci.

Skinner, F. A., and L. B. Quesnel (eds.), *Streptococci*, Academic Press, New York, 1978. A recent symposium on a wide variety of topics concerning the streptococci.

Articles and Reviews

Freimer, E. H., and M. McCarty, "Rheumatic Fever," *Sci. Am.*, 213:66–74 (December 1965). An early review of the evidence that relates rheumatic fever to streptococcal infections.

Wentworth, B. B., "Bacteriophage Typing of Staphylococci," *Bacteriol. Revs.*, 27:253–272 (1963). The Staphylococci can be separated into different types on the basis of the specificity of bacteriophages that infect them.

19

SPIROCHETES

Spirochetes are long, unicellular bacteria. Each spirochete has an outer envelope surrounding its coiled, protoplasmic cylinder (Figure 19–1). Between the cell's outer envelope and its wall are two or more endoflagella. These locomotor organelles enable spirochetes to move through liquid and semisolid media. The spirochetes are morphologically distinct bacteria, so they are classified in a single family, the Spirochaetaceae. This family is divided into five genera: *Spirochaeta, Cristispira, Treponema, Borrelia,* and *Leptospira*.

The spirochetes of these genera vary in size and in the tightness of the helical coiling of their protoplasmic cylinder. Because they are very narrow, many spirochetes pass through 0.22-μm membrane filters and are difficult to visualize in the bright-field

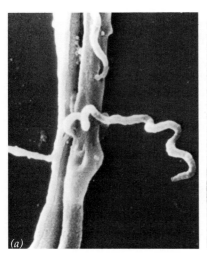

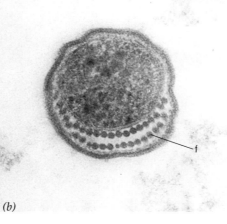

FIGURE 19–1

(a) Scanning electron micrograph of *Treponema pallidum* attached to testicular cell membranes. (Courtesy of Dr. J. B. Baseman. From N. S. Hayes, K. E. Muse, A. M. Collier, and J. B. Baseman, *Infection and Immunity,* 17:174–186, 1977, with permission of the American Society for Microbiology.) (b) Transmission electron micrograph of a cross section through the protoplasmic cylinder of a spirochete showing the location of the endoflagella (f). (Courtesy of Dr. M. A. Listgarten.)

microscope. One of the largest spirochetes is *Spirochaeta plicatilis*. It routinely grows to be 100 to 200 μm long; however, most spirochetes are only 5 to 20 μm long. Some spirochetes are tightly coiled *(Treponema)* and others are loosely coiled *(Cristispira)*. Other distinct morphological features are the pointed ends of the treponemes and the bent or hooked ends of the leptospiras.

MOTILITY

Spirochetes possess endoflagella composed of filaments, a hook, and a basal body (Figure 19–2). Each flagellum originates from an insertion point located at the end of a nondividing cell and extends to the midpoint of the helix. The outer envelope completely surrounds the cell and separates the endoflagella and the cell wall from the external environment. Except for the unique positioning on the protoplasmic cylinder, endoflagella are morphologically similar to the external flagella of eubacteria (see Chapter 3). In theory, the endoflagella rotate about their insertion point, which in turn propels the spirochete. When visualized in the microscope, the cell's movement appears as a corkscrew motion that is generated at the tail end of the cell.

Underlying the outer membrane and the endoflagella is the cell-wall, cytoplasmic-membrane complex. The cell walls of *Borrelia, Leptospira,* and *Treponema* are similar to other bacteria in that they contain peptidoglycan. Presumably, all spirochetes have a typical bacterial cytoplasmic membrane surrounded by a thin peptidoglycan-containing cell wall.

CLASSIFICATION

Spirochetes are classified into five genera based on their morphology, metabolism (where known), and pathogenicity. *Spirochaeta* are free-living, anaerobic bacteria found in ponds and streams. This is the only genus that does not contain parasitic spirochetes. *Cristispira* are found in the crystalline style of the digestive tract of freshwater and marine mollusks. They are microscopically visible in squashes of crystalline styles isolated from freshly harvested mollusks, but they have not yet been cultivated in

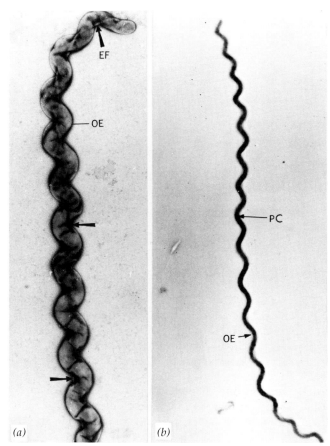

FIGURE 19–2
Electron micrographs of tightly wound leptospiras, negatively stained. (*a*) The endoflagella (EF) lie under the outer envelope (OE). 36,000X (*b*) The outer envelope (OE) and the protoplasmic cylinder (PC). (Courtesy of Dr. R. K. Nauman. From R. K. Nauman, S. C. Holt, and C. D. Cox, *J. Bacteriol.*, 98:264–280, 1969, with permission of the American Society for Microbiology.)

laboratory media. Spirochetes belonging to the genera *Treponema, Borrelia,* and *Leptospira* cause disease in humans.

TREPONEMES

Treponemes are narrow spirochetes (0.09 to 0.5 by 5 to 20 μm) with tight spirals that can be seen in the dark-field microscope. The cultivable treponemes are strict anaerobes that ferment amino acids or carbohydrates. Treponemes are found in the intestinal tract, oral cavity, and genitalia of animals including humans. *Treponema pallidum*, *T. petenue*, and *T. carateum* cause the human diseases of syphilis, yaws, and pinta, respectively.

Syphilis—*Treponema pallidum*

Syphilis is a venereal disease that was named after a mythical shepherd by Fracastorius in 1530. The origin of syphilis is unknown, but this illness appears to have been recognized under other names during ancient times. Europe experienced a significant epidemic of syphilis during the sixteenth century, and it was at this time that physicians recognized it as a venereal disease. The causative agent was first observed in 1905 when Schaudinn and Hoffman saw it in exudates from syphilitic lesions. Since that time, many microbiologists have attempted to grow *T. pallidum* in laboratory media—all without success. This bacterium can, however, be grown in rabbit testicles, which serve as a major source of *T. pallidum* for experiments and diagnostic techniques. Our knowledge of *T. pallidum* as a pathogen has been gained from studies of the organism grown in rabbit testicles and by studies of human syphilis.

Syphilis in humans. Venereal syphilis (Table 19–1) is transmitted between sexually active humans. It is caused by *T. pallidum*, which enters humans by penetrating skin or mucous membranes. This bacterium is an animal parasite that survives only for a short time outside its host, so it is transported only by direct contact. Infections most often occur in the genitalia, but can also occur in the mouth or rectum when these areas are exposed.

Primary syphilis. Following contact, viable cells of *T. pallidum* quickly reach the lymph nodes and/or bloodstream; from here they are disseminated to the remainder of the body. A primary lesion appears, usually at the site of initial contact, 10 to 30 days after infection. This lesion is a hard **chancre** or sore that contains motile spirochetes. The disease at this stage can be diagnosed both by serological and microscopic techniques. Patients are contagious during the primary stage of syphilis and should be treated. Human defense mechanisms do not necessarily cure a patient of syphilis, so untreated patients can progress to a more severe form of the disease.

Secondary syphilis. The chancre usually heals spontaneously and is gone completely within 4 weeks. During this time, the treponemes infect other parts of the body including the eyes, joints, bones, mouth, and the central nervous system. Treponemes can also be present in the blood. Between 2 and 12 weeks after the appearance of the chancre, a mild generalized body rash develops. This may be accompanied by cutaneous lesions (Color Plate 12) and/or

TABLE 19–1
Syphilis in Humans

Stage	Timing	Characteristics	Outcome
Primary	10 to 30 days after infection (average of 3 weeks)	Chancre at site of infection, contagious by sexual contact	Disappears within 4 weeks
Secondary	2 to 12 weeks after chancre	Generalized rash, cutaneous lesions, congenital syphilis, contagious	Many recover
Tertiary	Months or years after secondary, one-third of untreated patients develop tertiary symptoms	Slow progressive, destructive lesions, gummas, blindness, insanity	Gummas in soft tissue, heart, and nervous tissue contributing to possible death

lesions in the mucous membranes of the mouth and the genitalia. Patients with secondary syphilis are also contagious. The symptoms of secondary syphilis dissipate with or without treatment. Some patients recover, but a portion of the untreated patients later develop the symptoms of tertiary syphilis.

Tertiary syphilis. Approximately one-third of the patients with secondary syphilis are spontaneously cured; one-third have no symptoms, but are serologically positive for syphilis; and one-third display the symptoms of tertiary (late) syphilis. *T. pallidum* persists in the tissue of patients with tertiary syphilis where it forms soft lesions called gummas. A **gumma** is a nonspecific granulomatous lesion that may be microscopic in size or a large tumorous mass. Gummas cause little damage when they develop in the skin or bones; however, gummas that develop in the central nervous system, the eyes, or the heart can lead to insanity and blindness, and can eventually contribute to the patient's death. Tertiary syphilis is a slowly progressive inflammatory disease that can develop years after the initial infection.

Congenital syphilis. A fetus contracts **congenital syphilis** when it is infected (in utero) with *T. pallidum.* The fetus acquires the infection from its mother, who is usually in the secondary stage of syphilis. *T. pallidum* can cause local lesions in the fetus, or it can cause a generalized infection that results in a stillbirth. Congenital syphilis is not a genetic disorder as was once thought.

Immunity to syphilis. Patients develop a resistance to reinfection by *T. pallidum,* but they never become fully immune. Humans produce humoral antibodies that react specifically with treponemes and antibodies that react with by-products (cardiolipin) of the infection process. In some patients these immune reactions are protective; however, in patients with tertiary syphilis, *T. pallidum* persists even in the presence of the immune response. The lack of a cultivable strain of *T. pallidum* and the incomplete nature of the immune response to syphilis have dissuaded health professionals from developing vaccines against syphilis. Nevertheless, immune reactions are important for the diagnosis of syphilis.

Diagnosis of syphilis. The most straightforward means of diagnosing syphilis is the microscopic observation of spirochetes in material taken from a primary lesion. If present, *T. pallidum* can be seen in a dark-field microscope (Figure 19–3). Alternatively, they can be visualized in the bright-field microscope after they are stained with silver.

History—Wasserman complement-fixation test. The Wasserman complement-fixation test was once the major test for syphilis. It is a complement-fixation assay that detects the Wasserman antibody (also called reagin). At the turn of the century, cells of *T. pallidum* were not available even from animal sources. Therefore, Wasserman produced an antigenic preparation from extracts of the treponema-contaminated liver of a human fetus that had died of congenital syphilis. This antigenic preparation was then used to detect an antibody (Wasserman antibody) present in syphilitic patients. Later, the antigen was isolated from cardiac tissue and from normal human liver and was identified as cardiolipin (diphosphotidylglycerol). Cardiolipin is immunogenic in humans even though it is a normal human constituent. Presumably, cardiolipin is released by the destructive effects of the treponemes on mammalian tissue, so the detection of the Wasserman antibody is an indication of syphilis.

A sensitive complement fixation was developed to detect the Wasserman antibody. Wasserman used purified mammalian cardiolipin as the antigen in place of the unavailable treponemal antigens. The complex formed between the Wasserman antibody and cardiolipin fixes complement. The fixation of complement can be detected by observing the ability of unbound complement to lyse sensitized red blood cells. Historically, the Wasserman test for syphilis was very important, but it is no longer used because it often results in "biologic false positives" and because better tests are available.

Tests for syphilis. The standard screening tests for syphilis are the rapid plasma reagin (RPR) card test and the Venereal Disease Research Laboratories (VDRL) test. These tests detect serum antibody (reagin) that reacts with cardiolipin. The VDRL test is performed by mixing a suspension of cardiolipin-lecithin-cholesterol with the patient's serum on a microscope slide. Positive tests result in microscopically visible flocculation of the reagents. The inexpensive VDRL and RPR assays are accurate screening tests for syphilis—especially of patients with primary and secondary syphilis. Because they detect the nontreponemal antibodies (reagin) that react with cardiolipin, "biologic false positive" reactions do occur. Therefore, the specific treponemal tests are used to confirm positive RPR and VDRL tests.

The *T. pallidum* immobilization test (TPI) and the fluorescent treponemal antibody test (FTA) detect antibodies that react with *T. pallidum* and closely related strains. These tests use the Nichol strain of *T. pallidum*, which is cultivated in rabbit testicles. They are used to confirm positive RPR and VDRL results and to assess the adequacy of therapy.

TPI tests are done by suspending motile *T. pallidum* in a solution containing a patient's serum and guinea pig complement under anaerobic conditions at 37°C. After overnight incubation, the motility of the spirochetes in the test serum is compared to that in a control. A 50 percent drop in motility is indicative of a positive test for syphilis. The fluorescent treponemal antibody test is another direct test for treponemal antibodies (see Chapter 13).

Epidemiology. Syphilis is found only in primates, including humans. *T. pallidum* does not survive for long periods outside its host, so it is transmitted by direct contact with a syphilitic lesion. Since these lesions predominate in the genital region, syphilis is transmitted by sexual contact. Lesions in other body parts (mouth, skin, rectum) are also contagious. Congenital syphilis is a distinct form of syphilis caused by *T. pallidum* that is transmitted from the mother to her fetus. The fetus is infected in utero and is born with the disease.

During 1980, the incidence of primary and secondary syphilis per 100,000 people in the United States was 12 cases. This is much less than the current incidence of gonorrhea (443 cases per 100,000 persons

FIGURE 19–3
Dark-field micrographs of *Treponema pallidum*. (Courtesy of the American Society for Microbiology slide collection.)

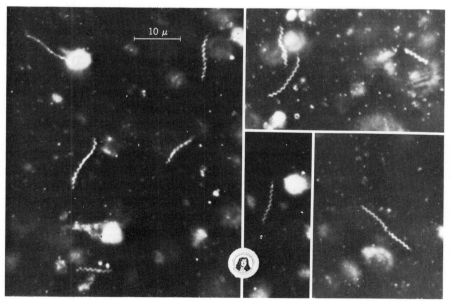

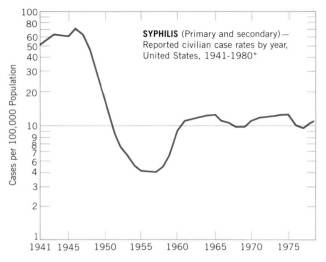

*1941-1946 Fiscal years: Twelve month period ending June 30 of year specified.
1947-1979 Calendar years.

FIGURE 19–4

Incidence of syphilis (primary and secondary) in the civilian population of the United States, 1941 through 1980. (Centers for Disease Control, "Annual Summary 1980: Reported Morbidity and Mortality in the United States," *Morbidity Mortality Weekly Report*, 29, No. 54, 1981.)

in 1980). The incidence of syphilis reached a peak during World War II (Figure 19–4), then declined dramatically following the widespread use of penicillin. The incidence of syphilis has remained constant during the 1960s and 1970s; however, the total number of cases has increased with the increase in the total U.S. population.

Treatment and prevention. Salvarsan (arsphenamine) was one of the first chemotherapeutic agents ever developed. It was used to treat syphilitic patients until antibiotics became available. Penicillin is now the drug of choice for treating patients with syphilis. Patients with allergies to penicillin are treated with erythromycin or tetracycline.

Preventing direct contact with a syphilitic person is the major means of controlling the spread of syphilis. An infected, promiscuous person can transmit this disease to numerous sexual partners. For this reason, syphilis is considered a social disease and it is necessary to treat syphilitic patients and to screen their known contacts for syphilis. Many states require a premarital test for syphilis as part of their public health screening program for syphilis. The social stigma associated with syphilis makes this a difficult disease to control.

Pinta—*Treponema carateum*

Pinta (Sp. *pinta,* blemish) is a nonvenereal skin disease caused by *Treponema carateum*. It is characterized by patches of discolored skin lesions. The treponemes are present in these lesions and can be seen in the dark-field microscope. *T. carateum* is morphologically indistinguishable from *T. pallidum*. Infected patients contain the Wasserman antibody, which can be detected in serological tests. Pinta occurs in rural populations of people living in the tropical climates of Central and South America.

Pinta is transmitted between all age groups by person-to-person contact. The infection begins as a papule at the site of infection and then spreads into a red patch (1 cm in diameter) in 4 to 5 weeks. The secondary lesions develop about 5 months later both at the site of the initial papule and elsewhere on the body. These secondary lesions become darkly pigmented and then undergo a gradual—over a period of 2 years—depigmentation. Penicillin is an effective drug for treating pinta.

Yaws—*Treponema pertenue*

Yaws is a nonvenereal disease that occurs in warm, humid climates in equatorial Africa, the tropical Americas, and tropical areas of the Far East. It is caused by *Treponema pertenue*, which in many respects is indistinguishable from *T. pallidum*. Humans infected with *T. pertenue* also produce the Wasserman antibody, which can be detected with serological tests.

T. pertenue infects humans through skin abrasions that usually occur on the legs or feet. A small, red papule with the appearance of a raspberry develops at the site of infection. The primary lesion appears 3 to 4 weeks after infection and progressively develops into an open lesion called a **yaw.** The yaw contains spirochetes and is contagious. The yaw eventually scabs over and heals. Six weeks to 3 months after the development of the yaw, secondary eruptions occur on the neck, the extremities, and at the juncture of the skin and mucous membranes (nose, mouth, anus).

Yaws occurs among primitive peoples in the tropics, where little protective clothing is worn and where the high humidity promotes the persistence of open skin lesions. The treponemes are transmitted by person-to-person contact and possibly by flies that feed on the open lesions. A single long-lasting injection of penicillin is an effective treatment for yaws.

BORRELIAE

Borreliae are anaerobic to microaerophilic, parasitic spirochetes that have coarse, uneven, or irregular coils (Figure 19–5). These spirochetes readily stain with aniline dyes and are large enough (0.2 to 0.5 by 3 to 20 µm) to be seen in the bright-field microscope. Borreliae live in mammals, insects, and birds. They have been cultivated in chick embryos and in young rats and mice. One spirochete, *Borrelia hermsii,* has been cultivated under microaerophilic conditions in a complex laboratory medium. It was viable and virulent for mice after 36 transfers. Since most borreliae have not been cultivated in the laboratory, they are assigned to species based on their vectors and the diseases they cause.

Relapsing fever

Relapsing fever is transmitted by either the human louse, *Pediculus humanus,* or by ticks of the genus *Ornithodoros.* **Louse-borne** (epidemic) **relapsing fever** is caused by *Borrelia recurrentis.* The louse is infected with *B. recurrentis* when it feeds on an infected human. The spirochetes penetrate the louse gut epithelium to multiply in their hemolymph. Spirochetes are transmitted back to humans only when the lice are squashed near broken skin. *B. recurrentis* is then

FIGURE 19–5

Photomicrographs of *Borrelia* in blood smears. (Courtesy of the American Society for Microbiology slide collection.)

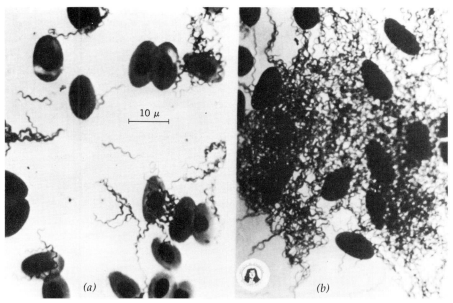

(a)   *(b)*

able to penetrate and infect humans who are the only animal reservoir for this bacterium. This spirochete is not passed transovarianly (via the egg of the parent) in lice, so it dies with its host louse.

Tick-borne *(endemic)* **relapsing fever** is transmitted to humans by ticks during feeding. The borreliae infect all tissues of the tick and are maintained in a tick population by transovarian passage. *Borrelia hermsii, B. turicatae,* and *B. venezuelensis* are major causes of relapsing fever in continental America. The clinical symptoms of both forms of relapsing fever are very similar, except that the tick-borne fever is less severe.

Relapsing fever in humans. The symptoms of relapsing fever begin with a sudden onset of fever that develops after an incubation period of 3 to 10 days. The fever continues for about 10 days, during which time the borreliae are easily demonstrated in the blood and urine. As the fever subsides, the spirochetes in the blood decrease and become less motile. After 3 to 10 days the fever recurs, and once again the patient's blood is teeming with borrelias. Tickborne relapsing fever progresses through three to ten sequential fever-relapse cycles, with each febrile stage becoming less severe.

The borreliae present in the blood during each febrile stage are antigenically different from those found in the previous febrile stage. The spirochetes mutate at a fairly high and constant rate to cause the relapsing nature of the disease. Antibodies are formed against the new antigens and again the infection subsides. Eventually the host manufactures enough varied antibodies to prevent the recurrence of borrelial multiplication.

Prevention and treatment. Relapsing fever is treated with penicillin, tetracycline, or chloramphenicol. Tick-borne relapsing fever occurs at a very low incidence in the southern and western parts of the United States. Control of relapsing fever is attained by limiting the distribution of the ticks and lice and by preventing humans from interacting with these arthropods.

LEPTOSPIROSIS

Leptospiras are free-living or parasitic spirochetes found in ponds, streams, or infected animals. They are distinct from other spirochetes in that leptospiras are aerobic and they have one or more hooked ends. They cause leptospirosis, which is primarily a zoonosis of wild and domestic animals.

Many leptospiras have been grown in artificial media containing heated rabbit serum or albumin. The media must also contain long chain fatty acids because pathogenic leptospiras are unable to manufacture long chain fatty acids de novo; these compounds also serve as a necessary oxidizable energy source. Leptospiras can be selectively isolated in the presence of 5-fluorouracil. This uracil analogue causes lethal mutations when it is incorporated into the nucleic acids of organisms that assimilate it. Leptospiras, however, are not affected by 5-fluorouracil because they are unable to metabolize purines present in their growth medium.

Leptospiras are 0.1 μm wide by 6 to 20 μm long. The spirals are tightly coiled and terminate in one or two hooked ends (Figure 19–6). The leptospiras present in samples of blood or urine taken from infected animals can be seen using a dark-field microscope. Although there are many serotypes, leptospiras are classified as two major species: *Leptospira interrogans* includes all the organisms that are pathogenic for animals, and *Leptospira biflexa* includes the nonpathogenic leptospiras. Serological differences within these species are used in the technical literature to designate leptospiral serotypes.

Leptospirosis in lower animals

Rodents and domestic animals are the major reservoirs of the pathogenic leptospiras. After they infect an animal, they establish a primary infection in the kidneys. In the mammalian kidney, they grow in the proximal, convoluted tubules and are excreted in high concentration in the urine. The excretion of leptospiras in the urine of cattle, swine, and dogs has been observed to last for 3.5 months, 11 months, and over 4 years, respectively. Leptospirosis is one

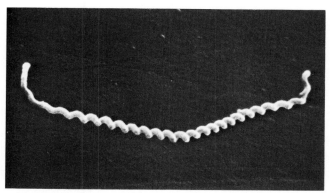

FIGURE 19–6
Scanning electron micrograph of *Leptospira interrogans* showing the helical coiling of a typical spirochete. (Courtesy of Dr. N. Charon. From O. Carleton, N. Charon, P. Allender, and S. O'Brien, *J. Bacteriol.*, 137:1413–1416, 1979, with permission of the American Society for Microbiology.)

of the most widely occurring zoonoses. Infected animals experience a mild, sometimes lifelong disease, but they rarely die of leptospirosis.

Leptospirosis in humans

Most cases of leptospirosis occur in young males during the summer or early autumn. Ninety percent of the cases of leptospirosis are mild illnesses, whereas the remainder are serious illnesses with jaundice that are known as **Weil's disease.** The leptospiras enter the host through abrasions on the skin or through mucous membranes that come in contact with contaminated soil or water. Following an incubation period of 6 to 12 days, the patient develops a high fever followed by nausea, headache, muscular pain, and nosebleeds. The leptospiras are present in the blood, the cerebrospinal fluid, and, during the later stages of the disease, the kidneys. Infection of the kidneys correlates with the excretion of the spirochetes in the urine. The immediate cause of human death from leptospirosis appears to be kidney failure. Fatality rates in humans have varied in different epidemics from 4.6 to 32 percent of those infected. Patients who recover possess a solid immunity to subsequent infection.

Epidemiology and treatment

Leptospirosis is a zoonosis that predominates in rodents and domestic animals. Dogs are a major carrier of leptospiras in the United States. Many animals are lifelong carriers of leptospiras and excrete them in their urine. The leptospira can survive for up to 15 days in warm, moist soil. Humans are infected through skin abrasions or mucous membranes by direct contact with contaminated soil or water. The number of reported human cases per year is usually less than 100 in the United States.

Treatment of leptospirosis remains unsatisfactory even with antibiotics. In the early stages of leptospirosis, the infection responds to penicillin or tetracyclines. Antibiotic treatment is less effective in the later stages of the disease, when most cases are diagnosed.

SUMMARY

Spirochetes are morphologically distinct from other bacteria in their size, shape, and means of motility. Their coiled cells are propelled by endoflagella that extend from the ends of the spirochete toward the center of the bacterium. An outer envelope covers the protoplasmic cylinder and the endoflagella. Most spirochetes are so thin that they pass through 0.22 μm membrane filters, and they can be viewed only in dark-field microscopes. There are five genera of spirochetes: three genera contain human pathogens (Table 19–2).

Treponema pallidum is the etiological agent of syphilis, which is primarily a venereal disease. The treponemes penetrate the mucous membranes, invade the lymph nodes, and then form a primary chancre at the site of infection. The spirochetes are found throughout the body during the secondary stage, which is characterized by cutaneous lesions and a skin rash. Gummas develop during tertiary syphilis months or years after the secondary stage. Gummas in the nervous tissue or heart often contribute to the death of the patient. The RPR and the VDRL tests for reagin are used to screen patients for syphilis. These tests can result in "biologic false positive" re-

TABLE 19–2
Disease Caused by Spirochetes

Disease (Epidemiology)	Etiological Agent(s)	Symptoms	Diagnosis and (Treatment)
Syphilis (venereal)	*Treponema pallidum*	Chancre, body rash, cutaneous lesions, gummas in tertiary stages	RPR, VDRL, TPI, FTA, and spirochetes in lesions (penicillin)
Pinta (direct contact)	*Treponema carateum*	Discolored patches on skin, cutaneous lesions	Tests for Wasserman antibody, spirochetes in lesions (penicillin)
Yaws (direct contact—flies?)	*Treponema pertenue*	Papule at site of inoculation, open lesion (yaw)	Tests for Wasserman antibody, spirochetes in lesions (penicillin)
Relapsing fever (tick-borne, louse-borne)	*Borrelia recurrentis, B. hermsii*	Spirochetes in blood and urine, recurring fever, antigenic change	Spirochetes in blood (penicillin, tetracycline, chloramphenicol)
Leptospirosis (animal urine)	*Leptospira interrogans*	High fever, nausea, headache, leptospira in urine	Serological tests, leptospiras in urine (antibiotics in early stages)

actions, so the TPI and the FTA tests are used to confirm the screening tests.

Treponema pertenue and *T. carateum* cause yaws and pinta, respectively. These skin diseases are prevalent in tropical regions. *T. pertenue* infects the skin to cause an open lesion called a yaw. *T. carateum* causes pinta, which is characterized by patches of discoloration on the skin. Patients with either yaws or pinta produce the Wasserman antibody, which can be detected serologically. Penicillin is an effective treatment for all three of the treponemal diseases.

Humans are the reservoir for *Borrelia recurrentis*, which is the causative agent of louse-borne relapsing fever. The borrelias multiply in the louse and infect the human when the louse is squashed near an abrasion. *B. recurrentis* is not perpetuated in the louse by transovarian passage. Tick-borne relapsing fever is caused by species of *Borrelia* that are transmitted by tick bites. These borrelias are maintained in the tick population by transovarian passage. Relapsing fever is characterized by alternating febrile and recovery stages that are correlated with the appearance of new antigenic variants of the infecting borrelias.

Leptospirosis is a zoonosis found in rodents and domestic animals (especially dogs). Leptospiras infect the blood, cerebrospinal fluid, and the kidneys; they are excreted in the urine of infected animals. Humans are infected by *Leptospira interrogans* when they come in direct contact with contaminated animals, soil, or water. Leptospirosis can be treated in its early stages with antibiotics, but treatment after the organism has infected the human kidney is unsatisfactory.

QUESTIONS AND TOPICS FOR STUDY AND DISCUSSION

Questions

1. Describe the unique morphology of the spirochetes. How is morphology used to classify these bacteria into genera?
2. Describe the clinical signs associated with the three stages of human syphilis. During which of these stages is the patient infectious?

3. Describe the transmission and symptoms of congenital syphilis.
4. Describe the Wasserman complement-fixation test. Why is the Wasserman test positive for infections of *T. pallidum, T. carateum,* and *T. pertenue?*
5. What are the biological and epidemiological characteristics of endemic and epidemic relapsing fever?
6. What biological mechanisms are involved in the dynamic relationship established between *Borrelia* and the humans they infect?
7. Explain the use of 5-fluorouracil in the isolation of leptospiras.
8. How do humans contract leptospirosis? How is leptospirosis prevented and/or treated?

Discussion

1. What physiological information concerning *Treponema pallidum* would help microbiologists grow this organism? Are there indirect ways of obtaining this information?
2. In Michigan, 16 cases of syphilis were detected by the 173,000 syphilis tests performed in 1979. These tests were required by the 1937 law that prohibits granting a marriage license without first submitting the results of a test for syphilis. Should this law be repealed? Should other laws be enacted to control the spread of venereal disease?

FURTHER READING

Books

Felsenfeld, O., *Borrelia, Stains, Vectors: Human and Animal Borreliosis,* Warren H. Green, St. Louis, 1971.

Johnson, R. C. (ed.), *The Biology of the Parasitic Spirochetes,* Academic Press, New York, 1976. A well-organized collection of articles with extensive coverage of the biology of the spirochetes.

Articles and Reviews

Fitzgerald, T. J., ''Pathogenesis and Immunology of *Treponema pallidum,*'' *Ann. Rev. Microbiol.,* 35:29–54 (1981). A review of the pathogenesis of *T. pallidum* and the human immune response to infections caused by this bacterium.

Holt, S. C., ''Anatomy and Chemistry of Spirochetes,'' *Microbiol. Revs.,* 42:114–160 (1978). The anatomy of the spirochetes is reviewed with the extensive use of superb electron micrographs.

Johnson, R. C., ''The Spirochetes,'' *Ann. Rev. Microbiol.,* 31:89–106 (1977). A review of the structure, composition, distribution, and nutrition of the spirochetes.

20

OBLIGATE PARASITIC BACTERIA: RICKETTSIAE AND CHLAMYDIAE

The rickettsiae and the chlamydiae are obligate intracellular parasites of animal tissue. These infectious agents were believed originally to be viruses, but now it is clear that they are bacteria. They have a typical Gram-negative cell wall, they contain both DNA and RNA, they possess a semipermeable cytoplasmic membrane, and they divide by binary fission (Figure 20–1). The obligate intracellular parasitic bacteria are collectively referred to as the **rickettsias.**

Human rickettsial pathogens are classified into two families: **Rickettsiaceae** and **Chlamydiaceae.** Rickettsiaceae are Gram-negative, nonmotile, coccoid or rod-shaped bacteria that multiply only inside host cells. They infect numerous wild and domestic animals, and many can grow in insect or arthropod vectors. Numerous species of *Rickettsia* and *Coxiella burnetii* cause human disease. Most species of *Rickettsia* multiply in the cytoplasm of their host cell (Table 20–1). This is also true for *Coxiella burnetii;* however, coxiella grows within a cytoplasmic vacuole (Figure 20–2). Only two species of the genus *Chlamydia,* family Chlamydiaceae, are known. These bacteria are "energy parasites" that depend on their

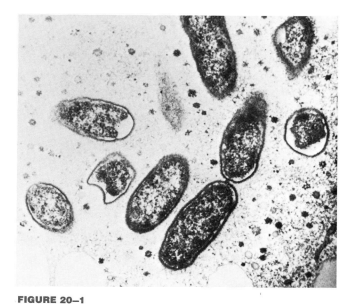

FIGURE 20–1

Electron micrograph of *Rickettsia* growing in the cytoplasm of a malpighian tube cell of *Dermacentor andersoni.* The rickettsia at the lower right is dividing by binary fission. (Courtesy of Dr. W. Burgdorfer. From W. Burgdorfer, "Introduction to the Rickettsia" in W. T. Hubbert, W. E. McCullock, and P. R. Schnurrenberg, eds., *Diseases Transmitted from Animals to Man,* 6th, ed. Copyright © 1979, Charles C Thomas.)

TABLE 20–1
Classification of the Human Rickettsial Pathogens

Family, *Genus*	Major Characteristics
Rickettsiaceae	
Rickettsia	Multiply in cytoplasm (rarely in nucleus) of host, not cultivable in absence of host cells
Coxiella	Multiply in host cytoplasmic vacuoles, resistant to physical and chemical agents, endosporelike structure seen in electron micrographs
Chlamydiaceae	
Chlamydia	Unique growth cycle, multiply within vesicle, host cell provides ATP (energy parasites), glucose metabolized

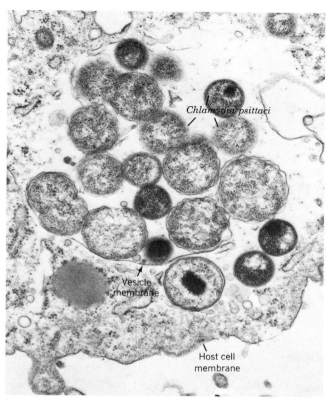

FIGURE 20–2
Electron micrograph of *Chlamydia psittaci* growing in a ruptured vacuole (↑) in the cytoplasm of a McCoy cell. (Courtesy of Dr. R. C. Cutlip. From R. C. Cutlip, *Infection and Immunity* 1:499–502, 1970, with permission of the American Society for Microbiology.)

host cells to provide them with ATP. Another distinguishing characteristic of the chlamydiae is that they have a unique reproductive cycle.

Rickettsiae and chlamydiae are perpetuated in animal reservoirs. Many rickettsiae are transmitted between hosts by arthropod vectors belonging to the class *Insectia* (fleas, lice) or *Arachnidia* (mites, ticks). Sometimes the vector is also the reservoir. Rats and rodents can be rickettsial reservoirs, whereas humans are the only reservoir known for the rickettsia that causes epidemic typhus. Because these bacteria are obligate intracellular parasites, their distribution corresponds to the geographical locale in which the vector and the primary host reside. On the other hand, there are no vectors involved in the transmission of the chlamydiae to humans. The *Chlamydia* species that exist in human reservoirs are transferred by direct contact, whereas those that exist in birds or mammals are transmitted in aerosols.

Rickettsial physiology

Rickettsiae are difficult to work with because of their obligate parasitism. The rickettsiae must be grown in the cells of animals or of tissue cultures. These eu-

caryotic host cells often interfere with experimental assays done on rickettsial cells. In addition, many of the rickettsiae readily infect humans, so working with them is dangerous. Nevertheless, research on the physiology of rickettsial parasitism has been remarkably successful.

Rickettsial growth. Rickettsiae are isolated from nature by injecting contaminated material into a host animal, usually a guinea pig or a mouse. When the infected animal becomes sick, it is killed and the rickettsiae are isolated with the animal's infected tissues (spleen is often a primary site of infection). These infected tissues are inoculated into embryonated eggs or animal cell tissue cultures that in turn yield sufficient rickettsial cells to perform physiological studies.

Physiology of *Rickettsia* and *Chlamydia*. Isolated *Rickettsia* species will perform metabolic reactions even though they will not grow outside of animal tissue. They are able to metabolize both glutamate and glutamine, which are structurally related amino acids (see Appendix 1 for structural comparison). When cells of *Rickettsia* are incubated in the presence of oxygen and glutamate, they produce ATP. They are presumed to have a respiratory electron-transport chain because their ability to produce ATP is inhibited by cyanide. Rickettsiae are unable to utilize glucose or amino acids other than glutamate and glutamine as substrates.

Rickettsia species are plasmolyzed by high concentrations of sucrose, NaCl, and KCl; so they possess a semipermeable cytoplasmic membrane. Some early evidence suggested that these membranes were leaky to some large, essential, cellular metabolites. For example, NAD, coenzyme A (CoA), and ATP get into these cells from the medium and are able to stimulate certain metabolic activities in their cytoplasm. This "leaky membrane theory" was once used to explain the obligate parasitism of the rickettsiae by suggesting that the rickettsiae depended on their host cell to provide them with NAD, CoA, and ATP. More recent evidence indicates that the rickettsial cytoplasmic membrane is tight, not leaky. Apparently, the observed stimulation of metabolic activities by ATP in rickettsiae is caused by one or more unusual transport systems that transfer ATP, and possibly NAD, and CoA from the host cell's cytoplasm into their cytoplasm.

Chlamydiae are energy parasites. These bacteria cannot manufacture ATP, so they rely on their host cell to provide them with this essential metabolite. The chlamydiae are further distinguished from the other rickettsiae because they can use glucose as a substrate and have a unique growth cycle.

RICKETTSIA

Rickettsiae multiply within the cytoplasm (or rarely in the nucleus) of certain vertebrate or arthropod cells (Figure 20–1). They are coccoid to rod-shaped organisms that do not grow outside their host cells. In fact, they are very unstable when separated from animal tissue and are rapidly inactivated at 56°C. The rickettsiae that cause human disease are transmitted from their animal reservoir to humans by an arthropod vector. Depending on the species of *Rickettsia*, humans are either a necessary or an incidental host.

Mice are the best experimental animal for isolating rickettsiae and for studying rickettsial diseases. All species of *Rickettsia* cause disease in mice when sufficient bacteria are injected intravenously. These bacteria cause a dramatic increase in the permeability of the vascular system that can lead directly to the death of the mouse within 1 to 8 hours. Rickettsiae enter the vascular epithelium—by an as yet unknown mechanism—where they grow and multiply. When they infect humans, they have a similar preference for growing in human vascular epithelium.

Five species of *Rickettsia* are major causes of human disease (Table 20–2). They are organized as the typhus group and the spotted fever group. Infections result in headache, fever, and a rash that is an important clinical sign of the infection. Rickettsial diseases are diagnosed by the clinical symptoms, the patient's history of exposure to vectors, and the seasonal and geographical incidence of the diseases. The isolation of the causative agents and serological tests for rickettsial infections have a minor impact on diagnosis. This is because serological evidence of infection develops late in these diseases, and the isolation of the rickettsiae is a specialized and potentially dangerous task.

Rickettsia: typhus group diseases

The major species of the *Rickettsia* are grouped into three biotypes based on the types of human diseases they cause (Table 20–2). Typhus fevers are rickettsial diseases found worldwide and are characterized by

TABLE 20–2
Human Diseases Caused by *Rickettsia*

Biotype	Typhus Group			Spotted Fever Group	
Disease	Epidemic Typhus	Endemic (murine) Typhus	Scrub Typhus	Rocky Mountain Spotted Fever	Rickettsialpox
Causative Agent	*R. prowazekii*	*R. typhi*	*R. tsutsugamushi*	*R. rickettsii*	*R. akari*
Growth Location in Cell	Cytoplasm	Cytoplasm	Cytoplasm	Cytoplasm, nucleus	Cytoplasm, nucleus
Natural Cycle					
Reservoir	Human	Small rodents	Rodents	Wild rodents	House mouse
Vector	Body louse	Rat flea	Mite	Tick	Blood-sucking mite
Rash	Trunk to extremities	Trunk to extremities	Trunk to extremities	Extremities to trunk	Vascular, trunk to extremities
Distribution	Worldwide (rare in U.S.)	Worldwide	Pacific islands, Asia, Australia	Western Hemisphere	Europe, N. America

a headache, a rash, and a stupor that arises from a fever (Gr. *typhus,* cloud). The three types of human typhus fever (Table 20–2) are caused by closely related species of *Rickettsia* that have different reservoirs, vectors, and geographical distributions.

Epidemic typhus. *Rickettsia prowazekii* causes epidemic typhus in humans who serve as the natural reservoir for these bacteria. This disease is transmitted between humans by the body louse, *Pediculus humanus.* The louse is infected by *R. prowazekii* when it feeds on a rickettsemic human. The louse eventually dies of this infection and is unable to pass its disease onto its offspring. The bacteria multiply in the louse-gut epithelium and are excreted in the louse feces. Humans are infected through abrasions in the skin caused by scratching the lice-infested area. The bacteria grow in the epithelial layer of the vascular system and cause severe changes in vascular permeability. Lice infestations spread rapidly between humans who are crowded together. Lice prefer temperatures of 37°C, so when a human becomes febrile or dies, the lice leave the body to seek another human host.

Lice infestations occur in areas of high population densities regardless of socioeconomic conditions.

Even though lice infestations still occur in the United States, louse-borne typhus does not. The last case was reported in 1950, which means that few, if any, humans (the only reservoir) are infected. Epidemic typhus is of historical significance because it causes severe morbidity and mortality during wars and famines. Major epidemics occurred during World War I and in concentration camps during World War II.

Symptoms of epidemic typhus. The incubation period of epidemic typhus is between 1 and 2 weeks. This illness begins with a sudden onset of chills, fever, headache, generalized aches, pains, and exhaustion. Body temperature can reach 40°C. A macular rash usually appears on the trunk (see Color Plate 14) after 4 to 7 days and then spreads to the extremities. Prostration, stupor, and delirium develop in severe cases. Prior to chemotherapy, the fatality rate was between 20 and 70 percent; however, now patients recover after early diagnosis and treatment. Persons who recover have lasting immunity to both epidemic typhus and the closely related endemic typhus.

Brill-Zinsser disease. Humans are the only reservoir of *R. prowazekii,* so these bacteria must remain in a living human carrier. Recurrent infections by *R.*

prowazekii appear as Brill-Zinsser disease, which is a mild illness resembling typhus fever. This disease is different from typhus because (1) no louse infestation is required, (2) no rash appears, (3) the clinical symptoms are less severe than in epidemic typhus, and (4) the serological reactions (Weil-Felix) associated with these diseases are different. Patients with Brill-Zinsser disease rapidly develop antibodies to *R. prowazekii* (within 3 to 4 days), and most patients have previously been ill with typhus fever. It is now clear that Brill-Zinsser disease develops from a latent infection of *R. prowazekii* in persons who act as carriers (human reservoirs) of epidemic typhus. Most cases in the United States occur in immigrants from Eastern Europe who were infected during World War II.

Treatment and control. Epidemic typhus can be prevented by controlling lice infestations, whereas the only control of Brill-Zinsser disease is to prevent the primary infection. Lice cannot move far after feeding on blood (1 yard at most), so they nest in a person's clothes. General insecticides such as DDT can be used to delouse large human populations by spraying each individual's clothes. Persons in crowded conditions where cleanliness of body and clothes is impossible are susceptible to lice infestations. These conditions rarely occur today. Persons infected with *R. prowazekii* are treated with tetracycline or chloramphenicol.

Endemic (murine) typhus. Endemic (murine) typhus occurs worldwide among persons who come in close contact with rats. Humans are incidental hosts for *Rickettsia typhi,* which causes endemic typhus fever in humans. This bacterium is very similar to *R. prowazekii;* however, rats and other rodents (not humans) are its primary reservoir. The infection is spread among rats by the rat flea or possibly the rat louse. Rat fleas are highly susceptible to infection, but appear to be unharmed by the process. *R. typhi* infects the flea's gut epithelial cells and is excreted along with these cells in the flea's feces. Humans are infected through skin abrasions. Neither the rat nor the rat flea succumb to the infection, so they constitute the reservoir of this disease.

Endemic typhus in humans. This human disease (Color Plate 14) is clinically similar to epidemic typhus. The symptoms of endemic typhus are milder, but otherwise the clinical symptoms and the diagnostic serology (see following) are the same. Recovery from endemic typhus provides protection against epidemic typhus because of the antigenic relatedness of these rickettsiae.

Control and treatment. Endemic typhus can be controlled by eliminating the rat population. An insecticide should be used prior to killing the rats to prevent the rat fleas from seeking a human host after the death of their rat host. Although endemic typhus is a worldwide problem, it is found in geographically isolated, infected rodent populations. In the United States, endemic typhus is geographically isolated in Texas, where 61 of the 81 cases reported in 1980 occurred. Patients with endemic typhus are treated with tetracycline or chloramphenicol.

Scrub typhus. Geographically isolated areas in Asia, the Pacific islands, and Australia harbor wild rodents infected with mites that carry scrub typhus. This disease is caused by *Rickettsia tsutsugamushi* (Japanese, *tsutsu,* something small and dangerous; *mushi,* mite). The bacteria live in both the rodents and in red mites *(Leptotrombidium);* it is not clear which is the more important reservoir. Mites spread the disease within the rodent population. Humans are incidental hosts that become infected when the mite larvae (chigger) attach to human skin and suck blood.

Scrub typhus in humans. Chills, fever, and intense headache develop 6 to 20 days after a human is bitten by an infected mite. An indurated papule often forms at the site of the mite bite. Pneumonitis and a rash develop, and the patient may suffer stupor and prostration. Immunity to the infecting strain develops on recovery from scrub typhus. This immunity does not extend to the many different strains of *R. tsutsugamushi,* so persons can get scrub typhus more than once. Treatment of patients with tetracycline is highly effective in curing the infection. Only Americans who travel to the Pacific islands, Australia, or Asia are exposed to scrub typhus. Most recent American cases occurred among military personnel serving in Southeast Asia.

Rickettsia: Spotted fever group diseases

The rickettsiae are named in recognition of the pioneering work on Rocky Mountain spotted fever done by H. T. Ricketts. The spotted fever group (Table 20–2) includes *Rickettsia rickettsii*, which causes Rocky Mountain spotted fever, and *Rickettsia akari,* which causes rickettsialpox in humans. These rickettsiae grow in both the cytoplasm and the nucleus of animal cells. Ticks and mites are the vectors for these bacterial diseases.

Rocky Mountain spotted fever. *Rickettsia rickettsii* is naturally found in ticks, which are the vector for the transmission of Rocky Mountain spotted fever in humans. The bacterium is found only in the Western Hemisphere, where it is maintained in the tick population by transovarian passage. Natural infections of rabbits, opossums, dogs, and rodents have been observed. Humans are incidental hosts who contract the disease during the bite of an infected tick.

Disease in humans. Rocky Mountain spotted fever is a seasonal disease that coincides with the tick season. The symptoms of this disease appear 1 to 2 weeks after the tick bite. The patient develops a fever, chills, prostration, and a rash. Unlike the rash in other rickettsial diseases, this rash begins on the extremities (ankles, wrists) and then spreads to the trunk. Recovery from Rocky Mountain spotted fever results in a solid immunity against reinfection. Patients may be effectively treated with chloramphenicol or tetracyclines.

Epidemiology, prevention, and control. Rocky Mountain spotted fever is the most significant rickettsial disease in the United States. It was first recognized in the Western Mountain States of Idaho and Montana, where the wood tick, *Dermacentor andersoni,* was found to be the vector and reservoir of the disease. Now, 50 to 69 percent of the cases of Rocky Mountain spotted fever occur in the south-eastern United States (see Figure 14–4), where the dog tick, *Dermacentor veriabilis,* is the major vector for transmitting this disease to humans.

Rocky Mountain spotted fever fatality rates in the different regions of the United States have varied from as high as 90 percent in the Bitterroot Valley of Montana to 25 percent in eastern Long Island, and to only 5 percent in the Snake River Valley of Idaho. The reason for these differences in virulence between strains of *R. rickettsii* is unknown. Now that Rocky Mountain spotted fever can be cured with antibiotics, the fatality rate is low (3 to 10 percent), and death is usually associated with a delay in diagnosing the disease.

R. rickettsii grow in many organs of the infected tick including the salivary glands and the ovaries. Infected ova give rise to infected larvae that metamorphose into adult ticks over a 2-year period. The infected adult ticks appear to be unharmed by the bacteria and can survive for as long as 4 years after infection. *R. rickettsii* is maintained in all reproductive stages of the tick by transovarian passage.

Rocky Mountain spotted fever is prevented by avoiding tick-infested areas and by observing tick bites for signs of inflammation. Rocky Mountain spotted fever can be successfully treated with tetracyclines and chloramphenicol when the disease is recognized at an early stage.

Rickettsialpox. *Rickettsia akari* is the obligate intracellular parasite of the spotted fever group that causes rickettsialpox in humans. The causative agent of rickettsialpox is a natural parasite of the house mouse that is transmitted by blood-sucking mites to humans who are incidental hosts (Figure 20–3).

Disease in humans. After an incubation period of 10 to 24 days, there is a sudden onset of fever accompanied by chills, sweating, headache, and backache. Within the next 1 to 4 days, a rash develops as a single crop of papules. These vesicular skin lesions are not present in any other rickettsial infections. An eschar develops at the site of the mite bite (Figure 20–4). This lesion is painless and lasts 3 to 4 weeks. Untreated patients usually recover within 1 to 2 weeks, whereas patients treated with chlorotetracyc-

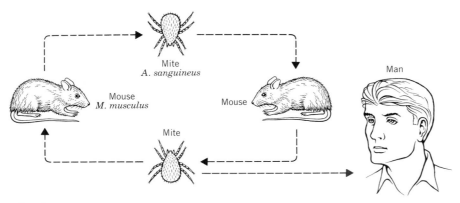

FIGURE 20–3
Maintenance of *Rickettsia akari* in nature. (Courtesy Dr. D. B. Lackman. From D. B. Lackman, *Clinical Pediatrics*, 2:296–301, 1963. Copyright © 1963, Lippincott.)

FIGURE 20–4
Rickettsialpox eschar formed at the site of an infection. (Courtesy Dr. D. B. Lackman. From D. B. Lackman, *Clinical Pediatrics*, 2:296–301, 1963. Copyright © 1963, Lippincott.)

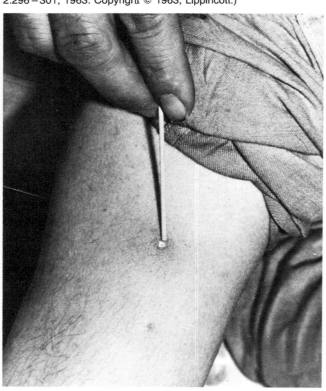

line or oxytetracycline usually recover within 48 hours.

Epidemiology. *R. akari* lives in the house mouse (*Mus musculus*) and is spread to other mice by mites (*Allodermanyssus sanguineus*). Humans are an incidental host. When mouse populations are high, the mites are content to live on their host mouse. As the mouse population drops, the mites seek another host, which may be a human. Prevention of rickettsialpox is accomplished by controlling the interactions between house mice and humans.

Diagnosis of rickettsial infections. Rickettsial infections elicit the formation of antibodies in the infected animal. By some quirk of nature, the rickettsial antigens that elicit these antibodies cross-react with antigens found in certain strains of *Proteus vulgaris*. *P. vulgaris* is an easy-to-grow, free-living bacterium, so it is an ideal source of these antigens. Three antigenically different strains of *P. vulgaris* are used in the Weil-Felix reaction to detect the cross-reacting antibodies in the rickettsial patient's serum (Table 20–3). Sera of patients infected with either *R. prowazekii* or *R. typhi* will agglutinate *Proteus* OX-19; however, the sera of patients with Brill-Zinsser disease are variable in their ability to agglutinate *Proteus* OX-19. Nevertheless, this disease appears to be a la-

TABLE 20–3
The Weil-Felix Reaction

Patient's Disease	Etiological Agent	Species of Proteus (Antigen)		
		OX–19	OX–2	OX–K
Epidemic typhus	R. prowazekii	+ + +[a]	–	–
Brill-Zinsser disease	R. prowazekii	–/+[b]	–	–
Endemic typhus	R. typhi	+ + +	–	–
Rocky Mountain spotted fever	R. rickettsii	+ + +	+ + +	–
Rickettsialpox	R. akari	–	–	–
Scrub typhus	R. tsutsugamushi	–	–	+ + +

[a]Indicates ability of patient's sera to agglutinate Proteus strains.
[b]Variable response.

tent infection of *R. prowazekii*. Rocky Mountain spotted fever patients contain antibodies that agglutinate both *Proteus* OX-19 and OX-2. This reaction differentiates infections of *R. rickettsii* from both the typhus group and from *R. akari*. Infections by *R. akari* do not elicit the formation of antibodies against any of the *Proteus* OX strains. Finally, *R. tsutsugamushi* infections elicit antibodies that agglutinate *Proteus* OX-K. Fluorescent antibody-staining techniques are used to detect the presence of specific *Rickettsia* in tissue samples (Figure 20–5). These serological tests can be used to distinguish the infectious agents involved in the rickettsial diseases.

COXIELLA BURNETII

The causative agent of Q fever is *Coxiella burnetii*, which was named after H. Cox. It is enzootic in a number of domestic animals including cattle, sheep, and goats and is found worldwide wherever these animals are domesticated. The genus *Coxiella* contains a single bacterium that is distinct from the other rickettsiae because it is remarkably resistant to chemical and physical agents; humans are infected by direct contact with contaminated fomites.

Coxiella grows in animal cells inside specialized vacuoles known as phagolysosomes. The phagolysosomes increase in size as the bacteria grow. Coxiella are released from infected animals in saliva, na-

sal secretions, and in the afterbirth of delivering animals. Outbreaks of Q fever correspond with the lambing season in areas where lambs are raised. Coxiella is amazingly resistant to desiccation, heat, and many chemical agents. In addition, it can survive in dried blood or on wool for more than 6 months, whereas cultures stored in skim milk at 15 to 20°C have survived for more than 2 years. Because coxiella are also very heat resistant, they are

FIGURE 20–5
Fluorescent antibody stain of *Rickettsia akari* in infected tissue culture cells. (Courtesy of Dr. D. B. Lackman).

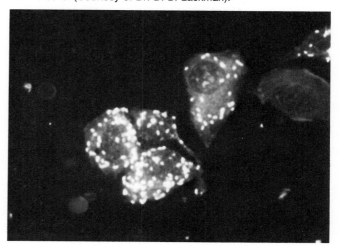

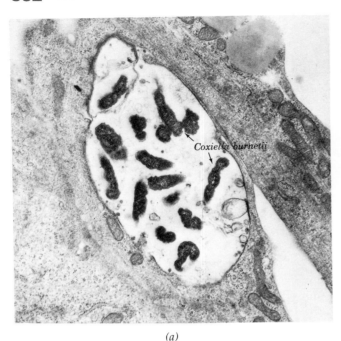
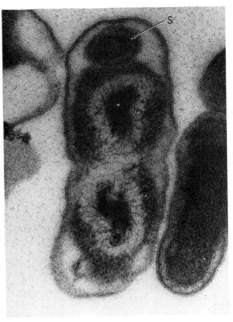

(a)
(b)

FIGURE 20–6

(a) *Coxiella burnetii* growing inside a vesicle of an infected L cell. (Courtesy of Dr. F. Eb. From F. Eb, J. Orfila, and J-F. Lefebure, *J. Microscopie Biol. Cell.*, 25:107–210, 1976.) (b) Formation of an endospore (s) by a cell of *Coxiella burnetii*. (Courtesy of Dr. J. C. Williams. From T. F. McCaul and J. C. Williams, *J. Bacteriol.*, 147:1063–1076, 1981, with permission of the American Society for Microbiology.)

used as the indicator organism for pasteurization. These unique characteristics may be explained by the recent observation that *Coxiella burnetii* form endosporelike structures during their intracellular growth (Figure 20–6).

Q fever

Coxiella burnetii causes a pneumonial (without a rash) disease in humans known as Q fever (Q for "query"). The bacterium is transmitted to humans in aerosols, not by arthropod vectors. In nature, however, the infection is transmitted between animal reservoirs by ticks. The disease manifests itself with a sudden onset of fever and chills. The organisms infect the human lungs where they cause symptoms resembling "atypical pneumonia." The human illness is readily cured with tetracyclines.

Q fever occurs worldwide. The organism is enzootic in domestic animals, which do not display outward signs of illness. Natural infections have been observed in large numbers of wild mammals and birds as well as in human body lice and ticks. Coxiella can be maintained in a tick population by transovarian passage. Domestic animals shed large numbers of these bacteria in milk, excreta, and placentas. Because of the mild nature of the human disease and the widespread infection of domestic animals, no major effort has been made to eradicate the causative agent.

CHLAMYDIA

Chlamydiae are nonmotile, spherical bacteria that are obligate intracellular parasites of animal cells (Figure 20–7). They have a unique reproductive cycle during which they grow in cytoplasmic vesicles of animal cells. Chlamydiae are dependent on their host cell to provide them with ATP. For this reason they are termed energy parasites. They metabolize glucose (Table 20–1), which further differentiates them from other rickettsias.

Growth of *Chlamydia*

Chlamydiae have a complex reproductive cycle that progresses through distinct stages. The **elementary body** (Figure 20–7) is the only growth stage of chlamydiae that is infectious. Elementary bodies are small cells packed with ribosomes. They have a thick, multilayered cell wall and contain RNA and

DNA in a ratio of 1:1. The elementary body is phagocytized by the host cell in a fashion that forms a vesicle in which the bacteria reproduce. In this vesicle, the elementary body changes into a larger thin-walled **reticulate (initial) body,** the chlamydial cell stage that grows and replicates by transverse fission (Figure 20–8). The ratio of RNA to DNA in the initial body is 4:1, which is indicative of protein synthesis. The process of infection, growth, and division takes between 24 and 78 hours. Initial bodies divide to form daughter cells that can change through the **intermediate body** (cells with dark centers) to form the condensed elementary bodies. The elementary body is the only infectious form of these bacteria and the only form to be released from the cell.

FIGURE 20–7

Electron micrograph of a Hela cell infected with *Chlamydia psittaci* that shows the three stages of the chlamydial reproduction cycle. The larger light bodies are the reticulate (R) cells, the large cells with dark centers are the intermediate (I) forms, and the smaller dark-staining cells are the elementary bodies (E). *Chlamydia* grow within a membrane-limited (↑) phagosome. 21,000X. (Courtesy of Dr. F. Eb. From F. Eb, J. Orfila, and J-F. Lefebure, *J. Microscopie Biol. Cell.,* 25:107–210, 1976.)

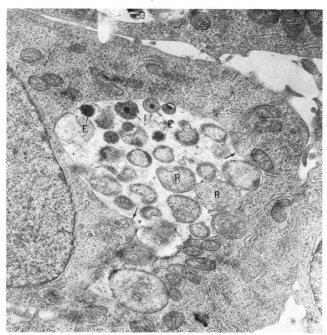

FIGURE 20–8

Electron micrograph of a Hela cell 24 hours after being infected with *Chlamydia psittaci.* Note the two dividing reticulate cells (▶◀). Elementary bodies (E) are more prevalent at this stage of infection. (Courtesy of Dr. F. Eb. From F. Eb, J. Orfila, and J-F. Lefebure, *J. Microscopie Biol. Cell.,* 25:107–210, 1976.)

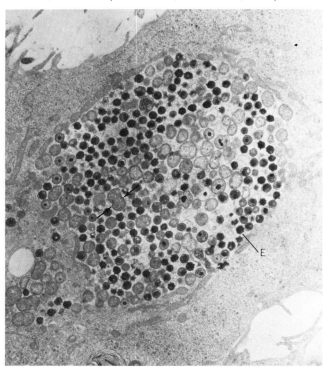

Chlamydial diseases in humans

There are two recognized species of *Chlamydia*, even though most experts presume that there are more because there are more than two human chlamydial diseases. Bacteria classified as *Chlamydia trachomatis* cause trachoma, nongonococcal urethritis, inclusion conjunctivitis, and lymphogranuloma venereum in humans (Table 20–4). Another species, *Chlamydia psittaci*, infects birds. Originally this species was isolated from parrots and other psittacine birds (Gr. *psittacus*, parrot), but now it is known to infect other birds as well. *C. psittaci* causes **psittacosis** (also known by the more general name—ornithosis) in humans.

Trachoma. The eye is unique in that the cornea and the underlying lens are avascular tissues. They contain no blood vessels to obstruct the passage of light, so these tissues derive all their nutrients from the eye's aqueous humor. *Chlamydia trachomatis* can infect the conjunctiva of the eye, causing a severe inflammation. In trachoma, lymphocytes, polymorphonuclear neutrophiles, and macrophages enter the area and form follicles beneath the conjunctival surface. These changes stimulate vascularization of the cornea, which can lead to permanent corneal scarring and blindness. Trachoma is a serious illness in the Middle East, where it is so prevalent that most children are infected during early childhood. The etiological agent is transmitted by direct contact or by towels and other inanimate objects. Trachoma is the leading cause of blindness in the world. It is estimated that 400 million people have this disease and more than 2 million people have been permanently blinded by it.

Trachoma can be treated with topical applications of sulfonamides and by systemic administration of tetracyclines. The host responds to this infection by producing immunoglobulins of the A class—secreted in the tears—and by developing a cell-mediated immune response. Reinfections or relapses do occur because immunity to trachoma is not long lasting.

Inclusion conjunctivitis. Inclusion conjunctivitis is clinically different from trachoma even though both diseases are caused by serologically related bacteria of the same species. Asymptomatic *C. trachomatis* infections of the adult female cervix appear to be epidemic in the developed countries. The eyes of newborns are infected with *C. trachomatis* during birth. This infection develops into inclusion conjunctivitis, which is many times more common than gonococcal ophthalmia neonatorum (see Chapter 18). The infection appears 2 to 25 days after birth and is recognized as an inflamed conjunctiva with a purulent ex-

TABLE 20–4
Human Diseases Caused by *Chlamydia*

Disease	Etiological Agent	Usual Mode of Transmission	Chemotherapy
Trachoma	*C. trachomatis*	Direct contact or via fomites	Sulfonamides, tetracyclines
Inclusion conjunctivitis	*C. trachomatis*	Newborns infected at parturition, fomites, unchlorinated swimming pools	Topical tetracyclines
Nongonococcal urethritis		Adult sexual contact	Tetracyclines
Lymphogranuloma venereum	*C. trachomatis* (rare *C. psittaci*)	Sexual intercourse	Sulfonamides, tetracyclines
Ornithosis	*C. psittaci*	Inhalation of bird feces	Tetracyclines

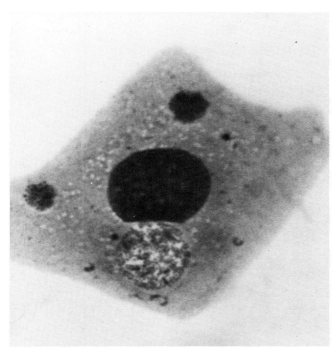

FIGURE 20–9
Chlamydial inclusion cell. A Giemsa stain of a conjunctival scraping from an infant with chlamydial conjunctivitis. 1000X. (Courtesy of Dr. N. M. Jacobs.)

udate. Inclusions of *C. trachomatis* cells are visible in Giemsa-stained conjunctival scrapings (Figure 20–9) and are used in diagnosis. The infection spontaneously clears over several months without permanent damage to the eye. Newborns can be treated with systemic antibiotics such as sulfonamides or erythromycin.

Inclusion conjunctivitis in adults begins in a clinical fashion similar to trachoma, but it never progresses to the chronic stage. Human eyes are infected when contaminated towels or fingers transfer *C. trachomatis* from exudates of the eye or the genitourinary tract to the eyes. Swimming in contaminated, unchlorinated pools is another source of the infection. Women are the natural reservoir of *C. trachomatis*, which is maintained and spread among humans by sexual contact. The disease causes in-

flammation of the conjunctiva, accompanied by a purulent exudate. No blindness results from this infection because vascularization of the cornea does not occur. Even though the disease is self-limiting, it is conveniently treated with systemic administration of tetracyclines or sulfonamides. Prevention is difficult because of the asymptomatic venereal nature of the infection in the human reservoir. Chlorination of swimming pools and good personal hygiene are important in controlling inclusion conjunctivitis.

Nongonococcal urethritis.   *C. trachomatis* causes venereal diseases that are remarkably similar to gonococcal infections. They are designated as *nongonococcal urethritis*. *C. trachomatis* causes urethritis and epididymitis in males, and it causes pelvic inflammatory disease in females. A large percentage of sexually active gonorrhea patients (30 to 50 percent) are coinfected with *C. trachomatis*. These patients are often incompletely diagnosed, which is a problem because the normal treatment for gonorrhea does not cure the patient of nongonococcal urethritis. This disease is a major problem in the United States in part because of the asymptomatic nature of this infection. Serious infections in females can lead to pelvic inflammatory disease. Tetracyclines are effective drugs for treating nongonococcal urethritis.

Lymphogranuloma venereum.   Certain serological strains of *C. trachomatis*, and more rarely *C. psittaci*, cause the venereal disease called lymphogranuloma venereum (LGV). This disease is recognized by the damage it causes to the regional lymph nodes of the groin. Transmission is restricted to sexual contact. After an incubation period of 3 days to 3 weeks, a vesicular lesion (similar to a herpes lesion) appears on the genitals. The vesicle is painless and soon heals without scarring. The bacteria infect the regional lymph nodes, which become enlarged, tender, and suppurative 1 to 2 months after infection. LGV can result in the permanent blockage of the lymphatic drainage from the groin. Between 199 and 756 cases per year were reported in the United States during the 1970s.

Diagnosis and treatment. LGV can be diagnosed by a complement-fixation test and by a clinical examination of the inguinal lymph glands for swelling. Patients are treated with tetracyclines or sulfonamides. Surgical drainage of enlarged lymph nodes (buboes) may be necessary to prevent them from rupturing.

Ornithosis (Psittacosis). Many species of birds are reservoirs for chlamydiae that cause ornithosis in birds and humans. Ornithosis occurs in flocks of domestic birds (such as turkeys) and in wild birds placed under stressful or crowded conditions. Ornithosis was first observed in parrots, so the causative agent was named *Chlamydia psittaci.* Diseased birds discharge the bacteria in their feces and in exudates from their noses and eyes. Widespread infection within a domestic flock has resulted in mortality rates as high as 30 percent.

Humans become infected by handling domestic or pet birds or by inhaling *C. psittaci* found in dried exudates or feces. The disease in humans can be asymptomatic, or it can develop into a severe and sometimes fatal pneumonia. The incubation period varies from 1 to 3 weeks. Human ornithosis begins abruptly with chills, fever, headache, and the symptoms of atypical pneumonia.

Ornithosis is diagnosed serologically by measuring an increasing titer of antibodies against chlamydia-family antigens using complement fixation or the fluorescent antibody techniques. The diagnosis is confirmed when chlamydiae from blood or sputum samples are grown in embryonated chicken eggs or tissue cultures. The pneumonial symptoms of human ornithosis can be eliminated by tetracycline therapy.

SUMMARY

Rickettsia and *Chlamydia* species are obligate parasitic bacteria that grow in animal tissue. Rickettsiae are able to produce ATP when they are incubated with

TABLE 20–5
Summary of Human Rickettsial and Chlamydial Diseases

Disease	Etiological Agent	Vector	Reservoir	Symptoms
Epidemic typhus	*R. prowazekii*	Body louse	Humans	Stupor, prostration, sudden fever, chills, rash on trunk
Endemic typhus	*R. typhi*	Rat flea	Rat	Same as above
Scrub typhus	*R. tsutsugamushi*	Mite	Rodent	Stupor, prostration, pneumonitis
Rocky Mountain spotted fever	*R. rickettsii*	Ticks	Ticks	Fever, chills, rash (extremities to trunk)
Rickettsialpox	*R. akari*	Mouse	Mites	Fever, chills, headache, rash, crop of papules
Q fever	*Cox. burnetii*	None	Aerosol	Fever, chills, pneumonia
Trachoma	*C. trachomatis*	Fomites	Humans	Inflammation of eyes, vascularized cornea
Inclusion conjunctivitis	*C. trachomatis*	Fomites, parturition, swimming pools	Humans	Inflammation of eyes of newborns and adults
Nongonococcal urethritis	*C. trachomatis*	Sexual contact	Humans	Urethritis, pelvic inflammatory disease
LGV	*C. trachomatis*	Sexual contact	Humans	Vesicular lesion, lymph-node swelling
Ornithosis	*C. psittaci*	Exudates	Birds	Mild to severe pneumonia

glutamate and oxygen. Chlamydiae cannot produce ATP, so they are energy parasites that depend on their host cell for energy. Because these bacteria are obligate parasites, they exist in an animal reservoir in nature; most are transmitted by arthropod or insect vectors.

The human rickettsial pathogens are classified in the genera *Rickettsia* and *Coxiella*. The *Rickettsia* that cause human diseases (Table 20–5) belong to the typhus group, the scrub typhus group, or the spotted fever group. *R. prowazekii* is transmitted between human reservoirs by lice and causes a severe form of typhus fever in humans. *R. typhi* is naturally found in rats and is transmitted to humans by the rat flea. Humans are incidental hosts for this bacterium, which causes endemic (murine) typhus. Scrub typhus is caused by *R. tsutsugamushi* and is limited to Asia and the Pacific islands. This bacterium exists in geographically isolated populations of rodents and is transmitted to humans by the chiggers of mites.

Rickettsia rickettsii causes Rocky Mountain spotted fever in humans. Ticks are both the reservoir and the vector for *R. rickettsii,* which is maintained in the tick population by transovarian passage. Humans are incidental hosts for *R. akari,* which causes rickettsialpox when it is transferred from its reservoir, house mice, to humans by mites. Rickettsial diseases are diagnosed by serology using the Weil-Felix test, by direct isolation in embryonated eggs or tissue culture, and by fluorescent antibody-staining techniques. The rickettsial diseases in humans are treated with chloramphenicol or tetracyclines.

Coxiella burnetii is remarkably resistant to physical and chemical agents, it grows in vacuoles, and it causes Q fever in humans. Endosporelike structures have been seen in electron micrographs of purified cell suspensions. Domestic animals are the natural reservoirs for *C. burnetii,* which is transferred to humans in aerosols.

Chlamydia trachomatis causes trachoma, inclusion conjunctivitis, nongonococcal urethritis, and lymphogranuloma venereum (LGV). *C. trachomatis* exists asymptomatically in the female cervix. Newborns are contaminated during birth, and adults are contaminated by direct contact with infected persons. Trachoma leads to vascularization of the cornea and blindness, whereas inclusion conjunctivitis is a less severe infection of the conjunctiva. Nongonococcal urethritis and LGV are venereal diseases that are caused by certain serotypes of *C. trachomatis*. Ornithosis is a bird disease caused by *C. psittaci* that can be transmitted to humans by the inhalation of dried, contaminated exudates and feces. Tetracyclines and sulfonamides are used in the effective treatment of chlamydial infections.

QUESTIONS AND TOPICS FOR STUDY AND DISCUSSION

Questions

1. Describe the physiological reasons behind the obligate parasitism of the rickettsiae and the chlamydiae.
2. How is *Coxiella burnetii* different from the other rickettsiae? How do these differences affect the diseases it causes?
3. Describe the different morphological stages in the growth cycle of *Chlamydia psittaci*.
4. What is Brill-Zinsser disease? How is this disease related to epidemic typhus?
5. Compare epidemic typhus to endemic typhus. Which is currently the more prevalent disease? Explain.
6. Why are reservoirs and vectors necessary for the perpetuation of the rickettsial diseases?
7. Are seasonal and geographic considerations important in diagnosing rickettsial diseases? Give examples to support your answer.
8. Explain how *Proteus* is used in the diagnosis of rickettsial diseases.
9. Describe the diseases of the eye caused by the chlamydiae.
10. What problems are associated with diagnosing nongonococcal urethritis?
11. How would you control the spread of psittacosis?

Discussion

1. The rickettsiae were once thought to be viruses. Do you think they are more like viruses or bacteria?
2. Is there a rationale for believing that there are more than two species of *Chlamydia*?

FURTHER READINGS

Books

Hubbert, W. T., W. F. McCulloch, and P. R. Schnurrenberger (eds.), *Diseases Transmitted from Animals to Man,* 6th ed., Charles C Thomas, Springfield, Ill., 1975. A collection of articles on the arthropod-borne bacterial diseases of humans written by experts in their respective fields.

Articles and Reviews

Becker, Y., "The Chlamydia: Molecular Biology of Procaryotic Obligate Parasites of Eucaryocytes," *Microbiol. Revs.,* 42:274–306 (1978). A review of the biology of the chlamydiae that details the life cycle of these bacteria.

Weiss, E., "Growth and Physiology of Rickettsiae," *Bacteriol. Revs.* 37:259–283 (1973). An early review of the growth and metabolism of selected members of the rickettsiae.

21

OTHER PATHOGENIC BACTERIA

The pathogenic bacteria that do not fit neatly into the other classification groups are for convenience described in this chapter. Some of them are listed as "of uncertain affiliation" in *Bergey's Manual*, and one was first described after the latest edition of the manual was published. The mycoplasmas, unique bacteria that permanently lack cell walls, are also discussed here.

Hemophilus, Bordetella, Francisella, and *Brucella* are short, Gram-negative, coccoid to rod-shaped bacteria that grow aerobically. The genus *Hemophilus* contains a number of pathogenic species that cause human diseases ranging in clinical severity from meningitis and pneumonia to conjunctivitis. Members of the genus *Bordetella* cause whooping cough in humans, whereas *Francisella tularensis* causes tularemia and species of *Brucella* cause brucellosis. Legionnaires' disease is a recently described human illness caused by *Legionella pneumophila*. Mycoplasmas are small, cell-wall-lacking bacteria. *Mycoplasma pneumoniae* is the major human pathogen in this group; it causes atypical pneumonia.

HEMOPHILUS

Species of *Hemophilus* are small, Gram-negative, coccoid to rod-shaped bacteria that cause disease only in humans. *Hemophilus* (Gr., *haemophilus*, blood-loving) is an appropriate name for these bacteria that grow on blood-based media. Many normal humans carry *Hemophilus influenzae* as a symbiont in their nasopharynx. It rarely causes disease in adults, but it is a major cause of meningitis in young children. Other pathogenic species of this genus include *H. ducreyi*, which causes the venereal disease known as chancroid, and *H. aegypticus*, which causes a highly contagious form of conjunctivitis.

Hemophilus influenzae

History and physiology.   For many years, *Hemophilus influenzae* was the bacterium commonly isolated from influenza patients; therefore it was thought to cause influenza. Following the discovery of the influenza virus, investigators realized that *H. influenzae*

359

does not cause influenza, but rather it is a secondary invader. *H. influenzae* also causes obstructive epiglottitis and is the most common cause of bacterial meningitis in toddler-aged children.

Hemophilus influenzae was first isolated in 1892 by Richard Pfeiffer, who grew it on a blood-based laboratory medium. This bacterium requires two blood factors for growth: the X factor and the V factor. The X factor can be replaced by hematin or hemoglobin, and the V factor can be replaced by NAD. All members of the *Hemophilus* genus are facultative anaerobes that can be grown on defined media containing the X and/or V factors. Some strains also require 5 to 10 percent CO_2 for growth. *Hemophilus* strains can be isolated on chocolate blood agar incubated at 37°C in an aerobic environment. Species within the genus *Hemophilus* are characterized by their requirements for the X factor, the V factor, and for CO_2.

The virulence of *H. influenzae* is directly related to the presence of a capsule. There are six (a to f) different capsular antigens. Almost all serious *H. influenzae* infections are caused by the strains with the type-b capsular antigen. Capsulated strains grow as smooth iridescent colonies.

Disease in humans. Between 30 and 50 percent of young children are asymptomatic carriers of *H. influenzae*. Most of these strains are noncapsulated avirulent strains; the few that are capsulated are almost always type b. The diseases caused by virulent strains often begin as nasopharyngitis that accompanies or follows a respiratory viral infection. Otitis media, sinusitis, pneumonia, and meningitis can follow *Hemophilus* nasopharyngitis. Meningitis is the most serious consequence of infections by this organism.

Hemophilus influenzae is the major cause of bacterial meningitis in children between the ages of 6 months and 1 year. The bacteria spread from the respiratory tract to the blood to the meninges. During the first 6 months of life, children possess circulating antibodies that are bactericidal for *H. influenzae* (Figure 21–1). These maternal antibodies disappear from the blood by the time the child is 6 months old, and they do not reappear until the child is about 3½ years old. The incidence of meningitis is greatest (6 to 18 months) when these circulating antibodies are absent from the blood. Fatality rates in untreated cases of *H. influenzae* meningitis are between 90 and 100 percent. Between 1500 and 2000 deaths caused by *H. influenzae* occur each year in the United States.

Ampicillin and chloramphenicol are effective chemotherapeutic agents for treating *Hemophilus* meningitis. Some strains are resistant to ampicillin because they produce β lactamase, so both ampicillin and chloramphenicol are recommended for initial therapy. The long-term sequelae of *Hemophilus* meningitis are of serious concern for the patients who recover. In one study of 40 patients, six patients were so severely affected that they required custodial care. Another one-third of the group suffered a wide variety of handicaps including behavioral problems, deafness, and speech impediments.

Hemophilus as a secondary pathogen. *Hemophilus* can cause bacterial pneumonia in debilitated influenza patients; it has also been isolated from patients with chronic bronchitis. Influenza is a viral disease (see Chapter 23) that greatly decreases a patient's ability to resist infection. Influenza patients are susceptible to secondary invasions by *H. influenzae*, which causes pneumonia. These infections contribute to the greater than normal mortality rate among the elderly from viral influenza. **Obstructive epiglottitis** is an infrequent disease that is caused by *H. influenzae*. In this disease, the bacteria spread from the pharynx to the epiglottis and then to the larynx. The swelling of the larynx obstructs the trachea to the extent that an emergency tracheotomy is often necessary to save the patient's life.

Immunity. Most persons develop an immune response to *H. influenzae* prior to adolescence. Normal adults possess bactericidal antibodies formed in response to trivial respiratory infections of *H. influenzae*. This immunity is normally directed against the type-b strain, which is the major etiological agent in *Hemophilus* infections.

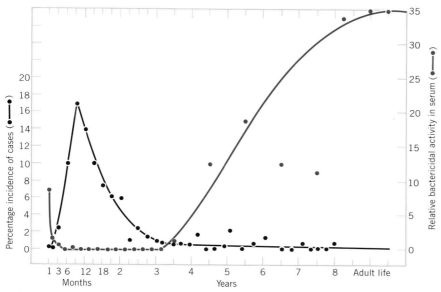

FIGURE 21–1

Relation of age to *Hemophilus influenzae* meningitis and the level of bactericidal antibodies in the blood. (From L. D. Fothergill and J. Wright, *J. Immunology*, 24:273–284, 1933. Copyright © 1933, The Williams & Wilkins Co.)

Other pathogenic *Hemophilus*

Hemophilus aegypticus is responsible for a purulent human conjunctivitis in hot climates. This pathogen is highly contagious and causes the disease commonly known as **pinkeye.** *Hemophilus aegypticus* is also known as the Koch-Weeks bacillus; however, it is so similar to *H. influenzae* that its status as a separate species is being questioned.

Hemophilus ducreyi causes a localized soft chancre in the genital region. This venereal disease is known as **chancroid** (soft chancre). It is most common among nonwhite, uncircumsized men: only about 10 percent of the cases occur in women. The infection begins as a lesion in the genital or perianal area and then spreads to the adjacent lymphatic glands. A diagnosis of chancroid is commonly made on clinical grounds, followed by the isolation of these bacteria on special media. Chancroid is treated with sulfoxazole or selected antibiotics.

BORDETELLA

Whooping cough in humans is caused by *Bordetella pertussis* and less commonly by *Bordetella parapertussis* (L., *pertussis*, severe cough). Jules Bordet and Octave Gengou first identified *B. pertussis* in 1900. This bacterium is morphologically similar to *Hemophilus*, but it requires neither the X nor the V factor for growth. Whooping cough is a serious disease of newborns who have no maternal antibodies against *B. pertussis*. Now whooping cough is controlled by the widespread use of the DTP vaccine.

Bordetella pertussis

Growth and physiology. *Bordetella pertussis* is a small, nonmotile, Gram-negative bacterium that grows aerobically on media with charcoal, starch, blood, or blood products. These additives protect the bacteria by inhibiting the toxic activity of unsaturated fatty acids. *B. pertussis* grows on potato-glyc-erol-blood agar into smooth, nearly transparent col-onies surrounded by a zone of hemolysis.

Newly isolated *B. pertussis* produces smooth colo-nies that contain encapsulated cells. During pro-longed laboratory cultivation, these bacteria lose their capsular antigens concomitantly with their change to a rough colonial morphology. The respi-ratory tract of humans is the only natural source of *B. pertussis*.

Whooping cough in humans. *Bordetella pertussis* in-fects the human trachea and grows preferentially on the ciliated epithelial cells of the bronchi (Figure 21–2). Infections are most prominent in children. The clinical symptoms that are observed after an average 10-day incubation period include a mild cough, sneezing, and inflammation of the nasal mucous membranes. During the next 10 to 14 days, the in-fection spreads to the lower respiratory tract. Pa-tients have a severe cough that is characterized by the whooping sound of inspired air. Vomiting is common. If sufficient mucus accumulates in the bronchi, the patient also suffers anoxia and even convulsions. During the later stages of whooping cough, lymphocytes are found in the bronchi. The whooping cough lasts approximately 2 weeks and is followed by a milder cough that lasts an additional 2 to 3 weeks.

Immunity. Recovery from whooping cough pro-vides resistance to subsequent infections, but recov-ery does not provide complete protection. Second attacks result in a less severe disease when they do occur. Active immunization of all children at 2 months is advocated because children have little or no maternal immunity against *B. pertussis*. Immuni-zation is effected by injection of killed cells of encap-sulated *B. pertussis* that are one component of the DTP vaccine. Three injections are given at 1-month intervals; then booster shots are given 1 and 5 years later.

Epidemiology and treatment. Whooping cough is a highly contagious disease that occurs throughout the world. Most nonimmunized individuals acquire

whooping cough during childhood. The mild form of this disease needs no specific treatment, whereas severe whooping cough is treated with erythromy-cin, chloramphenicol, or tetracycline. Antibiotic therapy rapidly renders the patient noninfectious even though the clinical symptoms usually persist.

There has been a steady decline in the incidence of whooping cough (Figure 21–3) since the wide-spread use of the pertussis vaccine began in the 1950s. Currently, there is a low but constant level of this disease in the United States.

FIGURE 21–2

Electron micrograph of *Bordetella pertussis* associated with cultured hamster tracheal cells. Note the 9 pairs plus 2 structure of the tracheal cilia. (Reprinted from A. M. Collier, L. P. Peterson, and J. B. Baseman, *J. Infect. Dis. Suppl.*, 136S:5196–5203, 1977, by permission of The University of Chicago Press.)

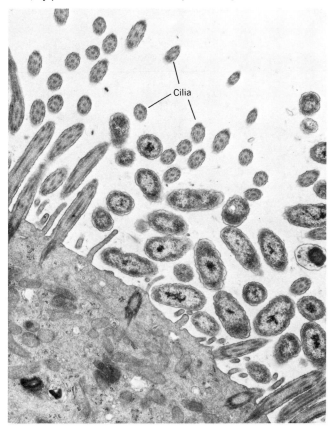
Cilia

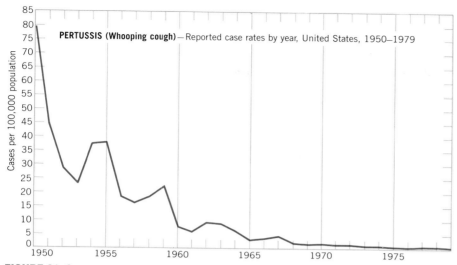

FIGURE 21–3

Incidence of whooping cough in the United States from 1950 to 1980. (Centers for Disease Control, "Annual Summary 1979: Reported Morbidity and Mortality in the United States," *Morbidity Mortality Weekly Report*, 28, No. 54, 1980.)

FRANCISELLA

A plaguelike disease in ground squirrels in Tulare County, California, led to the isolation of *Francisella tularensis* in 1912 by George McCoy and Charles Chapin. Edward Francis later did extensive field, laboratory, and clinical studies on this organism and described the human illness known as **tularemia**. *Francisella tularensis* is named after Edward Francis and Tulare County, California.

Francisella tularensis

Morphology and physiology. *Francisella tularensis* is a very small (0.2 by 0.2 to 0.7 μm), nonmotile, Gram-negative, coccoid to elipsoid rod that often shows bipolar staining. It grows aerobically on a complex medium and has a requirement for high amounts of cystine (see Appendix 1 for structure) in the medium. The slow-growing bacterium can be isolated on cystine-glucose-blood agar following 2 to 5 days of incubation at 37°C. Cells grown in culture are pleomorphic and possess cell morphologies that

range from spherical to bean-shaped to filamentous. *Francisella tularensis* is naturally found in stream water and in animals. Rabbits and ground squirrels are the natural carriers and are the major reservoir for human infections. Muskrats, beavers, opossums, coyotes, deer, red foxes, woodchucks, skunks, rats, mice, dogs, cats, and lambs are also known to be naturally infected.

Tularemia

Three clinical manifestations of tularemia occur in humans: ulceroglandular, pneumonic, and typhoidal. **Ulceroglandular tularemia** results from the primary infection of the skin. The skin is infected through the bite of a fly or tick—the known vectors—or by direct contact with the organisms present in infected animal tissue. Hunters and trappers are exposed to infection when they field-dress rabbits or skin small fur-bearing animals. *Francisella tularensis* establishes an infection after penetrating skin abrasions or mucous membranes. Ulceroglandular tularemia is characterized by an ulcerous papule that

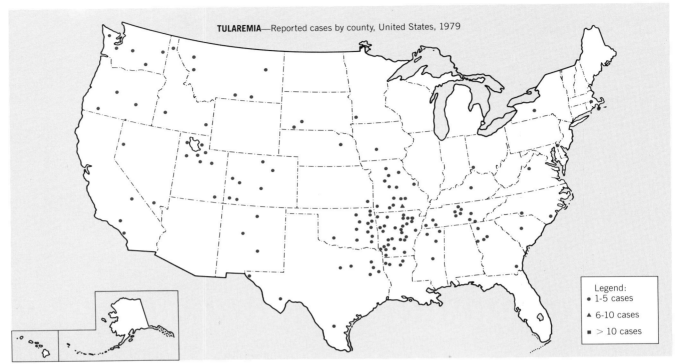

FIGURE 21–4
Geographical distribution of tularemia in the United States by county in 1979. (Centers for Disease Control, "Annual Summary 1979: Reported Morbidity and Mortality in the United States," *Morbidity Mortality Weekly Report*, 28, No. 54, 1980.)

forms at the site of entry. *Francisella tularensis* can also infect the conjunctiva to cause **ocularglandular tularemia.**

Disseminated tularemia is initiated by two distinct routes and can be caused by as few as 10 bacteria. **Pneumonic tularemia** is transmitted by inhalation of *F. tularensis* in aerosols. This disease is mainly an occupational hazard of laboratory personnel. **Typhoid tularemia** results from ingestion of improperly cooked contaminated meats.

After penetrating the skin or the mucous membranes of the oropharynx-gastrointestinal tract, the bacteria enter the regional lymph nodes. Infected lymph nodes become enlarged, tender, and suppurative. From the lymph nodes the bacteria enter the blood and cause a transitionary bacteremia. Next

these bacteria infect the lungs, liver, and spleen to cause the acute phase of disseminated tularemia. An incubation period of 3 to 10 days transpires prior to the appearance of the clinical symptoms of a headache, fever, and general malaise. Untreated tularemia has a greater fatality rate in the pneumonic and typhoid forms (30 percent) than in the ulceroglandular form.

Treatment and immunity.   Streptomycin is the antibiotic of choice for treating tularemia. Chloramphenicol and tetracycline are also effective, but they must be administered for a long period of time to eliminate recurrent infections. Recovery from tularemia results in partial protection against reinfection. A vaccine for preventing tularemia is available for protecting high-risk individuals, but even this is not completely satisfactory. On two occasions, vaccinated laboratory workers twice became ill with tularemia.

Epidemiology. The incidence of tularemia in the United States has decreased greatly since 2291 cases were reported in 1939. Between 129 and 234 cases per year were reported in the United States during the 1970s, and most of these cases occurred in Arkansas and Missouri (Figure 21–4). The incidence of tularemia is seasonal: it corresponds to winter rabbit-hunting season and the summer tick and fly seasons. One outbreak of tularemia in Vermont was traced to muskrats trapped or shot in three streams that feed into Lake Champlain. The 72 persons who became ill had each handled the pelts or the carcasses of skinned muskrats. Most cases of tularemia occur in the summer months, when humans spend time in the woods and fields where the vectors of *F. tularensis* (ticks and flies) live. Tularemia appears to be restricted to the Northern Hemisphere, for it has not been reported south of the equator.

BRUCELLA

The brucellae are natural parasites of domestic animals, which in turn are the major source of human brucellosis. The genus is named after Sir David Bruce, who first isolated *Brucella* from the spleens of British soldiers who had died of Malta fever. This febrile disease plagued the British troops stationed on the island of Malta. Bruce traced the source of the infection to the island's goat milk. As soon as the troops stopped drinking milk from the island's goat herd, Malta fever disappeared.

Brucellae are aerobic, Gram-negative, nonmotile, short, spherical to rod-shaped bacteria. They are morphologically similar to bacteria in the genus *Francisella* except that they do not show bipolar staining and pleomorphism is uncommon. They grow aerobically on laboratory media containing a variety of amino acids and vitamins. The major species that cause brucellosis in humans are differentiated by their metabolic and physiological reactions (Table 21–1). These bacteria infect domestic animals and preferentially grow in the uterus or the mammary glands of these animals. *Brucella melitensis* infects sheep and goats; *B. abortus* infects and causes abortions in cattle; *B. suis* infects domestic and wild pigs; and *B. canis* infects dogs.

Brucellosis

The incubation period for human brucellosis is usually several weeks or even months. The brucellae enter the body through broken skin, through the alimentary tract, or through the conjunctivae. They

TABLE 21–1
Metabolic Characteristics of *Brucella*

Biotype	Natural Host	CO$_2$ Required	H$_2$S Produced	Hydro-lysis Urea	Growth on Dye Media		Oxidative Metabolism		
					Thionine[a]	Basic Fuchsin[b]	Alanine	Ribose	Lysine
B. melitensis	Goats, sheep	−	−	Variable	−	+	+	−	−
B. abortus	Cattle	+/−[c]	+	Slow	−	+	+	+	−
B. suis	Swine	−	+/−	Fast	+	+/−	−	+	+
B. canis	Dogs	−	−	Fast	+	−	−	+	+

[a]Certified dye at a concentration of 1:25,000.
[b]Certified dye at a concentration of 1:50,000.
[c]+/− indicates variability among biotypes.

invade the lymphatic system, where they multiply within polymorphonuclear lymphocytes. At this stage of the disease, the bacteria either are destroyed or are carried from the lymphatics by the blood to infect the liver, spleen, bone marrow, and kidneys. In certain mammals, the brucellae are found in (a) mammary glands, where they are excreted in milk, and/or in (b) the uterus, where they cause abortions in pregnant animals. Brucellae have been isolated from the blood or urine of two human patients who had naturally aborted.

Brucellosis in humans. Clinical symptoms of human brucellosis appear gradually and include fever, chills, malaise, body ache, sweating, and headache. The presence of an intermittent fever has endowed this disease with the trivial name of **undulant fever.** The disease is diagnosed by cultivating the causative agent from the patient's blood, urine, or from a biopsy of liver, bone marrow, or lymph node. In humans, the illness lasts approximately 4 weeks and is similar in symptoms and duration regardless of the infecting species.

Epidemiology. Milk and milk products were once the major source of human brucellosis, so this disease occurred primarily among rural families who consumed unpasteurized dairy products. Currently, brucellosis is more prevalent among livestock handlers and workers in the meat-processing industry (Table 21–2).

The incidence of brucellosis in the United States has steadily dropped from a high of 6,321 cases in 1947 to between 183 and 310 cases per year during the 1970s. During a recent decade (1965 to 1974), 52.4 percent of the 2,047 cases reported in the United States were associated with the meat-processing industry (Table 21–2). Another 17.3 percent were associated with the livestock industry and 30.3 percent of the cases were associated with individuals in undesignated occupations. Only 9 percent of the cases of brucellosis could be attributed to dairy products as the probable source. This same study showed that 51 percent of the brucellae isolated from humans were *B. suis*, 20.9 percent were *B. abortus*, 10.8 percent were *B. melitensis*, and 2.6 percent were *B. canis*.

TABLE 21–2
Most Probable Source of Brucellosis

Source	Occupational Group		
	Meat-processing	Livestock Industry	Unassigned
Domestic animals			
Swine	702	54	39
Cattle	121	179	52
Swine or cattle	186	60	45
Sheep or goats	7	5	6
Unspecified animal	57	4	2
Dogs	0	0	6
Wild animals			
Caribou, moose			
Deer, feral swine	0	0	21
Accidents			
Vaccine	0	31	0
Laboratory	0	0	34
Milk products	0	9	182

Source: Cases reported in the United States, 1965–1974. Adapted from M. D. Fox and A. F. Kaufmann, *J. Infect. Disease*, 136:313–316, 1977.

Treatment and control. Streptomycin and tetracycline are effective antibiotics for treating brucellosis. Since streptomycin does not eliminate the organisms within the leukocytes, it is common practice to administer both streptomycin and tetracycline concurrently or to treat patients with tetracycline. The therapy should be continued for 3 to 4 weeks to assure against a relapse. Elimination of brucellosis from cattle, sheep, and goats can be accomplished by diagnosis and slaughter and/or by vaccination of all young animals. A cooperative state-federal brucellosis eradication program, in effect since 1931, is designed to control brucellosis in cattle. This program currently diagnoses and reports on brucellosis in herds of cattle, sheep, and goats.

LEGIONELLA

During July 1976, the American Legion held its 58th annual convention in Philadelphia. A significant number of legionnaires who attended became ill with a puzzling disease that was characterized by fever, coughing, and pneumonia. The illness appeared from the second day of the convention and continued into August. As reports of the illness became available to the Pennsylvania Department of Health and the news media, people realized that a major outbreak of an unexplained pneumonic disease had occurred. The news media labeled the illness legionnaires' disease; it is also referred to as **legionellosis.**

Legionella pneumophila

The causative agent of legionnaires' disease was finally isolated in January 1977. Investigators from the Centers for Disease Control inoculated guinea pigs with ground-up tissue from a diseased patient (Figure 21–5). These experiments were modeled after the isolation techniques used for *Coxiella burnetii,* which causes a similar febrile disease known as Q fever. A number of guinea pigs became ill with fever, and bacteria were visible in stained tissue samples from their spleens. The ground-up spleen tissue was inoculated into embryonated eggs. Yolk-sac membranes from these eggs contained an apparently pure culture of a rod-shaped bacterium (Figure 21–6).

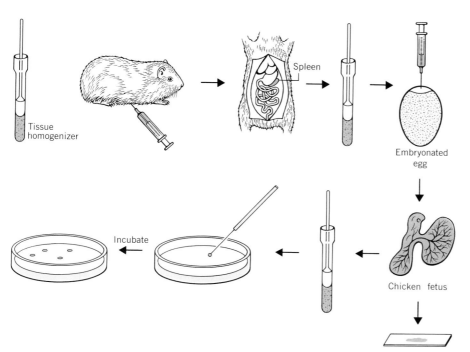

Tissue homogenizer

Spleen

Embryonated egg

Incubate

Chicken fetus

FIGURE 21–5
Initial isolation of *Legionella pneumophila.* A specimen from an infected patient was homogenized and then injected into a guinea pig. The spleen from an ill guinea pig was homogenized and used to infect an embryonated egg. The bacteria that grew in the chicken embryo could be seen in the light microscope. Colonies of *L. pneumophila* were then grown on Mueller-Hinton medium.

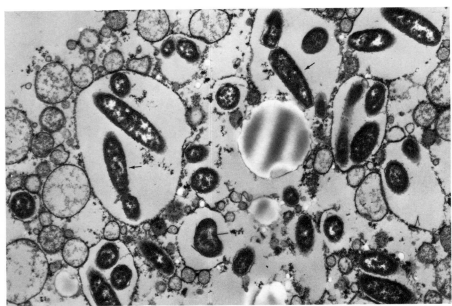

FIGURE 21–6
Electron micrograph of *Legionella pneumophila* (↑) growing in the yolk sac of an infected embryonated egg. (Courtesy of Dr. Francis W. Chandler, Centers for Disease Control, Atlanta.)

With the organism in hand, the CDC researchers tested the sera from legionnaires' disease patients for the presence of antibodies against their newly isolated organism. They used the indirect fluorescent antibody test and showed that patients with the disease had high titers of antibodies against their isolate. They named this newly isolated bacterium *Legionella pneumophila.*

Legionella pneumophila can be grown on a modified Mueller-Hinton agar that contains iron and high amounts of the amino acid cysteine. These bacteria form colonies on this medium when they are incubated aerobically in 2.5 to 5 percent CO_2 for 4 days. Morphologically (Figure 21–6), they are rod-shaped bacteria 0.3 to 0.4 μm wide and 2 to 3 μm long.

Legionnaires' disease in humans.

Legionnaires' disease begins 2 to 10 days after exposure with a general feeling of malaise accompanied by muscle ache and headache. The patient's temperature rises rapidly to between 38.9 and 40.5°C. This high temperature is accompanied by coughing, chest and abdominal pains, diarrhea, and shortness of breath. Chest roentgenograms show pneumonia in 90 percent of patients with legionnaires' disease. Untreated patients experience a progressive deterioration, and about 20 percent of them die from pneumonia and shock. The remaining patients gradually recover in 1 to 2 weeks. Most legionnaires' disease patients are hospitalized, and some require mechanical assistance in breathing and kidney dialysis.

Pontiac fever is a milder form of pneumonia that is also caused by *L. pneumophila.* In 1966, a pneumonic illness accompanied by a fever affected 95 out of the 100 persons who worked in one building at the Oakland County Health Department in Pontiac, Michigan. The symptoms of the illness included chest pains, coughing, sore throat, vomiting, diarrhea, and confusion. Patients were ill for 2 to 5 days before they spontaneously recovered. No causative agent was isolated at the time of the outbreak. However, serum samples from these patients were collected and preserved at the CDC. In 1978, these sera were tested for the presence of antibodies against *L. pneumophila*. Thirty of 37 sera from Pontiac fever patients were positive for antibodies against *L. pneumophila*, indicating that this bacterium also causes Pontiac fever.

Epidemiology. Why did such a high percentage of the legionnaires and of the Pontiac workers become infected? Apparently, the disease originates as a common-source epidemic and is spread in aerosols. *Legionella pneumophila* is able to grow in the water-cooling towers used to cool the refrigerant in air-conditioning systems. In the Pontiac epidemic, holes were discovered in the system that enabled mist from the water-cooling towers to be taken into a fresh air duct. This defect led to the circulation of *L. pneumophila* in an aerosol throughout the building. A similar problem existed in the air-conditioning system in the convention center hotel in Philadelphia in the 1976 epidemic.

Legionnaires' disease is not transmitted by person-to-person contact. This fact was apparent early in the CDC investigation because family members of the infected patients did not become ill. The bacteria are only spread by aerosols generated by contaminated water-cooling towers and/or by dust at construction sites. Now *L. pneumophila* has been isolated from many cooling towers and from mud sampled at numerous locations.

Prevention and treatment. Prevention of legionnaires' disease is a complex problem because of the widespread distribution of the bacterium. Special procedures have been developed for cleaning and decontaminating the water towers for air-conditioning systems. Once an outbreak occurs, it is necessary to discover the source of the infectious agent and to institute appropriate remedial actions to kill the *L. pneumophila*. Legionnaires' disease is treated with erythromycin or, in patients who do not re-

spond, with rifampin. The mild symptoms of Pontiac fever do not necessitate antibiotic therapy.

MYCOPLASMA

Mycoplasmas possess all the normal features of bacteria except for a cell wall. Mycoplasmas have DNA and RNA; they have bacterial ribosomes; and they are able to grow on special laboratory media. The outermost structure of the cell is their cytoplasmic membrane. They were initially identified as the causative agent of a lung infection of cattle known as pleuropneumonia. For these reasons, they were called the *pleuropneumonialike organisms,* or PPLO for short.

Mycoplasmas are grouped in a separate classification division because of their wall-less morphology. They have been isolated from plants, insects, and animals. Currently there are four recognized genera in this division. *Mycoplasma* and *Ureaplasma* are associated with human disease. *Mycoplasma pneumoniae* infects the human respiratory tract to cause atypical pneumonia, whereas *Ureaplasma urealyticum* has been implicated as a cause of nongonococcal urethritis.

Mycoplasma pneumoniae

Mycoplasma pneumoniae is a pleomorphic organism that can grow as filaments (Figure 21–7) or as spherical cells that average 0.3 to 1.0 μm in diameter. It grows on a beef heart infusion medium as a flattened colony with a raised center described as a "fried-egg" colony. The cytoplasmic membranes of the mycoplasmas contain sterols. Presumably, the presence of sterols strengthens the cytoplasmic membrane enough to resist the osmotic forces that otherwise would destroy the structural integrity of these cells. Mycoplasmas are unable to synthesize sterols from organic compounds, so a supply of sterols (such as cholesterol or unheated horse serum) must be available in their growth media. Mycoplasmas readily pass through small (0.22 μm) membrane filters because they lack a rigid cell shape. They are sensitive to a number of antibiotics, but they are re-

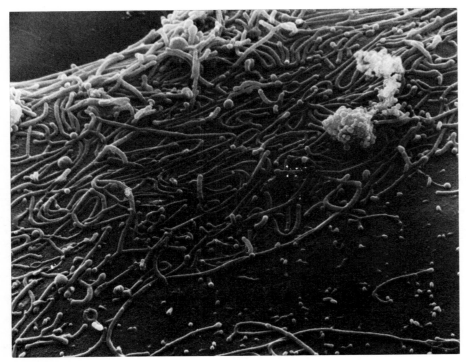

FIGURE 21—7
Scanning electron micrograph of *Mycoplasma*. (Photograph by Dr. David M. Philips, The Population Council.)

sistant to penicillins and other antibiotics that inhibit cell-wall synthesis.

Atypical pneumonia. Mycoplasmas were initially isolated in 1944 as filterable agents that caused atypical pneumonia in humans. When they were first isolated by serial passage in embryonated eggs, they were thought to be viruses; however, their sensitivity to antibiotics suggested that they were bacteria. It was not until 1961 that the bacterial nature of *Mycoplasma pneumoniae* was confirmed by their growth on laboratory media.

Mycoplasma pneumoniae infects the human lung to cause what is known as **atypical pneumonia.** The incubation period is 2 to 3 weeks, and infections are most prevalent among the 5- to 15-year age group. Outbreaks occur among close social groups such as

the family. A family outbreak is usually initiated by a school-age child and is transmitted among persons in close contact by respiratory secretions. *Mycoplasma pneumoniae* infects the surface epithelium in the tracheae and bronchi and inhibits the motility of the cilia. The disease is characterized by the common pneumonial symptoms of a fever, cough, and malaise; it is self-limiting in humans. Immunity is incomplete—reinfections are well documented.

Diagnosis and treatment. Mycoplasmas can be isolated in laboratory media after a 5- to 10-day incubation period. Infections can also be diagnosed by demonstrating a rise in serum antibody using a complement-fixation reaction. In severe cases, the presence of cold agglutinins are indicative of an *M. pneumoniae* infection. **Cold agglutinins** are antibodies that agglutinate type O human blood cells at 4°C but not at 37°C. Most cases are diagnosed by the clinical symptoms because of the delay necessitated by the just-cited assays. Mycoplasmal pneumonia can be effectively treated with tetracyclines or erythromycin. Other causes of atypical pneumonia include Q fever, ornithosis, legionnaires' disease, and viral pneumonia.

SUMMARY

Hemophilus influenzae causes meningitis, obstructive epiglottitis, and infections of the lung of debilitated influenza patients. *Hemophilus influenzae* is a normal inhabitant of the human nasopharangeal region in young children. Noncapsulated strains are avirulent, whereas encapsulated type-b strains are responsible for human illness. *Hemophilus influenzae* causes most

of the bacterial meningitis in children 6 months to 1 year old. Chancroid is the venereal disease caused by *H. ducreyi*. It predominates in uncircumcised males and is characterized by a soft chancre in the genital region. *H. aegypticus* is responsible for the contagious conjunctivitis commonly called pinkeye (Table 21–3).

Bordetella pertussis and *B. parapertussis* are morphologically similar to *Hemophilus* and cause whooping cough. These bacteria are found only in the human respiratory tract, where they grow preferentially on the ciliated epithelial cells of the bronchi. Children are actively immunized against *B. pertussis* with the DTP shots.

Tularemia is a disease of wild mammals that is transmitted to humans by flies or ticks or by direct contact with infected animals. *Francisella tularensis* enters the skin or mucous membranes and causes

TABLE 21–3

Summary of Other Pathogenic Bacteria

Disease	Bacterium	Symptoms	Particular Features
Hemophilus			
Meningitis	*Hemophilus influenzae*	Infection of spinal fluid	Prevalent in young children
Pneumonia		Infection of lung	Secondary invader, influenza
Epiglottitis		Swollen larynx	Emergency tracheotomy
Chancroid	*Hemophilus ducreyi*	Soft chancre in genitalia	Venereal transmission
Pinkeye	*Hemophilus aegypticus*	Inflamed conjunctiva	Highly contagious
Whooping cough	*Bordetella pertussis*	Severe cough	Immunize with DTP shots
(pertussis)	*B. parapertussis*		
Tularemia			
Ulceroglandular	*Francisella tularensis*	Fever, headache,	Wild animals are reservoir,
Pneumonic		general malaise	ticks and flies are vectors,
Typhoid			skinning fur-bearing
			mammals, infects via skin,
			lungs, or digestive tract
Brucellosis	*Brucella* sp.	Fever, chills, malaise,	Contaminated cattle, sheep,
(undulant fever)		undulating fever	goats, and swine, abortion in
			cattle
Legionellosis	*Legionella pneumophila*	Fever, cough, pneumonia	Aerosols from dust, air-
(Pontiac fever)			conditioning systems
Atypical	*Mycoplasma*	Infection of lung,	Cold agglutinins
pneumonia	*pneumoniae*	pneumonia	

fever, headache, and general malaise. Typhoid, pneumonic, and ulceroglandular tularemia are the three recognized forms of tularemia in humans. Most cases occur during the summer months, although outbreaks during the winter rabbit-hunting and muskrat-trapping seasons have been reported.

Brucellosis is prevalent in cattle, sheep, goats, and swine. The human disease is caused by *Brucella* species and is characterized by chills, malaise, body ache, sweating, and an undulant fever. Livestock handlers and meat processors have the highest incidence of brucellosis. The disease is controlled by the elimination of contaminated animals and by the vaccination of young livestock.

Legionnaires' disease is a febrile, pneumonic disease that occurs sporadically in humans as a characteristic point-source epidemic. The source of the causative agent, *Legionella pneumophila*, has been traced to air conditioning, water-cooling towers, and the dust generated at construction sites. Legionnaires' disease is a serious disease that usually requires hospitalization. Pontiac fever is a less severe disease that is also caused by *L. pneumophila*.

Mycoplasma pneumoniae is a cell-wall-lacking bacterium that causes atypical pneumonia. *Mycoplasma* can be grown on laboratory media containing sterols that are required for the synthesis of their cytoplasmic membrane. Mycoplasmal pneumonia is diagnosed by its clinical symptoms and can be treated with erythromycin or tetracycline.

QUESTIONS AND TOPICS FOR STUDY AND DISCUSSION

Questions

1. What is the derivation and significance of the name of the bacterium *Hemophilus influenzae*?
2. Why are infants between the ages of 6 and 12 months the group most susceptible to meningitis caused by *Hemophilus influenzae*?
3. Describe whooping cough as a disease and explain the steps taken to prevent this disease.
4. What persons are likely to be exposed to tularemia? Are there seasonal and geographical patterns associated with this disease? Explain.
5. What persons are most likely to contract brucellosis? How have public health measures changed the incidence and distribution of brucellosis in the United States? Explain.
6. Describe the epidemiology of legionellosis. How was Pontiac fever shown to be caused by *Legionella pneumophila*? (Pontiac fever occurred 10 years prior to the first reports of legionellosis.)
7. Assume that a patient is infected with both *Streptococcus pneumoniae* and *Mycoplasma pneumoniae*. What antibiotics would be effective against both bacteria? Explain.
8. What are cold agglutinins?

Discussion

1. Under what conditions can an airborne infectious agent, such as *Legionella pneumophila*, infect a large population of persons? How can this be prevented?

FURTHER READINGS

Articles and Reviews

Brooks, G. F., and T. M. Buchanan, "Tularemia in the United States," *J. Infect. Dis.*, 121:357–359 (1970). The epidemiology of tularemia in the United States during the 1960s, including a major outbreak in Vermont, is discussed.

Denny, F. W., W. A. Clyde, Jr., and P. Glenzen, "*Mycoplasma pneumoniae* Disease. Unusual Spectrum, Pathophysiology, Epidemiology, and Control," *J. Infect. Dis.*, 123:74–92 (1971). A review of the human morbidity caused by this bacterium.

Fox, M. D., and A. F. Kaufmann, "Brucellosis in the United States, 1965–1974," *J. Infect. Dis.*, 136:312–316 (1977). A review of the epidemiology of brucellosis in the United States.

Fraser, D. W., and J. E. McDade, "Legionellosis," *Sci. Am.*, 241:82–99 (October 1979). The story of the discovery of *Legionella pneumophila* as the causative agent of legionellosis.

Islur, J., C. S. Anglin, and P. J. Middleton, "The Whooping Cough Syndrome: A Continuing Pediatric Problem," *Clin. Pediatrics* (Phila.), 14:171–176 (1975). A review of the continuing incidence of whooping cough in both Canada and the United States.

Kendrick, P. L., "Can Whooping Cough Be Eradicated?" *J. Infect. Dis.*, 132:707–712 (1975). An analysis of the DTP vaccine on the incidence of pertussis.

Razin, S., "The Mycoplasmas," *Microbiol. Revs.*, 42:414–470 (1978). An extensive review of the bacteriology (including mycoplasma viruses) of the mycoplasmas.

Stanbridge, E. J., "A Reevaluation of the Role of Mycoplasmas in Human Disease," *Ann. Revs. Microbiol.*, 30:169–187 (1976). The importance of mycoplasmas in nongonococcal urethritis and other human illnesses is discussed.

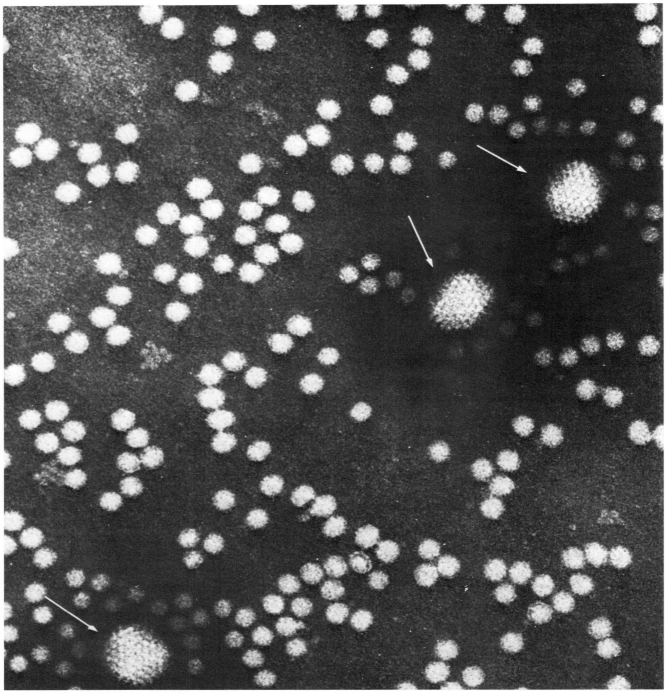

Electron micrograph of simian adenovirus SV15 (70 nm in diameter—white arrows) and the smaller adenosatellite virus. (Courtesy of Dr. H. D. Mayor. From H. D. Mayor "Picodnaviruses," in A. J. Dalton and F. Haguenau, eds., *Ultrastructure of Animal Viruses and Bacteriophages: An Atlas,* copyright © 1973, Academic Press.)

PART FOUR

SUBCELLULAR INFECTIOUS AGENTS

Humans are susceptible to a wide variety of viral diseases. Some viral infections, such as colds, are asymptomatic or only cause mild symptoms, whereas others can cause fatal illnesses. The clinical descriptions of many human viral diseases have been known for centuries; however, the techniques required to isolate and characterize the responsible viruses are relatively new. The tissue culture techniques that were a prerequisite for modern animal virology were developed during the early 1950s. Tissue culture technology and the maturation of molecular biology are two important reasons for the rapid progress in animal virology during the last three decades.

Human viral diseases remain a serious medical problem. Although the field of virology has expanded greatly, medical advances have had little effect on the control and prevention of viral diseases. Only a few viral diseases can be prevented with immunizations, and a few others can be treated with antiviral compounds. Most viral diseases, however, remain untreatable and run their course causing morbidity and, in some cases, mortality.

Part Four is devoted to the human animal viruses and the diseases they cause. Chapter 22 expands on the background presented on bacterial virology (Chapter 9) to provide a basic understanding of the principles of animal virology. This information is used in the discussions of the viral diseases that are presented in Chapters 23 through 26.

22

INTRODUCTION TO ANIMAL VIROLOGY

Animal viruses are self-replicating, intracellular parasites that are specific for the animals they infect. Humans and other vertebrates are susceptible to many different viral infections. A primary infection with most animal viruses causes a self-limiting, overt disease that can range in severity from asymptomatic to fatal. A few animal viruses are capable of establishing long-term latent infections, and the oncogenic animal viruses (none is known to cause human cancer) cause tumor formation.

Animal viruses are different from the bacteriophages (see Chapter 9) in a number of significant ways. The entire animal virus, instead of just the nucleic acid, usually enters the host cell. Animal viruses are decapsidated within the cell before they replicate within the cytoplasm or the nucleus of their host cell. Many enveloped animal viruses acquire their outer layer as they are released through the animal cell's cytoplasmic membrane. The specific characteristics of these phenomena and the basic concepts of animal virology are presented in this beginning chapter on animal virology.

CLASSIFICATION OF ANIMAL VIRUSES

Animal viruses are classified into families on the basis of their chemical composition and their morphology. This classification scheme is constructed without regard to evolutionary relationships because the origin of viruses is unknown. The purpose of classifying viruses is to assign each virus a specific name and to describe each virus in scientific terms.

Classification criteria

Before the molecular structures of the animal viruses were known, they were classified according to the hosts they infected and the diseases they caused. Now that many viruses have been isolated, they are characterized by their structure, size, and chemical composition. Using these data, virologists have constructed a modern viral classification scheme that groups animal viruses into 5 families of DNA viruses and into 10 families of RNA viruses (Table 22–1).

Viral nomenclature

Viral family names always have the ending -virus. The descriptive part of the family name sometimes connotes a characteristic of that viral family. For example, Picornavirus is a viral family that contains small (pico) RNA (rna) viruses. Myxoviruses infect the respiratory tract and cause the formation of mucus (Gr. myxa, mucus). Other family names have historical origins.

TABLE 22–1
Classification of Animal Viruses

Family[a]	General Characteristics	Typical Agents (infections)
RNA Viruses		
Arenaviridae (arenavirus)	Enveloped, helical nucleocapsid	Humans: lassa virus (rare, serious disease)
Bunyaviridae (bunyavirus)	Enveloped, helical nucleocapsid, segmented, ss,[b] minus RNA	Humans: bunyawera viruses (arthropod-borne)
Coronaviridae (coronavirus)	Enveloped, helical nucleocapsid, ss RNA, 80–120 nm particles, bulbous spikes	Humans: coronaviruses (cause common cold)
Orthomyxoviridae (orthomyxovirus)	Enveloped, helical nucleocapsid, segmented, ss, minus RNA	Humans: influenza A and B (infections in swine and birds)
Paramyxoviridae (paramyxovirus)	Enveloped, helical nucleocapsid, 18–1000 nm, ss, minus RNA	Humans: mumps, measles, and respiratory syncytial viruses
Picornaviridae (picornavirus)	Icosahedral, naked, ss, plus RNA, 27–35 nm capsid	Humans: poliovirus, coxsackie viruses, rhinovirus
Reoviridae (reovirus)	Icosahedral, naked, double-shelled virions; segmented (10 or more), ds[b] RNAs	Humans: gastroenteritis (infections of mammals and birds)
Retroviridae (retrovirus)	Enveloped, round particles approx. 100 nm diameter, helical nucleocapsid, two identical plus RNAs, reverse transcriptase	Mammals, birds; no known human viruses (oncogenic)
Rhabdoviridae (rhabdovirus)	Enveloped, bullet-shaped, 70 × 175 nm, ss, minus RNA, helical nucleocapsid	Humans: rabies virus (infections of insects and animals)
Togaviridae (togavirus)	Icosahedral, enveloped, ss, plus RNA, 50–70 nm capsid, 32 capsomeres	Humans: encephalitis, dengue, and yellow fever viruses (infections of insects, birds, and animals)
DNA Viruses		
Adenoviridae (adenovirus)	Icosahedral, naked, ds DNA (linear), 80 nm capsid, 252 capsomeres	Humans: adenovirus (causes upper respiratory diseases)
Herpetoviridae (herpesvirus)	Enveloped, icosahedral, ds DNA (linear), 100 nm capsid, 162 capsomeres	Humans: herpes simplex viruses, Epstein-Barr virus, varicella-zoster virus, and cytomegalovirus
Papovaviridae (papovavirus)	Icosahedral, naked, ds DNA (closed circle), 45–55 nm capsid, 72 capsomeres	Humans: warts (SV_{40} and polyoma viruses cause tumors in animals)
Parvoviridae (parvovirus)	Icosahedral, naked, ss DNA, 20 nm capsid, 23 capsomeres (all defective)	Humans: adeno-associated virus (needs helper virus)
Poxviridae (poxvirus)	Enveloped (ether-resistant), 160 × 200 nm "brick shape," ds DNA (linear), enzymes associated with virion	Humans: variola, vaccinia

[a]The vernacular name is in parentheses beneath the family name.
[b]ss = single-stranded; ds = double-stranded.

The International Committee on Nomenclature of Viruses is responsible for naming viruses. This committee has recommended the use of Latinized generic names for each virus, although the vernacular names are still widely used. Poliovirus type 1 and influenza virus are the vernacular names for *Entero-*

virus h-polio-1, and *Influenzavirus,* respectively. Acceptance of these generic names is still in a state of flux.

Common viral names were often derived from the name of the disease. Influenza is caused by the influenza virus; rabies is caused by rabies virus; and polio is caused by poliovirus. Some viruses are described by their classic names. Smallpox is caused by variola virus (L. *variola,* speckled); German measles is caused by rubella virus (L. *rubella,* reddish); and the common cold is caused by rhinoviruses (Gr. *rhino,* nose). Although the mixing of classic names with the Latinized viral nomenclature is confusing, it continues to be accepted because of its widespread use.

Chemical composition of animal viruses

The simplest animal viruses are composed of one type of nucleic acid surrounded by a proteinaceous capsid. The more complex animal viruses can contain enzymes, segmented nucleic acids, simple or complex capsids, and/or a lipid-containing envelope. Animal viruses can be as small as a ribosome (20 to 30 nm) or as large as a very small bacterium (1000 nm). The chemical composition of animal viruses can vary considerably from one group to another depending on the presence or absence of an envelope and the type of nucleic acid present.

Structure of animal viruses

Most animal viruses are either icosahedral or helical in shape (Figure 22–1); a few are pleomorphic; the poxviruses are brick-shaped; and the rhabdoviruses are bullet-shaped. Some animal viruses have envelopes, but they never have tails. Instead, they attach directly to the cytoplasmic membrane of their host cell (animal cells lack cell walls) through recognition sites on their outer envelope or capsid.

Viral capsids. The viral capsid is composed of capsomeres that surround the viral nucleic acid. **Capsomeres** are viral proteins that self-assemble into either a helical or an icosahedral structure. The capsid of an **icosahedral** virus is a symmetrical structure

composed of 20 equilateral triangles enclosing a central space (Figure 22–2). The size of an icosahedral viral capsid depends on the size of the capsomeres and on the number of capsomeres (*n*) on one side of each equilateral triangle in the icosahedron. The total number of capsomeres (*N*) is found by the formula, $N = 10 (n - 1)^2 + 2$. The number of capsomeres in a given icosahedral virus is constant and is used in viral classification.

Helical animal viruses always contain RNA as their sole nucleic acid. The capsomeres of a helical virus self-assemble to form a cylinder around the RNA, resulting in the formation of naked helical virions (Figure 22–1). The self-assembly of a helical virus is not constrained by geometric form, so individual helical capsids of the same virus can vary in length.

FIGURE 22–1
Diagrams of animal-virus structures.

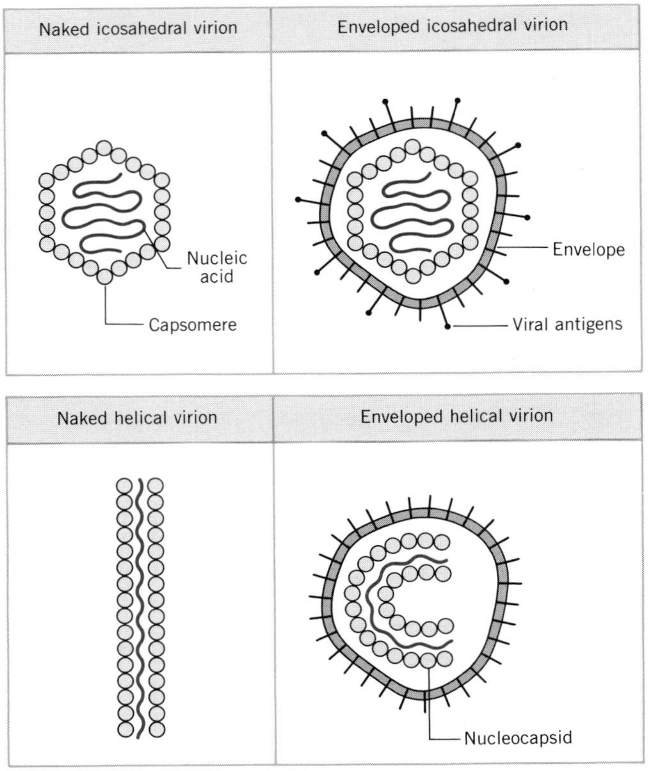

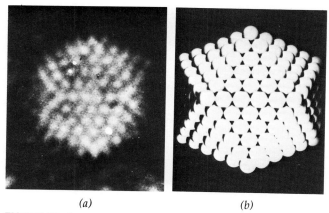

FIGURE 22–2

Electron micrograph of (*a*) adenovirus and (*b*) a model of its icosahedral capsid structure. (Courtesy of Dr. R. W. Horne. From R. W. Horne, S. Brenner, A. P. Waterson, and P. Wildy, *J. Mol. Biol.*, 1:84–86, 1959, copyright ©, Academic Press Inc., Ltd., London.)

Viral envelopes. Some helical and icosahedral capsids are surrounded by a lipid-containing membrane layer known as the **viral envelope.** The envelope is composed of lipid, carbohydrate, and protein and is derived from a membrane of the host cell. The capsid, nucleic acid complex of an enveloped virus is known as the **nucleocapsid** (Figure 22–1). In the simplest case, the nucleocapsid is surrounded by the envelope acquired when the virus is extruded from the cell (Figure 22–3). Other viruses acquire their envelope from the cell's nuclear membrane or endoplasmic reticulum. Enveloped viruses (except poxviruses) are inactivated by lipid solvents, such as ether, which destroy the lipid structure of the viral envelope. Sensitivity to ether is a widely used test for identifying enveloped viruses.

Viral nucleic acid. Animal viruses possess a viral genome composed of either DNA or RNA. This nucleic acid can be either single-stranded or double-stranded, linear or circular, monomolecular or segmented. By convention, single-stranded RNA that serves as a messenger RNA is designated as plus RNA (+RNA). Similarly, a single-stranded DNA molecule that serves as a template for transcribing

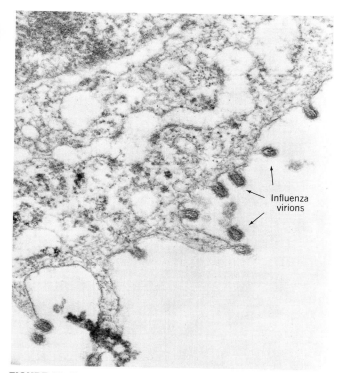

Influenza virions

FIGURE 22–3

Release of influenza virus from the surface of a chicken embryo fibroblast. (Courtesy of Dr. R. W. Compans. From R. W. Compans and P. W. Choppin, "Orthomyxoviruses and Paramyxoviruses," in A. J. Dalton and F. Haguenau, eds., *Ultrastructure of Animal Viruses and Bacteriophages: An Atlas*, copyright © 1973, Academic Press.)

mRNA is designated as minus DNA (–DNA). The complementary macromolecules are designated as minus RNA (–RNA) and plus DNA (+DNA). Most animal viruses contain only one nucleic acid molecule. Some of the RNA viruses, however, contain more than one RNA molecule, so they are described as having a **segmented genome.** These differences in viral nucleic acid are important characteristics for defining the different viral families (Table 22–1).

ENUMERATION OF ANIMAL VIRUSES

Experimental virology depends on the investigator's ability to detect and count specific viruses. Animal virologists have adapted the techniques of immunology, pathogenic bacteriology, and plaque assay to enumerate animal viruses. The most widely used technique is the tissue culture assay.

Tissue culture assays

The ability to propagate animal viruses in cell cultures was developed by John Enders and his colleagues in the late 1940s. They found that animal viruses grew in large numbers in excised animal tissues that were maintained in culture. Scientists are now able to culture many different animal cell lines in tissue cultures. The cells are grown in a complex culture medium that contains all the nutrients essential for cell growth.

Animal-cell cultures can be maintained through many aseptic transfers; however, these cells have an intrinsic age that prevents their perpetual reproduction. Tissue cultures derived from normal cells survive up to 50 transfers before they cease to propagate. In contrast, tissue cultures derived from malignant animal tissue can be maintained indefinitely. Most cultured animal cells possess the property of **contact inhibition,** which constrains their growth to a monolayer (one cell deep). They grow as a sheet of cells (Figure 22–4) over the surface of the culture dish.

Viruses often cause **cytopathic effects** (CPE) when they are grown in cultured animal cells or in embryonated eggs (Figure 22–4b). CPE appear as local necrosis or as a focus of transformed cell growth. Local necrosis is observed as cell lysis or cell death. **Transformed** animal cells grow in an unrestricted manner because they have lost their property of contact inhibition. Certain viruses cause transformation

FIGURE 22–4
Cytopathic effects of animal-virus growth. (a) Herpes simplex growing on WI38 cells in tissue culture. (Courtesy of Dr. N. Sharon). (b) Vaccinia virus growing on a chicken embryo. (Courtesy of Dr. L. LeBeau.)

(a)　　　　　　　　　　(b)

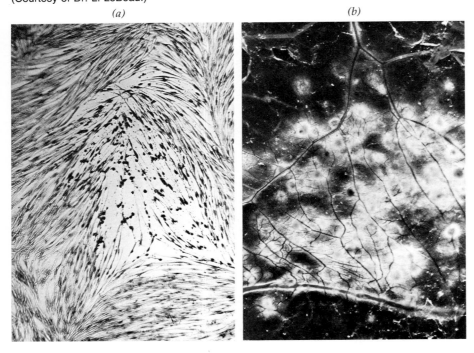

such that each infected cell grows into a visible, multilayered mass of cells. The number of foci of necrosis or transformation is equivalent to the number of infective viruses added to the culture. The actual effect observed is dependent on the cell line, the infecting virus, and the culture conditions.

Hemagglutination

Many animal viruses possess surface antigens that react with red blood cells. Hemagglutination occurs when enough viruses are present to cause the precipitation of red blood cells (agglutination). These viruses possess protein antigens called hemagglutinins (Figure 22–5). Hemagglutinins bind to specific receptors, usually surface glycoproteins, present on mammalian cell membranes. Red blood cells also possess hemagglutinin receptors. When a viral suspension is mixed with red blood cells, the viral hemagglutinins combine with the red-blood-cell receptors to cause clumping of the red blood cells. The greatest dilution of a virus that is able to agglutinate red blood cells is the end point, or titer, of the viral suspension.

Animal assays

The minimal dose of a viral preparation that causes disease in a susceptible animal can be used to quantitate virions in a suspension. The lethal dose that kills 50 percent of the animals (LD_{50}) is used as a quantitative measure of the viral population. These assays are performed with the techniques described (see Chapter 12) for determining the LD_{50} of a bacterial culture.

PROPAGATION OF ANIMAL VIRUSES

Vaccine manufacturers, viral diagnostic laboratories, and experimental virologists routinely grow animal viruses. Embryonated chicken eggs or one of a variety of tissue cultures are used as the animal host cells for viral propagation. The cell lines commonly used in diagnostic virology came from humans, monkeys, hamsters, or mice. A virologist must choose the specific cell line to be used in cultivating

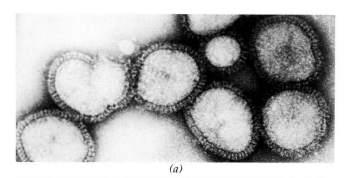

(a)

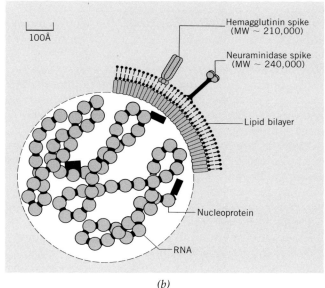

(b)

FIGURE 22–5

The surface of many enveloped viruses are covered by protein spikes that are involved in the adsorption of the virus to its host cell. (a) An electron micrograph of the influenza A virus and (b) a diagram of the hemagglutinin and the neuraminidase spikes attached to the viral envelope. (Courtesy of Dr. I. T. Schulze. From I. T. Schulze, *Virology*, 47:181–196, 1972, copyright © 1972, Academic Press.)

a given virus. There are approximately 25 cell lines that are commonly used to grow animal viruses. Although many different viruses may grow in a specific cell line, optimal viral growth is usually restricted to only a few.

Embryonated eggs contain a chicken embryo plus supportive tissues (see Figure 22–4b). Because they possess a variety of cell types, embryonated eggs are ideal culture environments for many different viruses. Viruses are inoculated into different parts of the egg after a hole is drilled in the egg's shell. The inoculated virus will then infect and grow in its specific host cells. Embryonated eggs are readily available, and they are easily maintained as self-contained virus cultures.

Diagnostic virology laboratories routinely use commercially available cell lines maintained in tissue cultures. A specimen is inoculated into the tissue culture, which is then incubated. Most human viruses grow at 36°C; however, the rhinoviruses, which cause human colds, have an optimum growth temperature of 33°C. The latent period for animal viruses in tissue cultures varies from a few hours to many hours, and many animal viruses take 6 days or longer to cause visible effects in tissue cultures. For this reason, diagnostic cultures are kept for 2 weeks before they are scored as negative.

Vaccines are manufactured from viruses grown in tissue cultures or in embryonated eggs. As an example, poliovirus is propagated in tissue cultures of monkey kidney cells for use in the Salk and the Sabin polio vaccines. Rabies virus is grown in duck embryos or in human diploid tissue cultures, and influenza virus is grown in embryonated chicken eggs. Vaccines are not available for all animal viruses, and, indeed, some animal viruses have never been grown outside their host.

REPLICATION OF ANIMAL VIRUSES

Animal viruses have a limited host range because they are specific for the cells they infect. Even within a given host, an animal virus will infect only certain cells. Viral infections occur in a two-step process that involves adsorption and entry. **Adsorption** is the process by which a virion binds to the cell's surface. Adsorption is followed by entry of the virion or its nucleic acid into the cell.

Viral adsorption

Approximately 1 in every 10,000 collisions between a host cell and a virion results in adsorption. Virions possess specific surface structures that recognize receptors on the cell's surface. For example, influenza virus contains protein "spikes" that extend from its envelope (Figure 22–5). These protein "spikes" are the hemagglutinins that are responsible for viral binding to the host cell's membranes. They are also responsible for agglutinating red blood cells. The binding proteins of naked virions are the exposed surfaces of the viral capsomeres.

The surface of the host cell's cytoplasmic membrane possesses viral receptors. Most of the known receptors are glycoproteins. The presence of a receptor on a cell surface is a key determinant for the adsorption of the virus to that cell. Measles virus infects many human cell types including those found in nasopharynx, lung, lymphatic, subcutaneous, testes, and nerve tissues. The host range of poliovirus is more limited. Poliovirus will infect only cells of primates, and in humans it will infect only cells of the nasopharynx, the intestinal tract, and the anterior horn cells of the spinal cord. Therefore, the nature of the viral binding proteins dictates, to a large extent, the cells that a virus can infect.

Viral entry into animal cells.

A virus, or at least the viral genome, must enter the cell's cytoplasm before it can establish an infection. Animal viruses enter their host cells by one of three poorly understood mechanisms.

Most nonenveloped animal viruses enter a host cell by the process of phagocytosis. The virus is taken into the cytoplasm in a vesicle whose outer layer is derived from the host cell's cytoplasmic membrane (Figure 22–6). Once inside the cell, the virus is released from this vesicle, presumably by enzymatic action. Another mechanism of penetration requires the viral envelope to fuse with the cell membrane. Fusion is followed by a mechanical rearrangement that permits the viruses to enter the cytoplasm of the cell. Still other viruses may enter their host cell as naked nucleic acid.

Once inside the cell, the viral nucleic acid becomes available to the biosynthetic machinery of the cell. Enveloped viruses undergo **decapsidation** (uncoating), presumably through the action of cellular enzymes. Virologists do not yet know how or where decapsidation occurs. Since RNA viruses repli-

(a) **PHAGOCYTOSIS**

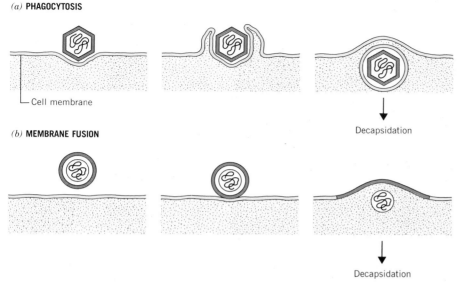

(b) **MEMBRANE FUSION**

Decapsidation

Decapsidation

FIGURE 22–6
Mechanisms of viral entry: (a) phagocytosis, (b) membrane fusion followed by mechanical rearrangement.

cate in the cytoplasm, this is the most probable location for them to be uncoated. Most DNA viruses replicate in the nucleus, so their DNA must be translocated to the cell's nucleus either before or after decapsidation.

Replication of the viral genome

DNA viruses (except the poxviruses) replicate their DNA in the nucleus of their host cell. They utilize the DNA precursors present in the cell's nucleotide pool; however, they do not mediate the degradation of the cell's DNA. The simpler DNA viruses utilize the cell's DNA polymerase(s) to synthesize viral DNA. The more complex viruses, such as the poxviruses and the herpesviruses, first synthesize polymerases before they manufacture viral DNA.

RNA viruses replicate their genome by making copies of their RNA genome. Single-stranded RNA viruses first make a **replicative RNA strand** from which they synthesize multiple copies of their genome. There are a few RNA viruses that make DNA as an intermediate in the synthesis of their RNA genome. These viruses are retroviruses.

Synthesis of viral mRNA

Most DNA viruses replicate in the nucleus of their host cell, which makes the nucleus the site of viral mRNA synthesis. Many of the posttranscriptional events of selection, processing, modification, and transport that affect host cell transcription and translation are also involved in the expression of viral DNA genes. For example, DNA viruses are able to form early and late messages that are translated into early and late proteins.

Double-stranded DNA viruses make mRNA directly from their minus DNA strand (Table 22–2). Single-stranded, plus DNA viruses must first make a minus DNA strand from which messenger RNA is formed. The enzymes necessary for forming the early mRNA from the viral DNA genome are present in animal cells. Posttranscriptional processes are involved in processing mRNA transcripts before they are translated on cytoplasmic ribosomes.

TABLE 22–2
Messenger RNA Formation by Viruses

Type	Example	Enzymes Required	Replication Strategy
ds DNA	Vaccinia	Cell enzymes	± DNA ⟶ → ―― mRNA ⟶
ss DNA	Parvovirus	Cell enzymes	+ DNA ⟶ → ± DNA → ―― mRNA ⟶
Plus RNA	Poliovirus	None required	Viral genome is mRNA
Minus RNA	Vesicular stomatis virus	Viral transcriptase	– RNA ⟵ → ―― mRNA ⟶
ds RNA	Reovirus	Viral transcriptase	± RNA ⟶ → ―― mRNA ⟶
Plus RNA	SV$_{40}$ (Retroviruses)	Viral transcriptase (reverse transcriptase)	+ + RNA ⟶ → ± DNA → ―― mRNA ⟶

Source: Adapted from D. Baltimore, "Expressions of Animal Virus Genomes," *Bacteriol. Revs.*, 35:235 – 241 (1971).

Animal RNA viruses are replicated in the cytoplasm of their host cells. Single-stranded, plus RNA genomes can serve directly as viral mRNA (Table 22–2). This is the simplest case of message formation because it requires no special enzymes. All other RNA viruses need to have an RNA transcriptase that must be present in the virion because animal cells do not contain these enzymes. The single-stranded, minus RNA viral genome serves as a template for making mRNA, as does the minus strand of the double-stranded RNA viral genome. Retroviruses are in a special group because they form a double-stranded DNA intermediate from which they make mRNA (Table 22–2). The retroviruses contain two identical plus RNA strands and an RNA-directed DNA polymerase (reverse transcriptase). These viruses make a double-stranded DNA intermediate that serves as the template for mRNA formation.

Synthesis of viral proteins

All protein synthesis, directed by viral nucleic acid, takes place on ribosomes in the cell's cytoplasm. Although the actual mechanism of translation is essentially the same for all viruses, significant differences between the strategies of viral protein synthesis exist.

The RNA genome of poliovirus is a single-stranded, 35S macromolecule that is translated as a single monocistronic message (Figure 22–7). The resulting giant polyprotein is approximately 250,000 daltons. This polyprotein is processed into shorter polypeptides by specific enzymes. The resulting viral proteins either have enzymatic activity, serve as capsid proteins (VP$_1$, VP$_2$, VP$_3$, VP$_4$), or are not utilized (N$_x$). Because all the viral protein is synthesized from one mRNA, there is no division between early and late protein synthesis. Apparently, the poliovirus genome lacks start and stop signals for the regulation of translation.

A second viral strategy is to synthesize multiple messages from a continuous genome or from a segmented genome. This mechanism necessitates the presence of an RNA-directed transcriptase that accompanies the virion into the cell. Vesicular stomatitis virus synthesizes multiple messages from a continuous, single-stranded, minus RNA genome (Figure 22–7). Each mRNA is derived from the single-stranded RNA genome, but it codes only for one functional protein.

The influenza virus has a segmented genome composed of eight different molecules of single-stranded minus RNA. Each molecule acts as a template for synthesizing a single mRNA. The seg-

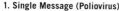

1. Single Message (Poliovirus)

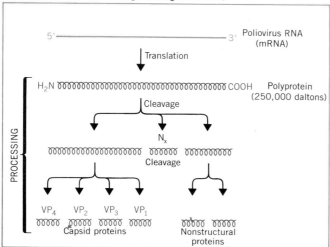

2. Multiple Messages

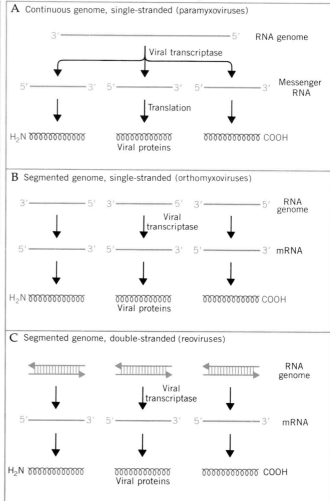

FIGURE 22–7

RNA viruses use various strategies for synthesizing proteins. A single polyprotein is made directly from the single-stranded, plus RNA genome of the poliovirus. The paramyxoviruses transcribe multiple messages from their single-stranded, minus RNA genome. The orthomyxoviruses have a segmented, single-stranded, minus RNA genome that codes for individual mRNAs. This is also the strategy used by the reoviruses, which have segmented double-stranded RNA genomes.

mented nature of the influenza genome is in part responsible for the antigenic changes (see Chapter 23) that occur in influenza viruses.

The nucleic acid of DNA animal viruses is replicated and the viral mRNA is made (transcription) in the nucleus of the host cell. This strategy is identical to the mechanisms used by eucaryotic cells: DNA synthesis and mRNA formation take place in the nucleus, whereas translation occurs in the cytoplasm. Viral DNA is transcribed into mRNA, which is then translocated to the cytoplasm. When this strategy is used, transcription can be regulated such that early and late proteins are synthesized.

Maturation and release

Complete virions are formed within the cell's nucleus or its cytoplasm, depending on the virus. Naked viruses self-assemble from preformed viral proteins and nucleic acids by a process that is governed by physicochemical forces. When aggregates of viral particles accumulate in the cytoplasm, they can be seen in electron micrographs (Figure 22–8). These aggregates are called **inclusion bodies** when they are visible in the light microscope. An example of this phenomenon occurs when the rabies virus accumulates in the cytoplasm of brain cells to form **Negri bodies.**

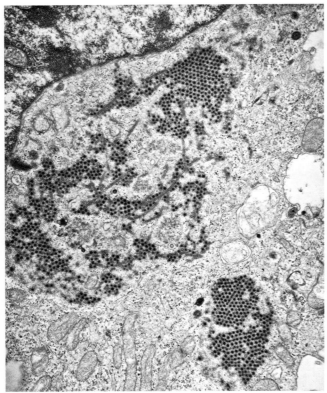

FIGURE 22–8
Intracellular inclusions of reovirus 12 hours after inoculation. Large aggregates of virus particles are present in the host cell's cytoplasm. (Courtesy of Dr. S. Dales. From S. Dales "The Structure and Replication of Poxviruses as Exemplified by Vaccinia," in A. J. Dalton and F. Haguenau, eds., *Ultrastructure of Animal Viruses and Bacteriophages: An Atlas,* copyright © 1973, Academic Press.)

Some animal viruses destroy their host cell when they are released into the extracellular environment. Other viruses are extruded through the cell's cytoplasmic membrane. Extrusion can result in the long-term production of virions by an infected cell.

Enveloped viruses acquire their outer coating as they are extruded through the membrane (Figure 22–9). The surface of the cell's membrane and the envelope of the virus are similar in chemical composition and structure, but they are not necessarily identical. Replicating viruses often produce viral proteins that become incorporated into the cell's cytoplasmic membrane. This process adds unique antigens to the cell's membrane, which in turn becomes the viral envelope (Figure 22–9). Cells that produce enveloped viruses do not lyse: they can extrude infective virions into the environment for long periods of time.

EFFECTS OF REPRODUCTION OF ANIMAL VIRUSES ON HOST CELLS

Animal viruses can affect their host cells in three distinct ways. Cytocidal viruses cause extensive cell damage, which results in the cell's death. Viruses can have an inductive effect on cells: the virus causes the cell to form both viral and cellular proteins that are not otherwise synthesized by the cell. Oncogenic viruses transform their host cell, which causes it to grow in an unrestricted manner.

Cytocidal effects

Cytocidal viruses take over the biosynthetic machinery of their host cell by inhibiting cellular protein synthesis. Soon after infection, cytocidal virions block the synthesis of ribosomal RNA and cellular mRNA; tRNA synthesis is not affected. Cellular DNA synthesis is also inhibited by some viruses soon after infection. Cytocidal viruses kill their host cell by taking over its synthetic machinery very much as the T-even phages commandeer the synthetic capacity of their *E. coli* host.

Inductive effects

Viruses induce host cells to manufacture viral proteins and other essential viral components required for virus propagation. In addition, some viruses induce cells to manufacture proteins that alter the cell's membrane structure. Since cells interact with neighboring cells via membrane contact, these changes in an infected cell's surface structure alter the cell's behavior. Viruses can also stimulate the cell to produce specific proteins (interferon) that interfere with viral replication in other cells.

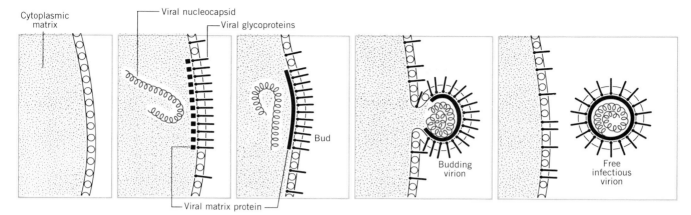

Cytoplasmic matrix — Viral nucleocapsid — Viral glycoproteins — Bud — Viral matrix protein — Budding virion — Free infectious virion

FIGURE 22–9
Budding of an enveloped virus. (Reproduced with permission. From B. D. Davis, R. Delbecco, H. N. Eissen, and H. S. Ginsberg, *Microbiology*, 3rd ed., copyright © 1980, Harper & Row.)

Interferons. Both living and ultraviolet-killed viruses induce many vertebrate cells to produce interferons. **Interferons** are a class of cellular proteins that protect other cells from viral infection. Their gross action can be measured by observing plaque reduction or virus-yield reduction when interferon-treated tissue culture cells are infected with a virus. Among the many animal cells that produce interferons are the mouse L cells and human fibroblast cells. These cell lines can be grown in tissue culture and serve as the source of experimentally produced interferon.

Human-fibroblast interferon is a glycoprotein (molecular weight 20,000 daltons). It is active at very low concentrations (10^{-11}M), which means that the infected cell needs to produce only a small quantity of interferon before it interferes with viral replication. The small quantities produced by a cell culture makes the purification of interferon a difficult task. Genetic engineering is probably the only economically feasible means of obtaining sufficient quantities of interferon to use it as a chemotherapeutic agent.

The exact mechanism by which a virus induces interferon production is not known. Once produced by an infected cell, the interferon leaves the cell and binds to the surface receptors on noninfected cells. This binding stimulates the cell to synthesize or to activate enzymes that inhibit viral reproduction. Interferon is currently the most general weapon known to combat viral infections.

Viral transformation

Oncogenic viruses induce tumor formation when they infect their host cells. This relationship between viruses and tumors is not a new concept. Ellerman and Bang (1908) and Peyton Rous (1911) were the first to report the transfer of cancer from one animal to another. Ellerman and Bang reported the transfer of chicken leukemia, and Rous demonstrated the transfer of chicken sarcoma (cancer of the connective tissue) from diseased to healthy chickens. The virus responsible for the chicken sarcoma was later identified and is now called Rous sarcoma virus (RSV). RSV is an RNA virus that is known for its ability to transform tissue culture cells. Oncogenic DNA viruses are also known. An oncogenic DNA virus was discovered in the rhesus monkey kidney tissue cultures used to grow poliovirus. It is named the simian (L. *simia*, ape) virus number 40 or SV_{40}.

Rous sarcoma virus. Domestic fowl can host a variety of viruses including the Rous sarcoma virus. Some strains of RSV are defective and are not able to produce progeny viruses. These defective Rous sarcoma virions transform their host cells, causing them to replicate in an uncontrolled manner.

RSV-transformed cells will propagate RSV particles if they are superinfected with a helper virus. This second virus provides genetic information essential for the replication of the Rous sarcoma virus. Each transformed cell, regardless of the number of generations after its initial infection, can be stimulated to produce progeny RSV particles by superinfection. Therefore, the transformed cells carry the RSV genome as a provirus just as the prophage is carried by lysogenized bacteria. Moreover, since RSV is an RNA virus, there must be mechanisms for maintaining an RNA genome in a host-cell line.

But a cell's genes are located in DNA and not in RNA. The only way that information encoded in RNA can be passed to progeny cells is to make it first into DNA (Figure 22–10). This concept was experimentally confirmed by the isolation of viral, RNA-directed DNA polymerase. RSV produces such

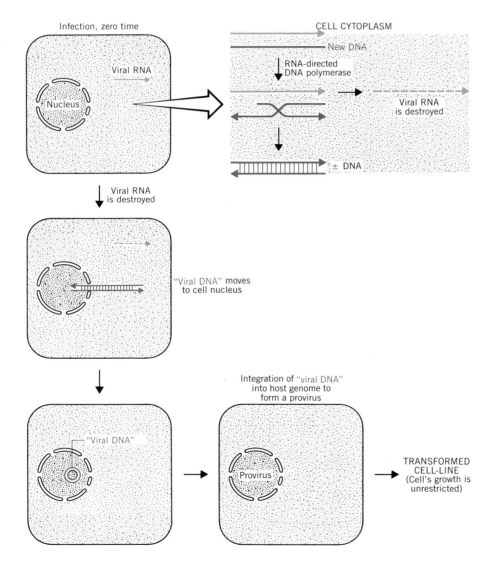

FIGURE 22–10
Transformation by Rous sarcoma virus. The initial replication of the viral RNA into double-stranded DNA occurs in the cell's cytoplasm. The double-stranded DNA replica then moves into the nucleus where it is incorporated into a cell chromosome as a provirus. The cell is now transformed and replicates in an unrestricted manner.

an enzyme, and it makes DNA from the viral RNA. This DNA is then incorporated into the host's genome, and the viral genes are passed on to progeny cells. In the process, the cell is transformed to replicate in an unrestricted manner.

SV$_{40}$ virus. This DNA virus was discovered as a passenger virus in the monkey kidney tissue cultures used to cultivate poliovirus. SV$_{40}$ produces tumors in baby hamsters. It transforms human embryonic cells and cultured hamster cells at a low efficiency. During a normal infection process, only 1 out of every 10,000 infected cells are transformed. When transformation occurs, the virus directs the synthesis of a new antigen that is incorporated into the cytoplasmic membrane. This antigen is the T antigen; it is used as a marker to identify SV$_{40}$-transformed cells.

SV$_{40}$ is an example of a DNA virus that can transform mammalian cell lines. Many oncogenic viruses are known, but to date only one human virus has been shown to be oncogenic. This virus is the Epstein-Barr virus, which has been isolated from Burkitt's lymphoma (see Chapter 25).

DIAGNOSTIC ANIMAL VIROLOGY

Viral diseases are diagnosed to enable the physician to administer treatment (if available), to provide an accurate prognosis to the patient, and to take steps to prevent the spread of the illness. Most viral diseases cannot be cured; however, there are a few exceptions. For example, postinfection rabies can be treated by active immunization because this disease has a long incubation period. A number of viral diseases in childbearing females jeopardize the health of the fetus if precautions are not taken. Other viral diseases are extremely contagious, and further illness can be decreased if proper preventative procedures are followed. The mental outlook of the patient is best served by an accurate prognosis of the disease. These aspects of a health care delivery system can be met only when an adequate viral diagnostic facility is available.

Many large hospitals and almost all state public health laboratories have viral diagnostic laboratories.

A modern virology laboratory is established to isolate viruses from patients to perform serodiagnostic tests, and to measure viral antigens directly. The state public health laboratory is likely to do the specialized virology tests. The Virology Division of the Centers for Disease Control tests specimens for the truly uncommon viral diseases, maintains a serological reference service for the identification of specific viruses, and conducts epidemiological investigations of major viral diseases.

Viral isolation

Many human viruses can be isolated by inoculating specimens into tissue cultures. Tissue cultures of monkey kidney, human embryonic kidney, and human embryonic lung cells are commercially available tissue cultures that are used to isolate human viruses. Clinical specimens are collected and transported using many of the techniques applicable to collecting bacterial specimens. After inoculation, cultures are incubated for an average of 5 days before 50 percent of the cultures are positive and an average of 10 days before 90 percent of the cultures are positive. Some cultures show positive viral growth within 1 or 2 days. Once a virus is grown in a tissue culture, the laboratory personnel identify it through serodiagnostic techniques.

Serodiagnostic virology

Immunological tests for viruses depend on the availability of the virus (antigen) or of a viral antibody that will specifically react with the virus. The level of antibody in a patient's serum can be determined using a specific antigen. Similarly, the kind of virus present in a tissue culture can be determined using a specific antibody. Standardized antigens and antibodies are available from commercial sources or from the CDC.

A variety of immunological tests are used to detect viruses. Hemagglutination, hemagglutination inhibition, complement fixation, fluorescent antibody techniques, and radioimmunoassays have been discussed previously (see Chapter 13). Each of these techniques has been adapted for use in virology.

CONTROL OF VIRAL DISEASES

Most human viral diseases are diagnosed by the clinical symptoms they cause. Some of these symptoms can be treated, but most viral diseases run their course without medical intervention. A few viral diseases can be treated with antiviral substances, by vaccination, or by passive immunization. Vaccines are the major weapon available for preventing viral infections, but they are available for only a few viral diseases.

Viral vaccines

Live-attenuated or killed virus preparations are used to immunize humans against specific viral diseases (Table 22–3). The vaccines are administered with a frequency and route that maximizes the human's immunological response. The measles, mumps, and rubella viruses are combined in a single vaccine, the MMR vaccine, which is administered once as a subcutaneous injection. This vaccine provides immunity against the diseases caused by these viruses. The polio vaccine (Sabin) contains three types of live, attenuated polio viruses. This vaccine is taken orally on two separate occasions. The Salk polio vaccine is a preparation of killed polio viruses that is injected intradermally. Vaccination against smallpox is now limited in use because of the eradication of the disease.

Yellow fever vaccine is given to persons in or traveling to areas where yellow fever is epidemic. This viral disease is transmitted by mosquitoes and is limited to tropical Africa, tropical South America, and the Caribbean. Influenza vaccine is produced from the type of influenza virus that is prevalent during a given influenza season. Influenza vaccine is administered to compromised patients and persons over 65. Rabies vaccine is given to persons who have been exposed to rabies. The incubation period of the rabies virus is sufficiently long to permit immunization against this disease even after infection.

Antiviral chemicals

Four major antiviral compounds are effective against a select group of human viral diseases (Table 22–4). The three nucleosides (Figure 22–11) are active against herpes simplex virus. Of the three, idoxuridine and cytosine arabinoside are prescription drugs used to treat herpes infections. Another prescription

TABLE 22–3
Virus Vaccines in Clinical Use

Vaccine	Description	Route	Frequency	Antibody Persistence
Measles	Attenuated virus	Subcutaneous	Once	12 years
Mumps	Attenuated virus	Subcutaneous	Once	8 years
Rubella	Attenuated virus	Subcutaneous	Once	8 years
Poliomyelitis (Sabin)	Attenuated viruses, three types	Oral	Three	10 years
Poliomyelitis (Salk)	Killed viruses, three types	Subcutaneous	Four	2 years
Vaccinia	Poxvirus, protects against smallpox	Intradermal	Every 3 years	3 years
Yellow fever	Attenuated virus	Subcutaneous	Once	10 years
Influenza	Influenza A and B (prevalent strains)	Subcutaneous	Twice a year	1 year
Rabies	Attenuated virus grown in duck embryos	Subcutaneous	Four times	1 year

TABLE 22–4
Antiviral Compounds Effective Against Human Viruses

Substance	Antiviral Activity	Applications	Mode of Action
Idoxuridine (Stoxil)	Herpes simplex	Topical	Inhibits or interferes with viral DNA and protein synthesis
Cytosine arabinoside (Cytarabine, Ara-C)	Herpes simplex	Intravenous	Inhibits or interferes with viral DNA and protein synthesis
Adenine arabinoside (Ara-A)	Herpes simplex	Intravenous	Inhibits or interferes with viral DNA and protein synthesis
Amantadine (Symmetrel)	Influenza A	Oral	Inhibits uncoating of influenza A virus

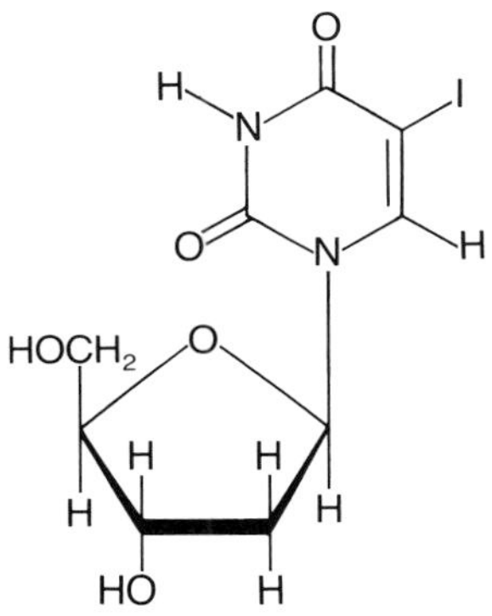

Idoxuridine
(5-iodo-2′-deoxyuridine)

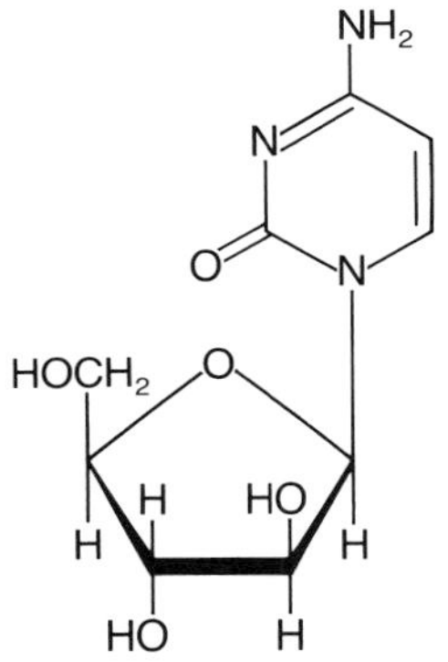

Cytosine arabinoside
(1-β-D-arabinofuranosyl-cytosine)

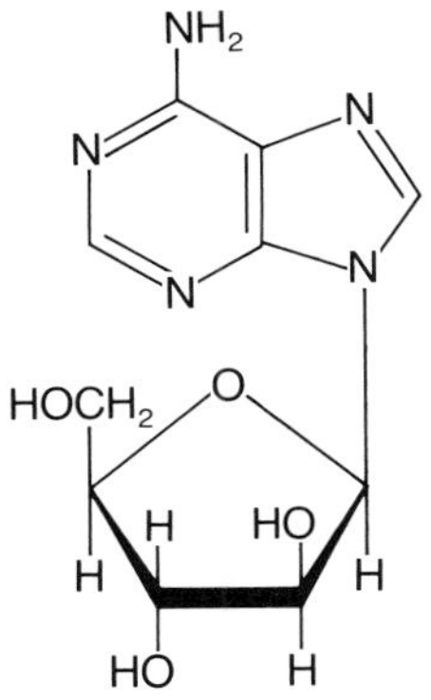

Adenine arabinoside
(9-β-D-arabinofuranosyl-adenine)

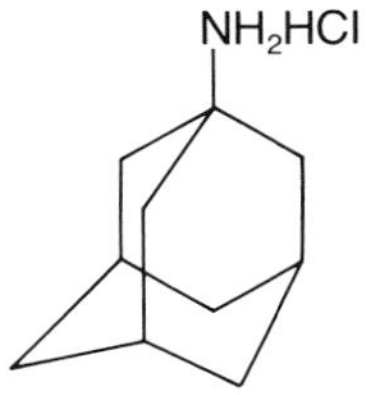

Amantadine
(1-aminoadamantane hydrochloride)

FIGURE 22–11
Antiviral compounds.

drug is amantadine, which is used to reduce the attack rate during influenza A epidemics. Amantadine decreases the symptoms of influenza caused by influenza A; however, it is ineffective against influenza B and C.

SUMMARY

All vertebrates are susceptible to viral infections. Animal viruses are classified on the basis of their structure, size, and chemical composition into 5 families of DNA viruses and 10 families of RNA viruses. Many animal viruses are named after the diseases they cause.

Animal viruses contain a nucleic acid (either RNA or DNA) surrounded by a protein capsid. Their morphology can be described as helical, icosahedral, brick-shaped, or pleomorphic. Many animal viruses are surrounded by an ether-sensitive, lipid-containing envelope that is derived from a host-cell membrane. The structure of viral nucleic acid can be segmented or continuous, linear or circular, single-stranded or double-stranded. In addition to nucleic acid, some capsids contain enzymes required for viral replication.

Animal viruses replicate in tissue cultures or in embryonated eggs; some animal viruses have not been cultivated outside their host animal. Infection occurs after a virus adsorbs specifically to a receptor located on the host cell's surface. Usually, the complete virus enters the cell's cytoplasm either by phagocytosis or membrane fusion. After entry, the viral nucleic acid is released from the virion by decapsidization (uncoating). RNA viruses are replicated in the cytoplasm of the cell, whereas the DNA of DNA viruses (except for the poxviruses) is transposed to and replicated in the cell's nucleus. DNA viruses utilize the cell's enzymes for the initial steps of this replication. The RNA viruses contain or manufacture specific enzymes that they use to replicate their RNA. These include the RNA-directed DNA polymerase made by retroviruses and the RNA transcriptase used to manufacture viral RNA.

Viral proteins are synthesized on cytoplasmic ribosomes by two basic strategies. The mRNA can be translated (1) as one long polypeptide that is later cleaved into functional viral proteins, or (2) as short segments of mRNA that are transcribed directly into viral proteins. DNA viruses produce mRNA in the nucleus, which is then translated on the cell's cytoplasmic ribosomes. Viral capsid proteins, essential viral enzymes, and viral nucleic acids accumulate in the host cell prior to self-assembly. Infective virions either accumulate in the cell, are released by extrusion through the cytoplasmic membrane, or are released on cell lysis. Enveloped virions acquire their outer layer, which is derived from a cell membrane either inside the cell or as the virion is extruded through the cell's cytoplasmic membrane.

Virus-infected cells are either killed, transformed, or induced to produce specific cellular proteins. Oncogenic viruses cause cell transformation. Transformed cells grow in an unrestricted fashion and create foci of transformation that can be seen in tissue cultures. Many viruses induce mammalian cells to produce interferon, proteins that inhibit viral replication in host cells. Vaccines and passive immunization are the major means of preventing and controlling human viral diseases. A small group of viral infections can be controlled or prevented by four known antiviral compounds.

QUESTIONS AND TOPICS FOR STUDY AND DISCUSSION

Questions

1. What are the major criteria used to classify animal viruses? Does this classification scheme indicate how viruses are related to each other? Explain.
2. Describe the organization of an enveloped virus by indicating the structure and chemical composition of its parts.
3. Define or explain the following.

capsid	nucleocapsid
capsomere	segmented genome
icosahedron	contact inhibition
envelope	transformation
$N = 10(n-1)^2 + 2$	viral hemagglutination
helical capsid	decapsidation

4. What effect did the development of tissue cultures have on the development of animal virology? Explain.

5. Describe three methods of enumerating animal viruses.

6. Compare the adsorption and entry of a typical animal virus to the same processes in a T-even bacteriophage.

7. What protein-synthesizing strategies are available to a plus RNA virus that are not available to a minus RNA virus?

8. Describe how the polycistronic message of the poliovirus is used to synthesize individual proteins. How does this system limit viral control over protein synthesis?

9. Do interferons have a potential use for treating viral infections? Explain.

10. What is an oncogenic virus? Give an example of an oncogenic virus and explain how it transforms its host cell.

11. How are viruses isolated? Are viruses isolated in the routine diagnosis of most viral infections? Explain.

12. What is/are the major method(s) used to control human viral diseases? Which diseases have been successfully controlled?

Discussion

1. Oncogenic viruses cause tumors in animals. Is it possible that viruses cause human cancer?

2. The ability to work with the viruses that cause human diseases developed about 50 years after the isolation of the majority of the bacteria that cause human diseases. What were the reasons for this delay?

3. Will interferons ever be as effective in treating viral diseases as antibiotics are against bacterial diseases?

4. What techniques will be used for the commercial production of interferons? Discuss.

FURTHER READINGS

Books

Davis, B. D., R. Dublecco, H. N. Eisen, and H. S. Ginsberg, *Microbiology*, 3rd ed., Harper & Row, New York, 1980. An advanced medical microbiology textbook with an extensive section on animal virology.

Luria, S. E., J. E. Darnell, Jr., D. Baltimore, and A. Campbell, *General Virology*, 3rd ed., Wiley, New York, 1978. An advanced, detailed textbook that covers all groups of viruses.

Mandel, G. L., R. G. Douglas, and J. E. Bennett, *Principles and Practice of Infectious Diseases*, vol. 2, Wiley, New York, 1979. An advanced reference book written for the medical practitioner that discusses each classification group of the human viruses.

McLean, D. M., *Virology in Health Care*, Williams & Wilkins, Baltimore, 1980. A concise presentation of clinical virology.

Watson, J. D., *The Molecular Biology of the Gene*, 3rd ed., Benjamin, Menlo Park, Calif., 1976. One of the best textbooks on the molecular aspects of biological systems. This book contains an entire chapter on viral replication and another on oncogenic viruses.

Articles and Reviews

Bishop, J. M., "Oncogenes," *Sci. Am.*, 246:80–92 (March 1982). Recent research on Rous sarcoma virus has led to the identification of both viral and animal genes that are involved in oncogenesis.

Burke, D. C., "The Status of Interferon," *Sci. Am.*, 236:42–50 (April 1977). A review of interferon research in the pre-biotechnology era.

Fenner, F., "The Classification of Viruses: Why, When, and How," *Austral. J. Exp. Bio. Med. Sci.*, 52:223–240 (1974). A description of the beginnings of the International Committee on Nomenclature of Viruses (ICNV) and the status of the classification of viruses at the committee's inception.

Gordon, J., and M. A. Minks, "The Interferon Renaissance: Molecular Aspects of Induction and Action," *Microbiol. Revs.*, 45:244–266 (1981). An update on the molecular biology of the synthesis and activity of interferons.

Simons, K., H. Garoff, and A. Helenius, "How an Animal Virus Gets Into and Out of Its Host Cell," *Sci. Am.*, 246:58–66 (February 1982). A detailed look at the entry, replication, and exit of an enveloped togavirus (Semliki Forest virus).

Spector, D. H., and D. Baltimore, "The Molecular Biology of Poliovirus," *Sci. Am.*, 232:24–32 (May 1975). The replication of this polycistronic, single-stranded, plus RNA virus is described and illustrated.

23

VIRAL DISEASES
OF THE
RESPIRATORY TRACT

Human viral diseases can be organized into groups based on the major target organ affected. This approach results in four groups of human viral diseases: respiratory tract diseases; dermatotropic diseases; blood, liver, and enteric diseases; and neurotropic diseases. Some viruses infect more than one organ in the human body, so their placement in one of these groups is partially subjective. The viruses belonging to these four groups of human diseases are discussed in four separate chapters.

VIRAL DISEASES OF THE UPPER RESPIRATORY TRACT

Many human viruses enter their host via the respiratory tract. Some of these viruses use this route of entry to cause diseases of the skin and the nervous system, whereas other viruses actually infect respiratory tract tissues. Viral infections of the upper respiratory tract can be asymptomatic to debilitating, but they rarely cause serious complications. A few respiratory tract viruses cause viremias (influenza and mumps viruses) that may lead to serious complications involving the central nervous system or to

secondary bacterial infections. Viral diseases of the human respiratory tract are transmitted by contaminated fomites, by person-to-person contact, and by viruses suspended in small-particle aerosols. Viral infections of the respiratory tract are among the most common human afflictions.

Coryza: the common cold

Coryza is the inflammation of the mucous membranes of the nasal passages that is commonly known as a head cold. Coryza results from a viral infection of the nasal membranes and is characterized by excessive mucous secretion. Common colds are debilitating viral diseases and are major causes of time lost from school and work.

Common cold viruses. Human head colds are caused by many different viruses. There are more than 89 types of rhinoviruses, at least 3 types of coronaviruses, 4 types of parainfluenza viruses, and 33 types of adenoviruses that cause common colds (Table 23–1). Indeed, there are so many viruses responsible for this disease that adults in the United States average two to four colds per year, and children average six to eight colds per year.

Rhinoviruses comprise the largest group of viruses that cause common colds in humans (Table 23–1). They are small, icosahedral, RNA viruses that belong to the Picornaviridae family. Rhinoviruses were first isolated from patients with head colds in 1959 by virologists who succeeded in growing them in tissue cultures. Unlike other viruses, the rhinoviruses have an optimum growth temperature between 33° and 35°C, which is within the temperature of the human nasal passages. They also require a growth medium with a low pH.

Eighty-nine antigenic types and one subtype of the rhinoviruses have been identified. Humans form antibodies (IgA) against each viral type. These antibodies are present in nasal mucus and protect against reinfection. Individuals experience multiple rhinovirus infections each year caused by the different antigenic types of rhinoviruses.

Coronaviruses are pleomorphic, enveloped, RNA viruses that possess petal-shaped structures projecting from their viral envelope (Figure 23–1). They belong to the Coronaviridae family. Each virus particle has the appearance of the sun surrounded by a corona; hence they are named coronavirus. Three im-

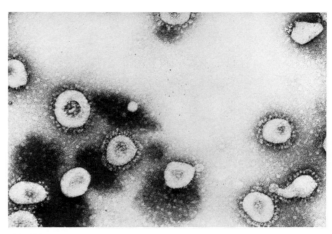

FIGURE 23–1
Human coronavirus from infected human embryonic tissue culture cells. The club-shaped projections emanating from the viral envelope have been likened to the sun's corona. (Courtesy of the Centers for Disease Control.)

portant human coronaviruses have been isolated. They cause mild upper respiratory tract infections in both children and adults. Coronaviruses are responsible for 2 percent or more of common colds in humans.

Cold symptoms also accompany certain viral infections of the lower respiratory tract. Human illnesses caused by parainfluenza virus, respiratory syncytial virus, influenza virus, and adenovirus infect the lower respiratory tract and cause cold symptoms (Table 23–1). Virologists estimate that between 30 and 40 percent of the viruses capable of causing coryza in humans have not been isolated.

Clinical symptoms. The incubation period for the common cold is between 2 and 3 days. Cold symptoms are readily recognized by most people and include sneezing, nasal discharge, sore-dry-scratchy throat, headache, cough, malaise, and chills. Initially, the nasal discharge is colorless and watery, but it later changes to a heavy, tan-colored mucus. Most cold patients maintain a near normal temperature and recover completely from these self-limiting diseases.

TABLE 23–1
Viruses Associated with the Common Cold

Virus	Antigenic Types	Percent of Colds
Rhinoviruses	89	25–30
	1 subtype	
Coronavirus	3 or more	2?
Parainfluenza virus	4	
Respiratory syncytial virus	1	10–15
Influenza virus	3	
Adenovirus	33	
Other viruses known		5
Other viruses (presumed)		30–40

Source: Adapted with permission from J. M. Gwaltney, Jr., "The Common Cold," in G. L. Mandell, R. G. Douglas, Jr., and J. E. Bennett (eds.), *Principles and Practice of Infectious Diseases*, Wiley, New York, 1979.

A few common cold patients (0.5 to 2 percent) develop bacterial sinusitis and/or otitis media (middle ear infection). Symptoms of these conditions are evident on a physical examination and are treated symptomatically. Respiratory syncytial virus and parainfluenza viruses (see following) infect young children and may lead to pneumonia, croup, and bronchiolitis. In the absence of these complications, the clinical symptoms of the common cold caused by rhinoviruses, coronavirus, parainfluenza virus, and respiratory syncytial virus are indistinguishable.

Epidemiology. The incidence of common colds in the United States rises during September to an elevated level that remains high through February. During March, April, and May, the incidence of the common cold gradually drops to its low summer level. There is no scientific explanation for the greater incidence of colds during the colder months. At one time people thought that "one caught a cold" by becoming chilled, but experiments have cast doubt on this belief. The susceptibility of a person to the rhinoviruses does not increase when a patient is chilled prior to exposure. Moreover, common-cold-causing viruses appear with their own seasonal fluctuations within the cold season. Coronaviruses cause more colds in the winter months, whereas outbreaks of rhinovirus-caused colds occur mainly in the early fall and in the spring.

The common cold viruses are transmitted by direct contact and by aerosols. Active viruses are secreted in mucus from the nasal passages and in sputum. When a patient uses a tissue or a handkerchief to clear the nose, the viruses are transferred to their hands. Hand shaking and other modes of direct personal contact are a major means of transferring cold viruses to other persons. Susceptible persons then infect their conjunctival mucosa or their nasal mucosa by direct contact. Transmission of the viral agents in aerosols, or as large particles of respiratory secretions suspended in air, probably occurs only over short distances. Experiments have demonstrated that rhinoviruses are not efficiently transmitted via air.

Prevention and treatment. Human colds can be prevented only by interrupting viral transmission. To avoid being infected, one should take extra care in washing one's hands after touching patients with colds and their contaminated clothes or tissues. Avoidance of cold patients is the only successful means of preventing the spread of these viruses.

The symptoms of coryza can be treated to decrease the patient's suffering. Phenylepherine (0.25 to 0.5 percent) and ephidrine (1 percent) are vasoconstrictors that decrease the swelling of the nasal membranes and permit the drainage of nasal secretions. Postnasal drip is relieved by administering nasal decongestants, which decrease the discharge of mucus into the pharyngeal region. This postnasal drip causes coughing, which can be suppressed by codeine. Aspirin is often taken to relieve the headaches and muscle pains that accompany the common cold.

Patients respond immunologically to the common cold viruses by producing immunoglobulin A. This protection must be developed against each cold virus, so humans may experience many head colds during a single year.

Respiratory infection caused by adenoviruses

Adenoids are lymphoid tissues located behind the uvula on the backside of the pharynx. Adenoviruses were originally isolated from human adenoid tissue that was removed during tonsillectomies. Thirty-five serotypes of adenoviruses have been identified; approximately half of these viruses cause human disease.

Virology of adenoviruses. Human adenoviruses are naked, icosahedral, double-stranded DNA viruses that belong to the Adenoviridae family. Their capsid is composed of 252 capsomeres, which are present in three distinct types (Figure 23–2). The majority of the capsomeres (240) are hexons that have six neighboring capsomeres. The 12 vertices of the icosahedron are occupied by pentons, which are capsomeres with five nearest neighbors. Each penton has a rodlike structure known as a fiber. Inside

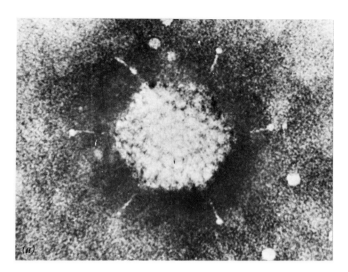

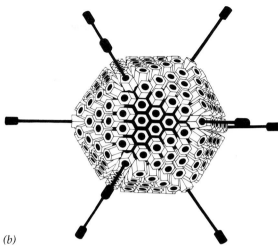

(b)

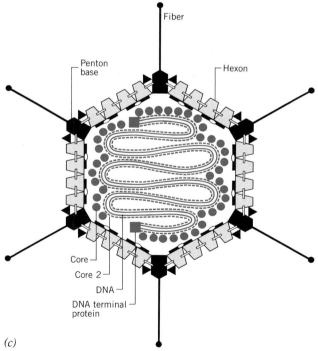

FIGURE 23–2

(a) Electron micrograph of adenovirus type 5 that shows its icosahedral structure and the fibers projecting from the penton bases. (Courtesy of Dr. H. G. Pereira. From R. C. Valentine and H. G. Pereira, *J. Mol. Biol.,* 13:13–20, 1965, copyright ©, Academic Press Inc., Ltd., London.) (b) Model of adenovirus type 5. (Courtesy of Dr. R. W. Horne. From R. W. Horne, I. P. Rohchetti, and J. M. Hobart, *J. Ultrastructure Res.,* 51:233–252, 1975, copyright © 1965, Academic Press Inc., Ltd., London.) (c) Diagram of human adenovirus illustrating the structure of the capsid and the positioning of the capsid proteins. (Courtesy of Dr. H. S. Ginsberg. From H. Fraenkel-Conrat and R. Wagner, eds., *Comprehensive Virology,* 13:409–457, 1979, Dover, New York.)

Adenoviruses cause cytopathic effects in tissue cultures of human epithelial cells (Figure 23–3). The infected cells round up and produce protoplasmic strands that connect adjacent cells. Infected cells also produce a virus induced T antigen, which becomes incorporated into the cell's plasma membrane. The presence of the T antigens on the surface of an infected cell can be demonstrated by immunofluorescent antibody techniques.

Adenoviruses can replicate in a normal lytic cycle, or they can cause chronic, latent infections of lymphoid tissue. These latent infections are normally asymptomatic in humans; however, adenoviruses

this capsid is the viral DNA that represents between 10 and 15 percent of the viral weight. Associated with the viral DNA are two core proteins and a DNA terminal protein.

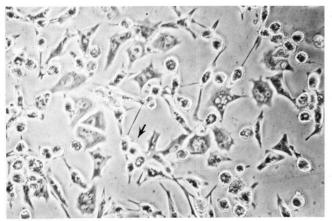

FIGURE 23-3
Cytopathic effects observed in a tissue culture of human epithelial cells infected with adenovirus. The flat, uninfected, multisided cells are distinct from the spherical, infected cells (↑) that possess interconnecting strands. (Courtesy of Dr. S. G. Baum, "Adenovirus," in G. L. Mandell, R. G. Douglas Jr., and J. E. Bennet, eds., *Principles and Practice of Infectious Diseases*, copyright © 1979, Wiley.)

do cause tumor formation in hamsters and other animals. These tumors are experimentally linked to adenovirus infections by the presence of the T antigen on the cell's surface. Adenoviruses are not known to be oncogenic in humans.

Diseases caused by adenoviruses. Adenoviruses are ubiquitous in humans and cause upper respiratory illnesses. These viruses cause coryza, pharyngitis, pharyngoconjunctival fever, acute respiratory disease, pneumonia, and epidemic keratoconjunctivitis. At least half of the human adenovirus infections are clinically insignificant. In infants, adenoviruses cause a mild to asymptomatic coryza and pharyngitis. All the adenoviral diseases are self-limiting, and death from them is extremely rare.

Pharyngoconjunctival fever. This disease occurs predominantly in children attending summer camps. It is spread by contaminated swimming water. The illness is characterized by slight fever and inflammation of the conjunctiva, the pharynx, and the nose. The symptoms develop rapidly after infection and last for 3 to 5 days. Patients recover from pharyngoconjunctival fever with no permanent eye damage.

Epidemic keratoconjunctivitis. Outbreaks of keratoconjunctivitis among adults have been traced to contamination of common towels and ophthalmic solutions. Adenoviruses have been identified as the etiological agent. The incubation period is 4 to 24 days, and symptoms may last for 1 to 4 weeks. The inflammation of the cornea (keratitis) develops after the inflammation of the conjunctiva dissipates. Keratitis is usually accompanied by distorted vision.

Acute respiratory illness. Acute respiratory illness is most common among military trainees. This disease is spread by aerosols and is prevalent among persons living in close quarters. Seasonal outbreaks occur between January and March in the Northern Hemisphere. The symptoms include fever, malaise, cough, sore throat, headache, and swollen neck lymph glands. Vaccines have been developed against adenovirus serotype 4 and 7. These vaccines were once administered to high-risk persons, but they are no longer used because of the potential of adenoviruses to act as oncogenic viruses.

VIRAL DISEASES OF THE LOWER RESPIRATORY TRACT

Influenza virus, parainfluenza virus, and respiratory syncytial viruses cause diseases of the human lower respiratory tract. The influenza viruses comprise the membership of the Orthomyxoviridae family. Parainfluenza viruses (croup) and respiratory syncytial viruses (bronchiolitis and bronchopneumonia) are members of the Paramyxoviridae family. These family names are derived from the word *myxo* (Gr. *myxa*, mucus).

Influenza

Human influenza is caused by influenza virus type A or influenza virus type B. These viruses sporadically cause severe human illness throughout the world. An influenza outbreak begins with the appearance of a new strain of the virus in a local geographical area. Influenza viruses are among the few infectious agents that can spread throughout the world's human population to cause a pandemic. The most severe influenza pandemic, during which 21 million people died worldwide and 549,000 people died in the United States, occurred in 1918–1919. Five major influenza pandemics have occurred since 1920; the most recent one occurred in 1977 (see Table 23–3). Influenza is a unique viral disease because the viral antigens have the propensity to change from one epidemic to the next. Infected humans build up an immunity against reinfection by the same influenza virus, but they are vulnerable to infections by each new influenza virus serotype.

Influenza viruses. The three known influenza viruses (type A, B, and C) are differentiated by their matrix protein and nucleoprotein. Type A and type B influenza virus cause human disease. Type A is responsible for pandemic human influenza; it also infects a variety of animals and birds. Type B influenza virus causes a milder form of human influenza, whereas influenza type C is rarely isolated from humans.

The influenza viruses are morphologically similar enveloped RNA viruses. Influenza viruses grown in tissue cultures are spherical to filamentous in shape (Figure 23–4). The spherical morphology predominates in laboratory stocks. The viral genome is composed of eight single-stranded minus RNA molecules. Each viral RNA molecule codes for one polypeptide (Table 23–2). The influenza virus contains a polymerase that makes plus RNA from the viral genome. Each plus RNA functions as an mRNA and codes for the synthesis of one viral protein.

Hemagglutinin, neuraminidase, and the matrix proteins are involved in the structure of the viral envelope (Figure 23–5). The hemagglutinin (HA) and the neuraminidase (NA) are formed inside the host cell. Both proteins have a hydrophobic end, which attaches them to the outside of the cell's plasma membrane. Matrix proteins and the nucleoproteins accumulate on the inner surface of the plasma membrane in regions that contain the HA and NA projec-

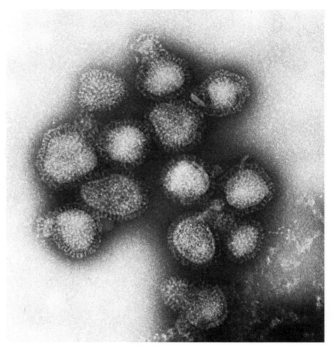

FIGURE 23—4
Electron micrograph of the spherical form of the influenza virus. (Omikron/Photo Researchers.)

FIGURE 23—5
Diagram of the influenza virus that shows the location of the viral antigens and the segmented nature of the viral genome. (Adapted from I. T. Schulze, *Advances in Virus Research*, 18:1–15, 1973, copyright © Academic Press.)

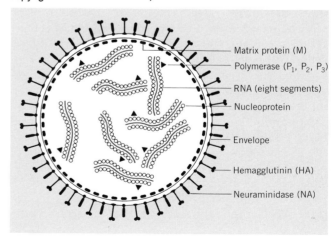

Matrix protein (M)
Polymerase (P_1, P_2, P_3)
RNA (eight segments)
Nucleoprotein
Envelope
Hemagglutinin (HA)
Neuraminidase (NA)

TABLE 23–2
Type A Influenza Viral Genome

RNA Segment Number	Gene Product (Designation)	Proposed Function of Viral Product
1	Polymerase (P_3)	Viral replication
2	Polymerase (P_1)	Viral replication
3	Polymerase (P_2)	Viral replication
4	Hemagglutinin (HA)	Attachment to cell membrane
5	Neuraminidase (NA)	Release from membrane: prevents viral aggregation
6	Nucleoprotein (NP)	Structural component of nucleocapsid
7	Matrix protein (M)	Structure of envelope
8	Nonstructural (NS)	Unknown

Source: Adapted with permission from R. Gordon Douglas, Jr., and Robert F. Betts, "Orthomyxoviridae," in G. L. Mandell, R. Gordon Douglas, Jr., and J. E. Bennett (eds.), *Principles and Practice of Infectious Diseases*, Wiley, New York, 1979.

tions. The adjacent cell membrane surrounds these viral components to form the outer envelope of the virus, and the virus is budded off into a distinct virion (see Figure 22–9).

Hemagglutinin and neuraminidase spikes. Protruding from the viral envelope are the hemagglutinin and neuraminidase spikes. Hemagglutinins recognize receptors on eucaryotic-cell surfaces. Both red blood cells and susceptible mammalian cells possess surface receptors that contain sialic acid residues attached to glycoproteins or glycolipids. The viral hemagglutinin binds to these red blood cell receptors, causing the agglutination of the red blood cells. The hemagglutinin also combines with receptor sites on susceptible cells. Binding of the influenza's hemagglutinin to a cell's receptor is the first step in viral infection.

Neuraminidase enzymatically cleaves the bond joining sialic acid to the cell receptor. This destroys the cell receptor in an irreversible way. The role of neuraminidase in viral propagation is not clear. Possible roles for neuraminidase are (1) to prevent virions from nonspecifically binding to mucins (glycoproteins) in the respiratory tract, (2) to prevent the virion from binding to its host cell's surface following release, (3) to decrease the tendency of the virions to form large aggregates, and (4) to hydrolyze mucin so that the virus can attach to the cell.

Antigenic structure. Hemagglutinin, neuraminidase, and nucleoprotein are the major antigens used to characterize influenza viruses. Each influenza subtype is designated by its nucleoproteins (as either type A, B, or C), the place (or animal) of initial isolation, and the antigenic composition of its hemagglutinin and neuraminidase. The different antigenic forms of hemagglutinin and neuraminidase are designated H_0, H_1, H_2, H_3, H_{sw}, and N_1, N_2. H_{sw} indicates the hemagglutinin found on the influenza virus isolated from swine. The influenza viruses are also designated A_0, A_1, A_2, A_3, etc. according to the sequence of their initial isolation.

Viral antigens have had a major effect on the severity of influenza epidemics (Table 23–3). A change from H_0N_1 to H_1N_1 resulted in a mild pandemic in 1947. This strain was prevalent until 1957, when the A/Singapore strain with its unique antigenic structure (H_2N_2) appeared and caused a severe pandemic. When a virus changes into a preexisting antigenic type, the resulting virus has a less drastic effect on the population. Influenza A/USSR has an antigenic subtype of H_1N_1 and caused only a mild disease when it appeared between 1977 and 1979.

Most viruses have stable surface antigens. The multiplicity of the antigenic strains of the influenza virus and their historical appearance make this virus unique. There are two theories to explain the antigenic multiplicity of the influenza virus: antigenic drift and antigenic shift.

Antigenic drift. A given influenza virus possesses one of five antigenic types of hemagglutinin and one of two antigenic types of neuraminidase. The change from one antigenic type to another occurs in nature with new antigenic types appearing over a period of years. Minor antigenic variations result from mutations in hemagglutinin and neuraminidase genes. Some of these mutant viruses will replicate in a host because they are not inactivated by the prevailing antibodies. **Antigenic drift** is the term used to describe this slow, sequential change in the antigenic structure of viral surface proteins. These antigenic changes occur only in the HA and NA antigens of the influenza virus: the type A, B, and C nucleoprotein antigens do not change.

Antigenic shift. Major antigenic changes have occurred in the influenza hemagglutinin and neuraminidase to create "new" viruses. The change is referred to as an **antigenic shift** when the amino acid sequence in the hemagglutinin and the neuraminidase differ greatly from the old forms of these antigens. These new influenza strains are responsible for the major influenza pandemics (Table 23–3). Antigenic shifts probably occur during the production of virions in cells infected with more than one influenza virus. Since each influenza surface antigen is coded for by an independent segment of RNA (Table 23–3), the reassortment of viral RNA segments during viral assembly in multiple infected cells could be responsible for the observed antigenic shifts. The "new" virus would be antigenically unlike either of its parent virions. Experiments with mixed influenza infections of swine and turkeys have provided experimental support for this theory.

Epidemic influenza. Influenza epidemics occur most frequently in the winter months. This respiratory illness occurs first among children in a given geographical local and then appears in adults. The illness usually affects between 10 and 20 percent of the population.

Pandemics occur following the emergence of a "new" influenza virus. This happens every 9 to 17 years, with a recent average of 12 years between pandemics (Table 23–3). During the intervals between pandemics, the human population builds up an immunity to the extant strain. Each new strain becomes widely disseminated when the majority of the human population is susceptible to it.

Influenza viruses are transmitted between persons by small-particle aerosols. The incubation period for

TABLE 23–3

Major Antigenic Subtypes of Influenza A Virus Associated with Pandemic Influenza

Year of Prevalence	Influenza A Subtype[a]	Antigenic Structure	Disease Characteristics
1918?	Swine	$H_{sw}N_1$	Severe
1933–1946	A_0/SW/33	H_0N_1	No pandemic
1947–1957	A_1/FM/47	H_1N_1	Mild
1957–1967	A_2/Singapore/57	H_2N_2	Severe
1968–1979	A_3/HongKong/68	H_3N_2	Moderate
1977–1979	A_1/USSR/77	H_1N_1	Mild

[a]Subtype/source/year.

influenza is between 18 and 72 hours. The viruses infect the patient's respiratory tract and grow in the epithelial cells of the tracheobronchial mucosa and the nasopharynx. At the onset of the clinical symptoms, the viruses are present in the patient's nasal discharges. They also become suspended in small-particle aerosols during coughing, sneezing, or talking. The major mode of transmission of influenza viruses is from person to person. Infection can occur by direct contact with an infected person; however, the rate of infection is much higher when subjects inhale the virus.

Clinical symptoms. Influenza is an acute febrile illness, which is usually self-limiting. The clinical symptoms include glazed mucous membranes of the nose and mouth; severe muscle pain (myalgia); weakness; fever (39° to 41°C); a dry, hacking cough; headache; and chills. The fever usually lasts 2 to 3 days, and a feeling of weakness may persist for 1 to 2 weeks.

Some patients experience a primary viral pneumonia. This syndrome follows the onset of the typical influenza symptoms accompanied by labored breathing (dyspnea), cough, and cyanosis. Viral pneumonia can lead to death, especially in compromised patients. Influenza patients are also vulnerable to secondary bacterial infections of the lungs. The bacteria commonly involved are *Streptococcus pneumoniae, Staphylococcus aureus,* and *Hemophilus influenzae.* The increased death rate in a human population (see Figure 14–1) above the expected threshold is attributed to influenza-caused viral pneumonia or to influenza-related bacterial pneumonia.

Diagnosis, treatment, and prevention. Influenza is diagnosed by isolating the virus during the initial outbreak. The virus can be grown in tissue cultures or in embryonated chicken eggs. Once the existence of an epidemic is established, influenza is routinely diagnosed by its clinical symptoms.

The antiviral drug **amantadine** is licensed in the United States for treating influenza type A. Amantadine inhibits the replication of influenza type A by

preventing viral uncoating. It is a specific drug that has little or no effect on the replication of influenza type B. This drug reduces the duration and the symptoms of influenza by approximately 50 percent. Its contraindications are insomnia, dizziness, and a loss of the ability to concentrate. The cold symptoms that accompany influenza can be treated with common cold remedies such as aspirin and phenylephrine. Pulmonary complications involving secondary bacterial infections are treated with appropriate antibiotics.

Influenza can be prevented by administering the appropriate inactivated virus vaccine. The influenza vaccines used in the United States are composed of inactivated type A and type B influenza viruses of the antigenic serotype that was prevalent during the previous year. The viruses are grown in embryonated chicken eggs and are administered preferentially to persons with chronic illness and to persons over 64 years of age.

Paramyxoviruses

Parainfluenza virus, respiratory syncytial viruses, and the mumps virus are members of the Paramyxoviridae family. They are spherical viruses composed of a nucleocapsid surrounded by an envelope (Figure 23–6). The nucleocapsid is composed of a linear RNA molecule surrounded by helically arranged nucleoprotein subunits. Their nucleocapsid is formed in the host cell's cytoplasm and accumulates near the plasma membrane. During maturation, the nucleocapsid is encompassed by the plasma membrane, which contains specific viral antigens. The paramyxoviruses contain hemagglutinin, and some contain neuraminidase. Their antigens are genetically stable.

Parainfluenza virus: croup. The three types of the parainfluenza virus cause respiratory illnesses in young children. They are distinguished by their complement-fixing and hemagglutinating antigens. Human types 1, 2, and 3 possess surface hemagglutinin, neuraminidase, and hemolysin. They can be

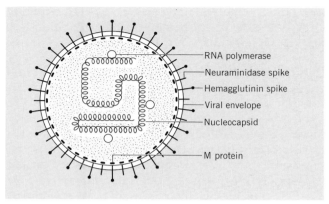

- RNA polymerase
- Neuraminidase spike
- Hemagglutinin spike
- Viral envelope
- Nucleocapsid
- M protein

FIGURE 23–6
Diagram of the nucleocapsid and the envelope of a paramyxovirus.

cultured in primary monkey kidney tissue cultures or in human embryonic tissue cultures.

Human illness. Parainfluenza viruses infect the respiratory tract of young children (Table 23–4). Croup is the most severe disease caused by the parainfluenza viruses. It occurs in children under 30 months of age who are infected with any of the three viral types. The symptoms of croup include a barking cough and hoarseness that may be accompanied by respiratory blockage. The most common form of the disease is a cold that is accompanied by bronchitis. The severity of croup depends on the specific virus and the immunological history of the patient. Most older patients have some immune resistance to the parainfluenza viruses.

Epidemiology. Parainfluenza viruses are transmitted by direct contact and by large droplets discharged from the respiratory tract. Type 1 parainfluenza virus is most frequently isolated in the fall and winter months, whereas type 3 is present at a low but persistent rate throughout the year. Young children are most often infected by type 1 and type 2 before they are 6 years old. Reinfections of older persons occur with all three types, but the symptoms are usually restricted to a cold and bronchitis, and the viruses are shed for only 1 to 3 days. There is no specific treatment for parainfluenza virus infections. The disease is self-limiting, and almost all patients recover.

Respiratory syncytial virus. Respiratory syncytial virus (RSV) is a major cause of bronchiolitis and pneumonia in young children. RSV is an enveloped RNA virus that is a paramyxovirus. Following its initial isolation from a chimpanzee, it was found to be widely distributed among humans. When RSV is grown in tissue culture, it coalesces the cells into a refractile mass referred to as a **syncytium,** for which it was named.

Outbreaks of RSV occur in the winter and spring. The virus is so prevalent that between 25 and 50 per-

TABLE 23–4
Parainfluenza Viral Infections of Children

Primary Infections	Usual Age at Onset	Clinical Symptoms	
		Severe	Mild
Type 1, Type 2	8 – 30 months	Croup	Cold, bronchitis
Type 3	1 – 24 months	Croup, pneumonia, bronchiolitis	Cold

Source: Modified from J. Owen Hendley, "Parainfluenza Virus," in G. L. Mandell, R. Gordon Douglas, Jr., and J. E. Bennett (eds.), *Principles and Practice of Infectious Diseases,* Wiley, New York, 1979.

cent of 1-year-olds and almost all 5-year-olds have specific antibodies against this virus. Symptoms of an RSV infection are nasal congestion, cough that can be accompanied by a sore throat, fever, conjunctivitis, and hoarseness. Primary viral infection or secondary bacterial infection of the middle ear (otitis media) is a common complication. The symptoms of bronchiolitis and pneumonia in young children are often caused by RSV infections. Most children recover and possess antibodies against RSV, even though reinfection may occur. Cardiopulmonary and/or congenital disorders are complications that may lead to the death of infected infants. There is no treatment for RSV infections; however, breast-fed infants are more resistant to infections of RSV than are bottle-fed infants.

Mumps

The massive swelling of the parotid glands is the unique clinical symptom that characterizes mumps. The clinical symptoms of this human viral disease were first reported in the fifth century B.C. writings of Hippocrates. The agent of mumps, however, was not demonstrated until 1934, when Johnson and Goodpasture reproduced the clinical symptoms of mumps in monkeys by inoculating animals with bacteria-free material. Eleven years later, the mumps virus was cultivated in chicken embryos, which led to the development of a killed virus vaccine in the 1950s. The mumps virus vaccine that is used today was first licensed in 1967. Mumps is discussed here because the mumps virus is a member of the Paramyxoviridae family and its port of entry is the respiratory tract.

Mumps virus. The mumps virus is morphologically and chemically similar to the parainfluenza viruses. Its nucleocapsid is composed of RNA and nucleoprotein combined with an RNA polymerase. The nucleocapsid is surrounded by an envelope that contains both hemagglutinin and neuraminidase (Figure 23–6). There is only one serotype of the mumps virus, and humans are its only natural host. The mumps virus can be grown in a variety of cell cultures and in embryonated chicken eggs. The mumps virus is detected by a hemadsorption inhibition test that uses chicken erythrocytes.

Clinical symptoms of mumps. The mumps virus enters humans via the respiratory tract, where it infects the epithelial cells. The virus replicates in the upper respiratory tract and lymph nodes prior to causing a generalized viremia. At the end of the 16- to 18-day incubation, the mumps virus infects the salivary glands. The swelling of the salivary glands (specifically the parotid glands) occurs over a 2- to 3-day period and is the first and most prominent clinical symptom of mumps. This swelling is often accompanied by an earache and a temperature of 37 to 40°C. All symptoms subside within the week following the maximum swelling.

The central nervous system and the gonads are often affected during a mumps infection. Meningitis is the most common central nervous system symptom and occurs in 1 to 10 percent of mumps patients. Recovery from mumps-associated meningitis is complete with no known sequelae. A small number (0.02 percent) of mumps patients have encephalitis (inflammation of the brain). **Orchitis** (inflammation of the testes) occurs in 20 to 30 percent of infected postpubertal males. The swelling and pain of orchitis disappear within 5 days with no long-term consequences (sterility is rare). **Oophoritis** (inflammation of the ovaries) occurs in 5 percent of infected postpubertal females.

Epidemiology and prevention. The mumps virus infects the respiratory membranes of susceptible patients via airborne droplet nuclei or via fomites. Before a live, attenuated mumps virus vaccine was licensed in the United States in 1967 (Figure 23–7), epidemics occurred from January through May in a 2- to 5-year cycle. The 5- to 9-year-olds were the major group affected, and mumps spread readily among school-age children. Mumps was less likely to spread among older groups that were composed of immune individuals who previously had a clinical or subclinical case of mumps.

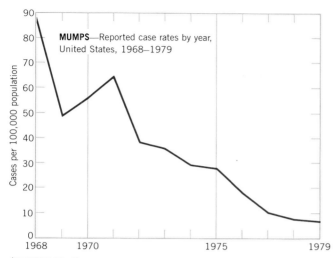

FIGURE 23–7

Reported case rates for mumps in the United States, 1968 through 1979. The mumps virus vaccine was licensed in December of 1967. (Centers for Disease Control, "Annual Summary 1979: Reported Morbidity and Mortality in the United States," *Morbidity Mortality Weekly Report,* 28, No. 54, 1980.)

The mumps vaccine is administered by a single subcutaneous inoculation. It is recommended for all children over 12 months of age. Current practice is to administer a combined measles-mumps-rubella vaccine (MMR) at 15 months of age. Introduction of the mumps vaccine in December 1967 has dramatically decreased the incidence of mumps in the U.S. population.

SUMMARY

The common cold is a viral infection of the mucous membranes of the nasal passages characterized by sneezing and a nasal discharge of watery to thick mucus. Rhinoviruses (89 types) and coronaviruses (3 types) are RNA viruses that cause the common cold (Table 23–5). Humans develop immunity to each infecting virus, but they remain susceptible to the others. Adults experience two to four common colds a year, whereas children have an average of six to eight colds a year. Colds predominate in fall and winter and are transmitted by direct contact or in aerosols. The symptoms of the common cold can be treated, whereas the only means of preventing colds is to avoid contact with cold patients.

Adenoviruses are DNA viruses that infect the human upper respiratory tract. Adenoviruses cause pharyngoconjunctival fever in summer camps, epidemic keratoconjunctivitis among adults, and acute respiratory illness among military trainees. At least half the human adenoviral infections are asymptomatic, and all are self-limiting diseases.

Lower respiratory tract infections caused by the influenza, parainfluenza, and respiratory syncytial viruses cause viral pneumonia, bronchiolitis, and bronchopneumonia. Influenza type A virus is responsible for pandemic influenza. Influenza viruses are segmented RNA viruses. Animals make antibodies against the hemagglutinin and neuraminidase surface antigens that inactivate the virus. The antigenic types of hemagglutinin and neuraminidase undergo modest changes by antigenic drift or major changes by antigenic shift. Major changes in the influenza antigens lead to influenza pandemics. The severe symptoms of influenza last 2 to 3 days; body weakness may persist for 1 to 2 weeks. Some patients die from primary viral pneumonia; others are debilitated by influenza that predisposes them to secondary bacterial infections. Bivalent influenza virus (types A and B) vaccines are used to prevent influenza in compromised patients and in persons over 65.

Parainfluenza viruses cause croup in young children. Croup is characterized by a barking cough and hoarseness emanating from a head cold and bronchitis. When adults are reinfected, the symptoms are milder than croup. The respiratory syncytial virus is a major cause of bronchiolitis in infants less than 2 years old. RSV is so prevalent that one-quarter of all 1-year-olds and almost all 5-year-olds have specific antibodies against it. Patients with cardiopulmonary or congenital disorders are especially vulnerable to RSV infections.

TABLE 23–5
Summary: Viral Diseases of the Respiratory Tract

Disease	Causative Agents	Clinical Disease	Transmission Prevention/Control
Coryza: common cold	Rhinoviruses: small, naked, single-stranded, RNA viruses, (89 antigenic types) Coronaviruses: pleomorphic, enveloped, single-stranded, RNA viruses	Sore throat, headache, cough, malaise, chills, nasal discharge	Avoid direct contact, treat symptoms
Upper respiratory illnesses	Adenoviruses: naked, double-stranded, DNA viruses	Pharyngoconjunctival fever, acute respiratory disease, pneumonia, pharyngitis, keratoconjunctivitis, latent infections of lymph tissue	Transmission by fomites, swimming water
Influenza	Influenza A, B, and C viruses: enveloped, RNA (8 single-strands of minus RNA), HA and NA surface antigens	Cold symptoms, headache, myalgia, fever, cough, chills, viral pneumonia (secondary bacterial pneumonia)	Immunization with inactive influenza A and influenza B vaccine, amantadine for influenza A
Croup	Parainfluenza viruses (3 types): enveloped, RNA nucleocapsid, HA and NA surface antigens	Barking cough, hoarseness, respiratory blockage	Affects young children, no specific treatment
Bronchiolitis	Respiratory syncytial virus: enveloped, nucleocapsid-RNA virus	Nasal congestion, cough, sore throat, fever, bronchiolitis, and pneumonia in children	Affects young children, no specific treatment
Mumps	Mumps virus: single-stranded, nucleocapsid-RNA virus, HA and NA surface antigens	Swelling of the salivary and parotid glands, earache. complications: meningitis, encephalitis, orchitis, and oophoritis	Live, attenuated virus vaccine

Mumps is caused by an RNA virus that infects the human respiratory tract prior to forming a viremia. The first clinical symptoms appear after a 16- to 18-day incubation period and include the swelling of the parotid glands. Complications of mumps include orchitis, oophoritis, meningitis, and encephalitis. Mumps is now controlled by the administration of a live, attenuated vaccine to children.

QUESTIONS AND TOPICS FOR STUDY AND DISCUSSION

Questions

1. Most human viral diseases do not recur because humans develop sufficient immunity against them. Why then do humans often contract more than one viral cold during a given year?

2. Describe the transmission and seasonal incidence of human head colds.
3. What diseases are caused by the human adenoviruses? Explain why the adenovirus vaccines are no longer recommended.
4. Describe the antigenic structure of the influenza type A virus. How are influenza type B and type C different from type A? Do these viruses also cause human illness? Explain.
5. What segment of the population is at the greatest risk from influenza? Explain.
6. Explain why the influenza type A virus is capable of causing pandemics.
7. What are antigenic drift and antigenic shift? What is the evidence for each type of antigenic change in influenza A virus?
8. How are infections of influenza prevented? What methods of treatment are available for influenza patients?
9. Describe the symptoms of croup. What virus causes this disease, and what segment of the population is most often affected?
10. What are the clinical signs of mumps? What other parts of the body can be affected by the mumps virus?
11. How is mumps transmitted, what is the incubation period, and how is this disease prevented?

Discussion

1. Can genetic engineering be used to develop an effective vaccine against all the antigenic varieties of the influenza virus?

2. Will modern technology ever be able to prevent the common cold?

FURTHER READING

Books

Fraser, K. B., and S. J. Martin, *Measles Virus and Its Biology,* Academic Press, London, 1978. A monograph on the biology of the measles virus and the disease it causes in humans.

Articles and Reviews

D'Allessio, D. J., J. A. Peterson, C. R. Dick, and E. C. Dick, "Transmission of Experimental Rhinovirus Colds in Volunteer Married Couples," *J. Infect. Dis.,* 133:28–36 (1976). A research paper on the transmission of two strains of rhinovirus.

Douglas, R. G., Jr., and R. F. Betts, "Influenza Virus," in G. L. Mandell, R. Gordon Douglas, Jr., and J. E. Bennett (eds.), *Principles and Practice of Infectious Diseases,* pp. 1135–1167, Wiley, New York, 1979. An informative article on the influenza virus written for the clinician.

Jackson, G. G., and R. L. Muldoon, "Viruses Causing Common Respiratory Infections in Man. V. Influenza A (Asian)," *J. Infect. Dis.,* 131:308–357 (1975). A detailed review of influenza A in outline form.

Laver, W. G., "The Polypeptides of Influenza Viruses," *Adv. in Virus Res.,* 18:57–103 (1973). A review of the structure and function of the influenza viruses.

24

VIRAL DISEASES OF THE HUMAN SKIN

Dermatotropic viruses infect humans via various routes, but ultimately they cause diseases of the human skin. These viruses cause skin infections that appear as maculopapular rashes, vesicular lesions, or warts. Maculopapular rashes are the spotty blemishes with raised inflamed centers that are characteristic of measles, German measles, and dengue.* These diseases are caused by RNA viruses belonging to three different viral families. Measles and German measles were once common childhood diseases, but now they are largely prevented by the use of vaccines.

Certain dermatotropic DNA viruses of the Herpetoviridae and the Poxviridae families cause vesicular skin lesions. Herpes simplex virus type 1 is primarily responsible for herpes labialis, whereas herpes simplex virus type 2 preferentially infects the ectodermal tissue of the urogenital region (urogenital herpes). Varicella-zoster virus, another member of the Herpetoviridae, is responsible for chickenpox and zoster. Smallpox (variola) is caused by a DNA virus belonging to the Poxviridae family, and warts

are caused by a single virus of the Papovaviridae family.

The current status of these viral diseases varies greatly. Measles and German measles are now controlled by administering the MMR vaccine to children. Smallpox (variola major) has been eradicated by worldwide surveillance by the World Health Organization (WHO) and vaccination. Chickenpox remains a mild childhood disease, whereas herpes viruses cause common and persistent human illnesses.

MACULOPAPULAR RASHES

Measles

Measles is a highly contagious human viral disease caused by the measles virus. Most people are infected during childhood; afterward, they recover and have lasting immunity against reinfection. Measles is now controlled by a vaccine that became available in 1963. Epidemiologists are hopeful that measles can be eradicated from the indigenous population of the United States in the near future.

Measles virus. The causative agent of measles is an enveloped, single-stranded minus RNA virus that

*Dengue is discussed in Chapter 26 with the other arthropod-borne viral diseases.

408

belongs to the Morbillivirus genus of the Paramyxoviridae family. The antigens of the measles virus include a hemolysin and a hemagglutinin that are associated with the viral envelope. The measles virus, however, lacks the neuraminidase that is present in the closely related mumps and parainfluenza viruses. The function of the measles hemagglutinin is to bind the virus to host cells, whereas the hemolysin functions in the fusion process of viral entry. Serodiagnosis can be made by hemagglutination inhibition or complement-fixing titrations. Even though the measles virus has been isolated in primary tissue cultures of human and monkey cells, isolation is rarely necessary for diagnosis because measles is easily recognized through its unique clinical symptoms.

Clinical symptoms. The highly contagious measles virus infects humans via the mucous membranes of the human respiratory tract and the conjunctiva. The virus is transmitted in secretions of the respiratory tract, in secretions of the eye, and in the urine from infected patients. There is an incubation period of 12 to 14 days before the clinical symptoms of measles begin (Figure 24–1). During the incubation period, the measles virus replicates within the human respiratory epithelium; then it infects the leukocytes of the reticuloendothelial system. Here the virus replicates again before it causes a generalized viremia. At this stage of the infection, viruses are found in the throat (Figure 24–1). The viremia coincides with the early symptoms of measles, which include fever, malaise, loss of appetite (anorexia), conjunctivitis, cough, and coryza.

Koplik spots appear on the inside of the cheek prior to the development of the measles rash. **Koplik spots** are bluish-gray specks highlighted by an inflamed background. They last for a few days, but disappear as the measles rash develops. The rash (Color Plate 15) first appears on the face, and then it spreads

FIGURE 24–1

Clinical symptoms of measles in humans. CF, complement-fixation antigen; HI, hemagglutination inhibition; NT, neutralizing antibody. (Reproduced with permission. From D. M. McLean, *Virology in Health Care*, p. 123, copyright © 1980, Williams & Wilkins.)

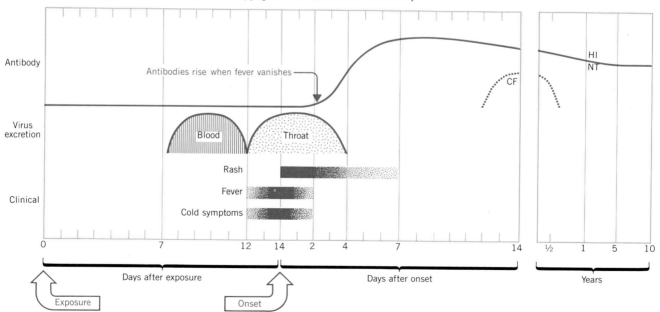

to the trunk and the extremities. The measles rash is initially spotty (maculopapular), but soon it becomes confluent over the neck and face. The patient may lose layers of skin (desquamation) as the rash dissipates. The major discomfort from this illness usually coincides with the second day of the rash. As the rash subsides about the fifth day, the virus disappears from the throat and the level of circulating antiviral antibody increases. Immunity from reinfection results following recovery from this illness.

Complications. Two neurological disorders may be complications of measles. **Subacute sclerosing panencephalitis** (SSPE) is a chronic degenerative neurological disease. Both the blood and the cerebrospinal fluid of SSPE patients have unusually high antibody titers against measles. This disease is slow to develop and occurs several to many years after a patient recovers from measles. **Multiple sclerosis** is a progressive, degenerative disease of the central nervous system that results in the loss of certain brain and spinal cord functions. Patients with multiple sclerosis have higher than normal measles-antibody titers in their spinal fluid. At present the link between measles infections and multiple sclerosis is considered to be tenuous. Less serious complications of measles are the secondary bacterial infections of the middle ear and the lungs. These secondary infections are routinely treated with antibiotics.

Epidemiology, prevention, and treatment. Prior to the introduction of the measles vaccine, measles was a childhood disease that occurred as cyclical epidemics every 2 to 5 years. These epidemics involved large groups of susceptible patients such as young children attending their first few years of school. The major epidemics of measles occurred in the winter months possibly because the measles virus is more stabile in dry air.

The incidence of measles in the United States dropped precipitously (Figure 24–2) following the introduction of the live, attenuated measles virus vaccine in 1963. This vaccine is routinely given to children over 12 months old. The incidence of measles in the United States dropped to a new low in

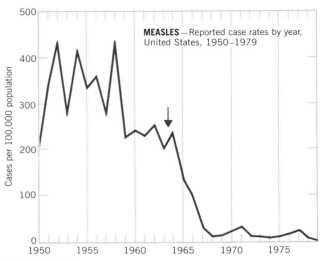

FIGURE 24–2

Measles cases reported in the United States by year from 1950 through 1979. The measles vaccine was introduced in 1963 (↓). (Centers for Disease Control, "Annual Summary 1979: Reported Morbidity and Mortality in the United States," *Morbidity Mortality Weekly Report*, 28, No. 54, 1980.)

1981 when less than 3100 cases were reported. This drop in the incidence of measles is the result of a national effort to eliminate indigenous measles from the United States by October 1982.

There is no specific treatment for measles except to make the patient comfortable. Hospitalized measles patients should be kept in respiratory isolation, and susceptible persons who are accidentally exposed should be vaccinated. Because the immunological response time to the vaccine is about 7 days, postinfection vaccination against the measles virus is an effective procedure.

Rubella (German measles)

Rubella (German measles) is an infectious viral disease that occurs only in humans. The symptoms of rubella are usually mild, especially in children. Congenital rubella is the most serious complication of rubella infections. It can develop in the fetus of a woman who contracts the disease during pregnancy. Today the incidence of rubella is greatly reduced because of the vaccination of prepubertal children.

Rubella virus. The rubella virus, first isolated in 1962, is a small (60 nm), enveloped RNA virus that possesses an envelope hemagglutinin, a complement-fixing antigen, and two precipitins. This virus is classified as the sole member of the Rubivirus genus in the Togaviridae family, but unlike other members of this family (see Chapter 26), the rubella virus is not transmitted by arthropod vectors. Instead, the virus is transmitted in aerosol droplets and infects the respiratory tract, where it is present in respiratory secretions. The rubella virus can be detected by hemagglutination, and a patient's immunity against the rubella virus can be measured by the hemagglutination inhibition activity of their serum.

Clinical symptoms. The severity of rubella is greatly dependent on the age of the patient. Infants and young children infected with the rubella virus experience a subclinical to mild illness. Adults usu-

ally experience the major clinical symptoms, which include fever, rash, and swelling of lymph nodes (lymphadenopathy), especially those in the back of the neck.

Incubation periods for rubella range from 12 to 22 days, with an average of 18 days. The rubella virus is present in the blood and the throat (Figure 24–3) prior to the appearance of the clinical symptoms. The clinical symptoms of fever, rash, and lymphadenopathy have a rapid onset after which they last for 4 or 5 days. Patients are most infectious during the height of the rash, but they shed rubella viruses from the throat prior to the onset of symptoms and for 10 to 15 days after onset. The increase in the antibody titer coincides with the abatement of the fever. Lifelong immunity against rubella develops in most patients following recovery from the illness.

Congenital rubella. The most serious complication from rubella occurs when pregnant women con-

FIGURE 24–3
Rubella (German measles) in humans. CF, complement-fixation antigen; HI, hemagglutination inhibition; NT, neutralizing antibody. (Reproduced with permission. From D. M. McLean, *Virology in Health Care,* p. 140, copyright © 1980, Williams & Wilkins.)

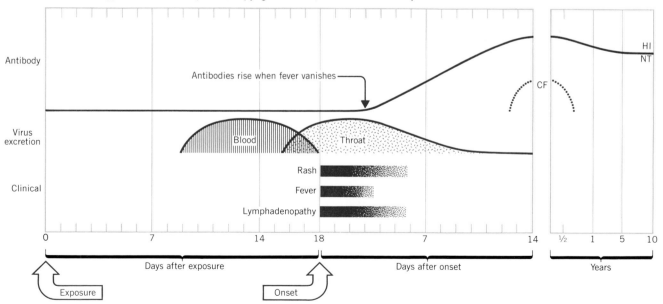

tract the disease and the rubella virus infects their fetus(es) to cause congenital rubella. This disease of the fetus can result in premature delivery, stillbirths, or in a variety of congenital defects.

The chance of a fetus contracting congenital rubella is dependent on the trimester in which the mother becomes infected. Mothers infected during the first 2 months of gestation have a 40- to 60-percent chance of bearing a fetus with multiple congenital defects. This probability drops to 30 to 35 percent if the mother is infected during the third month and to 10 percent if the mother is infected during the fourth month of gestation. Rubella infections occurring during the first trimester of pregnancy often result in spontaneous abortion. When congenital rubella develops during the third or fourth month of gestation, the outcome is usually a single congenital defect.

Permanent defects resulting from congenital rubella include hearing loss, cataracts, severe myopia, myocardial abnormalities, mental retardation, and diabetes mellitus. Temporary defects apparent at birth include low birth weight, meningoencephalitis, hepatitis, and pneumonia. Patients with congenital rubella are infected at birth and continue to shed the virus for many months. Why and how the rubella virus causes these severe defects is not known. The potential defects are so serious to the health of the child that mothers should seriously try to avoid contracting rubella during pregnancy.

Epidemiology of rubella. Infected persons shed rubella virus in respiratory secretions both before and after the onset of the symptoms. The virus is spread in aerosol droplets generated by the patient. Prior to the introduction of the rubella vaccine in 1969, rubella was most prevalent in young schoolchildren (ages 6 to 9). Now the disease occurs at a much lower frequency (Figure 24–4). During 1980, the 15-to-19 age group had the highest incidence of rubella followed by the 20-to-24 age group. These groups probably represented the only large group of nonimmune individuals in the population.

Rubella vaccine is now given to all prepubertal

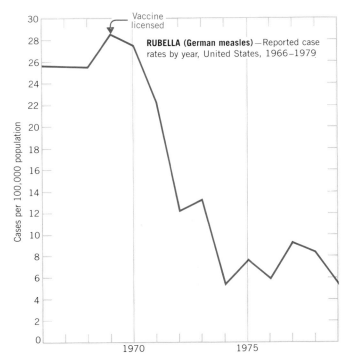

FIGURE 24–4
The effect of licensing the rubella vaccine on the incidence of rubella in the United States. (Centers for Disease Control "Annual Summary 1979: Reported Morbidity and Mortality in the United States," *Morbidity Mortality Weekly Report*, 28, No. 54, 1980).

children in the United States. Other countries vaccinate girls as they approach puberty, but do not vaccinate boys. Females of childbearing age are not vaccinated unless they are willing to practice some form of contraception for at least 3 months following vaccination. This is because the vaccine (RA 27/3) used in the United States is a live, attenuated strain of rubella that has the potential to cause congenital rubella in the fetus of pregnant women. However, recent studies conducted by the Centers for Disease Control indicate that the actual risk of congenital rubella occurring in the fetuses of vaccinated women is very low.

Use of the rubella vaccine has greatly reduced the incidence of congenital rubella. During the last major rubella epidemic, which occurred in 1964, 30,000 infants were affected by congenital rubella. Between 30 and 68 congenital rubella cases per year were reported to the Centers for Disease Control during the 1970s.

VESICULAR SKIN LESIONS

The viruses that cause vesicular lesions on human skin are all DNA viruses. The Herpetoviridae family contains the herpes simplex viruses (types 1 and 2) and the varicella-zoster virus. Varicella continues to cause major epidemics of chickenpox, and herpes simplex is a prominent and serious health problem. Vaccinia virus and the smallpox virus are two related human viruses belonging to the Poxviridae. Vaccinia virus is used to immunize humans against smallpox. Smallpox is caused by the variola virus (variola major), which has been eliminated for all practical purposes from the human population.

Herpesviruses

Four large, enveloped DNA viruses belonging to the family Herpetoviridae (Table 24–1) cause human disease. Epstein-Barr virus causes infectious mononucleosis, and cytomegalovirus causes diseases in newborns (see Chapter 25). Herpes simplex and varicella-zoster cause diseases of the human skin.

Herpes simplex viruses. Herpes simplex viruses (HSV) are large, enveloped, icosahedral DNA viruses. The capsid is composed of 162 elongated, hexagonal capsomeres each containing a central core (Figure 24–5). The capsid is surrounded by an envelope that is believed to be derived from the endoplasmic reticulum of the host cell's cytoplasm. Herpes simplex viruses are slowly released from their host cells by a process of reverse phagocytosis.

Herpes simplex viruses cause **herpes labialis** (cold sores) and the venereal disease known as **urogenital herpes.** HSV exists in two forms: HSV-1 is the major cause (80 to 90 percent) of herpes labialis, whereas HSV-2 is the virus isolated most often (70 to 90 percent) from urogenital herpes. These two Herpetoviridae are antigenically distinct and have distinctive growth characteristics in tissue cultures. Herpes simplex viruses are transmitted by direct contact between humans and pose a major threat to humans.

TABLE 24–1
Herpetoviridae and Poxviridae

Virus	Disease	Description
Herpetoviridae		
Herpes simplex type 1	Herpes labialis	Double-stranded DNA, 162 capsomeres, icosahedral, enveloped (180 – 200 nm)
Herpes simplex type 2	Urogenital herpes	As above
Varicella-zoster	Varicella and zoster	As above
Epstein-Barr virus	Infectious mononucleosis	As above
Cytomegalovirus	Disease of newborns	As above
Poxviridae		
Vaccinia	Cowpox	Double-stranded DNA, asymmetrical, brick-shaped, 250 – 390 by
Variola	Smallpox	200 – 260 nm, replicates in cytoplasm

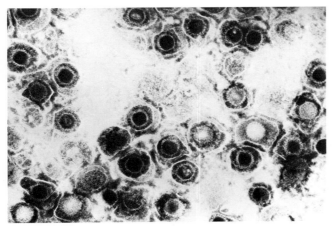

FIGURE 24–5
Electron micrograph of herpes simplex virus. (Courtesy of the Centers for Disease Control.)

Herpes infections. HSV-1 is most often associated with the lesions on the lips (Color Plate 16) known as **herpes labialis.** These lesions contain herpes viruses and can be transferred by autoinoculation either to one's hands or to one's eyes, where they cause keratitis (inflammation of the cornea). People in the medical professions and in contact sports experience a higher than normal incidence of herpes labialis. Dentists and respiratory care personnel are members of high-risk professions, and wrestling is an example of a close-contact sport with a higher than normal incidence of herpes infections.

HSV-2 causes **urogenital herpes,** which is transferred usually by sexual contact. Primary infection results in a vesicular lesion on the genitals of the male or female patient. The appearance of the lesion is often accompanied by malaise and fever. Although the lesion usually heals within a few days, the herpes simplex virus has a propensity to persist in a latent state.

All members of the Herpetoviridae family are able to establish latent infections in humans. The characteristic lesions of HSV-1 and HSV-2 infections may recur at any time, but usually they recur following stress, abrupt emotional change, exposure to sun, or menstruation. Recurrent herpes labialis begins with itching followed by the appearance of vesicles on the vermillion outer border of the lip. The lesions are usually crusted over within 48 hours, and they heal completely within 8 to 10 days. Genital herpes recurs as genital lesions in both male and female patients. Females may be asymptomatic even though they have cervical lesions. Patients with vesicular herpes lesions are infectious—they transfer the virus to others through direct personal contact.

Complications of herpes simplex. Neonatal infections caused by herpes simplex virus (HSV-2) can occur during delivery. The infection of the newborn can be localized or systemic; systemic infections are often fatal. An infected mother poses a 40-percent chance that her child will be infected. Many of the children who recover from a neonatal herpes infection develop long-term sequelae such as destructive encephalitis (inflammation of the brain). Women with genital herpes should be advised to have yearly Pap tests and, if pregnant, should inform their clinician of their history of genital herpes.

Diagnosis and treatment. Herpes can be diagnosed by culturing the virus in embryonated chicken eggs or in tissue cultures. Specimens are taken from a patient's vesicles and are promptly inoculated into eggs or tissue cultures. The viruses grow rapidly and can produce cytopathic effects within 24 to 48 hours if a large inoculum is used. Herpes infections can also be diagnosed by the cytological demonstration of multinuclear giant cells in the base of the vesicle.

There is no cure for recurrent herpes disease; however, accessible herpes lesions can be treated with topical antiviral agents. Infections of the cornea have been successfully treated with idoxuridine (5-iodo-2'-deoxyuridine) and cytosine arabinoside (1-B-D-arabinofuranosyl-cytosine). Other nucleoside derivatives* are being tested in the United States and elsewhere. The latent nature of recurrent herpes has curtailed the development of immunological approaches to controlling these viral infections.

Avoidance of direct contact with the herpes virus

---

*Acyclovir, 9-(2-hydroxyethoxymethyl) guanine, is now recommended by the CDC for treatment of genital herpes.

is the major means of preventing the spread of herpes. Medical and dental personnel should wear gloves when they come in contact with a herpes patient. Urogenital herpes is presently an incurable venereal disease. If a sexual partner has an active case or a history of recurrent urogenital herpes, there is a likelihood that he/she is infectious.

Urogenital herpes can be contracted by autoinoculation from fever blisters (HSV-1), so this disease does not presuppose sexual activity. Herpes simplex virus type 1 causes 10 to 30 percent of the cases of urogenital herpes—infections that presumably originate from autoinoculation. Herpes patients should recognize that these viruses can infect many skin areas and should avoid autoinoculation.

Varicella-zoster virus: chickenpox and zoster

Varicella (chickenpox) and zoster are two clinical diseases caused by a single virus, the varicella-zoster virus. The common etiology of these diseases was first recognized in 1892 by Von Bokay, who observed the occurrence of varicella in households where one or more zoster patients resided. **Chickenpox** is the result of an initial infection of the varicella-zoster virus. **Zoster** (shingles) results from the activation of latent infections of the same varicella-zoster virus.

Varicella-zoster virus. The varicella-zoster virus is a member of the Herpetoviridae family (Table 24–1). It is an enveloped, icosahedral DNA virus (Figure 24–6) that is morphologically identical to the herpes simplex viruses. The varicella-zoster virus is present in the fluid of the vesicular lesions it causes on human skin. The virus in these lesions can be grown in human-cell tissue cultures. There are no antigenic differences between the viruses isolated from varicella lesions and those isolated from zoster lesions.

Varicella (chickenpox). Humans are the only natural host for the varicella-zoster virus. Following infection, there is a relatively constant 14- to 15-day incubation period during which the virus is present in the blood and throat. The first clinical signs of

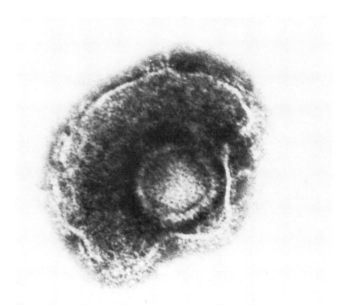

FIGURE 24–6
Electron micrograph of the varicella-zoster virus. (Courtesy of the Centers for Disease Control.)

chickenpox is a fever accompanied by a generalized eruption of vesicles on the scalp or trunk. The lesions spread centrifugally from the trunk to the extremities and may involve a major portion of the body surface. The fever lasts for 2 to 3 days, after which new lesions are rarely observed.

Varicella lesions begin as red spots, and then they vesicularize. Varicella-zoster virus is present in the vesicular lesions; the patient is infectious as long as the vesicular stage persists. Vesicularized lesions soon develop a crust and begin to itch. Crusted lesions can become infected by bacteria if the lesions are disturbed by scratching. Patients develop circulating antibody against the varicella-zoster virus concomitantly with the healing of the vesicles. Reinfection with varicella is rare; however, the varicella-zoster virus can establish a latent infection.

Varicella is a highly contagious viral disease that is transmitted in respiratory secretions and by direct contact. The illness occurs in yearly epidemics (Figure 24–7) and primarily infects young children. Epidemics occur in late winter through early spring and

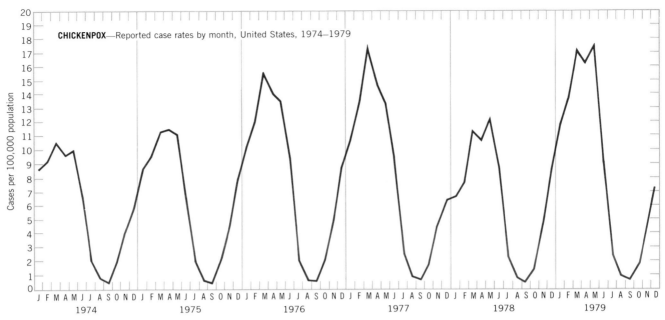

FIGURE 24—7

The cyclical nature of chickenpox in the United States. (Centers for Disease Control, "Annual Summary 1979: Reported Morbidity and Mortality in the United States," *Morbidity Mortality Weekly Report*, 28, No. 54, 1980.)

usually peak during April or May. Very few infections occur in July and August when the susceptible population of children is on summer vacation.

Zoster. Following the patient's clinical recovery from varicella, the varicella-zoster virus may establish a latent infection in the sensory nerve roots. Activation of the latent virus results in the disease known as zoster. Zoster occurs in patients of any age, but it is more prevalent in older persons. Unlike varicella, zoster occurs sporadically throughout the year. Zoster lesions appear in crops that erupt usually on the trunk (Color Plate 17), but also on the face, neck, and back. Most of these eruptions remain localized, although some patients develop disseminated zoster in which new lesions appear over the entire body about a week after the initial eruption. Zoster patients have a normal recovery if there are no exacerbating physical problems. Patients exposed to irradiation and immunosuppressive therapy are more apt to have zoster than are normal individuals.

Prevention and treatment. Varicella is a mild disease when it occurs in children, and most people contract varicella during childhood. Immunity against varicella is complete, although this immunity does not prevent the activation of latent varicella-zoster infections that result in zoster.

A live, attenuated varicella vaccine has been produced, but it is not used in the United States. Researchers are unsure of the viral vaccine's potential to cause latent infections. The immunity derived from the natural infection is currently preferable to the chance of significantly increasing the incidence of zoster by administering the live, attenuated viral vaccine.

Compromised and immunodeficient patients can be passively immunized with zoster-immune globulin. Passive immunization is only done for high-risk individuals. Normal varicella and zoster patients receive no special therapy. Calamine lotion can be applied to the itching rash, and oral trimeprazine is given occasionally to reduce the itching.

Poxviruses

Smallpox is a human disease that was known in China and India 2000 years ago. It was introduced into Europe between the fifth and seventh centuries A.D. and caused major epidemics in Europe during the Middle Ages. This dreaded viral illness was the first infectious disease to be controlled by vaccination, and the virus responsible was the first infective agent to be eradicated from the human population.

History of smallpox. Historical evidence suggests that immunizations against smallpox were practiced in China as early as the sixth century A.D. **Variolation** was the process by which individuals were inoculated with powdered smallpox crusts or fluid from the smallpox lesions as a prevention against smallpox. Variolation was widely practiced in China, elsewhere in Asia, and in Africa. The process was observed by Lady Mary Wortley Montague in Constantinople, and she introduced it into Europe in 1721. In Europe and in colonial America, material from the smallpox (variola minor) lesions were used to inoculate patients. Variolation was a controversial procedure because it disseminated smallpox into geographical areas where the disease was rare or absent, and because some people died from it.

Edward Jenner (1749–1823) was a British country doctor who attended to servants responsible for the care and milking of dairy cows. Dairy cows are susceptible to cowpox, which is caused by a virus related to the smallpox virus. Infected cows developed cowpox lesions on their teats. A number of Dr. Jenner's patients contracted cowpox, presumably from their contact with infected cows. When Jenner attempted the variolation procedure on these patients, they did not form the normal lesion at the site of inoculation. He further observed that these patients never contracted smallpox even when they were exposed to smallpox patients in their household.

From these observations, Jenner developed the process of smallpox vaccination that used material from cowpox lesions. An 8-year-old boy was vaccinated in May 1796 with material from the lesion of a cowpox. He experienced a mild illness, but recovered completely. That July, Jenner inoculated the same boy with material taken from a smallpox pustule. The boy remained healthy because he was immune to smallpox. Jenner's process was named **vaccination,** and it was the first recorded form of active immunization.

Smallpox: variola virus. The two major human poxviruses are vaccinia and the smallpox virus (variola). Originally, the vaccinia virus and the cowpox virus were presumed to be the same virus; however, now what we call the vaccinia virus is distinctly different from the cowpox virus and both are different from the variola virus. The origin of the vaccinia virus is unknown. At some time during the history of vaccination this virus appeared in vaccines; it has been perpetuated ever since. The poxviruses are large, brick-shaped DNA viruses (Figure 24–8). They are unique among the DNA viruses because

FIGURE 24–8

Purified vaccinia virus showing its brick-shape and its convoluted surface structure. (Courtesy of Dr. S. Dales. From P. Gold and S. Dales, *Proc. Natl. Acad. Sci. USA*, 60:845–850, 1968.)

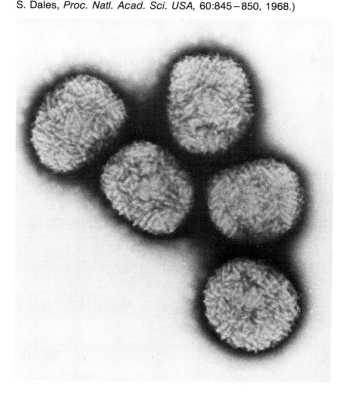

they replicate in the host's cytoplasm—most DNA viruses replicate in the cell's nucleus. There are two strains of the variola virus. **Variola major,** the most virulent strain, causes mortality in 20 to 50 percent of its hosts; **variola minor** causes a much lower (less than 1 percent) mortality rate.

Humans are the only host for the variola virus. The virus is transmitted by direct contact or by fomites and enters a patient via the respiratory tract. Here it multiplies in epithelial cells and in the regional lymph nodes before it establishes a viremia. Following a second replicative cycle, the virus infects the lymphatics, the internal organs, and the skin. This marks the beginning of the clinical symptoms, which usually appear 12 days after infection.

Clinical symptoms of smallpox include a high fever and a maculopapular rash. The rash appears on the scalp and face before it spreads to the back, chest, arms, and legs. The macular rash develops into firm, distinct papules, which change into vesicles over a 24-to-48 hour period (Color Plate 18). The vesicles become pearly white pustules that dry up and scab over during the second week of the rash. Finally, the scabs drop off, leaving pitted scars.

Eradication of smallpox. Public health measures have brought about the eradication of smallpox (variola major). The last case of variola major on the American continent occurred in Brazil in 1971; the last reported case in the world was reported in October 1975. Variola minor is still known to occur in some African countries. Smallpox was a target for eradication because of the effectiveness of the vaccine and because humans are its only known host.

The vaccinia virus has been used to vaccinate humans against smallpox. The vaccine is prepared by scraping vaccineal lesions, formed by one of three strains of vaccinia approved by the World Health Organization, from the skin of calves. These vaccines are stable in a freeze-dried form that can be distributed around the world because they do not require refrigeration. The vaccine is administered by dipping a bifurcated needle into the reconstituted vaccine and then puncturing the skin five times in a perpendicular motion. A "major" response is signified by a pustular lesion 6 to 8 days after vaccination. Successful vaccination confers a high degree of immunity on the individual.

In 1967, the World Health Organization began its effort to eradicate smallpox (variola major) from the world. It mounted a massive surveillance program, which identified and then vaccinated every contact of all known smallpox patients. No attempt was made to vaccinate the world population. Indeed, the virus may be present in one or more humans in remote, isolated tribes where WHO surveillance is impossible. Nevertheless, for all practical purposes, smallpox (variola major) is no longer a threat to the human population, and persons in civilized societies are no longer vaccinated.

HUMAN WARTS

Human warts are benign tumors caused by the papillomavirus. Warts occur principally in children and young adults and are classified according to their location and appearance. **Common warts** are flesh-colored to brown growths that average 2 to 10 mm in diameter (Figure 24–9). Their growth is fed by capillaries whose ends give the surface of the wart a spotted or pitted appearance. **Flat warts** have smooth, rounded surfaces and are found on the face, hands, and legs. **Plantar warts** grow from the skin surface inward and are often found on the feet. Plantar warts are more painful and more difficult to control than are other human warts. **Venereal warts** (condyloma acuminata) occur on the genitalia or perineum as clusters (Figure 24–9) of pink to brown growths. Warts are annoying and sometimes painful afflictions, but usually they pose no long-term threat to a person's health. Condyloma acuminata, however, are known to become malignant.

Human wart virus

Human warts are caused by a single human wart virus, which is classified in the genus Papillomavirus of the Papovaviridae* family. This single virus is capable of causing the different types of human warts. It is an icosahedral, DNA virus with a 45 to 55 nm

*The polyoma virus and the SV$_{40}$ virus are known oncogenic viruses that belong to the Polyomavirus genus of this family.

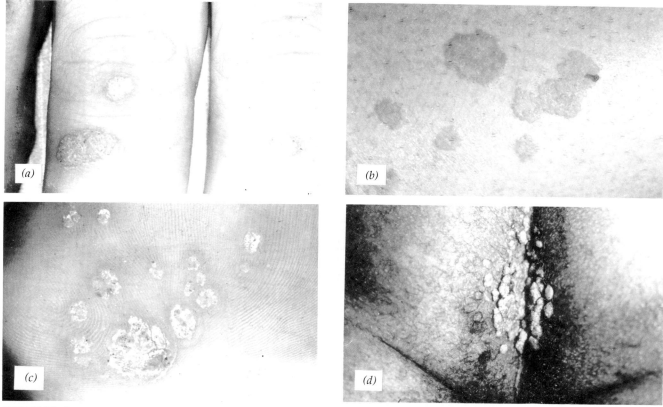

FIGURE 24–9
Human warts: (a) common wart on hand, (b) flat warts on thigh, (c) plantar warts, and (d) perianal condyloma acuminata. (Courtesy of Dr. K. E. Greer. From K. E. Greer, "Papovaviridae," in G. L. Mandell, R. G. Douglas Jr. and J. E. Bennet (eds.) *Principles and Practice of Infectious Diseases*, copyright © 1979, Wiley.)

capsid. The human wart virus penetrates through minor abrasions in the skin to infect a single epithelial cell. This cell is stimulated to divide, and after 1 to 6 months the benign growth is clinically recognized as a wart.

Treatment of human warts

Many warts spontaneously disappear, leaving no scar. Persistent warts can be treated surgically or chemically. Warts can be excised by electrosurgery, or the affected tissue can be destroyed by cryosurgery using liquid nitrogen (−196°C). Warts can be chemically treated by the topical application of sali-cylic acid or 5-fluorouracil. The severity of the treatment should be matched to the seriousness of the wart problem since the spontaneous regression of warts is a common occurrence.

SUMMARY

The maculopapular skin rashes of measles and rubella (German measles) are caused by RNA viruses. The measles virus is classified in the Paramyxoviridae family, whereas rubella is the sole member of the rubivirus genus of the Togaviridae family. Measles is a mild childhood disease (Table 24–2) that has

TABLE 24–2
Summary: Viral Diseases of Human Skin

Disease	Causative Agent	Symptoms	Complications	Prevention and Control
Measles	Measles virus	Fever, malaise, conjunctivitis, cough, coryza, Koplik spots, followed by a rash	Subacute sclerosing panencephalitis (multiple sclerosis?)	Vaccine, live attenuated virus
German measles (rubella)	Rubella virus	Rapid onset of fever, rash	Birth defects from congenital rubella	Vaccine, live attenuated virus
Herpes labialis (cold sores)	Herpes simplex type 1	Lesions on lips	Latent infection	Antiviral agents
Urogenital herpes	Herpes simplex type 2	Lesions in urogenital region	Latent infection	Antiviral agents
Chickenpox	Varicella-zoster (primary infection)	Fever, vesicles on scalp and trunk	Latent infection, scar tissue	None
Zoster	Varicella-zoster (latent infection)	Lesions on the trunk	None	None
Smallpox	Variola	High fever, vesicles on face, trunk, and legs	None	Vaccination with vaccinia virus
Warts	Human wart virus	Growths on skin (face, hands, legs, genitalia)	Condyloma acuminata, malignant transformation	Surgery (electro- and cryo-), chemical treatment

the potential to cause severe neurological disorders. The human respiratory tract and the conjunctiva are the portals of entry, and the virus is excreted in respiratory secretions, urine, and conjunctival fluid. The symptoms of measles include Koplik spots and a maculopapular rash. The incidence of measles in the United States has dropped dramatically following the introduction of a live-virus vaccine in 1963. The measles virus has been implicated in subacute sclerosing panencephalitis and multiple sclerosis. Rubella (German measles) is a mild childhood disease that can cause serious complications to the fetuses of pregnant women. Congenital rubella occurs when the rubella virus infects a fetus; the infection can result in abortion or serious birth defects. The risk of the fetus developing congenital defects from rubella is greatest during the first 2 months of pregnancy. Rubella is controlled by the immunization of prepubertal children with a live, attenuated rubella vaccine. Patients develop a persistent immunity against both the measles and the rubella virus.

The herpes simplex viruses and the varicella-zoster virus are DNA viruses belonging to the Herpetoviridae family. They cause vesicular skin lesions in humans. HSV-1 is primarily associated with herpes labialis (fever blisters). HSV-2 is the primary agent of the venereal disease urogenital herpes. HSV-2 also causes neonatal herpes when it is passed to the newborn during parturition. Herpes simplex viruses do exist in the latent state and can cause recurrent infections that are activated by stress, emotional changes, sun, or menstruation. These viruses are transmitted by direct contact between persons or by autoinoculation from one location to another. Initial infection by the varicella-zoster virus causes chickenpox. This is a highly contagious childhood disease that is easily recognized by its characteristic vesicular skin lesions. After the patient recovers, the varicella-zoster virus can establish a latent state. Zoster is the disease caused by the activation of this latent infection, which can occur months or years after recovery from chickenpox. Immunity against herpes simplex viruses or the varicella-zoster virus is at best incomplete.

Smallpox is a disease restricted to humans and is caused by variola major or variola minor. These are DNA viruses that replicate in the cytoplasm of the host cell. Smallpox caused by variola major has a high fatality rate and results in permanent pockmarks. Once this was a serious human disease, but now smallpox has essentially been eliminated from nature through the WHO program of worldwide surveillance and vaccination using the vaccinia virus. The last case of variola major was reported in 1975.

Papillomavirus is the human wart DNA virus that causes benign skin tumors. Many warts spontaneously regress; persistent warts can be treated chemically or by electro- and/or cryosurgery.

QUESTIONS AND TOPICS FOR STUDY AND DISCUSSION

Questions

1. Relate the evidence that links measles infections to long-term neurological disorders. Which disorders have been implicated, and what is the normal prognosis for the affected patient?
2. How has the use of the measles vaccine altered the incidence of measles? Is postinfection vaccination with the measles vaccine an effective treatment? Explain.
3. What is the most serious complication of a rubella infection? How is this complication prevented?
4. Explain the influence of the rubella vaccine on the changing incidence of this disease among different age groups.
5. What are the predominant characteristics of the herpes viruses? How do these characteristics affect the disease they cause? Explain.
6. What characteristics of urogenital herpes make this viral disease a serious public health problem with the prognosis that more and more humans will become infected in the years to come? Explain.

7. Why aren't people immunized against the varicella-zoster virus?
8. When and how was the smallpox vaccine developed? Is this vaccine still used today? Explain.
9. What is the etiological agent of human warts? How are warts treated?

Discussion

1. How are humans protected against the recurrence of chickenpox while they remain susceptible to zoster?
2. Will the widespread use of the measles vaccine shed any light on the etiological agent of subacute sclerosing panencephalitis and multiple sclerosis? What evidence will develop if these neurological disorders are caused by the measles virus?
3. Is it possible for the female partner of a married couple who have been faithful to each other for their 10 years of marriage to contract urogenital herpes caused by HSV-1? Explain.

FURTHER READING

Articles and Reviews

Baxby, D., "The Origins of Vaccinia Virus," *J. Infect. Dis.*, 136:453–455 (1977). An editorial dealing with the controversy over the biological "roots" of this virus, which played a central role in the elimination of smallpox.

Brunell, P. A., "Protection Against Varicella," *Pediatrics*, 59:1–2 (1977). A commentary on the use of a vaccine against chickenpox.

Henderson, D. A., "The Eradication of Smallpox," *Sci. Am.*, 235:25–33 (October 1976). An epidemiological report on the successful elimination of this serious human viral disease.

Langer, W. L., "Immunization Against Smallpox Before Jenner," *Sci. Am.*, 234:112–117 (January 1976). The history of variolation in England.

Wolontis, S., and S. Jeansson, "Correlation of Herpes Simplex Virus Type 1 and 2 with Clinical Features of Infection," *J. Infect. Dis.*, 135:28–33 (1977). A research report on the symptoms associated with more than 300 herpes simplex viruses isolated from human patients.

25

VIRAL DISEASES OF THE BLOOD, LIVER, AND ALIMENTARY TRACT

Viral infections of the human blood, liver, and alimentary tract cause a variety of human illnesses. Many of the viral agents responsible are well characterized; however, others have yet to be isolated and/or propagated in vitro. Among the well-characterized viruses are the Epstein-Barr virus and the cytomegalovirus. They are DNA viruses that belong to the Herpetoviridae family. Both can cause infectious mononucleosis; cytomegalovirus also causes congenital cytomegalic inclusion disease in newborns. Viral hepatitis is an ancient disease of the liver. It is caused by at least three viral agents. They have yet to be fully characterized, in part because they are difficult or impossible to cultivate in vitro.

A large group of enteric viruses causes acute gastroenteritis and neurotropic diseases in humans. Rotaviruses are the RNA viruses responsible for acute infantile diarrhea, whereas the Norwalk-like agents cause gastroenteritis. Other enteric viruses include the poliovirus and the ECHO viruses. Although these viruses infect the alimentary tract, they cause serious nervous system diseases, so they are discussed in the next chapter.

INFECTIOUS MONONUCLEOSIS

Infectious mononucleosis is an acute febrile illness of humans that is transmitted between people who come in close contact with each other. This viral disease is most prevalent among the 15- to 24-year-old age group. Adults with infectious mononucleosis have mild clinical symptoms, whereas the disease in young children is often asymptomatic. Infectious mononucleosis is caused by the Epstein-Barr virus and, less frequently, by the cytomegalovirus. This disease derives its name from the elevated level of white blood cells (leukocytosis) and the high number of atypical mononuclear leukocytes present in infected individuals.

Epstein-Barr virus

Historical perspective. Burkitt lymphoma is a cancer that occurs primarily in Africans and predominates in lymph tissue of the head and neck. Lymphoblasts from these tumors can be grown in tissue cultures. This is unusual because normal lymphocytes are in a terminal stage of cell differentiation, so they do not divide and cannot be cultured. Nevertheless, M. A. Epstein, B. A. Anchong, and Y. M. Barr (1964) were able to propagate lymphoblasts isolated from a Burkitt lymphoma; it was in cultures of these cells that they discovered the Epstein-Barr virus. Now it is experimentally possible to culture lymphoblasts that have been transformed by this virus. The Epstein-Barr virus is the first virus to be isolated from a human tumor.

The link between the Epstein-Barr virus and infectious mononucleosis was discovered accidentally. Immunological techniques for detecting specific EBV antibodies were developed soon after the virus's discovery. During these experiments, a laboratory technician became ill with infectious mononucleosis. Sequential blood samples taken from this patient's blood possessed increasing antibody titers against the EBV. This observation indicated a link between infectious mononucleosis and the Epstein-Barr virus. Subsequent epidemiological studies showed that between 80 and 90 percent of patients with infectious mononucleosis have antibody titers against the EBV. Other infectious mononucleosis patients possess neither anti-EBV titers nor the heterophile antibody (see following). These cases are caused by other viruses including cytomegalovirus.

Characteristics of EBV. Epstein-Barr virus is an enveloped DNA virus, belonging to the Herpetoviridae family, that infects humans and the higher primates. The Epstein-Barr virus has been cultivated, but only in B lymphocytes from its natural hosts. A small percentage of the B lymphocytes infected with EBV are capable of establishing permanent cell lines in tissue culture. In these cultures, the viral DNA is believed to exist as a plasmid within the cell. It is also possible that some viral DNA is integrated into one or more of the host cell's chromosomes.

Transformed B lymphocytes can be isolated from either infectious mononucleosis or Burkitt's lymphoma patients. These transformed cell lines can be induced to produce EBV by growing them in the presence of 5'-bromodeoxyuridine or 5-iodo-2'deoxyuridine or in arginine-free medium. These conditions stimulate the virus to initiate a lytic cycle, which demonstrates that the virus can exist in a latent form. This is the first human virus to be isolated from a human tumor that is able to transform human cells. Its role in the etiology of Burkitt's lymphoma is still unknown.

Diagnosis of infectious mononucleosis. J. R. Paul and W. Bunnell (1932) accidentally discovered that many patients with infectious mononucleosis possess high titers of antibodies against sheep red blood cells. These antibodies are called **heterophile antibodies** because they react with many antigens, including antigens found on sheep, horse, goat, or camel erythrocytes. Infectious mononucleosis patients possess heterophile antibodies against sheep erythrocytes that are not absorbed out by guinea pig kidney cells (contain the Forssman antigen) but are absorbed out* by beef erythrocytes (Table 25–1). The heterophile antibodies present in serum of normal patients and of patients with serum sickness are absorbed out by the guinea pig kidney cells. Ninety percent of infectious mononucleosis patients possess heterophile antibodies.

Mononucleosis **lymphocytosis** is a consistent clinical manifestation of infectious mononucleosis. At the peak of the illness, mononuclear lymphocytes comprise 50 percent of the white blood cell population. Between 10 and 30 percent of the white blood cells are enlarged atypical lymphocytes. Atypical lymphocytosis and the presence of heterophile antigens are diagnostic indicators of EBV-caused infectious mononucleosis. Detection of specific EBV antibodies is technically feasible, but it is not necessary except in atypical cases.

Clinical symptoms. Fever, sore throat, and lymphadenopathy are the three most common clinical symptoms of infectious mononucleosis. Patients often experience a rapid onset of these symptoms, which last for 10 to 14 days. Other infectious mononucleosis symptoms include malaise, headache,

---

*The patient's serum is mixed with specific cells. The cells and the antibodies that bind to them are removed by centrifugation.

TABLE 25–1
Diagnosis of Infectious Mononucleosis via the Heterophile Antibody

Patient's State	Agglutination of Sheep Erythrocytes[a] Treatment		
	Unabsorbed	Absorbed with Guinea Pig Kidney	Absorbed with Beef Erythrocytes
Healthy (Forssman antibody)	+	0	+
Serum sickness	+ + +	0	0
Infectious mononucleosis	+ + + +	+ + +	0

[a]Degree of agglutination is indicated as none (0) to strong (+ + + +).

muscle ache, hepatomegaly (enlarged liver), and splenomegaly (enlarged spleen). Hepatomegaly is present in about 15 percent and splenomegaly is present in 50 percent of the cases of infectious mononucleosis. Splenic rupture does occur, but it is a rare complication of this illness. Most patients recover without complications after a prolonged but relatively mild illness.

Epidemiology of EBV-infectious mononucleosis. EBV is shed from the oropharynx by 25 percent of seropositive healthy adults, 50 to 100 percent of infectious mononucleosis patients, and by some critically ill cancer patients. The virus is labile outside the body, so it is transferred presumably by intimate contact between persons. Children appear to have an asymptomatic disease, whereas persons infected during their second decade usually have the typical symptoms. Most diagnosed cases occur in the 15- to 24-year-old age group.

The symptoms of infectious mononucleosis are treated with aspirin or acetaminophen; the sore throat can be treated with a warm saltwater gargle. Corticosteroids have been advocated as a treatment for this disease, but their use remains controversial.

Cytomegalovirus-induced mononucleosis

Cytomegalovirus (CMV) is assigned to its own genus (Cytomegalovirus) in the Herpetoviridae family. This virus is named for its ability to form inclusion bodies in the cytoplasm of its host cell. CMV causes a major illness in newborns known as **congenital cytomegalic inclusion disease,** and it is responsible for some (between 10 and 20 percent) cases of infectious mononucleosis. Serological studies have shown that more than 40 percent of adult humans have experienced cytomegalovirus infections.

Cytomegalovirus. CMV is an enveloped DNA virus that is larger (180 to 250 nm) than the other Herpetoviridae. Humans are the only host for the human strain; however, many animal species are infected by other strains. CMV can be grown in cultures of human fibroblast cells in which they form distinctive cytoplasmic inclusion bodies. Antigenically, cytomegalovirus is distinct from the herpes simplex viruses and from the varicella-zoster virus. It is similar to these Herpetoviridae because CMV forms latent infections.

Clinical aspects of CMV infections. Congenital cytomegalic inclusion disease (CID) occurs in newborns and is characterized by jaundice, hepatosplenomegaly, and a rash. The nervous system is involved as is indicated by microcephaly and motor disability. Infected newborns are lethargic; they experience respiratory distress; and they have convulsive seizures. Many patients with CID die shortly after birth. Survivors may develop neurological sequelae such as microcephaly, mental retardation, and motor disability. The virus is transferred from infected women to their fetuses either by transplacental transfer or by vaginal transfer during birth. The incidence of bearing a CID child increases in mothers who contract primary cytomegalovirus infections during pregnancy. At present, there is insufficient evidence to determine the effect of the timing of maternal infection (trimester) on the incidence or the severity of this illness.

Postnatal acquisition of CMV infections results in an asymptomatic illness with no central nervous system or visceral organ involvement. Symptoms similar to CMV-induced mononucleosis may be present.

Symptoms of CMV-induced mononucleosis. Ten to twenty percent of the cases of infectious mononucleosis are caused by cytomegalovirus or by an unidentified virus. The symptoms are highlighted by a fever that lasts an average of 19 days and by lymphocytosis. Atypical lymphocytes are present in some patients. CMV-induced mononucleosis does not stimulate heterophile antibodies, so their absence is used to differentiate this illness from EBV-caused infectious mononucleosis. Patients normally recover from CMV-induced mononucleosis without complications.

Epidemiology. Cytomegalovirus causes latent infections and can be transmitted by various poorly understood mechanisms. There is presumptive evidence that cytomegalovirus is transmitted by direct sexual contact. Moreover, a small percentage of patients receiving blood transfusions become infected with CMV, and some patients contract CMV infections following transplant operations. A remarkably high number of CMV infections occur following renal and bone marrow transplants. The latent nature of CMV infections has clouded our understanding of the epidemiology of the diseases it causes.

VIRAL HEPATITIS

Since the Middle Ages, major epidemics of **infectious icterus** have occurred in both military and civilian populations. The disease results in liver damage, which in turn causes jaundice (icterus). The viral etiology of hepatitis was first recognized in the mid-1940s, when infectious icterus was transmitted with bacteria-free filtrates. An understanding of this illness has been hampered by the inability of virologists to cultivate the responsible filterable agents. Now at least three types of viral hepatitis are recognized by their differences in epidemiology, in clinical symptoms, and in the immunological properties of the viral agents (Table 25–2).

During the late 1960s and early 1970s, two distinct antigens were discovered to be associated with hepatitis. Antigen (A) was found in patients with **infec-**

TABLE 25–2
Agents of Human Viral Hepatitis

Agent	Characteristics	Disease	Transmission
Hepatitis A	Virus in feces, 3- to 6-week incubation period, small (27 nm), RNA virus, hepatitis A antigen	Infectious hepatitis: fever, acute onset, treated with pooled immunoglobulins, autumn and winter	Person-to-person contact, oral-fecal
Hepatitis B	Virus in blood, 5- to 10-week incubation period, 42 nm, DNA virus (Dane particles), hepatitis B surface antigen	Serum hepatitis: insidious onset, year-round, two forms: (1) persistent infection with continuous viremia, (2) self-limiting illness	Blood and blood products, infected needles, tattooing, ear piercing, drug abuse
Non-A, non-B hepatitis	Unidentified agent, 5-to-7 week incubation period	Hepatitis: indistinguishable from hepatitis A or B	Blood and blood products

tious hepatitis (hepatitis A); antigen (B) was found in patients with **serum hepatitis (hepatitis B)**. Both these viruses have been isolated from infected patients (feces or serum) and shown to be unrelated viruses. The third type of human hepatitis is caused by one or more agents possessing neither the A-antigen nor the B-antigen. This disease is called **non-A, non-B hepatitis.**

Hepatitis A: infectious hepatitis

Infectious hepatitis is caused by an RNA virus designated the hepatitis A virus (HAV). This virus resembles a picornavirus, although at this time it remains unclassified. The virus is transmitted via the oral-fecal route, and it causes outbreaks of illness among families or restaurant-goers who eat contaminated food. Recovery from infectious hepatitis is normally complete and results in immunity.

Hepatitis A virus. Infectious hepatitis occurs in humans, monkeys, and chimpanzees. The hepatitis A virus has recently been grown in fetal rhesus monkey kidney cells and in marmoset liver explant cultures. This technical advance, however, has not yielded sufficient viruses for biochemical studies. Our knowledge of this virus comes from studying the virus particles isolated from feces of infected humans and animals. Purified particles possessing the HA-antigen are 27 nm in diameter (Figure 25–1), and they possess single-stranded RNA that is susceptible to RNAase (but not to DNAase). Similar particles have been localized in the cytoplasms of liver cells of infected animals by an HA-antigen detecting immunofluorescent technique.

Infectious hepatitis in humans. Infectious hepatitis is transmitted by the fecal-oral route through direct contact between persons or by the consumption of contaminated food. The incubation period varies from 3 to 6 weeks. HAV particles are found in the feces for about 1 week prior to the appearance of the clinical symptoms of hepatitis (Figure 25–2). The virus particles in the feces appear to come from the liver via the bile duct. There is usually a rapid onset

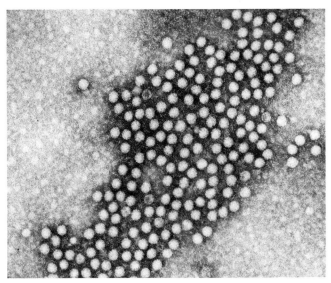

FIGURE 25–1
Hepatitis A virus particles measure 24 to 29 nm in diameter. (Reproduced with permission. From A. J. Zuckerman and C. R. Howard, *Hepatitis Viruses of Man*, copyright © 1979, Academic Press Inc., Ltd, London.)

of symptoms, which include fever, headache, anorexia, nausea, and vomiting. Hepatomegaly and elevated serum aminotransferases (glutamic oxaloacetic and pyruvic acid transaminases) precede jaundice by several days. These symptoms last for 8 to 13 days in children; in adults the jaundice may last for 30 days. Patients recover and have lasting immunity against future hepatitis A infections.

Diagnosis and prevention. Usually, infectious hepatitis is diagnosed by its clinical symptoms, although laboratory diagnosis is possible. The HA-antigen can be detected in fecal specimens by using immune electron microscopy or by detecting the antibody against the HA-antigen by using a radioimmunoassay. Infectious hepatitis can be prevented by interrupting the fecal-oral transmission of the virus and by passive immunization of susceptible persons. Foodborne outbreaks originate in family settings or from contaminated food served in restaurants. These

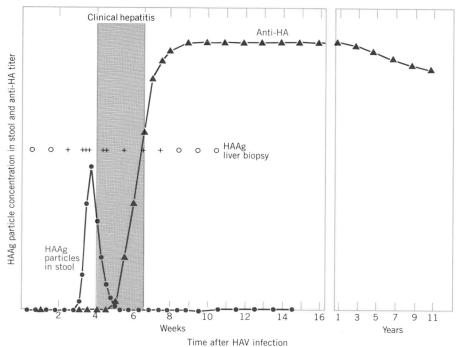

FIGURE 25-2

Course of hepatitis A virus infection. The clinical symptoms appear after a 3-to-6-week incubation period. Hepatitis A virus particles are excreted in feces and are present in the liver for 1 week before and 1 week after the clinical symptoms appear. (Courtesy of Dr. W. S. Robinson. From W. S. Robinson "Hepatitis A Virus," in G. L. Mandell, R. G. Douglas Jr., and J. E. Bennet, eds., *Principles and Practice of Infectious Diseases,* copyright © 1979, Wiley.)

outbreaks can be curtailed by identifying the source of the virus, which is usually a food-handler.

Passive immunization of select groups of persons with ordinary pooled human immunoglobulin* can be used to control infectious hepatitis. Persons in nursery schools, facilities for the mentally retarded, or psychiatric institutions have been passively immunized to control the spread of an infectious-hepatitis outbreak. Passive immunization of preexposed persons results in a significant reduction in the incidence of infectious hepatitis. Postexposure passive

immunization is also effective in limiting the spread and in lessening the symptoms of the illness. The long incubation period of this disease permits effective passive immunization of susceptible patients for up to 6 weeks after exposure.

Hepatitis B: serum hepatitis

Serum hepatitis is unrelated to infectious hepatitis in its viral etiology, persistence of infection, and mode of transmission. Serum hepatitis is a persistent infection caused by the hepatitis B virus (HBV) that is transmitted by blood and blood products. This illness poses a threat to persons receiving transfusions, so it is a major problem for blood banks.

*Pooled serum from adults contains anti-HAV antibodies because of the high incidence of infection with the hepatitis A virus.

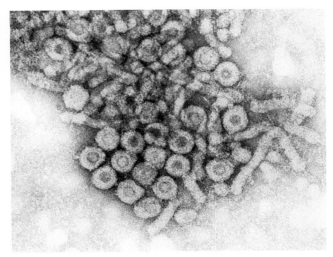

FIGURE 25-3
Electron micrograph of an aggregate of hepatitis B particles. Both spherical (42 nm) and tubular particles are present. (Reproduced with permission. From A. J. Zuckerman and C. R. Howard, *Hepatitis Viruses of Man*, copyright © 1979, Academic Press Inc., Ltd, London.)

Hepatitis B virus. The causative agent for serum hepatitis is the hepatitis B virus (HBV). This virus infects humans and other primates, but researchers have been unable to subculture it from cell cultures. Serum hepatitis is transmitted by a filterable agent; its symptoms develop coincidentally with the appearance of the hepatitis B surface antigen (HBsAg) in the patient's serum. This antigen is found on the surface of Dane particles (Figure 25-3). A **Dane particle** is composed of a core nucleocapsid (28 nm) surrounded by a lipid-containing outer envelope that is 42 nm in diameter. Dane particles are now considered to be the hepatitis B virus (HBV) even though they have never been propagated in vitro. The nucleocapsid core contains circular DNA that is double-stranded over two-thirds of its length. This unique DNA structure is not known to exist in other viruses, which is one reason that the HBV is still unclassified.

Serum hepatitis in humans. Infections with hepatitis B virus can develop into a self-limiting disease, or they can lead to a persistent viral infection that lasts for years. The **self-limiting infection** requires about 6 weeks before the HBsAg is detectable in the patient's blood (Figure 25-4). The Dane particles appear in the blood (they are not demonstrable in feces) after the 10th week, and symptoms of clinical hepatitis begin on the 14th week and last for about 4 weeks.

Persistent HBV infections have a longer incubation period and apparently last for years (Figure 25-5). The HBsAg appears in the serum about 15 weeks after infection and remains indefinitely. Dane particles are present in the serum 2 weeks later, and their concentration peaks as the clinical symptoms of hepatitis appear. In contrast to the self-limiting infection, anti-HBs antibodies are absent. Persistent HBV infections represent between 5 and 10 percent of the cases of acute hepatitis. Low infecting doses, a young age, and a mild or inapparent case of hepatitis favor the persistent form of HBV infections.

Clinical symptoms. Patients with hepatitis B have clinical symptoms that are indistinguishable from hepatitis A. Their symptoms include dark urine, malaise, anorexia, nausea, fever, vomiting, headache, and jaundice. The prolonged and severe symptoms of acute hepatitis from HBV infections are rare. Most HBV infections result in a mild illness, which can be subclinical. Serum hepatitis is diagnosed by the presence of the HBsAg in the serum and by the presence of high levels of serum aminotransferase activity.

Epidemiology of serum hepatitis. Most cases of serum hepatitis are derived from blood transfusions and administration of blood product. Infectious virus particles have also been demonstrated in human saliva and semen. To eliminate blood transfusions and blood products as a source of infection, the U.S. Food and Drug Administration has required that all blood donors be tested for the HBsAg. Infected persons are not allowed to donate blood. However, donors with low levels of HBsAg can be missed even when the most sensitive radioimmunoassay is used. Volunteer blood donors are preferred over paid donors because there is a higher incidence of HBsAg-positive persons in the latter group.

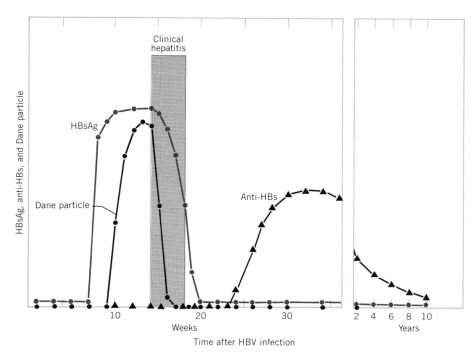

FIGURE 25–4
Course of self-limiting hepatitis B virus infection. Dane particles and HBs-antigen are present in the patient's blood during the later part of the 6-to-10-week incubation period. (Courtesy of Dr. W. S. Robinson. From W. S. Robinson, "Hepatitis B Virus," in G. L. Mandell, R. G. Douglas Jr., and J. E. Bennet, eds., *Principles and Practice of Infectious Diseases,* copyright © 1979, Wiley.)

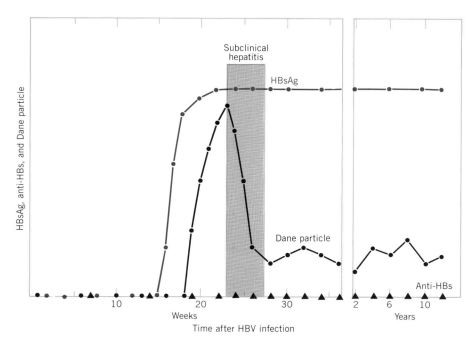

FIGURE 25–5
Persistent hepatitis B infection. The incubation period is longer than in other forms of viral hepatitis, and no antiviral antibodies are found in the patient's serum. (Courtesy of Dr. W. S. Robinson. From W. S. Robinson, "Hepatitis B Virus," in G. L. Mandell, R. G. Douglas Jr., and J. E. Bennet, eds., *Principles and Practice of Infectious Diseases,* copyright © 1979, Wiley.)

Infections with HBV have been attributed to hemodialysis, ear piercing, tattooing, drug abuse, and accidental punctures with contaminated needles. The virus can also infect humans through open skin abrasions and through direct contact with mucous membranes, but these sources of the infection are rare. Contaminated instruments and all samples taken from infected patients should be sterilized to prevent the spread of the virus.

Patients may be passively immunized with hepatitis B immunoglobulin, but this practice has limited application. The U.S. Food and Drug Administration recently approved a new vaccine for hepatitis B. The vaccine is produced from viral particles isolated from the blood of human carriers. This vaccine is expensive, so its use will be limited to high-risk persons.

Non-A, non-B hepatitis

Serum hepatitis (HAV) is diagnosed by the presence of HAAg in the patient's serum, and infectious hepatitis (HBV) is diagnosed by the presence of HBsAg. A third form of hepatitis is designated non-A, non-B hepatitis because neither of these antigens is involved. It causes an acute, chronic form of human hepatitis for which there is probably more than one etiological agent. This disease has been transmitted by transferring human plasma and serum to chimpanzees, so it is most likely an infectious viral disease.

Epidemiological evidence indicates that non-A, non-B hepatitis is transmitted primarily by blood and blood products. It is a major cause of posttransfusion hepatitis. The incubation period of non-A, non-B hepatitis is 4 to 5 weeks, which is intermediate to the incubation periods for hepatitis A and hepatitis B infections (Table 25–2). The clinical symptoms are the same for all types of acute hepatitis.

Specific immunological tests are not available for detecting non-A, non-B hepatitis. This infection is diagnosed by the absence of HAAg and HBsAg, by abnormal liver function, and by its clinical symptoms. The abnormal liver function is detected as elevated levels of serum aminotransferases and can persist for 1 year or longer. Currently, there is no effective treatment for non-A, non-B hepatitis. Preventive measures depend on selecting against blood donors who are potential carriers.

VIRAL GASTROENTERITIS

Rotaviruses and the Norwalk-like agents are responsible for nonbacterial gastroenteritis in humans. The Norwalk-like agents are presumed to be viruses even though they have never been isolated. They are associated with major outbreaks of gastroenteritis occurring among school or family groups. Rotaviruses cause mild gastroenteritis as well as acute infantile diarrheal disease.

Rotaviruses: acute infantile diarrheal disease

Rotaviruses (L. rota, wheel) have been detected microscopically in electron micrographs of stools from human diarrheal patients. Although they have been isolated from feces, they have not been propagated in vitro. The isolated viral particles contain 10 or more segments of RNA and are surrounded by a double-shelled, wheel-like capsid measuring 70 nm in diameter (Figure 25–6). The number of segments in the viral genome justifies their classification in their own genus, Rotavirus, in the Reoviridae family. A variety of animals including calves, mice, piglets, foals, lambs, rabbits, and antelopes are susceptible to rotaviral infections. Each of these viruses has a common complement-fixing antigen, but beyond that their similarities and differences remain unknown. There are two known serotypes of Rotavirus that cause illness in humans.

Clinical symptoms and treatment. Rotaviral infections vary from being asymptomatic to being a severe diarrheal disease. The illness begins with vomiting followed by diarrhea that lasts for a mean duration of 5 days. The degree of dehydration and the characteristics of the stools (watery/semisolid) vary with the severity of the illness. Infants between 6 and 24 months of age have the highest incidence

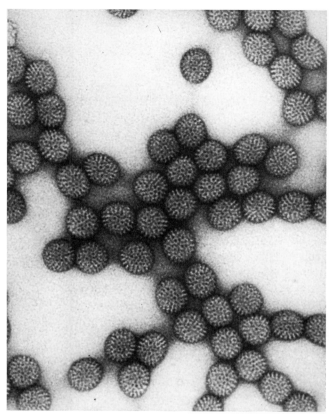

FIGURE 25–6
Electron micrograph of the human rotavirus, which is the cause of infantile gastroenteritis. (Courtesy of the Centers for Disease Control.)

of **acute infantile diarrheal disease.** A few infants have died from severe dehydration and electrolyte imbalance caused by this disease.

Rotavirus infections are treated by rehydrating the patient. This is accomplished by administering, orally if possible, electrolyte solutions containing glucose (sucrose can be used). When excessive vomiting occurs, the patient is rehydrated by intravenous therapy.

Epidemiology. Rotavirus infections occur in many parts of the world, and they are a major cause of infant morbidity and, probably, infant mortality. In temperate climates, these infections occur primarily during the cooler months, whereas in tropical climates they occur throughout the year. The mode of transmission is assumed to be by the fecal-oral route. Almost all children in the United States possess antibodies against rotaviruses before they are 3 years old. The widespread infection rate in this developed country suggests that adequate sewage facilities alone will not prevent the spread of rotaviruses. Presently, there are no vaccines against the human serotypes of rotaviruses.

Norwalk-like agents of gastroenteritis

Epidemic diarrhea, viral gastroenteritis, winter vomiting disease, and acute nonbacterial gastroenteritis are names for the diseases caused by Norwalk-like agents. These agents were first observed in electron micrographs of samples taken from patients involved in an epidemic in Norwalk, Ohio. The particles have yet to be isolated or grown in vitro. The Norwalk agents are visible in electron micrographs and appear to be viruses with a diameter between 25 and 27 nm in size. At least six similar agents have been identified from patients with vomiting or diarrheal diseases, and they are described as the Norwalk-like agents.

Norwalk-like agents cause an epidemic form of gastroenteritis. This illness begins with abdominal cramps and/or nausea after an incubation period of 24 to 48 hours. The symptoms, including vomiting, diarrhea, and a low-grade fever, last from 48 to 72 hours after which the patient recovers without sequelae. Norwalk-like illnesses predominate during the colder months of the year, have a short incubation period, and occur as outbreaks among groups of people in close personal contact. Researchers presume that these agents are transmitted by the fecal-oral route. Diagnosis is made on these epidemiological criteria together with the clinical symptoms of the illness. These illnesses usually are self-limiting and are resolved without treatment. A greater understanding of these diseases and their etiological agents is necessary before actions to prevent them can be taken.

TABLE 25-3
Summary: Viral Diseases of the Blood, Liver, and Alimentary Tract

Disease	Causative Agent	Clinical Symptoms	Transmission
Infectious mononucleosis	Epstein-Barr virus: Enveloped, double-stranded DNA virus	Fever, sore throat, lymphadenopathy, lymphocytosis, heterophile antibody	Person-to-person contact, intimate contact
	Cytomegalovirus: Enveloped, double-stranded DNA virus	Fever, lymphocytosis, no heterophile antibody	Blood transfusions, transplants, sexual contact
Congenital cytomegalic inclusion disease	Cytomegalovirus	Jaundice, hepatosplenomegaly, rash, microcephaly, motor disability	Mother to fetus, disease of newborns
Infectious hepatitis	Hepatitis A virus: Single-stranded RNA virus, 27 nm in diameter, unclassified	Jaundice, fever, headache, nausea, vomiting, hepatitis A antigen in feces, 3- to 6-week incubation	Oral-fecal route, contaminated food
Serum hepatitis	Hepatitis B virus: Circular, ⅔ double-stranded DNA, 47 nm diameter, unclassified	Same as hepatitis A, persistent infection, 6- to 10-week incubation, hepatitis B surface antigen (HBsAg)	Transfusions of blood and blood products, contaminated needles
Non-A, non-B hepatitis	One or more unclassified viruses	Indistinguishable from hepatitis A or B, 5- to 7-week incubation, absence of HA and HB antigens, high SGOT	Blood transfusions
Viral gastroenteritis	Rotavirus: 11 segments of double-stranded RNA, double-shelled capsid,	Vomiting and diarrhea, severe dehydration in young children	Fecal-oral route, prevalent in cold months
	Norwalk-like agents: Unclassified, many virus-like particles, 25 – 27 nm	Vomiting, abdominal cramps, nausea, diarrhea, low-grade fever	Fecal-oral route, prevalent in cold months

SUMMARY

Infectious mononucleosis is an acute febrile illness caused by the Epstein-Barr virus and, less frequently, by the cytomegalovirus (Table 25–3). The EBV and CMV are both enveloped DNA viruses that belong to the Herpetoviridae family. Clinical symptoms of infectious mononucleosis include fever, sore throat, lymphadenopathy, and lymphocytosis. Heterophile antibodies are present in the serum of most patients infected with EBV, but not in those with CMV-induced infectious mononucleosis. Most cases of infectious mononucleosis occur in 15- to 24-year-olds and are caused by the EBV. Transmission of this disease is by direct contact. CMV also causes congenital cytomegalic inclusion disease in newborns.

Viral hepatitis occurs in three distinct forms: infectious hepatitis caused by hepatitis A virus; serum hepatitis caused by hepatitis B virus; and non-A, non-B hepatitis caused by one or more currently uncharacterized agents. Infectious hepatitis has a short incubation period, is transmitted by the fecal-oral route, is caused by an unclassified RNA virus, results in immunity, and can be prevented by passive immunization. Serum hepatitis often causes persistent infections recognized by the presence of the HBsAg in the blood. This illness is caused by an unclassified DNA virus that is transmitted to susceptible persons in blood transfusions and blood products. The hepatitis B virus is transmitted by punctures with contaminated needles and other instruments. Non-A, non-B hepatitis is transmitted by blood and by blood products and is believed to be a viral disease. Its symptoms are identical to those of acute hepatitis.

Rotaviruses and Norwalk-like agents are responsible for most cases of nonbacterial gastroenteritis. Rotaviruses are segmented RNA viruses that are transmitted by the fecal-oral route. Rotaviral infections vary from being asymptomatic to being a severe diarrheal disease. They occur worldwide and are a major cause of infant morbidity. They can cause infant mortality associated with severe dehydration and electrolyte imbalance. Norwalk-like agents are viruslike particles (25 to 27 nm) associated with an epidemic form of acute gastroenteritis. These agents cause nausea and/or vomiting, stomach cramps, and diarrhea following a short incubation period. Epidemics caused by these agents occur among school and family groups.

QUESTIONS AND TOPICS FOR STUDY AND DISCUSSION

Questions

1. Describe the etiological agents responsible for infectious mononucleosis. Explain a serological assay used to diagnose this disease.
2. From what human tissue was the Epstein-Barr virus first isolated? What significance is attached to the initial isolation of the Epstein-Barr virus? How was this virus implicated in infectious mononucleosis?
3. Describe the clinical symptoms of infectious mononucleosis. What groups of people are most apt to contract this disease?

4. Compare congenital cytomegalic inclusion disease in newborns to congenital rubella. How are these diseases different from herpes infections of the newborn?
5. Describe the epidemiology of the three types of viral hepatitis. What steps can be taken to prevent the spread of these viruses?
6. How do we know that infectious hepatitis and serum hepatitis are caused by different viruses? What are the physical characteristics of these viruses?
7. What human disease is caused by rotaviruses? How serious are these infections and how are they treated?
8. What clinical signs indicate infection by the Norwalk-like agents?

Discussion

1. The new hepatitis B virus vaccine uses virus material purified from humans. Are there long-term problems that could develop from using this new type of vaccine?
2. The Epstein-Barr virus was originally isolated from a human lymphoma and is now grown in B lymphocytes. Is it possible that oncogenic viruses are important causes of human cancer? If so, why have virologists not demonstrated their etiological role?

FURTHER READING

Books

Zuckerman, A. J., and C. R. Howard, *Hepatitis Viruses of Man,* Academic Press, London, 1979. A comprehensive account of the history, epidemiology, and important advances in viral hepatitis.

Articles and Reviews

Alter, H. J., P. V. Holland, R. H. Purcell, and H. Popper, "Transmissible Agent in Non-A, Non-B Hepatitis," *Lancet,* 459–463 (March 1978). The first report of the transmission of non-A, non-B hepatitis to chimpanzees.

Brodsky, A. L., and C. W. Health, Jr., "Infectious Mononucleosis: Epidemiologic Patterns at United States Colleges and Universities," *Am. J. Epidemiol.,* 96:87–93 (1978). An epidemiological study conducted during the 1969–1970 academic year.

Epstein, M. A., B. G. Achong, and Y. M. Barr, "Virus Particles in Cultured Lymphoblasts from Burkitt's Lymphoma," *Lancet*, 702–703 (March 1964). The first report of the isolation of an oncogenic virus from human tissue.

Melnick, J. L., G. R. Dreesman, and F. B. Hollinger, "Viral Hepatitis," *Sci. Am.*, 237:44–52 (July 1977). Discussion of the epidemiology and immunology of viral hepatitis.

Rakela, J., and J. W. Mosley, "Fecal Excretion of Hepatitis A Virus in Humans," *J. Infect. Dis.*, 135:933–938 (1977). A research paper that demonstrates viral excretion in feces prior to the appearance of hepatitis symptoms.

Weller, T. H., "The Cytomegaloviruses: Ubiquitous Agents with Protean Manifestations," *N. Engl. J. Med.*, 285:203–214 (1971). An early review of these important herpesviruses.

26

VIRAL DISEASES OF THE NERVOUS SYSTEM

A number of human nervous system infections are caused by viruses. The seriousness of these infections cannot be understated—many cause permanent damage or even death. Untreated rabies, for example, is almost always fatal; and paralytic polio can kill or permanently maim its victims. Other neurotropic illness, such as aseptic meningitis and viral encephalitis, can progress rapidly from mild disorders of the nervous system to coma and death.

These neurotropic viruses enter the human body via the normal portals of entry before they infect the nervous system. Poliovirus and the other enteric viruses are spread by the oral-fecal route and establish an infection in the human gastrointestinal tract. Rabies is an enzootic disease that is transmitted to humans by the bite of infected animals. Aseptic meningitis and viral encephalitis are transmitted from animal reservoirs to humans by mosquitoes and ticks. The diverse epidemiologies of the diseases caused by the neurotropic viruses necessitate individual approaches to their prevention and control.

THE CENTRAL NERVOUS SYSTEM

The brain, the spinal cord, the cranial nerves, and the spinal nerves comprise the human central nervous system. The spinal cord and the brain are surrounded by one or more membranes referred to as the **meninges.** The space between the meninges and the nervous tissue is occupied by the cerebrospinal fluid (CSF). This fluid supplies nutrients to the brain. The nutrients are transferred to the CSF through an extensive array of blood vessels. These blood vessels also function as the blood-brain barrier that prevents blood cells and many proteins, such as immunoglobulins, from entering the CSF.

Most neurotropic pathogens damage the blood-brain barrier before they are able to infect the tissue of the central nervous system. This barrier is impermeable to viruses, bacteria, human cells, and/or immunoglobulins unless it has been damaged. Most neurotropic viruses enter the central nervous system via the blood; however, a few viruses infect the central nervous system from peripheral nerves by the process of **neurotropic spread.** The clinical symptoms and the severity of the neurotropic viral infections depend on the specific nervous tissue affected.

ENTEROVIRUSES: POLIOVIRUS

The small RNA viruses of the Picornaviridae family are classified in two genera, Enterovirus and Rhinovirus (Table 26–1). The rhinoviruses infect the human respiratory tract (see Chapter 23), whereas the enteroviruses infect humans via their respiratory tract or their intestinal tract. The enteroviruses include poliovirus, coxsackievirus group A, coxsackievirus group B, and the echoviruses. Unlike many human viruses, the enteroviruses are stable between pH 3 and pH 10 and are not inactivated by the acidity of the human stomach.

Poliomyelitis

Poliomyelitis (Gr. *polios*, gray; and *myelos*, spinal cord) is usually a mild asymptomatic disease, but in a small percentage of cases it causes permanent paralysis and deformities. Historically, poliomyelitis was known to the early Egyptians, who depicted polio victims in their sculptures. The infectious nature of polio was first demonstrated in 1909 by Landsteiner and Popper, who infected monkeys with human polio. The virus responsible was discovered 1 year later (1910) by S. Flexner and P. A. Lewis. Almost 40 years elapsed before John Enders and his colleagues (in 1949) were able to culture poliovirus in tissue cultures. Enders' group developed techniques for growing cultures of human embryonic tissue that, in turn, enabled virologists to propagate poliovirus under controlled conditions. Their contributions initiated the technology required to produce viral vaccines.

Poliovirus. The polioviruses are small (20 to 30 nm), nonenveloped, icosahedral RNA viruses. Their viral RNA (plus RNA) functions as the viral messenger RNA and codes for one giant polypeptide (see Figure 22–7). This peptide is subsequently cleaved into functional proteins. There are three distinct polioviruses that are recognized by immunological techniques. Each type elicits an immunological response in humans, so all three serotypes are used in the polio vaccines.

Poliomyelitis in humans. The polioviruses are transmitted between humans by the oral-fecal route. The viruses infect and multiply in the mucosa of the oropharynx and the intestine before they spread to the lymphoid tissue. Infections that never progress past this stage result in a mild form of polio known as **inapparent poliomyelitis** (Figure 26–1). Inapparent poliomyelitis is the most common outcome of a poliovirus infection: it represents between 90 and 95 percent of the known cases. Inapparent poliomyelitis can be detected by isolating the virus from the throat or feces or by detecting a rising antibody titer.

Other polio infections progress to a viremic stage following the replication of the virus in the lymph tissue. Polio viremia is accompanied by minor clinical symptoms including headache, fever, sore throat, anorexia, vomiting, and abdominal muscle pain. These symptoms begin 2 days after infection and last for 2 to 3 days (Figure 26–1). Complete recovery follows these minor clinical symptoms in 4 to 8 percent of the known polio cases. This form of the disease is termed **abortive poliomyelitis** because the poliovirus does not affect the central nervous system.

TABLE 26–1
The Picornaviridae Family

Group	Viruses	No. of Serotypes	Host Range, Growth
Enterovirus	Polioviruses	3	Primates, humans
	Coxsackievirus Group A	24	Humans, suckling mice
	Coxsackievirus Group B	6	Humans, suckling mice, cell cultures
	Echoviruses	34	Humans
Rhinovirus	Rhinoviruses	89	Humans

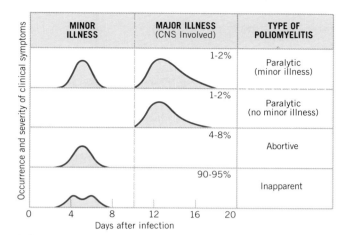

MINOR ILLNESS	MAJOR ILLNESS (CNS Involved)	TYPE OF POLIOMYELITIS
	1-2%	Paralytic (minor illness)
	1-2%	Paralytic (no minor illness)
	4-8%	Abortive
	90-95%	Inapparent

FIGURE 26–1

Types of poliovirus infections in humans. The occurrence of each type of polio within a nonimmunized population is indicated as a percentage. (Modified from D. M. Horstmann, *Yale J. Biol. Med.*, 36:5, 1963.)

Paralytic poliomyelitis develops in only 1 to 2 percent of the polio cases. The symptoms appear about 10 days after infection either with or without the precursory symptoms of the abortive illness. The symptoms of paralytic poliomyelitis show central nervous system involvement; they include meningitis, headache, fever, malaise, stiff neck, and vomiting. The presence of muscle pain, most commonly in the neck or lumbar spinal region, occurs as a precursory symptom of paralysis. If the minor illness occurs (Figure 26–1), the patient appears to recover for 2 to 5 days prior to the onset of the paralytic symptoms.

Unlike other neurological spinal disorders, paralytic polio is characterized by the asymmetric distribution of the muscle groups affected by paralysis. A patient's legs are more often involved than arms, and the proximal muscles of the extremities are more often involved than the distal muscles. The onset of paralysis can be very rapid (hours), but usually paralysis develops over a period of several days. The ability to swallow and breathe can also be impaired if the virus affects the ninth and tenth cranial nerves. The frequency of these symptoms has varied in different epidemics and is more common among

adults. Respiratory distress resulting from this form of poliomyelitis requires immediate attention.

Epidemiology of poliomyelitis. During the early decades of this century, infants less than 5 years of age were the primary victims of paralytic polio, and the disease was known as "infantile paralysis." We now have evidence that infection with poliovirus was widespread; however, most persons had a mild form of polio and paralysis was rare. The situation changed in the late 1940s when children 5 to 9 years old became the major victims. The incidence of paralytic polio increased, and major epidemics occurred in the developed countries. These epidemics were common in the summer and fall months of the late 1940s and the early 1950s. From 1951 to 1955 there were between 10,000 and 21,000 yearly cases of paralytic poliomyelitis reported in the United States.

Jonas Salk introduced the first polio vaccine in 1955. A second vaccine, the attenuated oral polio vaccine (OPV), was introduced in 1962. These vaccines significantly decreased the incidence of paralytic polio (Figure 26–2). Today, almost all paralytic polio has been eliminated; however, in 1979 there were still 26 cases reported in the United States. Eleven of these cases developed after administration of the OPV and are classified as vaccine-associated cases. Thirteen cases occurred in a single outbreak that developed in a nonvaccinated Amish community. These cases highlight the two major problems of controlling paralytic poliomyelitis: vaccine-associated cases and polio occurring among communities of unvaccinated persons.

Poliovirus vaccines. The Salk poliovirus vaccine is composed of the three serotypes of poliovirus, which have been killed by formalin treatment. This **inactivated polio vaccine** (IPV) is effective in eliciting circulating antibodies against all three serotypes (Table 26–2) and has a zero risk of transmitting paralytic polio. Its disadvantages are its high cost, its requirement for multiple injections, the necessity for assuring complete inactivation, and the inability of this vaccine to stimulate secretory immunoglobulins in the intestine.

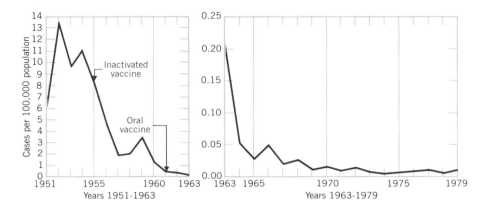

FIGURE 26–2
Number of cases of paralytic poliomyelitis reported per year in the United States from 1951 to 1979. The scale is changed after 1963 to reflect the lowered incidence of this disease after this date. (Centers for Disease Control, "Annual Summary 1979: Reported Morbidity and Mortality in the United States," *Morbidity Mortality Weekly Report,* 28, No. 54, 1980.)

The Sabin vaccine is composed of attenuated (living) strains of the three poliovirus serotypes and is called the **trivalent oral polio vaccine** (TOPV). The oral administration of the vaccine initiates an active poliovirus infection that results in an asymptomatic to mild illness. During the infection, polioviruses are excreted in the feces of the patient. The vaccine stimulates the patient to develop an immunity against all three serotypes of poliovirus. The advantages of the TOPV vaccine are its easy administration, its low cost, its stability without refrigeration, and its ability to elicit the formation of both secretory and circulating antibodies. The incidence of paralytic poliomyelitis associated with TOPV, although low, is a major disadvantage.

The United States recommends the administration of the TOPV to most infants beginning at 2 months of age. The IPV is recommended for immunizing immunodeficient children, for immunosuppressed patients, and for immunizing adults who are being vaccinated for the first time. Some countries use the IPV exclusively. There is an ongoing scientific discussion over the relative merits and ethics of which polio vaccine should be used.

ENTEROVIRUSES: COXSACKIEVIRUS AND ECHOVIRUS

In 1948, Dalldorf and Sickles isolated a new virus from the feces of two children who were suffering poliolike symptoms. The children lived in Coxsackie, New York, so the virus was named the **coxsackievi-**

TABLE 26–2
Polio Vaccines

Type	Advantages	Disadvantages
Inactivated polio vaccine (IPV), also called the Salk vaccine	No risk of polio from vaccine	Multiple injections, boosters needed, relatively high cost, no secretory immunity in intestine
Trivalent oral polio vaccine (TOPV), also called the Sabin vaccine	Both secretory and cellular antibodies, lifelong immunity, oral administration, low cost, stable without refrigeration, prepared in human cells	Risk of paralytic polio, chance of mutant virus, little efficacy in warm climates

rus. Subsequently, many strains of coxsackievirus were isolated in suckling mice. Following the development of tissue culture techniques in the 1950s, investigators isolated other viruses from the feces of healthy children. These viruses caused cytopathic effects in tissue cultures; however, they would not grow in suckling mice. They were called "orphan" viruses because they apparently caused no clinical symptoms. Now they are called the **echoviruses,** which is short for enteric cytopathic human orphan viruses. Virologists have now identified 29 serotypes of coxsackievirus and 31 serotypes of echovirus. Each is a small RNA virus that infects humans via the mouth or nose and is transmitted by the oral-fecal route. The coxsackieviruses and the echoviruses are members of the enterovirus group of the Picornaviridae family (Table 26–1).

Most coxsackievirus and echovirus infections result in asymptomatic or mildly febrile illnesses in humans. Sometimes, however, these viruses cause clinical symptoms that vary from mild head colds to serious aseptic meningitis or myocarditis. The coxsackieviruses and the echoviruses are discussed with the neurotropic viruses because certain serotypes can cause aseptic meningitis.

Aseptic meningitis: enteroviruses

Over half the cases of human viral meningitis (aseptic meningitis) are caused by coxsackieviruses or echoviruses. The term **aseptic meningitis** refers to an inflammation of the meninges not caused by bacteria. The cerebrospinal fluid (CSF) of patients with aseptic meningitis is free of bacteria; however, it often contains lymphocytes whose presence indicates this disease. The causative virus can often be isolated from the CSF during the days immediately after the onset of clinical symptoms. There are 3 serotypes of coxsackievirus and 26 serotypes of echovirus that cause aseptic meningitis (Table 26–3). This syndrome can also be caused by other viruses including mumps virus, flaviviruses, alphaviruses, bunyaviruses, and herpes viruses.

TABLE 26–3
Clinical Symptoms Caused by Coxsackieviruses and Echoviruses

Clinical Symptoms	Coxsackievirus Group A	Coxsackievirus Group B	Echoviruses
Asymptomatic infection	All	All	All
Febrile illness without coryza	All	All	All
Aseptic meningitis	A9	B2, B5	All (except 24, 26, 27, 29, 32)
Hand-foot-and-mouth disease	A16 (Also A5, A10)	B2, B5	None
Myopericarditis	Some	B2, B3, B4, B5	Some
Rubelliform	A9	None	Especially 9
Suspected Clinical Symptoms			
Diarrhea	+	+	+
Guillain-Barré syndrome	+	−	−
Reye's syndrome	+	+	+
Mononucleosis-like syndrome	+	+	−
Diabetes mellitus	−	+	−

Source: Modified from N. A. Young, "Coxsackievirus and Echovirus," in G. L. Mandell, R. G. Douglas, Jr., and J. E. Bennet, eds., *Principles and Practice of Infectious Diseases,* Wiley, 1979.

Echoviruses are the most common cause of aseptic meningitis, followed by type B and then type A coxsackievirus. These viruses cause aseptic meningitis predominantly in children less than 1 year of age. The symptoms of these infections include nausea and vomiting and are often accompanied by a sore throat. These symptoms last for a few days to 1 week, after which the patient recovers without sequelae. The symptoms are more severe in newborns who are irritable, drowsy, and reluctant to feed. Newborns may develop permanent neurological sequelae following aseptic meningitis.

Other symptoms of coxsackievirus and echovirus infections

Rashes. Certain serotypes of coxsackieviruses and echoviruses can cause skin rashes or lesions that may be clinically confused with the symptoms of other viral diseases. Echovirus type 9 is often associated with a **rubelliform rash**. The rash, accompanied by a fever, begins on the face (Color Plate 20) and then spreads to the neck and trunk. This rash can be confused with the clinical symptoms of rubella. Echovirus type-9 infections are different from rubella symptoms because they occur in the summer and they do not cause lymphadenopathy in patients.

Coxsackieviruses type A16 and, to a lesser extent, B2 and B5 cause vesicular skin lesions that resemble the lesions caused by the herpes simplex or the varicella-zoster viruses. The virus causes **hand-foot-and-mouth disease,** which is characterized by the presence of lesions in the mouth, on the hands (Color Plate 19), and on the feet. Hand-foot-and-mouth disease can be distinguished from chickenpox (varicella-zoster virus) by the distribution of the lesions (hands, feet, and mouth) and by the failure of the lesions to scab over or scar.

Muscle infections. Coxsackievirus types B2, B3, B4, and B5 are prone to cause infections of the muscle. They can infect the heart tissue to cause **myopericarditis**—an inflammation of heart muscle (myocarditis) and of the pericardium (pericarditis). The incidence of myopericarditis is twice as great among adult males as among adult females. The most common symptoms are chest pain, labored breathing, fever, and malaise. These patients are treated by bed rest.

Myocarditis in newborns is a more serious infection. The group B coxsackieviruses can be acquired from the mother or from hospital personnel. The onset of symptoms is rapid and may result in heart failure. About 50 percent of infected newborns die during the week following the onset of symptoms.

The numerous immunotypes of the coxsackieviruses and the echoviruses combined with the variety of clinical symptoms they cause make these infections difficult to diagnose. In addition to the known clinical syndromes caused by these viruses, their involvement is suspected in other human diseases (Table 26–3). One or more of these enteroviruses has been implicated in Guillain-Barré syndrome, Reye's syndrome, mononucleosis-like syndrome, diarrhea, endocarditis, and diabetes mellitus. The demonstration of a specific etiological agent in these human diseases must await further experimental evidence.

RHABDOVIRUSES: RABIES VIRUS

Rabies is a disease of domestic and wild animals; it rarely occurs in humans. The rabies virus infects the nervous tissue of animals and causes the animal to go mad (L. *rabidus*, mad). The saliva of the infected animal contains the rabies virus, which is transmitted between animals and humans by animal bites. Rabies has been known since ancient times. For centuries this disease was treated by cauterizing the site of the animal bite. In 1885, Pasteur introduced a rabies vaccine that consisted of attenuated rabies virus grown in dog brains. The immunization of rabies victims is still practiced; however, now the rabies vaccine is prepared in human cell cultures.

Rabies

There is only one rabies virus, and it is classified in the Rhabdoviridae family. This virus is a bullet-shaped (Figure 26–3) RNA virus. The chemical composition of this virus is complex. It contains at least four proteins, lipids, one single-stranded minus RNA molecule, and some carbohydrates. The spike-

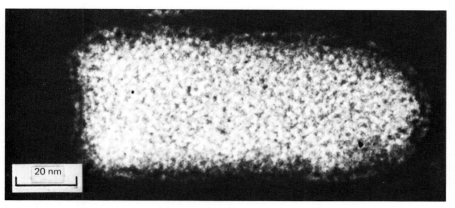

FIGURE 26—3
Electron micrograph of the bullet-shaped rabies virion. (Courtesy of Drs. K. Hummeler and N. Tomassini. From K. Hummeler and N. Tomassini, "Rhabdoviruses" in A. J. Dulton and F. Haguenau, eds., *Ultrastructure of Animal Viruses and Bacteriophages: An Atlas,* copyright © 1973, Academic Press.)

like structures extruding through the viral envelope function to bind the virus to the host cell. The glycoprotein in these spikes is the major viral immunogen and elicits the formation of neutralizing antibodies.

Animal rabies. Rabies is an enzootic disease of both domestic and wild mammals. The highest incidence of rabid animals in the United States is found among skunks, raccoons, and foxes. Coyotes, bobcats, weasels, and bats can also be infected. Among domestic animals, dogs and cats are most often involved in transferring rabies to humans; however, cows, horses, and pigs are also sources of human infection.

Infected animals secrete rabies virus in their saliva before the clinical symptoms appear, so they are infectious before they appear rabid. Asymptomatic virus secretion lasts up to 3 days in dogs, up to 2 days in cats, and up to 18 days in skunks. Cats and dogs that have bitten a human should be confined for 10 days to determine if they develop symptoms of rabies.

Rabies in humans. Most human rabies cases develop following direct contact with the saliva of a rabid animal. A few cases have been traced to viral aerosols produced in laboratories or in bat caves. The rabies virus infects the muscle and connective tissue at the site of entry. During a long incubation period, the virus multiplies, enters nervous tissue, and then physically moves within the long nerve axon to infect the ganglion of the central nervous system. There is little or no hematogenous spread of the rabies virus. Once in the central nervous system, the virus is thought to travel to the salivary glands in the efferent (away from the brain) neurons.

Incubation period. The infection remains localized for days or months before it infects nervous tissue to cause the clinical symptoms of rabies. The incubation period depends on the number of virions in the inoculum and the closeness of the wound to the central nervous system. Observed incubation periods have varied from 25 and 48 days, for a bite on the head, to 46 and 78 days for bites on an arm or a leg. The incubation period for most rabies cases is long enough to allow for postexposure immunization.

Clinical symptoms of rabies. Initial symptoms of human rabies include fever, nausea, vomiting, headache, malaise, hydrophobia (Gr. *hydrophobia,* fear of water), and lethargy. These symptoms last for 2 to 10 days before the neurological symptoms appear. Neurological signs of rabies include hyperactivity, disorientation, hallucinations, seizures, and/or paralysis. The acute neurological phase lasts 2 to 7 days and is followed by coma. Rabies patients may remain in a coma for a few hours to 14 days before they die from the degeneration of the spinal cord and brain. Although the incidence of rabies in humans is low, the majority of humans with diagnosed rabies die. Only three persons with it have survived, and each of them received either postexposure or preexposure prophylaxis.

Prevention and treatment. Vaccination against rabies is recommended for all persons exposed to rabies. Exposure is determined by finding signs of rabies in the animal involved. These animals are confined and observed for 10 days. Animal rabies is confirmed by the histological demonstration of **Negri bodies** (Figure 26–4) in tissue sections taken from the brain of sacrificed animals. If the animal is not caught, the decision to vaccinate depends on the known incidence of rabies in that species living in the geographical area of the incident.

Postinfection vaccination is effective in preventing the symptoms of rabies and is done if there is any indication of exposure. The **human diploid cell vaccine** (HDCV) was approved in 1980 for use in the United States and is now recommended for postexposure rabies treatment. Patients are given an injection of rabies immune globulin together with one dose of the vaccine. This is followed by doses of the vaccine on days 3, 7, 14, and 30. The HDCV is easily administered, effectively prevents rabies, and has no neurological side reactions. The HDCV replaces the duck embryo rabies vaccine that was used through the 1970s.

Epidemiology. The incidence of human rabies in the United States has fallen dramatically since 1951 (Figure 26–5) to an average of less than five cases per year. The widespread immunization of domestic dogs and cats has greatly reduced their involvement in transmitting rabies. Animal rabies is still prevalent

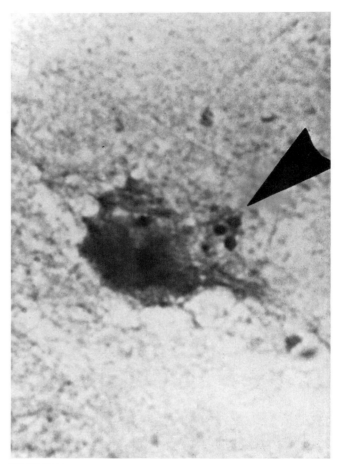

FIGURE 26–4
Negri bodies in brain tissue are diagnostic of rabies. (Courtesy of Dr. L. LeBeau.)

in the United States with between three and five thousand cases in animals per year. Wild animals (especially skunks) are currently the most common animals infected.

ARTHROPOD-BORNE HUMAN VIRAL INFECTIONS

Birds and animals serve as reservoirs for a number of neurotropic viruses that are transferred to hu-

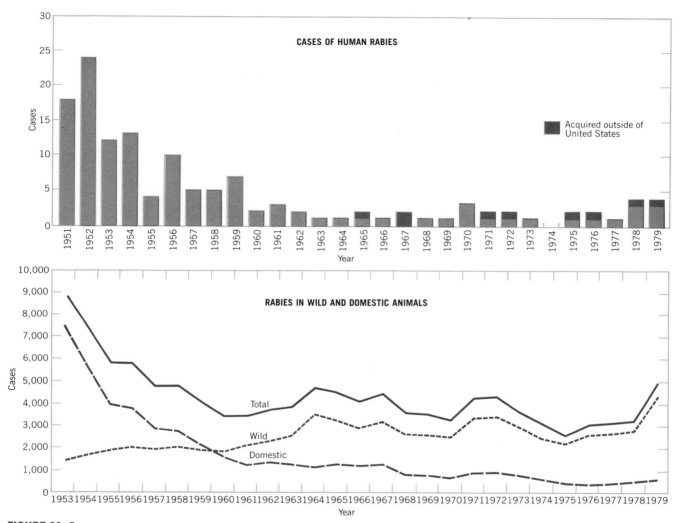

FIGURE 26–5
Rabies cases reported in the United States from the early 1950s through 1979. (Centers for
Disease Control, "Annual Summary 1979: Reported Morbidity and Mortality in the United
States," *Morbidity Mortality Weekly Report,* 28, No. 54, 1980.)

mans by arthropod vectors (either ticks or mosquitoes). The human diseases caused by these viruses
can be severe, even though humans are usually incidental or dead-end hosts for them. The incidence
of these diseases is restricted to certain seasons and

geographical areas because of the life cycles and distribution of the vectors and reservoirs.

Arthropod-borne viruses are classified in one of
three families (Table 26–4) according to their size,
structure, and chemical composition. Viruses of the

TABLE 26–4
Classification of the Arthropod-borne Animal Viruses

Family	Bunyaviridae	Togaviridae		Reoviridae
Genus	Bunyavirus	Alphavirus	Flavivirus	Orbivirus
Morphology	Spherical	Spherical	Spherical	Icosahedral (32 to 92 capsomeres)
Nucleocapsid	Helical	Cubic	Cubic	N. A.
Envelope	Yes	Yes	Yes	No
Size	90 –100 nm	45 – 75 nm	37 – 50 nm[a]	65 – 80 nm
Nucleic acid	Segmented ss (−) RNA	ss (+) RNA	ss (+) RNA	Segmented, ds RNA

[a]Yellow fever virus is smaller (29 – 31 nm).

Bunyaviridae and the Togaviridae families are enveloped, single-stranded RNA viruses. Viruses of the Reoviridae family are nonenveloped, icosahedral viruses that possess segmented, double-stranded RNA. Rubella virus, a member of the Reoviridae family, is discussed in Chapter 24.

Bunyaviridae

The bunyaviruses are a large group of mosquito-borne, enveloped RNA viruses. They are differentiated from the togaviruses by their larger size and because they have segmented RNA. In North America, the medically important Bunyaviridae belong to the **California encephalitis virus** group that causes human encephalitis.

Epidemiology. The California encephalitis group viruses are transmitted to humans by the *Aedes* mosquitoes (Table 26–5). The medically predominant virus in this group is the **LaCrosse encephalitis** (LE) **virus.** Its principal vector is the forest-dwelling mosquito *Aedes triseriatus,* which is found in the north-central and eastern United States. The LE virus is maintained within the mosquito population by trans-

TABLE 26–5
Classification, Vectors, and Reservoirs of Arthropod-borne Viruses

Family	Virus	Reservoir	Vector
Bunyaviridae	California encephalitis viruses	Ground squirrel, chipmunks	*Aedes triseriatus, A. melanimon*
Togaviridae			
Alphavirus	Eastern equine encephalitis virus	Wild birds	*Culiseta melanura*
	Western equine encephalitis virus	Wild birds	*Culiseta melanura Culex tarsalis*
	Venezuelan equine encephalitis virus	Rodents and horses	*Culex* sp.
Flavivirus	St. Louis encephalitis virus	Perching birds	*Culex tarsalis C. pipiens C. nigripalpus*
	Dengue virus	Humans	*Aedes aegypti*
	Yellow fever virus (epidemic)	Humans	*Aedes aegypti*
Rubivirus	Rubella virus	None	None
Reoviridae	Colorado tick fever virus	Ground squirrel, chipmunks	*Dermacentor andersoni*

ovarian passage and winters over in infected eggs. During the summer months, infected mosquitoes transmit the LE virus to chipmunks and squirrels. The virus replicates in these animals and causes an asymptomatic viremia. The distribution of the virus is amplified as the mosquitoes transmit the virus among the local animal population. Humans who live near forests or who enter the woods for recreational purposes are the people most often infected. In 1978, 109 cases of viral encephalitis caused by the California encephalitis group were reported in the United States. The majority of these cases occurred in the north-central states (Michigan, Wisconsin, Minnesota, and Iowa).

Clinical manifestations. The California encephalitis viruses cause human diseases that vary from mild febrile illnesses to severe forms of encephalitis. The most common clinical symptom is an acute viral encephalitis that is difficult to differentiate from other viral caused central nervous system disorders. Initial symptoms of infection include headache, fever, chills, vomiting, and nausea. These symptoms may be accompanied by convulsions (especially in children), a stiff neck, and paralysis. Most patients recover completely without sequelae.

Prevention. Limiting human exposure to mosquitoes is the only means of preventing these infections. Insecticide spraying of infected areas can be done to decrease the risk of human exposure. At present there are no antiviral agents or vaccines available. Patients are treated with supportive therapy and intensive nursing care.

Togaviridae

The Togaviridae family is organized into three genera: Alphavirus, Flavivirus, and Rubivirus. Alphaviruses and flaviviruses are almost identical (except for size) mosquito-borne, enveloped RNA viruses (Table 26–4). The reservoirs for these viruses include horses and wild birds, whereas humans are the reservoir for the dengue virus. The alphaviruses (especially Western equine encephalitis and Eastern equine encephalitis) cause severe cases of encephalitis;

the flaviviruses cause a wider array of illnesses. The third genus, Rubivirus, contains the nonarthropod-borne rubella virus (see Chapter 24).

Alphaviruses. The alphaviruses are spherical, enveloped RNA viruses that are approximately 45 to 75 nm in diameter. They are classified on the basis of their complement-fixing and hemagglutinating antigens. The three major alphaviruses are the Western equine encephalitis (WEE) virus, the Eastern equine encephalitis (EEE) virus, and the Venezuelan equine encephalitis (VEE) virus. These viruses were isolated from the brains of horses (equines) suffering from encephalitis. The horse plays a role in the transmission of the VEE virus, but both horses and humans are dead-end hosts (Figure 26–6) for the WEE or EEE viruses.

Equine encephalitis viruses. The **Eastern equine encephalitis** virus is transmitted between many species of wild birds by the swamp mosquito, *Culiseta melanura*. Horses, humans, domestic pheasants, and quail are incidental hosts that can become infected during an epidemic. The incidence of equine encephalitis viral infections in northern climates peaks between late summer and early autumn, which coincides with the population peak of the vector.

The **Western equine encephalitis** virus is maintained in a bird-mosquito cycle very similar to the EEE virus. The two viruses can coexist in the same geographical location where they use the same vectors and host birds. In the eastern United States, the vector is *Culiseta melanura,* whereas in the western United States the vector is *Culex tarsalis,* a mosquito that lives in irrigation ditches.

South America, Central America, and the southern United States harbor species of the *Culex* mosquito that transmit the **Venezuelan equine encephalitis** virus. Venezuelan equine encephalitis is a serious disease in horses; it is rare in humans. Horses and rodents are the reservoir for the VEE virus. Mosquitoes transmit the virus between horses and rodents and, on occasion, to humans (Figure 26–7). Venezuelan equine encephalitis is rare in the United States, although a major outbreak in 1971 took the lives of more than 10,000 Texan horses.

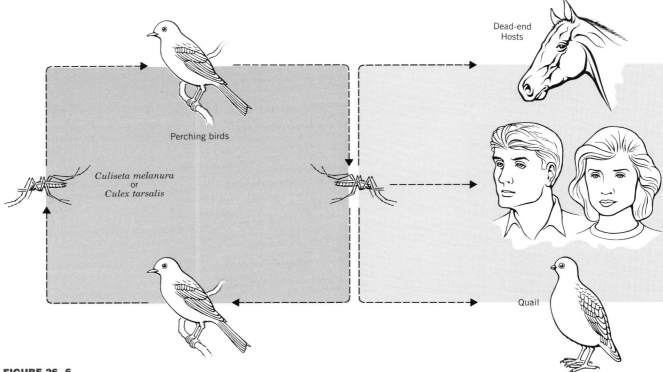

FIGURE 26–6
Epidemiology of Western equine encephalitis and Eastern equine encephalitis. Horses, humans, and domestic quail are dead-end hosts for these viruses.

Clinical manifestations. The alphaviruses cause a viremia accompanied by fever, chills, and aches. The severity of the encephalitis that follows depends on the infecting virus. EEE virus causes a serious encephalitic disease with a fatality rate of 70 percent. WEE virus causes a milder disease in adults; however, children are more susceptible to serious illness. Children infected by the EEE or the WEE virus may have sequelae that include behavioral changes, convulsive disorders, and paralysis. VEE is primarily a fatal disease of horses. The symptoms of VEE in humans can be subclinical, or they may cause severe encephalitis with a rapid progression to shock, coma, and death. As with the WEE virus, children are more likely to have severe central nervous system involvement than are adults.

Diagnosis and prevention. The presence of the virus is suspected on clinical and epidemiological grounds. A diagnosis is made by isolating the virus or by demonstrating an increasing antibody titer against the suspected virus. There are no specific treatments available for persons with the illness; however, the spread of the disease can be curtailed by controlling the vectors. Vaccines for EEE, WEE, and VEE are available and are recommended for laboratory workers—they are not recommended for the general population.

Flavivirus

Flaviviruses are smaller than the alphaviruses, but otherwise they are structurally and chemically similar (Table 26–4). In the United States, the most important flavivirus is the St. Louis encephalitis virus, which is transmitted from its natural avian reservoir to humans by mosquitoes of the *Culex* genus. Dengue is a human viral disease prevalent in Southeast

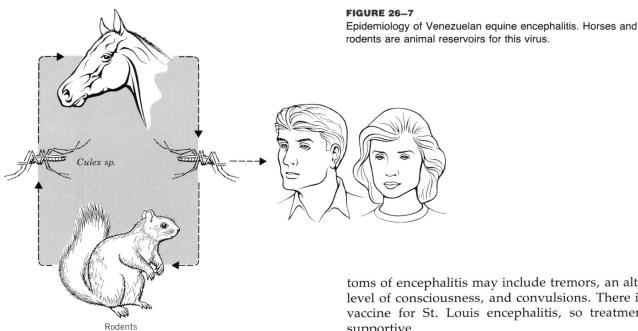

FIGURE 26-7
Epidemiology of Venezuelan equine encephalitis. Horses and rodents are animal reservoirs for this virus.

Asia. It is caused by the dengue virus, which is transmitted between humans by *Aedes aegypti*. This species of mosquito also transmits the yellow fever virus. Yellow fever and dengue can be transmitted from human to human without an intervening animal reservoir (Table 26–5).

St. Louis encephalitis virus. This virus is transmitted from its reservoir in perching birds to humans by *Culex* mosquitoes that are found in the states of the Ohio-Mississippi Valley, Florida, Texas, California, and Washington. Major human epidemics of St. Louis encephalitis occur during the mosquito season in late summer and autumn. The last major epidemic in the United States occurred during August and September in 1975 when 1815 cases resulting in 140 deaths were reported. In a normal year, fewer than 400 cases are reported in these prime months. Insecticides are used to control the mosquitoes that transmit this form of encephalitis.

The St. Louis encephalitis virus can cause a mild disease, aseptic meningitis, or encephalitis. The incubation period is 4 to 21 days. The illness is monitored by the progression of the symptoms and by the duration and height of the fever. Clinical symp-

toms of encephalitis may include tremors, an altered level of consciousness, and convulsions. There is no vaccine for St. Louis encephalitis, so treatment is supportive.

OTHER ARTHROPOD-BORNE DISEASES

Dengue (deng' ee) is an arthropod-borne disease that is characterized by a maculopapular rash on the skin. It is discussed here because it is an arthropod-borne viral disease. The yellow fever virus is the one species of the Flavivirus genus that causes jaundice in humans. Both the dengue virus and the yellow fever virus are transmitted between humans by *Aedes aegypti* without the intervention of a reservoir.

Dengue and hemorrhagic disease

Dengue and hemorrhagic disease are mosquito-borne viral diseases of humans that occur in Asia, tropical Africa, the Southwest Pacific (including Hawaii), the Caribbean, Central America, and South America. Humans are the primary reservoir for the dengue virus, and *Aedes aegypti* is the major vector. *Aedes aegypti* nests in standing water close to human habitation. The mosquito becomes infected with the dengue virus when it takes a blood meal from an infected human. The virus multiplies in the mosquito's tissues and is present in high titers in the mosquito's salivary glands. Humans are infected by the

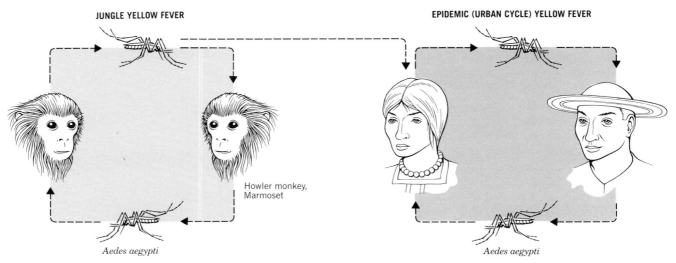

FIGURE 26–8
Epidemiology of yellow fever.

virus when the mosquito feeds. *A. aegypti* does not live in the continental United States; however, American cases of dengue do occur in Hawaii and among travelers who have visited endemic areas.

Dengue virus. Dengue is caused by one of four serotypes of the dengue virus that belongs to the Flavivirus genus of the Togaviridae family. The dengue virus is a small (45 nm), enveloped RNA virus.

Clinical symptoms. "Dengue" is a pathological term that describes an infectious, eruptive fever of warm climates. Dengue patients develop a sudden fever following an incubation period of 5 to 8 days. The fever is accompanied by a frontal headache; pain in the back, limbs, joints, and behind the eyes (retro-orbital); and lymphadenopathy. A maculopapular rash begins on the chest and spreads outward in two-thirds of the cases of dengue. The fever is often biphasic (peak-remission-peak) and lasts from 3 to 5 days. Dengue is diagnosed by the presence of these clinical symptoms.

Hemorrhagic dengue has been reported in Southeast Asia since 1958 and from islands in the Southwest Pacific since 1971. Patients with this syndrome suffer visible signs of hemorrhage in addition to the just-cited clinical symptoms. Hemorrhages in the skin (purpura), blood in the urine (hematuria), gastrointestinal hemorrhage, and varying degrees of shock are clinical symptoms of hemorrhagic dengue.

Dengue is endemic in tropical regions inhabited by mosquitoes (principally *A. aegypti*). Epidemics occur during the rainy season in the tropics, especially when a new serotype of the virus is introduced into an isolated region. People living in endemic areas can reduce their risk of acquiring dengue by wearing protective clothing and by using mosquito repellent. Live, attenuated viral vaccines have been developed for each of the four serotypes and are currently being evaluated.

Yellow fever

The wild yellow fever virus is enzootic in tree-dwelling monkeys (howler monkeys and marmosets) of tropical climates. Humans contract **jungle yellow fever** when they enter a tropical jungle and are bitten by infected mosquitoes (Figure 26–8). Yellow fever also occurs in an **epidemic** or **urban, cycle** that does not have a wild animal reservoir. Instead, the yellow fever virus is transmitted from human to human by *Aedes aegypti*.

Historical perspective. Epidemics of yellow fever were first seen in the seventeenth century coincident with expanding trade between the colonists and the countries of South and Central America. Yellow fever was introduced into urban ports when infected sailors came home. Colonial Americans quarantined these returning ships as the only means of preventing epidemic yellow fever. The threat of yellow fever persisted until the early 1900s when Major Walter Reed and his Yellow Fever Commission demonstrated that yellow fever was a mosquito-borne viral disease. The control of the mosquito population in Cuba, and subsequently in other parts of the world, resulted in a significant reduction in the epidemic disease. Now the incidence of yellow fever is limited to tropical areas of Africa, South America, and Central America (Figure 26–9).

Yellow fever virus. There is only one serotype of the yellow fever virus. It is a small, enveloped RNA virus that belongs to the Flavivirus genus of the Togaviridae family. The virus can be propagated in embryonated chicken eggs.

The disease in humans. *Aedes aegypti* is the only vector involved in the spread of yellow fever between humans. The yellow fever virus multiplies within the human, causing a viremia 4 to 5 days after infection. Mosquitoes feeding on infected humans are themselves infected. The virus grows in the mosquitoes' salivary glands. The mosquito remains infectious throughout its lifespan (6 to 8 weeks). The symptoms of yellow fever can be a denguelike or an influenzalike illness lasting 1 week, or it can cause jaundice and fever. Yellow fever patients have a rapid onset of chills and fever followed by headache, backache, nausea, and vomiting. Jaundice, when present, appears after a brief recovery.

FIGURE 26–9

Yellow fever endemic zones. (From World Health Organization, Geneva.)

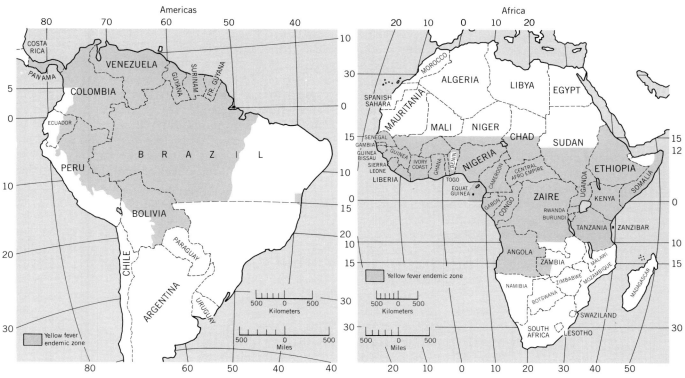

During this stage, the heart may be affected and, in fatal cases, the central nervous system is affected. Fatality rates vary with the geographical distribution of the illness and range from 10 to 60 percent of yellow fever patients.

Prevention and control. The spread of yellow fever is prevented by the yellow fever vaccine and by control of the mosquito population. Mosquito control has been effective in urban areas where the jungle yellow fever cycle does not exist. Vaccination is used to protect persons who enter epidemic areas. A live, attenuated yellow fever virus vaccine produced in chicken embryos provides long-lasting protection.

Colorado tick fever

Colorado tick fever is a viral disease that occurs in the mountainous regions of the western United States and Canada where the tick vectors reside. The virus can winter over in the nymph and adult forms of the tick. The nymphs infect rodents when they take a blood meal before initiating their reproductive cycle. Ground squirrels are the major reservoir for this virus. Infected squirrels become viremic after infection and pass the virus to other ticks in a spring amplification cycle. Humans, who are dead-end hosts for the virus, are infected when adult ticks take a blood meal. The virus is a double-stranded RNA virus that belongs to the Orbivirus genus of the Reoviridae family (Table 26–4).

Colorado tick fever in humans. After a 3- to 6-day incubation period, the patient experiences a sudden onset of fever, chills, headache, ocular pain, nausea, and vomiting. The acute phase of the illness lasts 7 to 10 days, with half the patients having a "saddleback" fever. Recovery is usually complete.

Residents of enzootic areas who work in outdoor professions or who pursue recreational activities in the Rocky Mountain states are the persons most likely to get Colorado tick fever. The disease can be prevented by the use of insect repellents and protective clothing and by the removal of ticks before they attach and feed. Campers and campsite planners should avoid areas where Colorado tick fever is a known problem.

SLOW-DEVELOPING NEUROLOGICAL DISEASES

Kuru and Creutzfeldt-Jakob Disease

Kuru and the Creutzfeldt-Jakob disease (CJD) are slow-developing degenerative diseases of the human central nervous system. Both diseases have been transmitted by a filterable agent to chimpanzees; however, the etiological agents have not been determined. They may be viral agents or they may be other infectious agents.

Kuru. This disease was restricted to the Fore tribe who live in the mountainous highlands of eastern New Guinea. When this disease was discovered in the 1950s, kuru was causing 200 (1 percent of the tribe) deaths per year. Kuru occurred among adults and preadolescents and affected three times as many adult women as adult men. Transmission of kuru was traced to the cannibalistic custom of consuming dead tribe members as a rite of mourning. The women and small children were the main participants in this ceremony. It was postulated that the victims infected themselves and that the infectious agent entered through cuts or mucous membranes. The disease symptoms did not occur until 5 to 20 years after infection. This long incubation period has given the "slow virus" label to the etiological agent.

Kuru has a sudden onset of symptoms characterized by cerebellar ataxia and shivering tremors of the head, trunk, and extremities. The symptoms progress until the patient is unable to walk and cannot move without suffering uncontrolled tremors. The patient usually dies 3 to 9 months after the initial onset of symptoms. Kuru has declined since 1965, when the ritual of cannibalism ceased. Kuru is no longer seen in either children or adolescents; however, it still occurs in adults—a fact that attests to the long incubation period of kuru.

Creutzfeldt-Jakob disease. This illness is an uncommon dementing illness of humans that has a worldwide distribution. It occurs with equal frequency among men and women, and it generally affects persons between 50 and 70 years old. There may be a genetic predisposition to Creutzfeldt-Jakob disease. Among a group of Libyan Jews who had migrated to Israel, the incidence of CJD was 30 times higher than the incidence of CJD in the general population.

Creutzfeldt-Jakob disease has a rapid onset in late middle-aged people characterized by profound dementia and diffuse, rapid muscle spasms (myoclonus). The patient progresses through a period of behavioral changes, loss of memory and reasoning, and a loss in visual acuity. The patient's health deteriorates rapidly, resulting in delirium, coma, and, invariably, death. The etiology and epidemiology of CJD disease is unclear. The disease has been transmitted to chimpanzees; however, the nature of the etiological agent is still unknown.

SUMMARY

The neurotropic enteroviruses that belong to the Picornaviridae are the polioviruses, the coxsackieviruses, and the echoviruses. The polioviruses (Table 26–6) are transmitted by the fecal-oral route and cause inapparent, abortive, and paralytic poliomyelitis in humans. Paralytic poliomyelitis (1 to 2 percent of polio cases) causes paralysis of the limbs and can affect the patient's ability to breathe and swallow. Poliomyelitis is now prevented by using the TOPV or the IPV vaccine. Coxsackieviruses and echoviruses are responsible for more than half the proven cases of aseptic meningitis. The symptoms of aseptic meningitis caused by these viruses are more severe in children than in adults. Echoviruses and coxsackieviruses also cause other clinical illnesses, including a rubelliform rash (especially echovirus type 9), hand-foot-and-mouth disease (coxsackievirus B2, B5, A16), and myopericarditis (coxsackievirus B2 through B5).

Rabies is enzootic in wild animals; it rarely occurs in humans. Skunks, raccoons, and foxes are the wild animals most often found to be rabid. Human rabies is usually acquired when the saliva of a rabid animal enters muscle tissue. The rabies virus multiplies in the muscle before it travels to the brain by neurotropic spread. Postexposure vaccination with the human diploid cell vaccine is effective in treating rabies because of the disease's long incubation period. Untreated human rabies is always fatal.

Viruses belonging to the Bunyaviridae, the Togaviridae (except rubella), and the Reoviridae families exist in natural animal reservoirs and are transmitted by arthropod vectors. The LaCrosse encephalitis virus is the most important member of the California encephalitis group viruses that cause human encephalitis. *Aedes triseriatus* is a forest-dwelling mosquito that transfers the LaCrosse encephalitis virus from its reservoir in chipmunks and squirrels to humans. This virus is a major cause of encephalitis and infects persons primarily in the north-central United States during the late summer and early autumn.

The alphaviruses and the flaviviruses also cause encephalitis in humans. The EEE virus and the WEE virus are transferred from their reservoirs in wild birds by *Culiseta melanura*. Humans, horses, and domestic quail are dead-end hosts for these viruses. VEE virus is present in wild rodents and is transmitted to horses and humans by species of the *Culex* mosquito. St. Louis encephalitis virus belongs to the Flavivirus genus and causes either a mild disease, aseptic meningitis, or encephalitis. Perching birds are its natural reservoirs, and species of the *Culex* mosquito are its vector.

The tropical mosquito *A. aegypti* is the vector for the dengue virus and the yellow fever virus—both are flaviviruses. Dengue is an endemic viral disease characterized by a maculopapular rash, a fever, and severe pains in the joints and muscles. Jungle yellow fever exists in tropical forests in a cycle involving the howler monkey and *A. aegypti*; humans are incidental hosts. Epidemic (urban cycle) yellow fever is transmitted between humans by *A. aegypti*. Yellow fever has a rapid onset of denguelike or influenzalike symptoms. Jaundice may appear after a brief recovery. Ticks and ground squirrels are the reservoirs, and ticks are the vectors, for the Colorado tick fever virus. Infected humans, the dead-end hosts for this virus, become sick with fever, nausea, and vomiting for 7 to 10 days before they recover completely.

TABLE 26–6
Summary: Viral Diseases of the Nervous System

Disease	Viral Agent	Symptoms	Epidemiology	Control
Poliomyelitis	Poliovirus (3 serotypes)	Inapparent illness, abortive illness, paralytic illness with CNS involvement	Fecal-oral route	TOP or IP vaccines
Aseptic meningitis	Coxsackievirus (A9, B2, B5) Echoviruses (all except 5)	Nausea, vomiting, neurological sequelae in newborns	Fecal-oral route	Supportive treatment
Myopericarditis	Coxsackievirus (B2–B5)	Inflammation of heart muscle and pericardium	Transmitted by infected persons	Supportive treatment
Hand-foot-and-mouth	Coxsackievirus (A16, B2, B5)	Vesicular lesions on hands, feet, and mouth	Fecal-oral route	Supportive treatment
Rubelliform	Echovirus type 9 Coxsackievirus A9	Fever; rash on face, neck, trunk	Fecal-oral route	Supportive treatment
Rabies	Rabies virus	Nausea, vomiting, hydrophobia, headache, malaise, fever, seizures, and paralysis	Bite of rabid animal (virus in saliva)	Human diploid cell vaccine (postexposure use is effective)
Encephalitis	Many (see Table 26–5)	Fever, headache, vomiting, nausea. Severe form: convulsions, stiff neck, paralysis, coma, and death	Arthropod-borne (mosquitoes)	Mosquito control supportive treatment
Yellow fever	Yellow fever virus	Influenzalike, jaundice, CNS involvement in fatal cases	Arthropod-borne (*Aedes aegypti*)	Yellow fever virus vaccine
Dengue	Dengue virus	Eruptive fever; pain in back, limbs, joints; maculopapular rash; possible hemorrhages	Arthropod-borne (*Aedes aegypti*)	Mosquito control, supportive treatment
Colorado tick fever	Colorado tick fever virus	Fever, chills, ocular pain, headache, nausea, vomiting	Bite of infected tick	Removal of ticks from body
Kuru	Unknown	Cerebral atoxia, shivering, and uncontrolled tremors	Cannibalism (5- to 20-year incubation)	Prohibition of cannibalism
Creutzfeldt-Jakob disease	Unknown	Profound dementia, rapid muscle spasms	Unknown	No known treatment

Kuru and the Creutzfeldt-Jacob disease are caused by slow-acting, as yet uncharacterized etiological agents. Kuru is a progressive, debilitating neurological disease that has an incubation period of 5 to 20 years. It occurs among the Fore tribe in New Guinea and is transmitted by the cannibalistic custom of consuming dead tribemembers. Creutzfeldt-Jakob disease is an uncommon, dementing human illness that strikes elderly people. It is characterized by profound dementia and diffuse, rapid muscle spasms.

QUESTIONS AND TOPICS FOR STUDY AND DISCUSSION

Questions

1. Describe the natural barriers that prevent infectious agents from entering the human central nervous system.
2. Describe the three possible clinical outcomes of a poliovirus infection. What are the most serious consequences of polio, and how are they treated?
3. Name, describe, and compare the use and effectiveness of the two poliovirus vaccines.
4. List and describe the key characteristics of the viruses that can cause aseptic meningitis.
5. Coxsackieviruses and echoviruses cause clinical signs that can be confused with two childhood diseases. Explain.
6. Rabies is an epizootic disease. How does it affect humans?
7. What steps are taken to prevent human rabies, and how is the disease in humans treated?
8. Which arthropod-borne viral diseases are important to humans living in North America? Describe the clinical nature of these diseases, their reservoirs and vectors, and their seasonal and geographical incidence.
9. Was yellow fever ever a significant disease in the continental United States? Explain.
10. Describe a slow-developing neurological disease. Have the etiological agents been identified? Are they viruses?

Discussion

1. The Sabin vaccine is used in the United States for immunizing children against polio. Should physicians in this country change this practice and use the Salk vaccine? Explain.
2. There is a low incidence of human rabies in the United States. If the practice of vaccinating dogs and cats against rabies were abolished, would you expect increased human rabies?
3. RNA viruses mutate at faster rates than do DNA viruses because there are fewer mechanisms in animal cells to correct for mistakes in RNA replication. Discuss why this is the case. Can this situation explain why there are more RNA animal viruses than DNA animal viruses?

FURTHER READING

Books

Baer, G. M. (ed.), *The Natural History of Rabies,* vols. 1 and 2, Academic Press, New York, 1975.

Paul, J. R., *A History of Poliomyelitis,* Yale, New Haven, 1971. A comprehensive history of polio.

Articles and Reviews

Gajdusek, D. C., "Unconventional Viruses and the Origin and Disappearance of Kuru," *Science,* 197:943–960 (1977). The Nobel lecture of Carleton Gajdusek delivered when he accepted the Nobel Prize in Physiology and Medicine.

Kaplan, M. M., and H. Koprowski, "Rabies," *Sci. Am.,* 242:120–134 (January 1980). A review of the history of this viral disease.

Miller, G. D., "Hand-foot-and-mouth Disease," *JAMA,* 203:827–830 (1968). The case histories of 11 cases of hand-foot-and-mouth disease caused by coxsackievirus A16.

Salk, J., and D. Salk, "Control of Influenza and Poliomyelitis with Killed Virus Vaccines," *Science,* 195:834–847 (1977). A review article that presents scientific data in support of the use of the Salk vaccine in preference to the use of the TOPV.

Smith, W. G., "Coxsackie B Myopericarditis in Adults," *Am. Heart J.,* 80:34–46 (1970). A detailed clinical report on 42 adult patients.

Wilfert, C. M., B. A. Lauer, M. Cohen, M. L. Costenbader, and E. Myers, "An Epidemic of Echovirus 18 Meningitis," *J. Infect. Dis.,* 131:75–78 (1975). A research paper describing an outbreak of meningitis in North Carolina.

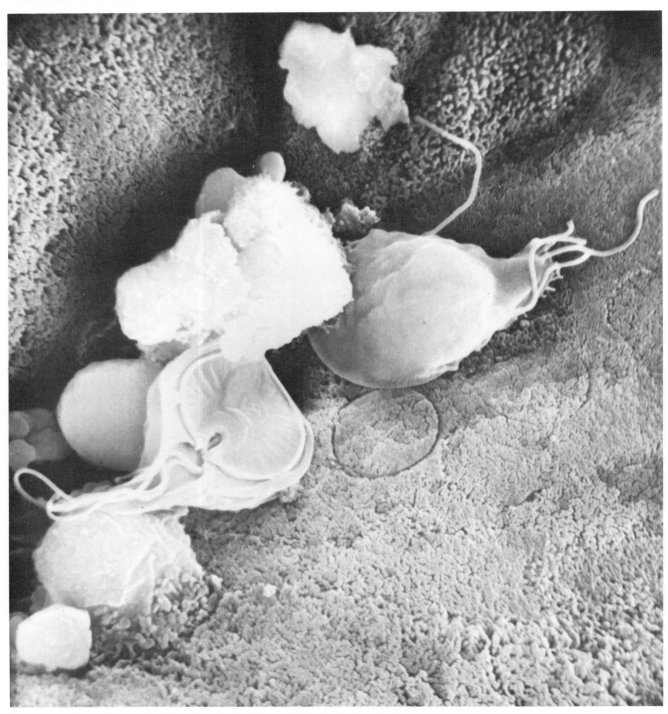

Scanning electron micrograph of dorsal and ventral views of *Giardia* trophozoites in mouse. (Courtesy of Dr. R. L. Owen. From R. L. Owen, P. C. Nemanic, and D. P. Stevens, *Gastroenterology,* 76:757 – 769, 1979.)

PART FIVE

EUCARYOTIC PATHOGENS

The eucaryotic microorganisms that can cause infectious diseases include a select group of fungi and protozoa. In size, they can be as small as a large bacterium or large enough to be visible under a strong magnifying glass. A basic feature of eucaryotic cells is that they possess more than one chromosome, therefore they are genetically more complex than procaryotic cells. The chromosomes of eucaryotic cells are organized in a nucleus and are replicated during mitosis. In addition to the nucleus, eucaryotic cells can possess mitochondria, chloroplasts, and complex organelles of locomotion.

Biologists have intuitively thought of organisms as being either animals or plants: animals being the motile heterotrophs and plants being the sessile phototrophs. The eucaryotic microorganisms do not fit easily into these groupings. Protozoa are similar to animals because they are motile; however, some have plantlike cell walls and some possess chloroplasts. Algae are studied by botanists because they are phototrophs; however, many are motile or have motile stages during their life cycle. Fungi have plantlike cell walls, but they are nonphotosynthetic. For these reasons, eucaryotic microorganisms represent the middle ground of the living world, which makes their classification a perplexing problem. A reasonable solution was first proposed in 1866 by E. H. Haeckel. His proposal placed protozoa, algae, fungi, and bacteria into a third kingdom that he called *Protista*. The modern form of this proposal assigns the bacteria to the *lower protists*, while the eucaryotic microorganisms including the protozoa, algae, and fungi comprise the *higher protists*.

27

MEDICALLY IMPORTANT FUNGI

The higher protists are found throughout the world in soil, water, aerosols, and on vegetable matter. The algae are photosynthetic organisms that fall into the realm of botany; no algae are known to cause infectious human diseases. Protozoa usually exist in aquatic environments. Most protozoa are innocuous to humans, although a few cause serious human disease. Some examples of protozoan diseases of humans are described in Chapter 28. The fungi are higher protists with some representatives that are beneficial and others that are harmful to humans. Mycologists are scientists who study the fungi and their field of study is called *mycology.*

Fungi (sing. fungus; Gr. *sphongos,* sponge) are spore-bearing, achlorophyllous, and usually nonmotile higher protists that possess a cell wall. The fungi are a morphologically diverse group of organisms. Many fungi are microorganisms that grow as single cells, known as yeast cells, or as filaments known as hyphae. All fungi reproduce asexually, and most fungi also replicate by sexual reproduction. The large, visible fungi that produce fruiting bodies are known as mushrooms and toadstools.

Fungi are ubiquitous in soil, decaying plant material, aerosols, and aquatic environments. Fungi benefit the human race by recycling plant material. Some are eaten by animals as food, and many form symbiotic relationships with plant roots. Other fungi are important to humans because of the compounds they produce. For example, *Penicillium* produces the antibiotic penicillin; *Saccharomyces* is used in the manufacture of both alcoholic beverages and bread; and certain fungi are used to manufacture cheeses. Other fungi pose serious problems for humans. Fungi are responsible for the majority of plant diseases. There are fungi capable of destroying food, fabrics, and leather, and some fungi produce potent animal toxins. About 100 of the known fungal species cause disease in humans and animals.

FUNGAL MORPHOLOGY

The fungi are structurally more complex and are generally larger than the bacteria. The term **fungus** encompasses both the filamentous, tubular molds and the single-celled yeasts. The tubular protoplasmic structure of the molds is known as a **hypha** (Gr. *hyphe,* web). The presence of hyphae differentiates the molds from the single-celled yeasts. A given fungus may have a predominant structure (yeast or mold); however, intermediate structures (pseudohyphae) and the ability of a fungus to grow as either a mold or a yeast (dimorphism) complicate morphological identification.

Unicellular morphology

The term **yeast** is used to describe a single, oval, or spherical fungal cell that reproduces asexually by budding or fission (Figure 27–1). Microscopically, a budding yeast cell is characterized by the presence of attached buds and by the unequal size of the daughter cells. Some yeasts grow as elongated, attached single cells known as **pseudohyphae,** which are intermediate forms between the morphologies of yeasts and molds. *Saccharomyces cerevisiae* is the common yeast that is widely used in the brewing and baking industries.

Filamentous morphology

Many fungi grow as an extensive, multibranched, interwinding mat known as a **mycelium** (Gr. *mykes,* mushroom, fungus). This mat is composed of hyphae (Figure 27–2) surrounded by the fungal cell wall. Some hyphae are divided into compartments by cross-wall structures called **septa** (sing. septum;

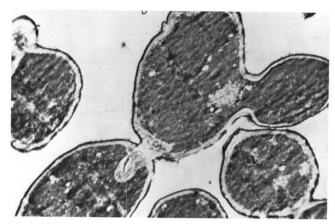

FIGURE 27–1
Electron micrograph of budding yeast cells. (Courtesy of the American Society for Microbiology Slide Collection.)

L. *septum,* hedge, partition); nonseptate fungi lack these cross-walls. The compartments (cells) can be uninucleated, binucleated, or multinucleated. The septate fungi have cross-wall pores (Figure 27–3), which are usually large enough to permit the movement of nuclei from one compartment to the next.

FIGURE 27–2
Electron micrograph of a longitudinal section of a hypha of *Pythium aphanidermatum* showing its eucaryotic cell structure. This section of the coenocytic hypha contains numerous nuclei (n). (Courtesy of Dr. C. E. Bracker. From S. N. Grove and C. E. Bracker, *J. Bacteriol.,* 104:989–1009, 1970. With permission of the American Society for Microbiology.)

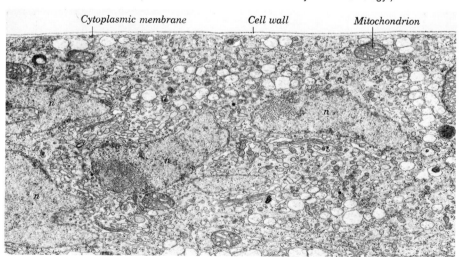

Cytoplasmic membrane   Cell wall   Mitochondrion

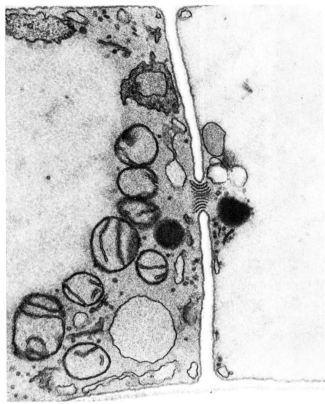

FIGURE 27–3
Electron micrograph of a longitudinal section through a fungal septum showing a central pore. (Courtesy of Dr. C. E. Bracker. Reproduced with permission, from *Annual Review of Phytopathology*, 5:343 – 374, copyright © 1967, Annual Reviews Inc.)

Organisms possessing a multinucleated protoplasm are described as being **coenocytic,** which literally means "common cell" (Gr. *koinos,* common; and *kytos,* a hollow vessel).

Molds, yeasts, and dimorphism

The colony morphologies of the medically important fungi grown on laboratory media is an aid to fungus identification. Molds grow as dry, cottonlike masses of protoplasm (Figure 27–4). These filamentous fungi produce aerial hyphae that may support terminal spores, surface hyphae that laterally extend the colony, and submerged hyphae that extract sustenance from the substratum. Yeasts grow as moist, opaque, pasty, or creamy colonies. Morphological observations further aid in the identification of fungal isolates. Fungi are morphologically characterized according to their size, presence of capsules, cell-wall thickness, pseudohyphae, and by the types of spores they form.

Some molds are dimorphic: they grow either as single cells or as hyphae, depending on the growth environment. Most dimorphic fungi grow as yeast cells in tissue and at 37°C, but as molds (mycelia) when they are cultured at room temperature. Dimorphism adds a degree of complexity to fungal identification.

Growth and reproduction

Vegetative growth of the mycelium occurs when the fungus increases the mass of its protoplasm. The diameter of the hypha remains essentially constant, while the mycelium increases in mass by elongation and branching. The nuclei in these cells divide by the normal process of mitosis, even in the absence of septa formation.

Fungi are broadly characterized as parasites when they obtain their food from living tissue or as **saprobes** (Gr. *sapros,* rotten; and *bios,* life) when they obtain their food from dead organic matter. The medically important fungi are primarily saprobes that become parasites when given the opportunity. For this reason, most pathogenic fungi can be grown on defined media containing salts, NH_4^+ or NO_3^- as their source of nitrogen, vitamins (biotin and/or thiamine), and a sugar. They are aerobic heterotrophs that will grow at various pHs (2.0 to 10), even though they prefer an acid pH (4.0 to 6.0). Their preference for an acid pH enables mycologists to selectively grow them in the presence of bacteria, most of which do not grow at acid pHs. Most pathogenic fungi grow on Sabouraud's medium, which contains peptone and glucose adjusted to pH 5.0. Another way to prevent the rapid growth of bacteria during

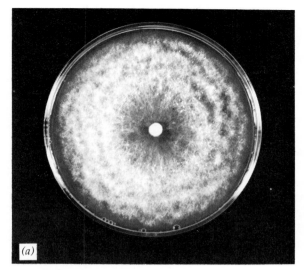

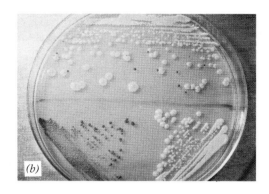

FIGURE 27—4

(a) Filamentous growth of a fungal mycelium on an agar plate after 7 days of growth. Photograph by R. W. Scheetz. (Courtesy of C. J. Alexopoulos and C. W. Mims, *Introductory Mycology*, Wiley, 1979.) (b) Separation of yeast colonies on bromcresol green agar. Photo by Phoebe Rich. (Courtesy of M. C. Campbell. From M. C. Campbell and J. L. Stewart, *The Medical Mycology Handbook*, copyright © 1980. Reprinted with permission of John Wiley & Sons, Inc.)

fungal isolation is to add antibiotics, such as chloramphenicol and penicillin, to the isolation media. The combined effects of antibacterial agents and a low pH prevent bacteria from overgrowing the fungi.

Fungi grow over a narrower temperature range than do bacteria. Their normal temperature range is between 0 and 35°C with an optimum between 20 and 30°C. The temperature maximum for thermophilic fungi appears to be 50°C. Because many pathogenic fungi take a long time to grow, cultures with no growth should be incubated for at least 2 and usually 6 weeks before they are discarded. The morphology of a dimorphic fungus depends primarily on the growth temperature and the medium used for its cultivation.

Pathogenic fungi can be grown in the ordinary microbiology laboratory; however, certain precautions should be strictly observed. Since inhaled fungal spores can cause infections, fungal cultures should never be smelled, and petri dishes containing fungal cultures should be opened only in a well-vented hood. Stock cultures can conveniently be maintained on slants in screw-cap tubes. Since many fungi grow in soil and are transmitted with dust, a laboratory should be kept dust-free, and potted plants should never be permitted in the laboratory. Old cultures are destroyed routinely by autoclaving and should not be allowed to accumulate.

Asexual reproduction. Fungal spores produced by sexual and asexual processes are the basis for the classification of most fungi. The production of spores is the most common form of asexual reproduction. Asexual spores produced in a sporangia are called **sporangiospores,** whereas asexual spores produced at the end of a hypha are referred to as **conidia** (sing. conidium; Gr. *konis,* dust). Macroconidia are large, multicellular conidia; small, unicellular conidia are known as microconidia. **Chlamydospores** are surrounded by a thick, double-walled spore coat and are formed either on the hyphal tip or within the hypha (Figure 27–5). **Arthrospores** are produced within the hyphae by septation, whereas **blastospores** are budlike projections formed by yeasts. The morphology of the asexual spores varies greatly and is used in identification.

Asexual fungal spores are dispersed to new locations by air currents after they break off from their parental hypha. When appropriate nutrients are available, a spore will germinate and develop into a new mycelium. Humans are continuously exposed to aerosols of fungal spores. These spores can cause asthma attacks in allergic persons, and the inhalation of the spores of certain pathogenic fungi can cause pulmonary infections.

Sexual reproduction. In addition to asexual spore formation, many fungi can reproduce by the fusion of gametes in a process of sexual reproduction. Sexual reproduction is an advantage to a species because it generates individuals with new genotypes. This form of genetic transfer in fungi has been used to understand the basic nature of genes (see *Neurospora*, Chapter 6).

Sexual reproduction occurs when two nuclei (gametes) of the same species fuse. These nuclei can come from reproductive structures on the same fungus, or they can come from reproductive structures produced by different mating types of the same species. Sexual reproduction begins when two fungal elements join. Next, the nuclei from the two different mating types fuse. This fused structure proceeds to undergo meiosis (reductive division), which is usually accompanied by the reassortment of chromosomes.

The structures observed in sexual reproduction are morphologically distinct (Figure 27–6) and are used to identify the subdivisions of the perfect fungi. **Oospores** and/or **zygospores** are sexually produced by Mastigomycotina and Zygomycotina; **ascospores** are sexually produced by Ascomycotina; and **basidio-**

FIGURE 27–5
Asexual fungal spores. (a) Arthrospore formation in *Coccidioides immitis*, (b) chlamydospores and blastospores of *Candida albicans*, (c) conidia of *Aspergillus fumigatus*, (d) macroconidia of *Microsporum*, and (e) sporangiospore of *Absidia*.

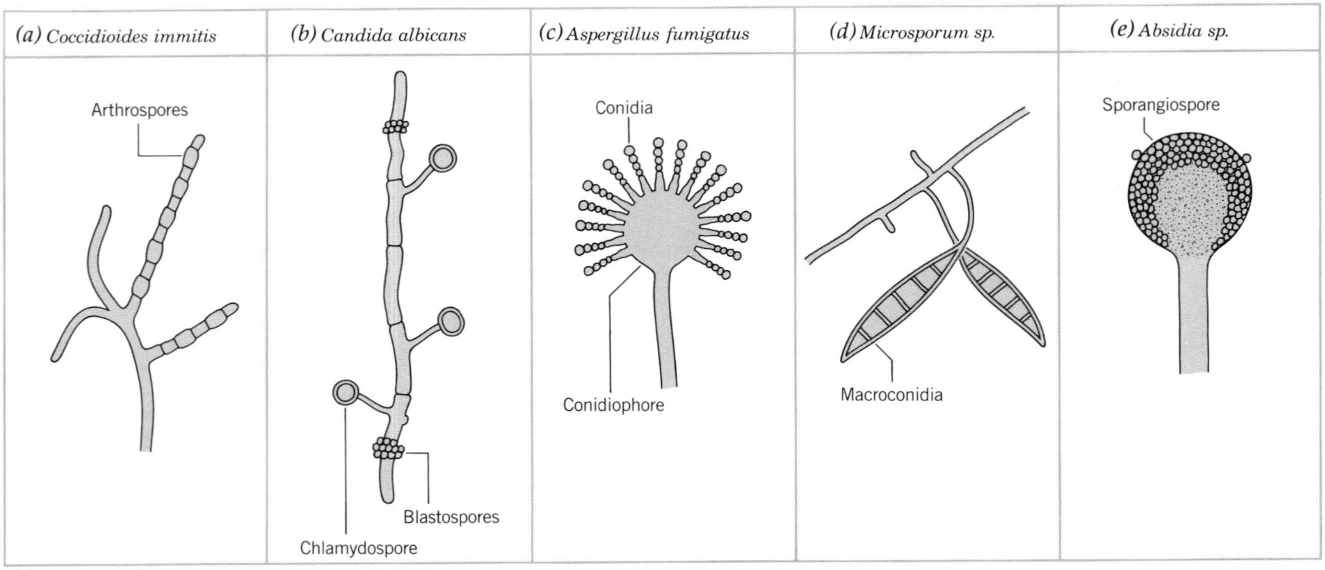

| (a) Coccidioides immitis | (b) Candida albicans | (c) Aspergillus fumigatus | (d) Microsporum sp. | (e) Absidia sp. |

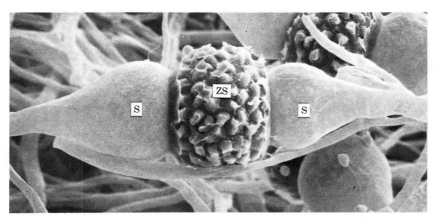

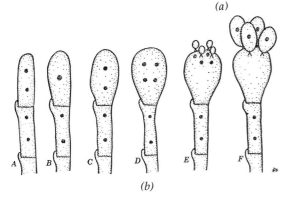

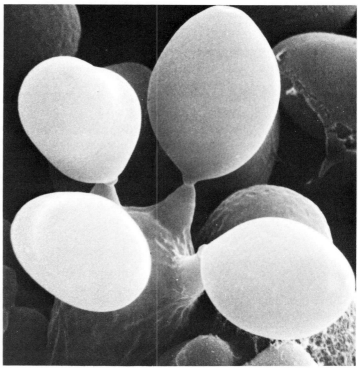

FIGURE 27–6
Sexual reproduction in fungi. (*a*) Scanning electron micrograph of a mature zygosporangium (zs) between two tong-shaped suspensors (s) of *Gilbertella persicaria*. (Courtesy of Dr. K. L. O'Donnell. From K. L. O'Donnell et al., *Can. J. Bot.*, 55:662-675, 1977. By permission National Research Council of Canada.) (*b*) Six successive stages in the formation of a basidium and (*c*) a scanning electron micrograph of a basidium bearing four basidiospores. (Photograph by S. L. Flegler. Courtesy of Dr. C. J. Alexopoulos and C. W. Mims, *Introductory Mycology*, Wiley, 1979.)

spores are sexually produced by Basidiomycotina. Sexual spores are blown on the wind to new locations and function as a major means of dispersing a fungal species. Once in an appropriate environment, the sexual spores germinate to form a vegetative mycelium.

Classification

The true fungi are grouped into five subdivisions of the division Eumycota (Table 27–1). They are distinguished by sexual and asexual reproductive processes and by the presence or absence of septa. *Neurospora* produces sexual spores in a saclike structure

TABLE 27–1
Subdivisions of the True Fungi (Eumycota)

Subdivision	Asexual Spores	Sexual Spores	Mycelium	Representative Genera
Ascomycotina	At ends or sides of hyphae	Ascospores in asci	Septate	*Neurospora*
Basidiomycotina	At ends or sides of hyphae	Basidiospores on surface of basidium	Septate	*Filobasidiella*
Mastigomycotina[a]	In sacs	Oospores	Nonseptate	*Pythium*
Zygomycotina[a]	In sacs	Zygospores	Nonseptate	*Absidia, Mucor, Rhizopus*
Deuteromycotina (fungi imperfect)	At ends or sides of hyphae	Absent	Unicellular or septate	*Candida, Coccidioides, Sporothrix, Epidermophyton*

[a]Formerly classified as the lower fungi in the class Phycomycetes.

called an **ascus** and belong to the subdivision **Ascomycotina.** Mushrooms produce basidiospores and are classified in the subdivision **Basidiomycotina.** Fungi that do not demonstrate a sexual form of reproduction are classified as imperfect fungi in the class **Deuteromycotina.** Fungi in the **Mastigomycotina** and the **Zygomycotina** have nonseptate mycelia and possess asexual spores that are always formed within a saclike structure, either a zoosporangium or sporangium. Oospores are the sexual spores formed by fungi of the subdivision **Mastigomycotina,** whereas zygospores (Figure 27–6) are formed by members of the subdivision Zygomycotina.

Sexual reproduction in many of the pathogenic fungi either is unknown or has only recently been discovered. Demonstrating sexual reproduction in a given isolate is not always easy: it often necessitates that the investigator isolate both mating types of the fungus. When sexual reproduction of a Deuteromycotina is discovered, by definition the organism must be reclassified. The old (anamorphic) names are still used because they are so ingrained in the medical vocabulary. The perfect (teleomorphic) names assigned to these organisms (Table 27–2) indicate the correct fungal classification based on current taxonomic principles.

TABLE 27–2
Perfect Stages of Pathogenic Fungi

Old (Anamorphic) Name (Imperfect Fungi)	Perfect (Teleomorphic) Name (Subdivisions)
Blastomyces dermatitidis	*Ajellomyces dermatitidis* (Ascomycotina)
Cryptococcus neoformans	*Filobasidiella neoformans* (Basidiomycotina)
Histoplasma capsulatum	*Ajellomyces[a] (Edmonsiella[a]) capsulatum* (Ascomycotina)
Microsporum gypseum	*Nannizia gypsea, N. incurvata* (Ascomycotina)
Trichophyton mentagrophytes	*Arthroderma benhamiae* (Ascomycotina)

[a]Considered to be the same genus by M. R. McGinnis and B. Katz, *Mycotaxon,* 8:157–164 (1979).

THE PATHOGENIC FUNGI

Only about 100 of the more than 50,000 species of fungi cause disease in humans. Most of the pathogenic fungi are incidental or opportunistic pathogens whose normal habitat is soil or vegetable matter. Only a few pathogenic fungi are naturally found associated with animals.

Mycoses are diseases caused by pathogenic fungi. For convenience, we will divide the fungal diseases into three major groups. **Systemic** or **deep mycoses** are fungal infections of internal organs that usually begin as pulmonary lesions. Systemic mycoses are caused by soil fungi that are inhaled by humans. In their chronic form, these infections spread from the lungs to other internal organs. Soil fungi or fungi associated with vegetable matter cause **subcutaneous mycoses** when they infect the skin, subcutaneous tissue, connective tissue, and/or bone. These diseases are prevalent in tropical regions where people are infected through puncture wounds by a contaminated splinter, thorn, or soil. **Cutaneous mycoses** are fungal infections of the keratinous structures found in human hair, nails, and epidermis. **Dermatophytes** (Gr. *derma*, skin) are the fungi responsible for cutaneous mycoses. Most cutaneous mycoses are caused by fungi that are associated with humans; a few are contracted from animals.

Diagnosis and treatment of fungal diseases

Fungal infections are usually diagnosed by the microscopic identification of the etiological agent in lesions, exudates, hair, or in scrapings from the infected tissue. Exposure of specimens to warm alkali (10 percent NaOH or KOH) followed by staining is one method in common use (Figure 27–7). The alkali destroys the structure of the human tissue, while the morphology of the fungus is retained because it possesses an alkali-resistant cell wall. Usually the reproductive structures of the fungus are observable only after culturing the fungus in the laboratory.

Final identification of the etiological agent of a fungal infection may take several weeks because many pathogenic fungi grow very slowly on laboratory media. Standard isolation media include blood

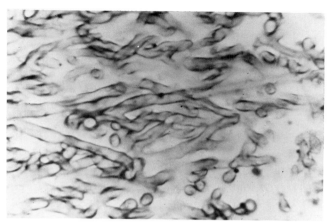

FIGURE 27–7
Stained preparation of nonseptate hyphae of *Mucor pusillus*. (Courtesy of Dr. C. W. Emmons.)

agar, Sabouraud agar, birdseed agar, and yeast extract agar. Antibacterial antibiotics can be added to media to prevent bacteria from overgrowing the fungi. Nutrient-limited media are also used when the stimulation of spore formation is desired.

Immunological techniques applicable to fungal infections. Immunological techniques are available for the detection of certain fungal infections. Persons exposed to a given fungus often develop a sensitivity to that fungus. This sensitivity can be demonstrated following an intradermal injection of a specific fungal extract. Sensitized patients have a delayed-type hypersensitivity reaction that is similar to the positive tuberculin reaction. **Histoplasmin** prepared from *Histoplasma capsulatum*, **blastomycin** prepared from *Blastomyces dermatitidis,* and **coccidioidin** prepared from *Coccidioides immitis* are preparations that have been used for skin testing.

A positive skin test indicates that the patient has been exposed to that fungus. These tests have some value in epidemiological studies; however, they are of limited diagnostic value. Their role in diagnosis is limited by the following: (1) histoplasmin and blastomycin have a high degree of cross-reactivity when tested against each other; (2) skin testing with histoplasmin has the ability to convert a seronegative person to seropositive, which interferes with other serological tests for histoplasmosis; and (3) there is a high incidence of healthy seropositive individuals in areas where these fungi are endemic.

More sophisticated serodiagnostic tests are available for diagnosing a select group of systemic mycoses. These include complement fixation, immunodiffusion, and latex agglutination tests. In the latex agglutination test, antifungal antibodies from immune serum are attached to small latex beads. When a specimen from a patient contains the specific fungal antigen, the specimen will cause the latex beads to agglutinate.

Chemotherapy. There are a variety of antifungal agents available for treating human fungal infections. The antifungal antibiotics include griseofulvin, and the polyene antibiotics, amphotericin B, nystatin, and pimaricin. In addition, the synthetic imidazoles, ketoconazole, miconazole, and clotrimazole, and the synthetic antimetabolite 5-fluorocytosine are used as antifungal chemotherapeutic agents.

Griseofulvin is an antifungal antibiotic produced by *Penicillium griseofulvum*. It inhibits fungal growth presumably by interfering with the function of microtubules during mitosis. Griseofulvin is effective in preventing subcutaneous mycoses in keratinous tissues (hair, nails, and the cornified layer of the epidermis). This antibiotic must be taken over a long period of time in order to be effective. It accumulates in keratinous tissue, where it prevents the growth of pathogenic fungi.

Antifungal polyene antibiotics interfere with fungal cell membranes by binding to membrane sterols. **Amphotericin B** is a polyene antibiotic produced by *Streptomyces nodosus* that is widely used for treating systemic mycoses. Even though it has serious side effects, amphotericin B has been used to treat what would otherwise have been fatal fungal infections. **Nystatin** is another polyene antibiotic that interferes with fungal cell membranes. Nystatin, which is produced by *Streptomyces noursei,* was named for the New York State laboratory in which it was discovered. It is applied topically to treat superficial my-

coses, taken as a lozenge for thrush, and used as a suppository for treating candida vaginitis.

Clotrimazole and **miconazole** are two of the imidazole antifungal agents now in use. Both act on a wide range of fungi and are considered broad-spectrum agents. They are used in the topical treatment of infected smooth skin and vaginal infections. Micronazole has limited use as an intravenous infusion for treating systemic fungal diseases.

Ketoconazole is a new, promising antifungal agent belonging to the imidazole group. It is a broad-spectrum agent that is active against many pathogenic fungi. Ketoconazole has the following advantages: (1) it can be taken orally, (2) it is virtually nontoxic to humans, (3) it is rapidly absorbed into target tissues, with the exception of cerebrospinal fluid, and (4) it is effective against many of the pathogenic fungi that cause systemic mycoses. This drug appears destined to make a major impact on the future treatment of fungal diseases.

SYSTEMIC MYCOSES

Systemic mycoses are the most serious of the human fungal diseases—some untreated systemic mycoses can have a fatal outcome. The distribution of the specific diseases is restricted by the geographical habitat of the responsible fungi. These fungi naturally live in soil, and many grow well in bird droppings or in soil enriched with bird droppings. Humans are infected when they inhale the fungal spores. The fungus can then establish a primary lung infection prior to being disseminated to other body organs and tissues. The systemic mycoses and their etiological agents are listed in Table 27–3.

Cryptococcosis (*Cryptococcus neoformans*)

Cryptococcosis is caused by *Cryptococcus neoformans* when it establishes an infection in the human lungs. Most cases are asymptomatic; however, the fungus can spread from the lung to other visceral organs, the central nervous system, and sometimes skin and bones to cause serious disseminated disease.

The typical encapsulated yeast morphology of *Cryptococcus neoformans* is observed when the fungus is growing in infected tissue or in cultures at 23°C

TABLE 27–3
Systemic Mycoses

| Disease | Fungus | Morphology in | | Ecology (Distribution) |
		Infected Tissue	Culture 23°C	
Cryptococcosis[a]	*Cryptococcus neoformans*	Yeast (encapsulated)	Yeast (encapsulated)	Soil, pigeon droppings (worldwide)
Blastomycosis	*Blastomyces dermatitidis*	Yeast	Mycelium	Soil? North America
Histoplasmosis	*Histoplasma capsulatum* (*H. duboissii* in Africa)	Yeast	Mycelium	Soil, droppings of bats, starlings, and chickens (Mississippi and Ohio river valleys, Africa)
Coccidioidomycosis	*Coccidioides immitis*	Sporules	Mycelium	Desert soils (northern Mexico, southwestern United States)
Paracoccidioido-mycosis	*Paracoccidioides brasiliensis*	Yeast	Mycelium	Natural habitat undiscovered (South America, Mexico)

[a]Known as *European blastomycosis* in the European literature.

and 37°C (Table 27–3). The capsule is the most distinctive feature of this yeast (Figure 27–8). It can be seen in india ink preparations, and it reacts specifically with antisera against it in the Quellung reaction. Until recently, *C. neoformans* was classified as an imperfect species. Now that its sexual phase has been discovered, it is recognized as a Basidiomycotina (Table 27–2) assigned to the genus *Filobasidiella*.

Disseminated cryptococcosis. The disseminated forms of cryptococcosis are serious diseases characterized by the presence of fungal lesions in visceral organs, the central nervous system, skin, and/or bones. Chronic meningitis is the most common disseminated form of cryptococcosis. In this disease, the fungus infects the cerebrospinal fluid; it can also form brain lesions that result in meningoencephalitis. This disease is diagnosed by the presence of the encapsulated yeast cells of *C. neoformans* in cerebrospinal fluid. In addition, the capsular antigen can be detected in spinal fluid, urine, or serum by a latex agglutination test. Systemic cryptococcosis is often a fatal illness if patients are not treated with amphotericin B.

Cryptococcosis is a disease that occurs throughout the world; approximately 300 cases per year are reported in the United States. *Cryptococcus neoformans* is present in soil, especially soil contaminated with pigeon droppings, which provides an ideal growth environment for this fungus. Human-to-human

FIGURE 27–8
Electron micrograph of *Cryptococcus neoformans* showing the capsule (c), cell wall (cw), nucleus (n), and emergent bud. (Courtesy of Dr. E. Peterson.)

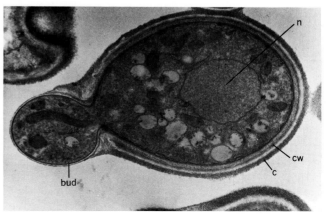

transmission of cryptococcosis has never been observed.

Blastomycosis (*Blastomyces dermatitidis*)

Blastomycosis is a chronic infection of the lungs, skin, bones, and genitourinary tract caused by *Blastomyces dermatitidis*. This fungus is dimorphic: it grows as a yeast in infected tissue and as a mycelium at room temperature (Table 27–3). The yeast form is multinucleated, has a thick cell wall, and divides by budding. The perfect stage of this fungus was discovered in 1968; the fungus is now assigned to the genus *Ajellomyces* (Table 27–2). Mycologists presume that *B. dermatitidis* exists in soil, even though its natural reservoir is unknown.

Humans are infected when they inhale spores of *B. dermatitidis*. There is no evidence for human-to-human transmission. Blastomycosis occurs in areas of North America including southern Manitoba, the Mississippi, the Ohio, and the St. Lawrence river valleys, the mid-Atlantic United States, and the southern United States. Sporadic cases have occurred in Africa, South America, and Mexico.

Blastomycosis is a chronic infection in which the fungus establishes itself in the lungs before it spreads, via the blood and lymph, to the skin, bones, and genitourinary tract. Skin lesions arise either by metastasis from the primary lung infection or occasionally by direct infection through skin abrasions. Lesions in bones and skin develop in a high percentage of infected patients. The male genitourinary tract can be involved, however this occurs with a lower incidence. Blastomycosis occurs far more frequently in males than in females.

Blastomycosis is highly suspected when the clinical symptoms affect combinations of the skin, lungs, bones, and the urinary tract. The presence of the yeast form of *B. dermatitidis* in exudates of lesions or in histological sections of affected tissue supports the clinical diagnosis. A confirmed diagnosis is attained by isolating the fungus; however, cultivation and identification of *B. dermatitidis* takes 4 weeks or longer.

A presumptive diagnosis is sufficient to warrant treatment with amphotericin B. Although blastomycosis occasionally remits, the disease is usually a debilitating illness that is fatal if not treated. Amphotericin B is effective against all forms of blastomycosis and is given intravenously on alternate days in small doses (adult dose is 50 mg per day) until a total of 2.0 g is administered. The death rate is greatly reduced (to about 10 percent) when this regimen is followed.

Histoplasmosis (*Histoplasma capsulatum*)

Histoplasmosis is a fungal infection of the human lungs, caused by *Histoplasma capsulatum*, that is prevalent in the Ohio and Mississippi river valleys. The perfect stage of *H. capsulatum* was discovered (1972) to be *Ajellomyces (Emmonsiella) capsulatum*, which is classified in the subdivision Ascomycotina (Table 27–2). *Histoplasma capsulatum* grows as a budding, noncapsulated (species designation is a misnomer) yeast in infected tissue and as a mycelium (Table 27–3) in cultures at room temperature. The yeast form of the fungus is present in extracellular tissue spaces or inside macrophages.

Diagnosis. Histoplasmosis is diagnosed by the clinical symptoms, the presence of the yeast form of *H. capsulatum* in sputum or biopsied tissue, roentgenograms of the chest, and cultivation of the fungus. *H. capsulatum* produces thick-walled, asexual spores with distinctive spiny projections (Figure 27–9) when cultures are grown at room temperature. Histoplasmin skin tests are used in young children to detect the asymptomatic forms of histoplasmosis. Complement fixation and other serodiagnostic tests are also available.

Epidemiology. The incidence of histoplasmosis is greatest in the Ohio and Mississippi river valleys. Epidemiologists have estimated that as many as 40 million Americans would be positive if they were skin-tested with histoplasmin. Histoplasmosis also occurs in Africa, where the causative agent is *H. duboissii*. *Histoplasma capsulatum* is found in soil, where it can persist for months or years. Its growth is stimulated by the presence of bird droppings. Epidemics

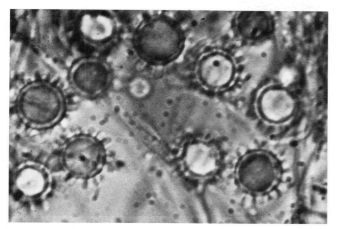

FIGURE 27–9
Microconidia of *Histoplasma capsulatum*. (Courtesy of Dr. C. W. Emmons.)

of histoplasmosis have been traced to exposure to the soil in dirt-floor chicken houses, soil under blackbird roosts, and soil contaminated with bat excretia. *Histoplasma capsulatum* does not appear to infect birds, presumably because the fungus is unable to grow at a bird's high body temperature; however, it does grow in guano-enriched soil. In contrast to birds, bats are infected by *H. capsulatum* and disseminate the fungus in their excreta. Epidemics of histoplasmosis have occurred among groups of persons who were exposed to bat excreta in bat caves.

Histoplasmosis in humans. Children and infants often acquire asymptomatic pulmonary histoplasmosis. Symptomatic pulmonary histoplasmosis can be mild or severe depending on the degree of exposure. Patients have a fever and a cough that in severe cases can appear as a case of influenza. The incubation period is 3 to 20 days, and lung lesions may persist for 2 or 3 months. Patients normally recover from this form of histoplasmosis even without chemotherapy.

Chronic pulmonary histoplasmosis and progressive disseminated histoplasmosis are serious illnesses requiring chemotherapy. The symptoms of chronic pulmonary histoplasmosis resemble pulmonary tuberculosis. This disease occurs predominantly in male patients (the ratio of affected men to women is 10:1) with an average age of 50. Patients have serious pulmonary malfunctions caused by the extensive lesions that progressively destroy the lungs. Chemotherapy does not improve pulmonary function, but it can limit the progression of the disease. Histoplasmosis can disseminate to other tissue including the larynx, mouth, nose, and pharynx. Both chronic pulmonary and disseminated histoplasmosis are treated with ketoconazole or amphotericin B.

Coccidioidomycosis (*Coccidioides immitis*)

The etiological agent of coccidioidomycosis was first classified as a protozoan and named "immitis," which means nonmold. This mistake was corrected when the mycelial phase of *Coccidioides immitis* was grown in culture. This fungus is found in the soil of arid regions of North and Central America. In the United States, its natural habitat is the seven southwestern states. *Coccidioides immitis* causes coccidioidomycosis, which in its mild form resembles an upper respiratory tract infection.

Mycology of *C. immitis*. This fungus exists in soil as a mycelium that forms barrel-shaped arthrospores. These arthrospores are often dispersed by the wind and can be inhaled by humans. Once in the lungs, the arthrospores grow and develop into a complex structure known as a **spherule** (Figure 27–10), which contains as many as 800 endospores. Endospores released from this structure can grow into a new spherule. The presence of spherules in infected tissue is diagnostic of coccidioidomycosis.

Coccidioides immitis can be selectively cultured on Sabouraud's medium containing chloramphenicol and cycloheximide. It can be identified by the arthrospores it forms on Sabouraud's medium and by the spherules it produces when grown on Converse (or other media) medium in an atmosphere of 5 percent CO_2 incubated at 37°C. Extreme care must be taken in handling this fungus because the arthrospores are highly infectious.

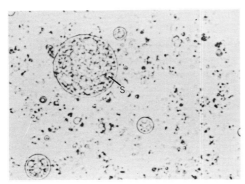

FIGURE 27–10
KOH-treated sputum preparation containing spherules (s) of *Coccidioides immitis*. (Courtesy of M. C. Campbell. From M. C. Campbell and J. L. Stewart, *The Medical Mycology Handbook*, copyright © 1980. Reprinted with permission of John Wiley & Sons, Inc.).

Coccidioidomycosis in humans. About 60 percent of persons infected with *C. immitis* have a benign respiratory infection. Others develop a primary infection involving the lower respiratory tract. The disease resembles a severe form of pneumonia with chest pain, cough, malaise, fever, chills, and sputum production. After recovery, some patients retain a pulmonary nodule or cavity. Other outcomes of *C. immitis* infections include an often fatal progressive pneumonia, chronic pulmonary disease, and/or disseminated (extrapulmonary) disease. These forms of coccidioidomycosis occur in less than 5 percent of infected patients. They are serious diseases that require chemotherapy.

Diagnosis and therapy. Coccidioidomycosis is provisionally diagnosed on epidemiological grounds, clinical manifestations, and the patient's response to skin testing with coccidioidin. A definitive diagnosis is made by demonstrating spherules in sputum or tissue. Patients recover without treatment when the infection is confined to the lungs. Ketoconazole and amphotericin B, which is moderately effective, are used to treat disseminated coccidioidomycosis.

Paracoccidioidomycosis (*Paracoccidioides brasiliensis*)

South American blastomycosis (paracoccidioides) is caused by *Paracoccidioides brasiliensis*. This organism was first isolated in Brazil and is restricted to Latin American countries from Mexico south to Argentina. *Paracoccidioides brasiliensis* is a dimorphic fungus that grows as variable-size budding yeast cells in cultures at 37°C and in tissue samples. It causes ulcers of the mucous membranes of the mouth and nose that often spread into cutaneous lesions of the face. The disseminated disease causes difficulty in swallowing and respiratory distress and is treated with ketoconazole or amphotericin B. The epidemiology of paracoccidioidomycosis is not well understood because the natural habitat of this fungus is still unknown.

MYCOSES CAUSED BY OPPORTUNISTIC FUNGI

A number of fungi that are normal inhabitants of the human body or human living environs are opportunistic pathogens (Table 27–4). They include *Candida* and *Aspergillus* of the subdivision Deuteromycotina and several species in genera of the subdivision Zygomycotina. The diseases caused by these fungi usually begin as inapparent, superficial ailments; however, they can eventually develop into systemic mycoses.

Candidiasis (*Candida albicans*)

Seven species of *Candida* have been isolated from humans. In nature they are believed to grow in association with humans and other animals, although occasionally they are found in contaminated food and fomites. The most important human pathogen is *Candida albicans*.

Mycology. *Candida albicans* is a dimorphic fungus that grows either as a yeast cell or as an elongated cell called a pseudohypha (Figure 27–11). No sexual reproduction has been observed in *Candida* species, so this genus is classified in the subdivision Deuteromycotina. The yeast cells reproduce by budding, whereas the pseudohyphae can reproduce by bud-

TABLE 27—4
Systemic Mycoses: Opportunistic Fungi

Disease	Fungi	Morphology in Tissue	Tissue and Organs Affected
Candidiasis (systemic)	*Candida albicans*	Yeast and hyphae	Mouth, vagina, skin, gastrointestinal tract, heart
Aspergillosis	*Aspergillus fumigatus*	Mycelia	Lung, ears, eyes, nervous system
Mucormycosis	Mucorales (order), *Absidia, Rhizopus, Mucor, Mortierella*	Mycelia	Lung, nervous system, gastrointestinal tract

ding to form blastospores or they can fragment to form chlamydospores.

Candidiasis in humans. *Candida albicans* is a normal inhabitant of the human mouth, gastrointestinal tract, and vagina. It causes disease when the normal ecological balance of these environments changes. Species of *Candida* are often responsible for the vaginal infections seen in pregnant women, in diabetic women, and in women on antibiotic therapy. *Can-*

FIGURE 27—11
Pseudohyphae of *Candida albicans* with two types of asexual spores: chlamydospores (c) and blastospores (b). (Courtesy of Dr. N. L. Goodman.)

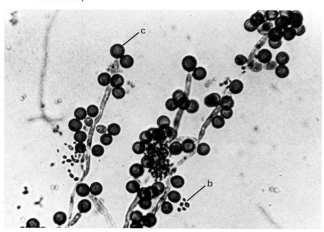

dida infections of the mouth occur in newborns, and infections of the esophagus and stomach occur in cancer patients.

Thrush, or **oral candidiasis,** is an infection of the mouth that appears as white patches (composed of fungal mats) on the mucous membranes and the tongue. Newborns are particularly susceptible to thrush, which they contract from their infected mothers as they pass through the birth canal. This is one of the few mycoses that is passed between humans. Probably the most common form of vaginal infection is *Candida*-**induced vaginitis.** This venereal disease is transmitted by sexual contact and is usually characterized by a thick curdlike vaginal discharge. *Candida albicans* also infects epidermal tissue, especially if the tissue remains moist. Folds of the skin in obese persons, tissue that remains wet from occupational activities, and skin covered by wet diapers are primary sites of infection.

Disseminated *Candida* infections can affect the nervous system to cause *Candida*-induced meningitis, and the heart to cause myocarditis, pericarditis, and endocarditis.

Diagnosis and treatment. Microscopic examination of lesions or exudates, clinical symptoms, and isolation of the fungus are all used to diagnose *C. albicans* infections. *Candida* grows on a variety of laboratory media to form smooth, creamy, bacterialike colonies. Cells from these colonies stain Gram-positive and have a typical yeast cell structure. Systemic candidiasis is treated with ketoconazole or amphotericin B, whereas nystatin is used to treat the benign forms of candidiasis such as thrush and candida-induced vaginitis. Nystatin is available as throat lozenges for treating thrush and as suppositories for treating vaginitis. Accessible cutaneous infections of candida are treated with creams containing either nystatin or amphotericin B; ketoconazole is also effective.

Aspergillosis (Aspergillus fumigatus)

Aspergillus is ubiquitous in most countries of the world. It grows only as a mycelium (Figure 27–12) and is found on vegetable matter including hay and stored grains. *Aspergillus* reproduces asexually by producing conidia; it is classified in the subdivision Deuteromycotina. Some species of *Aspergillus* produce toxins. For example, *A. flavus* is a common contaminant of stored grain in which it can produce **aflatoxin**. This toxin causes serious illness in fowl that eat these contaminated grains; it is also a potential carcinogen for humans.

Aspergillus fumigatus is the causative agent of most human aspergillosis. This fungus establishes an in-fection in the human lungs following the inhalation of its conidia. Aspergillosis occurs most often in compromised patients usually as pulmonary aspergillosis. *Aspergillus fumigatus* can invade the central nervous system, and it can cause a superficial eye infection known as keratomycosis.

Aspergillosis is diagnosed by the presence of its mycelia in lesions or exudates (Figure 27–12). Aspergillosis is treated with amphotericin B.

Mucormycosis

Mycoses caused by members of the order Mucorales are referred to as the **mucormycoses**. Members of the genera *Absidia*, *Mucor*, *Mortierella*, and *Rhizopus* are opportunistic human pathogens (Table 27–4). They cause diseases in compromised patients, especially those with acidosis (resulting from diabetes mellitis), impaired phagocytosis, and patients being treated with corticosteroids. These fungi infect human tissue via the mucous membranes of the nose and palate. They can invade nervous tissue, the lungs, and the gastrointestinal tract. Prevention of mucormycoses depends on the control of the predisposing condition. Amphotericin B can be used to treat mucormycosis.

SUBCUTANEOUS MYCOSES

Fungal diseases of the epidermis usually result from infections of abrasions and wounds of the skin. Subcutaneous mycoses are most prevalent in the tropics, where humans wear a minimum of protective clothing. Sporotrichosis, chromomycosis, and maduromycosis are three major subcutaneous mycotic diseases (Table 27–5).

Sporotrichosis (Sporothrix schenckii)

Sporotrichosis is an infection of the skin caused by *Sporothrix schenckii* (Figure 27–13) that begins as an ulcerous lesion. The human epidermis is infected by the fungus when a contaminated splinter or thorn penetrates the outer layer of the skin. After a 1- to 2-week incubation, a painless papule develops at the

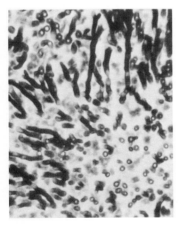

FIGURE 27–12
Aspergillus hyphae in bronchial washings. (Courtesy of M. C. Campbell. From M. C. Campbell and J. L. Stewart, *The Medical Mycology Handbook*, copyright © 1980. Reprinted with permission of John Wiley & Sons, Inc.)

TABLE 27–5
Subcutaneous Mycoses

Disease	Fungal Agents	Morphology	Distribution	Clinical Manifestations
Sporotrichosis	*Sporothrix schenckii*	Dimorphic cells	Worldwide	Cutaneous and subcutaneous lesions
Chromomycosis	*Cladosporium carrionii, Phialophora verrucosa*	Round cells	Tropics	Lesions on legs and feet
Eumycetoma[a]	*Petriellidium boydii, Madurella mycetomi,* other soil fungi	Dark grains (colonies) in exudate	U.S., Canada, Africa, India	Local lesions on feet or hands

[a]Actinomycetes (see Chapter 17)—including species of *Actinomadura, Nocardia,* and *Streptomyces*—cause similar infections known as actinomycetomas.

inoculation site. This papule enlarges to become an ulcerated lesion. **Lymphocutaneous sporotrichosis** occurs when the fungus forms multiple nodules af-

FIGURE 27–13
Typical morphology of conidia of *Sporothrix schenckii.* (Courtesy of Dr. C. Emmons.)

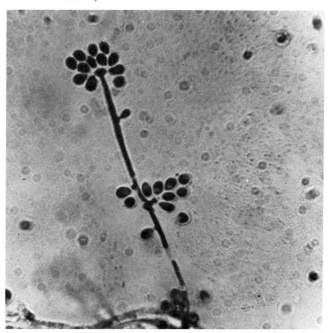

ter being spread by the draining lymph channels. These nodules can also ulcerate. Spontaneous recovery is rare, and untreated lesions remain for years.

Other forms of this disease are cutaneous sporotrichosis and extracutaneous sporotrichosis. **Cutaneous sporotrichosis** affects the skin without involving the lymphatics. **Extracutaneous sporotrichosis** is a rare fungal infection of the lungs, eyes, or central nervous system. Sporotrichosis occurs sporadically among farmers and gardeners in North America and other parts of the world.

Sporothrix schenckii is a dimorphic fungus that is a common inhabitant of soil and vegetable matter. The yeast form is present in tissue and in cultures grown at 37°C, whereas the filamentous form occurs at 25°C. Positive cultures of the causative fungus (Figure 27–13) are diagnostic of all types of sporotrichosis. Cutaneous sporotrichosis is treated by giving iodides (KI) in milk or juice; extracutaneous sporotrichosis is treated with amphotericin B. Recovery from cutaneous sporotrichosis following iodide treatment is usually complete; the prognosis for recovery from extracutaneous sporotrichosis is still poor.

Chromomycosis

A number of darkly pigmented fungi (Table 27–5) cause **chromomycoses,** which are chronic, localized fungal infections of the skin. The causative agents include *Cladosporium carrionii, Phialophora verrucosa,* and other species of the genus *Phialophora.* These fungi are found in the soil and decaying vegetation of tropical and subtropical climates. The fungi enter a skin wound and cause the development of a wart-like, scaly nodule or a small, firm tumor. The painless lesions become unsightly as they continue to develop. Patients who seek medical treatment usually do so for cosmetic reasons or because of secondary infections.

Chromomycosis is diagnosed by the observation of the pigmented mycelia in histological sections or scrapings of the lesions. Usually the infection can be treated by surgical excision. Most chemotherapeutic agents are ineffective, presumably because their access to these lesions is limited; however, ketoconazole is effective.

Eumycetomas

Mycetoma is a general term that refers to an infection caused either by fungi or by a bacterium classified in the subdivision Actinomycetes. The "true" mycetomas, **eumycetoma,** are caused by fungi (Table 27–5). *Petriellidium boydii* causes eumycetomas in the United States and Canada, whereas mycetomas in the tropical regions of Africa and India are caused by *Madurella mycetoma.* **Actinomycetomas** are caused by species of *Nocardia* and *Streptomyces* (see Chapter 17).

Mycetomas were first described in the district of Madura in India and were originally called **maduromycoses.** Eumycetomas (madura foot) are chronic, local subcutaneous infections of the foot and, occasionally, of the hand. They are progressive, destructive infections that destroy muscle, bone, and connective tissue. Eumycetomas occur most often in male farmers in rural areas of the tropics. The infections originate from penetrating wounds of the feet often caused by thorns and splinters. A suppurative lesion develops at the site of infection. The causative agents can be seen as dark grains within the pus-containing exudate. The body responds to the infection by forming scar tissue, which causes local disfigurement. The disease progresses slowly and is

TABLE 27–6
Cutaneous Mycoses (Dermatomycoses)

Disease	Most Common Causative Agent	Primary Reservoir	Affected Tissue
Tinea corporis	*Trichophyton rubrum*	Anthropophilic	Body (except head, groin, feet)
	Trichophyton mentagrophytes	Anthropophilic	
	Microsporum canis	Zoophilic	
Tinea cruris	*Epidermophyton floccosum*	Anthropophilic	Groin
	Trichophyton rubrum	Anthropophilic	
	Trichophyton mentagrophytes	Anthropophilic	
Tinea pedis	*Trichophyton rubrum*	Anthropophilic	Feet
	Trichophyton mentagrophytes	Anthropophilic	
	Epidermophyton floccosum	Anthropophilic	
Tinea capitis	*Microsporum canis*	Zoophilic	Scalp
	Microsporum audouinii	Anthropophilic	
	Microsporum sp.	Anthropophilic	
	Trichophyton sp.	Anthropophilic	
Candidiasis	*Candida albicans*	Anthropophilic	Diaper area, skin, hands, feet, face, and scalp

usually not life threatening. There are no spontaneous recoveries from eumycetoma and no dependable chemotherapeutic treatments.*

CUTANEOUS MYCOSES (DERMATOMYCOSES)

Cutaneous mycoses are fungal infections of the keratinous tissues found in nails, hair, and the outer cornified layer of human skin (stratum cornium). The keratinous material is often nonviable except for a germinative zone in the nail plate or the hair follicle. **Dermatophytes** are fungi that infect and grow in these nonviable keratinous tissues. The human dermatophytes belong to the genera *Epidermophyton, Microsporum,* or *Trichophyton.* They are identified by the morphology of their asexual conidia. Dermatophytes are also grouped according to their primary natural reservoirs, which include humans (anthropophilic), animals (zoophilic), and soil (geophilic).

Cutaneous mycoses often appear in the shape of a ring caused when the dermatophyte grows outward from the infection site. These infections were originally thought to be caused by worms and are still called **ringworm** or **tinea** (L. *tinea,* worm). More than one fungus is able to infect a given anatomical location (Table 27–6), so the diseases have anatomical designations. The human diseases are designated ringworm of the body, **tinea corporis;** of the groin, **tinea cruris** (jock itch); of the head, **tinea capitis;** and of the feet, **tinea pedis** (athlete's foot).

Dermatophytes

Trichophyton. Thirteen species of *Trichophyton* cause cutaneous mycoses in humans. This genus is identified by its smooth-walled macroconidia (Figure 27–14). Species of *Trichophyton* cause tinea pedis, tinea capitis, and infections of human hair.

Microsporum. Nine species of *Microsporum* cause human dermatomycoses. Many of these are carried

*Actinomycetomas can be treated with sulfa drugs.

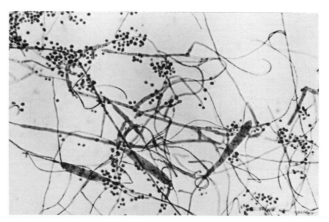

FIGURE 27–14
Micro- and macroconidia of *Trichophyton mentagrophytes.* 552X. (Courtesy of Dr. L. Ajello, Mycology Division, Centers for Disease Control and the American Society for Microbiology.)

in animal fur, for example, *M. canis,* and infect humans who pet fur-bearing animals. *Microsporum* species are characterized by their rough-walled macroconidia (Figure 27–15). *Microsporum* is a major cause of hair loss observed in the disease tinea capitis.

FIGURE 27–15
Rough-walled macroconidia of *Microsporum canis.* (Courtesy of Dr. L. Ajello, Mycology Division, Centers for Disease Control and the American Society for Microbiology.)

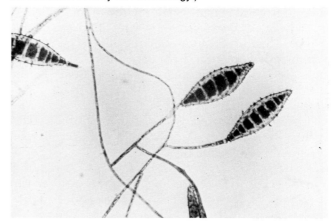

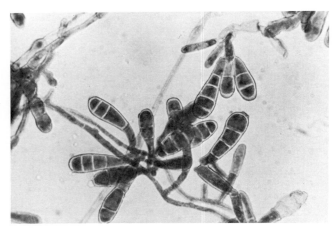

FIGURE 27-16
Clusters of smooth macroconidia of *Epidermophyton floccosum*. 552X. (Courtesy of Dr. L. Ajello, Mycology Division, Centers for Disease Control and the American Society for Microbiology.)

Epidermophyton. *Epidermophyton floccosum* (Figure 27-16) is the sole species of this genus. It is isolated exclusively from humans in whom it infects the epidermis (not hair or nails) to cause athlete's foot or jock itch.

Diseases in humans

Tinea corporis. This dermatophytic infection of the skin (excluding the head, scalp, feet, beard, and groin) occurs worldwide; however, it is most common in tropical climates. The causative fungi include *T. rubrum*, *T. mentagrophytes*, and *M. canis* (Table 27-6). The infection usually begins as a papule, which grows to form an anular lesion. Many other diseases have similar clinical manifestations, so the diagnosis of tinea corporis is difficult without microscopic examination of scrapings from the lesion. Tinea corporis is treated with topical antifungal ointments: the imidazoles (miconazole and clotrimazole) are the most effective fungicides.

Tinea cruris. Ringworm of the groin, or jock itch, is caused by *E. floccosum*, *T. rubrum*, and *T. menta-* *grophytes*. Tinea cruris is most common in males but does occur in females. Moisture in the groin region from a wet bathing suit, athletic supporter, tight-fitting slacks, pantyhose, and obesity predispose an individual to these fungal infections. Tinea cruris is effectively treated with imidazoles administered as powders.

Tinea pedia. Athlete's foot occurs worldwide, but it is primarily a disease of people who wear shoes. The causative agents grow between human toes, where they cause inflammation and desquamation (loss of skin). The infection is commonly spread through the use of common shower facilities. The causative agents (Table 27-6) are all anthropophilic and include the same species that are responsible for tinea cruris. Treatment is the same as for tinea corporis. **Tinea manuum** is a dermatomycosis of the hands (palms) caused by fungi that also cause tinea pedis.

Tinea capitis. Many anthropophilic dermatophytes of the genera *Microsporum* and *Trichophyton* cause infections of scalp hair in humans. The infection begins in the stratum cornium (outer layer of the scalp) with hyphae extending into the opening of the hair follicle. These hyphae penetrate the hair near the bulb and extend into the hair shaft. As their growth proceeds, they form spores near the surface of the hair shaft. The presence of the fungus weakens the hair such that a plucked hair will break off next to the scalp. Hair loss (alopecia) is a common result of tinea capitis infection, especially when it is accompanied by a major inflammatory response that destroys the hair follicle. Alopecia may be localized and spotty or it may involve large areas of the scalp. This form of tinea capitis can be treated with oral griseofulvin.

A few species of *Trichophyton* cause an infection of the hair shaft without destroying the hair follicle. These fungi form arthrospores in the hair shaft that greatly weakens the hair, causing it to break off just below the follicle's surface. The resulting cavity soon fills with bacteria and debris to give the scalp a black-dot appearance that is characteristic of this form of tinea capitis. Griseofulvin taken orally can be used to treat this infection.

SUMMARY

Fungi are unicellular or multicellular heterotrophs that belong to the higher protists. Most fungi are microorganisms; however, some produce visible fruiting bodies (mushrooms and toadstools). The morphology of the fungal structures involved in asexual and/or sexual reproduction are used as one basis for fungal classification.

Fungal diseases are categorized as systemic mycoses, subcutaneous mycoses, and cutaneous mycoses. Most pathogenic fungi are natural inhabitants of soil or vegetable matter and are opportunistic or incidental pathogens. Humans are infected by inhaling spores, by penetrating injuries caused by contaminated plant material (thorns, splinters), and by direct contact with infected humans or fur-bearing animals. Fungal infections are diagnosed by the microscopic demonstration of the fungus in exudates or scraping of the infected tissue, by growing the fungus in laboratory media, and/or by serodiagnostic techniques.

Systemic mycoses (Table 27–7) are initiated by the inhalation of fungal spores and are treated with the intravenous administration of antifungal agents such as amphotericin B. Cryptococcosis occurs throughout the world and is caused by *Cryptococcus neoformans*, which grows in soil, especially soil enriched with pigeon droppings. Disseminated cryptococcosis affects the visceral organs, the central nervous system, and, sometimes the skin and bones. Blastomycosis is caused by *Blastomyces dermatitidis* and occurs in North America. It is a chronic infection of the lungs, skin, bones, and, sometimes, the genitourinary tract. Blastomycosis is a debilitating illness that can be fatal. Histoplasmosis is prevalent in the Ohio and Mississippi river valleys, where *Histoplasma capsulatum* is present in soil enriched with bird and bat excreta. Histoplasmosis occurs as an influenzalike pneumonia or as a chronic pulmonary disease that can spread to the larynx, nose, and mouth. *Coccidioides immitis* is found in the arid regions of North and Central America and causes coccidioidomycosis. *Coccidioides immitis* forms spherules in the lungs, where it causes a benign pneumonia. Paracoccidioidomycosis is a similar systemic fungal disease that is restricted to countries in South America.

Species of *Candida* are opportunistic pathogens that cause thrush, candida-induced vaginitis, skin infections, and infections of the gastrointestinal tract. Nystatin is used to treat most forms of candidiasis. *Aspergillus flavus* causes pulmonary aspergillosis, infections of the nervous system, and infections of the eyes. Mucormycosis is caused by fungi of the order Mucorales and occurs in compromised hosts.

Sporotrichosis and chromomycosis are subcutaneous mycoses that are initiated by skin-penetrating injuries and are caused by soil fungi that contaminate splinters, thorns, and dirt. Sporotrichosis begins as a painless papule and develops into a ulcerative lesion; spontaneous recovery is rare. Chromomycosis is caused by darkly pigmented fungi that cause wartlike, scaly nodules or small tumors to develop at the site of infection. These growths are surgically removed for cosmetic reasons. Eumycetomas are progressive, destructive fungal infections that destroy the muscle, bone, and connective tissue of the feet and, occasionally, the hands. The host responds to the infection by forming scar tissue that in turn causes local disfigurement.

The dermatophytes infect keratinous tissue including hair, nails, and stratum cornium to cause cutaneous mycoses. The fungi involved belong to the genera *Epidermophyton*, *Microsporum*, and *Trichophyton*, which have reservoirs in humans, animals, or soil. Dermatomycoses are popularly known as ringworm (tinea) and are grouped by the anatomical location of the infection. Common cutaneous mycoses include tinea corporis, tinea cruris, tinea capitis, and tinea pedis. They are treated with topical antifungal creams and powders containing imidazoles and/or with griseofulvin.

TABLE 27–7
Summary: Medically Important Fungi

Disease	Etiological Agent(s)	Source	Distribution	Treatment
Systemic Mycoses				
Cryptococcosis	*Cryptococcus neoformans*	Soil, bird droppings	Worldwide	Amphotericin B
Blastomycosis	*Blastomyces dermatitidis*	Soil?	North America	Amphotericin B
Histoplasmosis	*Histoplasma capsulatum*	Soil, droppings of birds and bats	Mississippi and Ohio river valleys	Amphotericin B, ketoconazole
Coccidioidomycosis	*Coccidioides immitis*	Desert soils	Southern U.S. and northern Mexico	Amphotericin B, ketoconazole
Paracoccidioido-mycosis	*Paracoccidioides brasiliensis*	Natural habitat undiscovered	South America, Mexico	Amphotericin B, ketoconazole
Candidiasis	*Candida albicans*	Humans (opportunistic)	Worldwide	Nystatin, amphotericin B, ketoconazole
Aspergillosis	*Aspergillus fumigatus*	Soil, vegetation	Worldwide	Nystatin, amphotericin B
Mucormycosis	*Absidia, Rhizopus, Mucor, Mortierella*	Widely dispersed	Worldwide	Prevent predisposing conditions, amphotericin B
Subcutaneous Mycoses				
Sporotrichosis	*Sporothrix schenckii*	Soil, vegetation	Worldwide	Amphotericin B
Chromomycosis	*Cladosporium carrionii, Phialophora verrucosa*	Soil, vegetation	Tropics, subtropics	Surgical excision, ketoconazole
Eumycetoma	*Petriellidium boydii, Madurella mycetomi*	Soil, vegetation	Tropics	No good treatments
Cutaneous Mycoses (Dermatomycoses)				
Tinea corporis	One or more of the following	Humans, animals	Worldwide	Imidazoles
Tinea cruris	*Trichophytom* sp.,	Humans	Western cultures	Imidazoles
Tinea pedis	*Microsporum* sp.,	Humans, animals	Shoed peoples	Imidazoles
Tinea capitis	*Epidermophyton floccosum*	Humans	Worldwide	Griseofulvin
		Humans		
Candidiasis	*Candida albicans*	Humans	Worldwide	Nystatin

QUESTIONS AND TOPICS FOR STUDY AND DISCUSSION

Questions

1. Describe and compare the morphologies of a filamentous fungus and a yeast cell. What mechanism do these cells use to reproduce?

2. Define or explain the following

hyphae	ringworm
mycelium	parasite
coenocytic	septa
saprobe	

3. What is meant by fungal dimorphism, and what impact does dimorphism have on medical mycology?

4. Draw diagrams and label the following.

pseudohyphae	sporangiospores
ascospores	spherule
basidiospores	conidia
chlamydiospores	zygospores

5. Outline the classification of the fungi. Weigh the importance of sexual versus asexual reproduction in this approach. Explain.

6. What techniques are used to diagnose fungal infections?

7. Construct a chart of the major antifungal agents that includes their source, the site of action, and the infections they are effective against.

8. Describe a systemic mycosis that is common in the continental United States. What epidemiological factors affect the high incidence of the disease you described?

9. Where is *Coccidioides immitis* found? Describe the clinical and epidemiological characteristics of the disease caused by this fungus.

10. Describe the different human diseases caused by *Candida albicans*. Why is *C. albicans* an opportunistic pathogen?

11. What is the common means of acquiring subcutaneous mycoses? How are these infections recognized, and how are they treated?

12. Describe the clinical signs of four common dermatomycoses. How are these infections prevented and treated?

Discussion

1. Mushrooms and toadstools are classified as fungi. Should these organisms be classified with the microscopic molds and yeasts? What reason can you present to justify your answer?

2. Do humans mount an immunological response to a systemic mycotic infection? What is the evidence for this response, and does it justify the production and use of vaccines against fungal infections.

3. Many people are allergic to molds. Discuss the conditions under which allergic persons would be exposed to molds. What steps can be taken to decrease this exposure?

4. Discuss the beneficial uses of the fungi.

FURTHER READINGS

Books

Ainsworth, G. C., and A. S. Sussman (eds.), *The Fungi, An Advanced Treatise*, vols. 1–4, Academic Press, New York, 1965. A recognized authoritative series on the biology and classification of the fungi.

Alexopoulos, C. J., and C. W. Mims, *Introductory Mycology*, 3rd ed., Wiley, New York, 1979. An advanced textbook that is an excellent reference for the biology of the nonpathogenic fungi.

Beneke, E. S., and A. L. Rogers, *Medical Mycology Manual With Human Mycoses Monograph*, 4th ed., Burgess, Minneapolis, 1980. A manual that can be used in the clinical laboratory and in medical mycology courses.

Campbell, M. C., and J. L. Stewart, *The Medical Mycology Handbook*, Wiley, New York, 1980. A laboratory handbook for the identification of the pathogenic fungi.

Emmons, C. W., C. H. Binford, and J. P. Otz, *Medical Mycology*, 3rd ed., Lea & Febiger, Philadelphia, 1977. A classic approach to the biology and laboratory diagnosis of the pathogenic fungi.

28

MEDICALLY IMPORTANT PROTOZOA

Protozoa—literally meaning the "first animals"—are the simplest forms of animal life known. These microscopic organisms were first described by Anton van Leeuwenhoek in his famous "Letter on the Protozoans" that he sent to the Royal Society of London in 1676. This letter contains the first written description of *Daphnia,* a common crustacean, and of the common protozoa *Vorticella* and *Monas.* Five years later Leeuwenhoek observed the pathogenic protozoan *Giardia lamblia* in his own stools. There are now at least 45,000 known species of these single-celled microscopic animals.

Protozoa are free-living animals residing in oceans, freshwater, and soil, or they are symbionts of animals. The free-living protozoa can be heterotrophs or photoautotrophs; the latter do not cause disease. Other protozoa form symbiotic relationships with their host that can be beneficial, commensal, or harmful. Parasitic protozoa cause a wide variety of animal diseases. Certain protozoa infect humans and are a major cause of morbidity and mortality in the world, especially in tropical countries.

BIOLOGY OF THE PROTOZOA

Single-celled animals are the large group of complex microorganisms that are classified in the phylum **Protozoa.** The complex morphologies of these single-celled animals are amazing. Many have specialized organelles for the acquisition of food and for motility. In addition, many protozoa utilize unique processes for nuclear division and/or have complex life cycles. Others divide by simple fission. Protozoa are classified by the types of organelles involved with their locomotion and food acquisition and by their methods of reproduction.

Locomotor organelles

Motility of protozoa involves four basic organelles: cilia, flagella, undulating ridges and membranes, and pseudopodia. The **axoneme** is the core structure of cilia and flagella and is composed of a group of microtubules present in the 9 pairs plus 2 arrangement common to eucaryotes (see Chapter 3). The axoneme is surrounded by a unit membrane that is

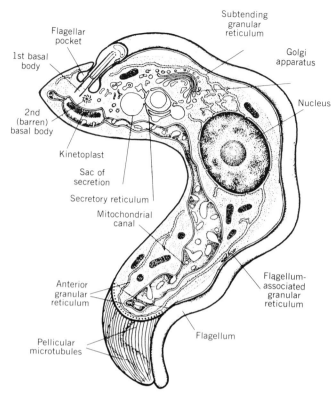

FIGURE 28–1

Internal structure of a *Trypanosoma* showing the DNA-rich kinetoplast, mitochondrial canal, flagellar pocket, and the flagellum attached to an undulating membrane. (Courtesy of Dr. K. Vickerman. From K. Vickerman, *J. Protozoology*, 16:54 – 69, 1969.)

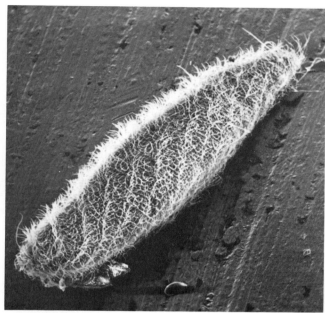

FIGURE 28–2

Scanning electron micrograph of the ciliate *Paramecium*. (Photo by E. Vivier, from W. J. Wagtendonk, ed., *Paramecium*, Elsevier North Holland Bio-Medical Press, New York, 1974.)

contiguous with the cell membrane. In many protozoa the entire flagellum is free to whip about in the medium, whereas in others the axoneme is a part of an undulating membrane that lies along the outside of the animal. Sporozoans contain less obvious locomotor organelles. These organisms' gliding motility is attributed to undulating ridges beneath their outer membrane. Movement and food acquisition in amebas are mediated by the temporary organelles known as pseudopodia.

Flagella and cilia. Flagella are complex organelles found in the flagellates. The axoneme of a flagellate originates in the basal body located in the flagellar pocket (Figure 28–1). The basal body is composed of microtubules with the conformation of a small centriole. Protozoa can have one or more flagella arranged in a variety of conformations.

The cilia of protozoa are similar in structure to flagella; however, they beat with a rhythmic, coordinated motion. Each cilium has an axoneme, a basal body, and a surrounding membrane. Cilia are always found in groups or rows (Figure 28–2). The basal bodies of each cilium are joined by interconnecting fibers known as **kinetodesma**. These fibers are responsible for coordinating the characteristic rhythmic motion of cilia.

Pseudopodia. Pseudopodia are temporary protoplasmic extensions found in ameba. Pseudopodia are classified into four major morphological groups: lobopodia, filopodia, rhizopodia, and axopodia (Figure 28–3). Lobopodia are encountered in pathogenic amebas that use them for locomotion and food ac-

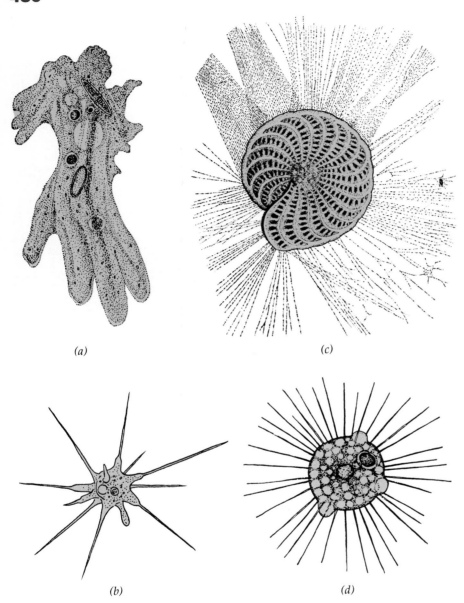

(a)

(c)

(b)

(d)

FIGURE 28—3
Types of pseudopodia. (*a*)
Lobopodia, (*b*) Filopodia, (*c*)
Rhizopodia, and (*d*) Axopodia.
(From R. Kudo, *Protozoology*, 5th
ed., 1966. Courtesy of Charles C
Thomas, Publisher, Springfield, Ill.)

quisition. The surface of the ameba is composed of a very flexible membrane, which is easily distorted by the streaming of the internal protoplasm. When the protoplasm streams in an outward direction, a pseudopodium is formed. This extension of the animal moves it toward its food. Once in contact with a food particle, the pseudopodium surrounds the food to form a phagocytic vacuole.

Undulating membranes and ridges. Some protozoa are moved by the wave motion generated in the finlike structure called an **undulating membrane.** In

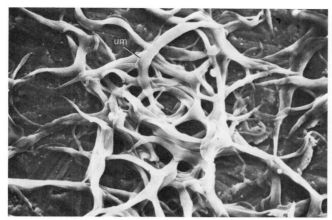

FIGURE 28–4
Scanning electron micrograph of trypanosomes. Note the distinctive undulating membrane (um) of these animals. (Courtesy of Father Francis X. Venuta, S.J., Ph.D.)

trypanosomes, the axoneme extends along the length of the animal and is a part of the undulating membrane (Figure 28–4). The basal body is closely associated with a mitochondrion that supplies ATP for flagellar motion. Mitochondria are present in many flagellates such as the trypanosomes; however, they are noticeably absent from other flagellates, for example, species of *Giardia* and *Trichomonas*. The dense-staining, DNA-containing structure at the flagellar end of the mitochondria is the **kinetoplast.** This organelle divides by binary fission during cell replication and gives rise to the cell's mitochondria.

Certain sporozoans contain **undulating ridges** lying just beneath the animal's cell membrane. These ridges are not obvious to the casual microscopist. They are formed by submicroscopic contractile structures whose composition and mechanism of action is unknown. Apparently, their contractions propagate a surface-wave motion that enables them to move with a gliding motility.

Food acquisition and nutrition

Parasitic protozoa are heterotrophs that gain food by a variety of mechanisms including permanent cytostomes (mouths), phagocytosis, pinocytosis, and membrane transport. Many protozoa can grow on

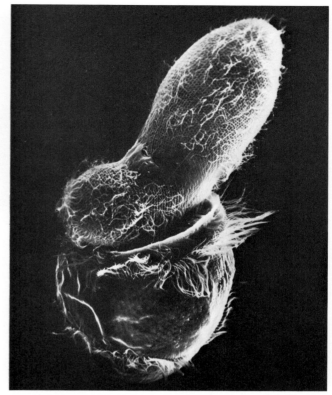

FIGURE 28–5
Scanning electron micrograph of a *Paramecium* being engulfed by a *Didinium*. (From H. S. Wessenberg and G. Atipa. *J. Protozoology*, 17:250 – 270, 1970.)

simple carbohydrates under anaerobic conditions or by aerobic respiration. The nutritionally less fastidious species are routinely grown in laboratory cultures. Ciliates have a permanent cytostome through which large particles or entire microorganisms can be engulfed (Figure 28–5). The cilia surrounding the cytostome set up currents that propel food into the cytostome. Once inside the cell, the food is digested in a cytoplasmic food vacuole. Amebas use their pseudopodia to capture food and to form food vacuoles by the mechanisms of phagocytosis. Protozoa also take up nutrients directly from the environment by pinocytosis, diffusion, facilitated transport, and active transport.

Protozoa exist within their hosts as extracellular or intracellular parasites. The extracellular parasites are found in the intestine, blood, and other organs of infected animals. Parasitic protozoa may multiply within erythrocytes or in phagocytic cells of higher animals. Other protozoa actively penetrate their host cell's membrane using a boring action. Once inside, the protozoa multiply at the nutritional expense of their host cell.

Reproduction

Protozoa reproduce by both asexual and sexual processes. In some species, only one form of reproduction occurs, whereas others have distinct life cycles in which asexual and sexual processes alternate. As in other eucaryotic cells, mitosis is used by protozoa to duplicate and distribute their genetic information. Protozoa use many variations on the classic process of mitosis, and sometimes not all the classic steps are represented. Mitosis does, however, result in the replication and distribution of the chromosomes to daughter cells.

Asexual reproduction. Asexual reproduction occurs by binary fission, budding, or multiple fission, depending on the species of protozoa. Binary fission is transverse in ciliates and longitudinal in flagellates. Budding results in the formation of two daughter cells of unequal size. Multiple fission, or **schizogony**, is an asexual process of reproduction used by sporozoans. The dividing cell is called a **schizont;** it repeatedly divides its nucleus and other organelles prior to cell division (Figure 28–6). The resulting daughter cells are known as **merozoites.** They eventually break away from the parent cell to begin another cycle of schizogony or sexual reproduction.

Sexual reproduction. The first stage of sexual reproduction is the formation of gametes during **gametogenesis.** The animal undergoes meiosis (reductive division) to form haploid cells called **gametes** or to form haploid nuclei. The gametes produced by a protozoan can be morphologically similar **(isoga-**

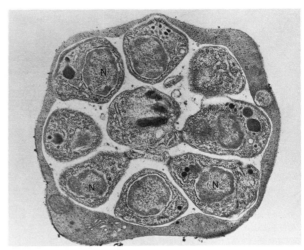

FIGURE 28–6
Electron micrograph of the late schizont stage in the development of *Plasmodium cathemerium*. The individual nuclei (N) of the developing merozoites that are formed from the mother schizont are readily apparent. (From M. Aikawa, *Am. J. Trop. Med. Hyg.*, 15:449–471, 1969.)

metes) or different **(anisogametes).** Anisogametes usually vary in size, so they are designated as macrogamete and microgametes. The second stage of sexual reproduction is the formation of a diploid zygote. The **zygote** is formed on the union of two isogametes from different mating types or the union of a microgamete and a macrogamete. When the zygote undergoes multiple fission, the process is called **sporogony** and the daughter cells are known as **sporozoites.** Still another way by which protozoa exchange genetic information is conjugation, which is observed in ciliates.

Encystment

Trophozoites (Gr. *trophe,* food, nourishment) are the feeding (vegetative) form of a protozoan. The trophozoites of certain protozoa form cysts when they encounter adverse environmental conditions. These cysts are resting forms of the animal that are able to withstand harsh environmental conditions. The cyst is the infectious form of certain species of parasitic protozoa. The protozoa excyst when they encounter

TABLE 28–1
Classification of the Protozoa

Taxonomic Group	Description	Representative Genera	Human Diseases
Sarcodina	Form pseudopodia, binary fission	*Entamoeba*	Amebiasis (dysentery)
Mastigophora	Flagellates		
	Phytoflagellates	*Euglena*	None
	Zooflagellates	*Giardia*	Giardiasis
		Trichomonas	Vaginitis
		Leishmania	Leishmaniasis
		Trypanosoma	Chagas' disease, African sleeping sickness
Ciliophora	Rows of cilia, sexual conjugation	*Balantidium*	Dysentery
Sporozoa	No obvious locomotor organelle, alternate sexual and asexual reproduction, all parasitic	*Plasmodium*	Malaria

favorable growth conditions to form trophozoites, which feed, grow, and reproduce asexually. In sporozoans, the cysts originate from zygotes called **oocysts.** Multiple fission within oocysts results in daughter cells known as **sporozoites.**

Classification

Locomotion can be used as the major criterion for classifying the protozoa. Under this scheme, the phylum Protozoa is divided into four taxonomic groups: *Sarcodina, Mastigophora, Ciliophora,* and *Sporozoa* (Table 28–1).

Sarcodina. Single-cell organisms that produce pseudopodia (Figure 28–3) for locomotion and food gathering are classified in the taxonomic group Sarcodina. They divide by binary fission: no sexual reproduction is known. Amebas form pseudopodia in response to an external stimulus. Amebas ingest food by forming food vacuoles around large particles of food, such as bacteria, or by endocytosis. *Entamoeba histolytica* is the pathogenic sarcodine that causes amebic dysentery in humans.

Mastigophora. Unicellular flagellates comprise a large group of organisms that are subdivided into phytoflagellates and zooflagellates. The **phytoflagellates** are unicellular animals that possess chlorophyll-containing chloroplasts. *Euglena* is an example (Figure 28–7). **Zooflagellates** are unicellular heterotrophs that vary greatly in size, shape, position, and form of flagella, and in their internal organelles (Figure 28–8). Trichomoniasis, leishmaniasis, giardiasis, and trypanosomiasis are human diseases caused by zooflagellates. Protozoologists have evidence that the zooflagellates evolved from phytoflagellates, so on evolutionary grounds both groups are classified in the Mastigophora.

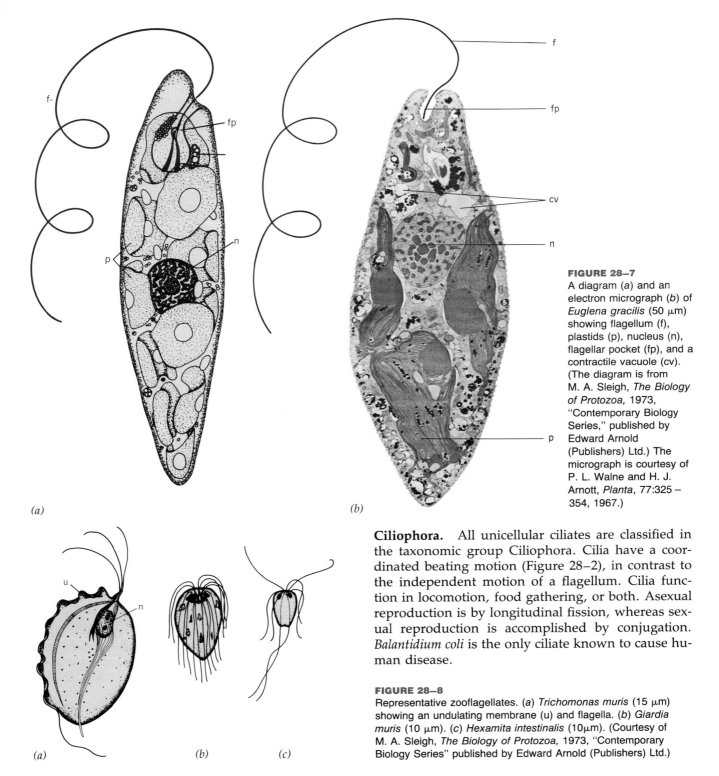

(a)

(b)

FIGURE 28–7
A diagram (a) and an electron micrograph (b) of *Euglena gracilis* (50 μm) showing flagellum (f), plastids (p), nucleus (n), flagellar pocket (fp), and a contractile vacuole (cv). (The diagram is from M. A. Sleigh, *The Biology of Protozoa*, 1973, "Contemporary Biology Series," published by Edward Arnold (Publishers) Ltd.) The micrograph is courtesy of P. L. Walne and H. J. Arnott, *Planta*, 77:325 – 354, 1967.)

Ciliophora. All unicellular ciliates are classified in the taxonomic group Ciliophora. Cilia have a coordinated beating motion (Figure 28–2), in contrast to the independent motion of a flagellum. Cilia function in locomotion, food gathering, or both. Asexual reproduction is by longitudinal fission, whereas sexual reproduction is accomplished by conjugation. *Balantidium coli* is the only ciliate known to cause human disease.

FIGURE 28–8
Representative zooflagellates. (a) *Trichomonas muris* (15 μm) showing an undulating membrane (u) and flagella. (b) *Giardia muris* (10 μm). (c) *Hexamita intestinalis* (10μm). (Courtesy of M. A. Sleigh, *The Biology of Protozoa*, 1973, "Contemporary Biology Series" published by Edward Arnold (Publishers) Ltd.)

(a)

(b)

(c)

Sporozoa. The Sporozoa contain all the endoparasitic, nonmotile (lacking motile appendages) protozoa, all of which have complex life cycles. They form spores or cysts and are infective as sporozoites. They reproduce with an alternation of sexual and asexual mechanisms. The most important human pathogens in this group belong to the genus *Plasmodium* and are the causative agents of malaria.

HUMAN PROTOZOAN DISEASES

Protozoan diseases in livestock and humans take an immense toll on human welfare. Many protozoa cause debilitating illness and even death, especially among persons less than 5 years old. The agricultural productivity in many parts of the world is seriously limited because of the destructive nature of these microbes. For example, only certain breeds of cattle can be raised in the tsetse-fly belt of Africa because of the presence of trypanosomes. The incidence of protozoan diseases depends on the distribution of the etiological agent, the resistance of the population to the infectious agent, and, in some diseases, the distribution of the vectors and reservoirs. Selected protozoan diseases of humans are described in the sections that follow.

Sporozoa

Malaria: *Plasmodium.* For centuries, malaria has been associated with swamps and night air (It. *mal aria,* bad air). The disease was known to the early Egyptians (1550 B.C.) and continues even today to be devastating. The species of *Plasmodium* that cause human malaria are widely distributed in the tropical regions of the world (Figure 28–9) and cause what

FIGURE 28–9
Areas of risk for malaria, December 1977. (WHO Weekly Epidemiological Record No. 22, 1979.)

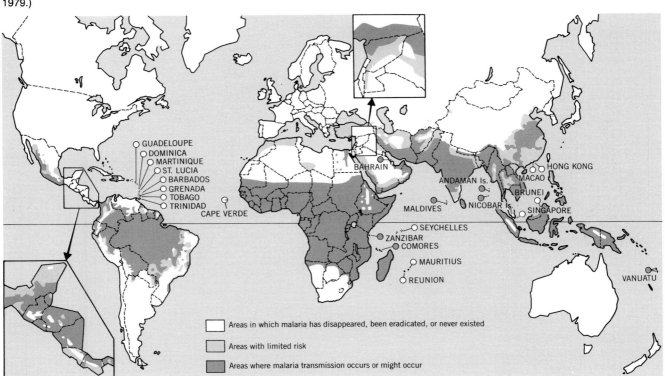

GUADELOUPE
DOMINICA
MARTINIQUE
ST. LUCIA
BARBADOS
GRENADA
TOBAGO
TRINIDAD
CAPE VERDE
BAHRAIN
ANDAMAN Is.
HONG KONG
MACAO
BRUNEI
MALDIVES
NICOBAR Is.
SINGAPORE
SEYCHELLES
ZANZIBAR
COMORES
MAURITIUS
REUNION
VANUATU

Areas in which malaria has disappeared, been eradicated, or never existed

Areas with limited risk

Areas where malaria transmission occurs or might occur

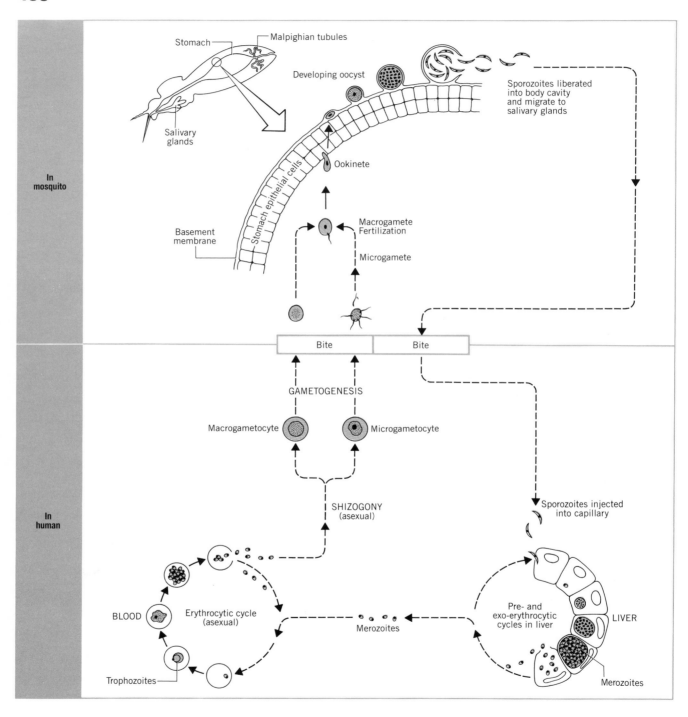

is probably the most common infectious disease of humans. Plasmodia have a complex life cycle that requires both a vertebrate and an invertebrate host. Anopheles mosquitoes are invertebrate hosts and vectors for plasmodia. They transmit plasmodia to reptiles, birds, and mammals, which are vertebrate hosts.

Life cycle of *Plasmodium* sp. Many sporozoans, including species of *Plasmodium*, reproduce by both sexual and asexual mechanisms. The sporozoites of *Plasmodium* sp., present in an infected mosquito's salivary glands, are transferred to humans when the mosquito takes a blood meal (Figure 28–10). The sporozoites are transported in the human blood to the liver, where they grow as trophozoites. The trophozoites grow in the liver cells for about 1 week prior to schizogony, an asexual process of multiple fission that results in the formation of numerous **merozoites.** The merozoites either infect other liver cells or they infect erythrocytes. Once in the erythrocyte, they grow as trophozoites (Color Plate 21) before they again reproduce by schizogony. The merozoites produced from erythrocyte schizogony (Color Plate 22) are released into the blood at synchronized intervals. After one or more cycles of erythrocyte schizogony, the merozoites enter other erythrocytes to begin the process of sexual reproduction. During the process of gametogenesis, the trophozoite changes into a gamete known as a **gamont** (Figure 28–11, Color Plate 23). Both microgamonts (microgametes) and macrogamonts (macrogametes) are produced in infected erythrocytes. These gamonts remain within their erythrocyte until they are ingested by a female mosquito.

Once in the stomach of the mosquito, the gamonts emerge from the erythrocyte. Next, fertilization takes place and a diploid zygote is formed. The zygote quickly differentiates into an **ookinete.** The oo-

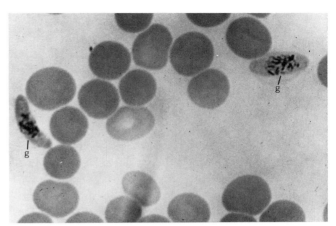

FIGURE 28–11
Plasmodium gamonts (g) seen in a blood smear. (Courtesy of Dr. I. Armstrong.)

kinete penetrates through the midgut wall into the coelom, where it becomes an oocyst (Figure 28–10). The zygote in the oocyst undergoes meiosis and then sporogony to produce infective sporozoites. These sporozoites are released into the hemocoel. From here they spread through the mosquito and eventually reach the salivary glands. A new reproduction cycle is initiated when the sporozoites in the mosquitoes' salivary glands are again injected into a human.

Malaria in humans. Malaria is characterized by cycles of chills and fever. The chills are followed by a fever during which the patient's temperature rises to 104 or 105°C. The patient feels unbearably hot during the peak of the fever and then begins to sweat as the fever declines. The cycle recurs on a systematic basis regulated by the synchronized release of merozoites from infected erythrocytes. There are four species of *Plasmodium* that cause human malaria. The cycle recurs every 48 hours in patients infected with *P. falciparum, P. ovale,* and *P. vivax*; and every 72 hours in patients infected with *P. malariae.* Untreated cases last for 3 to 6 weeks interspersed with periods of apparent good health. Relapses occur after a 2- to 10-month latency period, and complete recovery occurs only after 2 to 3 years. Falci-

FIGURE 28–10
The life cycle of *Plasmodium vivax.* Replication occurs in an invertebrate host (mosquito) and a vertebrate host. (From K. M. Adam, J. Paul, and V. Zaman, *Medical and Veterinary Protozoology. An Illustrated Guide,* Churchill Livingston, London, 1971.)

parum malaria is always serious, and it can be rapidly fatal.

Immunity to malaria. Humans develop a partial immunity to malaria. This immunity is short-lived and apparently depends on the ability of macrophages to phagocytize infected erythrocytes. In addition to this immunity, Negroes are less susceptible to vivax malaria than are Caucasians, and falciparum malaria is less severe in Negroes. *Plasmodium falciparum* is unable to replicate in sickle-cell erythrocytes, which provides resistance to malaria for persons with the sickle-cell trait.

Diagnosis and treatment. Malaria is diagnosed by observing the reproductive stages of *Plasmodium* in the blood (Figure 28–12). Enlargement of the spleen is another important diagnostic indicator of malaria, especially in persons with latent malaria.

For centuries, malaria has been treated with quinine extracted from the bark of cinchona trees. Quinine has served as a model compound for making synthetic antimalaria drugs, including chloroquine and quinacrine hydrochloride (Atabrine). Chloroquine can be used on an outpatient basis to treat all malarias except falciparum malaria. Patients with falciparum malaria are usually hospitalized and treated with a combination of drugs. Chloroquine can be used in chemoprophylaxis when it is given for 2 weeks before entering and for 6 weeks after leaving a malarious area.

Sarcodina

Amebas are found in soil, water, on plants, and in other organisms. The major human pathogenic ameba is *Entamoeba histolytica* (Figure 28–13), which causes amebic dysentery (amebiasis). The incidence of this disease is highest in the tropics, where the cysts of this animal are more likely to survive outside of their hosts. More than 40 percent of the population of some tropical countries are infected by *E. histolytica,* whereas only 3 to 4 percent of the population in the United States is infected. Most infections of *E. histolytica* are asymptomatic; however, serious dysenteric disease and even death can result.

Characteristics of *Entamoeba histolytica*. This ameba grows and reproduces by binary fission in the human large intestine. *Entamoeba histolytica* is recognized by its large size (up to 50μm) and its granular cytoplasm, which often contains ingested erythrocytes (Figure 28–13). Its movement is mediated by its lobose pseudopodia. The trophozoites of *E. histolytica* are sensitive to the acid pH and the enzymes of the human stomach. Only the cysts survive outside their host's body.

Entamoeba histolytica has a simple life cycle during which the trophozoites, growing in the human colon, form cysts. During encystment, the amebas round up, lose their ingested food particles, and

FIGURE 28–12
Plasmodium trophozoites in erythrocytes of an infected human. (Courtesy of Dr. I. Armstrong.)

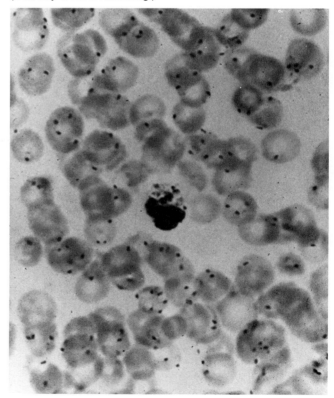

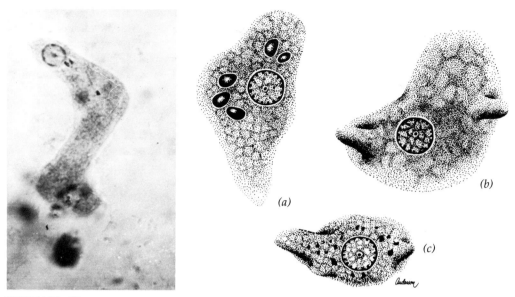

FIGURE 28–13
Micrograph and drawing of *Entamoeba histolytica* trophozoites: (*a*) ingested erythrocytes, (*b*) pseudopodia, and (*c*) ingested bacteria. (From J. W. Beck and J. E. Davis, *Medical Parasitology*, 3rd ed., Mosby, St. Louis.)

shrink in size. Cyst formation is completed when the animal forms a thin cell wall around itself and its nucleus divides twice to form four nuclei. These cysts are the infective form of *E. histolytica;* they can remain viable in water for up to 30 days and in moist, nontoxic soil for days or months. Ingested cysts are not affected by the pH and enzymes in the human stomach. Once in the intestine, the nuclei of the cyst again divide and eight trophozoites emerge through a hole in the cyst wall. These amebas invade the colon and the cycle repeats.

Amebiasis in humans. Most infections of *E. histolytica* are asymptomatic. Infected persons who become ill experience amebic dysentery characterized by abdominal pains and loose stools that may contain mucus and blood. *Entamoeba histolytica* can secrete proteolytic enzymes that enable it to invade the intestinal mucosa, where it forms lesions. The amebas cause extensive necrosis and grow by ingesting products of decomposed tissue, erythrocytes, and

bacteria. Infections confined to the intestine are not life threatening.

Extraintestinal amebiasis occurs when amebas penetrate the colon or blood vessels of the bowel. The penetration of the bowel and infection of the peritoneal cavity occurs in 3 to 4 percent of the patients with amebic dysentery. Amebas that invade the blood vessels of the bowel can be transported to the liver and from the liver to the lungs.

Epidemiology. The incidence of amebiasis parallels the sophistication that a community has in matters of sanitation and personal hygiene. Foreign visitors to tropical countries are often exposed to amebiasis because of the high incidence of asymptomatic carriers among the local population. Visitors become infected when they consume local water or eat contaminated raw vegetables. Amebiasis also occurs in northern climates: it is epidemic among some Eskimos. In order to eliminate the threat of amebiasis, water must be boiled for 10 to 15 minutes and vegetables should be treated with a strong detergent and then soaked in vinegar.

Diagnosis and treatment. Amebiasis is diagnosed by identifying *E. histolytica* in specimens taken from the patient. The size, the number of nuclei in the cysts, and the motility of the amebas all contribute to its identification. *Entamoeba histolytica* is morphologically very similar to common, nonpathogenic amebas, so experience in making the morphological diagnosis is very important.

A number of drugs are effective against amebiasis; however, no one drug prevails, and some of the effective drugs are not licensed in the United States. Tetracycline in combination with either diiodohydroxyquin or diloxoanide furoate has been used to treat asymptomatic infections of the colon lumen. Metronidazole (Flagyl) is recommended for treating symptomatic amebiasis.

Amebic meningoencephalitis. Free-living amebas found in soil and freshwater rarely cause human disease. However, about 100 cases of meningoencephalitis have been reported to be caused by amebas. Amebic meningoencephalitis occurs most often in children or young adults with a history of swimming in freshwater. This disease begins as a severe frontal headache with lethargy and fever and then progresses to confusion, convulsions, coma, and death. The disease is diagnosed by the presence of amebas and erythrocytes in the spinal fluid combined with an elevated protein and a decreased sugar level. The causative agent in most cases has been identified as an ameba belonging to the genus *Naegleria*. Successful treatment of *Naegleria*-induced meningoencephalitis has been accomplished with amphotericin B and miconazole; however, most cases are fatal.

Ciliophora

Balantidium coli (Figure 28–14) is the only ciliophoran known to cause human disease. It is a common inhabitant of swine, which are the major source of the human infection. Cysts of this ciliate are transmitted by the oral-fecal route. The ciliate emerges from the cyst and establishes an infection in the large intestine. This infection, called **balantidiasis,** is characterized by dysentery and, in some cases, appendicitis. The symptoms last 1 to 4 weeks, and they may recur. The causative agent is identified in feces or in scrapings from the ulcer formed in the colon. Several

FIGURE 28–14

The trophozoite and the cyst of the ciliate *Balantidium coli.* (From E. R. Noble and G. A. Noble, *Parasitology: The Biology of Animal Parasites*, 4th ed., Lea & Febiger, Philadelphia, 1976.)

Trophozoite

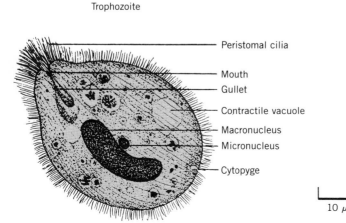

Peristomal cilia
Mouth
Gullet
Contractile vacuole
Macronucleus
Micronucleus
Cytopyge

10 μm

Cyst

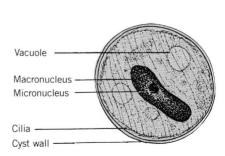

Vacuole
Macronucleus
Micronucleus
Cilia
Cyst wall

drugs are used to treat balantidiasis including tetracyclines and diiodohydroxyquin.

Mastigophora

Flagellated protozoa comprise a large group of organisms that include a number of zooflagellates that cause serious human illness. The pathogenic zooflagellates infect the human intestinal tract, the urogenital tract, or the blood. These protozoa are transmitted by blood-sucking insects, by direct contact, or by consuming infected food.

Trichomoniasis: *Trichomonas vaginalis.* In the United States, *Trichomonas vaginalis* is a common human pathogenic flagellate. An estimated 3 million American women are infected every year by this protozoan that is transmitted by sexual contact. The disease also occurs in males, but at a much lower rate (4 to 15 percent the incidence observed in females). Nonvenereal transfer does occur, but it does not have a major impact on the incidence of trichomoniasis.

Trichomonas vaginalis is a large (7 to 32 μm long by 5 to 12 μm wide), motile, pear-shaped flagellate (Figure 28–15), which divides by longitudinal fission. No sexual reproduction is known, and they do not form cysts. Each flagellate possesses an undulating membrane and four anterior flagella that arise from a single anatomical site. They have a characteristic twitching motility, which is used to identify them under the microscope. *Trichomonas vaginalis* is an anaerobic protozoan that grows on carbohydrates, bacteria, and erythrocytes. Mitochondria are notably absent.

Trichomonas vaginalis causes trichomoniasis (trich) when it multiplies in the vagina after an incubation period of between 5 and 28 days. The main symptoms are vulvovaginal soreness and vaginal discharge. These symptoms are usually exacerbated during the menstrual period probably because of the rapid replication of the pathogen at this time. Approximately 25 percent of infected females are asymptomatic. Infected males rarely have symptoms even when *T. vaginalis* is present in the urethra. The prostate and the epididymis are also sites of infection in males.

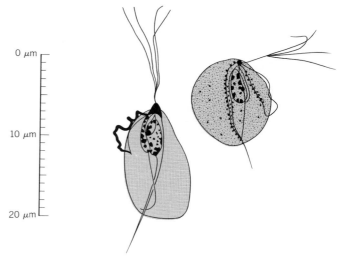

FIGURE 28–15
Trophozoites of *Trichomonas vaginalis.* (Courtesy of Dr. B. M. Honigberg. From B. M. Honigberg and V. M. King. *J. Parasitology,* 50:345 – 364, 1964, copyright © 1964, *The Journal of Parasitology.*)

Trichomoniasis is diagnosed by microscopically identifying the organisms in specimens from infected individuals. Infected patients and their sexual partners are treated with oral doses of metronidazole (Flagyl) in a 7-day regimen. Approximately 95 percent of the cases are cured with treatment. The disease will recur in patients who are reinfected.

Giardiasis. *Giardia lamblia* is the most common human intestinal flagellate. This pear-shaped flagellate has four pairs of flagella (Figure 28–16), which arise from the anterior, posterior, caudal, and ventral surfaces of the animal. Giardia attaches to its host cell by a flattened adhesive disk found on its ventral surface. *Giardia lamblia* divides by binary fission.

Giardia lamblia causes giardiasis in humans when it is ingested as a cyst. The trophozoite attaches by its adhesive disk to the cells lining the duodenum. Here they consume mucous secretions and replicate. After an incubation period of approximately 15 days, the patient experiences the sudden onset of watery, foul-smelling diarrhea, abdominal distension, flatulence (gas), nausea, and anorexia. Blood and mucus are rarely present in the stools. The acute stage lasts

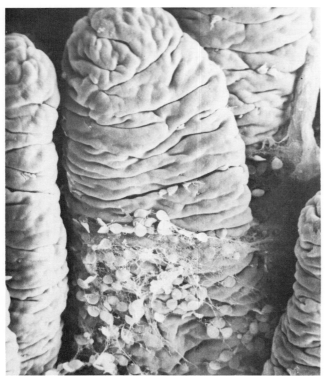

FIGURE 28–16
Giardia trophozoites adhering to the microvillous surface of the villi in the mouse jejunum. (Courtesy of Dr. R. L. Owen. From R. L. Owen, P. C. Nemanic, and D. P. Stevens, *Gastroenterology*, 76:757–769, 1979.)

3 to 4 days. The presence of trophozoites or cysts of *G. lamblia* in the stools is diagnostic of giardiasis. Patients are treated with atabrine or metronidazole.

The extent of *G. lamblia* infections in humans runs from low (2 to 5 percent) to high (60-plus percent) depending on the geographical region. Most infections are asymptomatic; however, outbreaks of giardiasis do occur, and in recent years giardiasis has been a major cause of waterborne epidemics in the United States (see Table 14–4). Epidemics have been reported from a number of western states, New York, and New Hampshire. Hikers camping in remote areas of the Rocky Mountains have also contracted giardiasis, suggesting that animals also serve as a reservoir. Beavers, associated with an outbreak

in Camus, Washington, have been the only animal shown to carry this protozoan; however, other species of *Giardia* infect dogs, cats, rodents, and cattle.

Mastigophora: arthropod-borne

Leishmania sp. and *Trypanosoma* sp. are flagellated, pathogenic protozoa that are transmitted between humans, or to humans from animal reservoirs, by blood-sucking insects. These protozoa are most prevalent in the tropical climates of the world. Species of *Trypanosoma* cause African sleeping sickness and Chagas' disease, whereas species of *Leishmania* cause kala-azar, cutaneous leishmaniasis, and mucocutaneous leishmaniasis.

Leishmaniasis: kala-azar. The major form of leishmaniasis in India is kala-azar, which means "black fever." In 1903, Leishman and Donovan independently reported oval parasites in macrophages taken from kala-azar patients. When cultured, these oval parasites developed into flagellated organisms. They were named *Leishmania donovani* and were classified as Mastigophora.

Leishmania donovani is an obligate parasite whose prominent reservoirs are humans, dogs, and foxes. Sandflies of the genus *Phlebotomus* (Table 28–2) are the intermediate host and vector of this parasite. In humans, *L. donovani* is an intracellular parasite that multiplies in the cells of the reticuloendothelial system. In its host, it is a nonmotile, 2- to 3-μm oval cell. The flagellated form is present in the laboratory cultures and in the intestine of infected sandflies.

Kala-azar occurs in Asia, Europe, Africa, and in South and Central America. Depending on the geographical location, dogs, foxes, rats, rodents, and humans are important reservoirs for *L. donovani*. The vectors are sandflies that live on flat plains, usually above 2000 feet in altitude. The female sandflies produce eggs after a blood meal and lay their eggs in soil, leaf litter, and/or animal feces. The female sandfly is infected when she takes a blood meal from an infected reservoir. The protozoa replicate in the sandfly before they are transmitted to humans by the bite of the fly.

TABLE 28–2
Arthropod-borne Protozoan Diseases

Disease	Etiological Agent	Reservoirs	Vectors	Distribution
Leishmaniasis	*Leishmania* sp.			
Kala-azar	*L. donovani*	Dog, fox, human	*Phlebotomus* sp.	Asia, Europe, Africa, China,
Cutaneous	*L. tropica*	Gerbil, dog, cat		Asia Minor, Africa, South
leishmaniasis				and Central America
Mucocutaneous	*L. braziliensis*	Dog, rat, cat,	*Lutzomyia* sp.	South America
leishmaniasis	*L. mexicana*	horse		
Trypanosomiasis	*Trypanosoma* sp.			
Chagas' disease	*T. cruzi*	Cat, dog	Reduviidae	Central and South America
African sleeping	*T. brucei*	Human	*Glossina palpalis*	Western Africa
sickness	*gambiense,*		(tsetse fly)	
	T. brucei	Human, antelope,	*Glossina morsitans*	Eastern Africa
	rhodesiense	wild hog	(tsetse fly)	

Kala-azar is an insidious disease whose symptoms usually develop after a 2-week to 15-month incubation period. Patients suffer vague discomfort, diarrhea or constipation, low-grade fever, and anorexia. Another form of the disease has an acute onset characterized by a high fever and chills. During the later stages of the disease, the abdomen becomes extended because of the enlarged liver and spleen. The skin at this stage becomes a characteristic gray, the sign from which the disease derived its name, kala-azar. The patient deteriorates gradually with prolonged symptoms of fever, weight loss, weakness, splenomegaly, and hepatomegaly. Patients may succumb to secondary bacterial infections.

Kala-azar is diagnosed by the clinical syndrome and by the presence of *Leishmania* sp. in host spleen or bone marrow samples. Leishmaniasis is treated with either pentavalent organic antimonials and/or the more effective aromatic diamidines. Amphotericin B is also effective, but it is a secondary drug because of its toxicity.

Cutaneous leishmaniasis. *Leishmania tropica* exists in dog, cat, and rodent reservoirs and causes cutaneous leishmaniasis when it is transmitted to humans by infected sandflies. A papule forms at the inoculation site following an average 2- to 6-month incubation period. The ulcer that forms at this site usually heals spontaneously over a period of several months. Patients develop a permanent immunity following recovery. The infection can be treated with antimony compounds.

Mucocutaneous leishmaniasis. This disease causes facial disfigurement and occurs primarily in Brazil and Peru (Table 28–2). It is caused by *L. mexicana* or *L. braziliensis*, both of which are transmitted to humans by sandflies of the genus *Lutzomyia*. Ulcers usually develop in the oral or nasal mucosa. Facial disfigurement is caused by the destruction of tissue attacked by the spreading ulcer. The drugs used to treat kala-azar are applicable here also.

Trypanosomiasis. Many vertebrates are destroyed by diseases caused by trypanosomes. These arthropod-borne protozoa infect wild vertebrates as well as domestic livestock. Species of trypanosomes exist in more than 4.5 million square miles (larger than the continental United States) of Africa and seriously restrict the breeds of domestic animals that can be raised there. In addition humans are infected by trypanosomes that cause African sleeping sickness and Chagas' disease.

Species of the uniflagellated *Trypanosoma* are readily seen in blood and are identified by their morphological characteristics (Figure 28–17). The single fla-

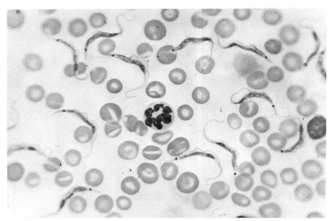

FIGURE 28–17
Micrograph of *Trypanosoma lewis* in blood. (Courtesy of Carolina Biological Supply Co.)

gellum is part of an undulating membrane that runs most of the cell's length (Figure 28–4). Each cell is between 15 and 40 μm long and divides by longitudinal fission. Nonflagellated forms are present in some infected tissues.

Chagas' disease. *Trypanosoma cruzi,* the cause of *Chagas' disease,* is found in South and Central America (Table 28–2), where it infects an estimated 12 million people. It is transmitted to humans by bloodsucking insects of the family Reduviidae, called the "assassin bugs," which live in the cracks and crevices of dwellings. The trypanosomes live and replicate in the gut of the insect and are excreted in the insect's feces. Humans are infected after the trypanosomes are deposited on the skin in the insect's feces. From the skin surface, they penetrate scratches and abrasions. They can also penetrate the mucous membranes of humans if they are transferred to the membranes by contaminated fingers. The trypanosomes are intracellular parasites that multiply in human lymphoid tissue. They then spread to the cells of the nervous system and muscle (mostly cardiac) fibers.

Chagas' disease occurs mainly in children and is largely restricted to persons living in primitive dwellings. Clinical symptoms include fever, malaise, anorexia, and edema. **Romana's sign** is caused by edema of the eyelid, which partially closes the eye.

This is present in about 50 percent of the acute cases. The mortality rate is 5 to 10 percent of the acute cases and results from heart failure or acute meningoencephalitis. These infections do not respond well to chemotherapy (Nifurtimox), apparently because the drugs do not kill the intracellular parasites.

African sleeping sickness. *Trypanosoma brucei gambiense* and *T. brucei rhodesiense,* the two races of *Trypanosoma brucei,* cause African sleeping sickness in West and East Africa respectively. Both species of *Trypanosoma* are transmitted by tsetse flies (*Glossina* sp.), and both sexes of these flies live on blood meals. *Glossina palpalis* is found in the western regions of tropical Africa, where it breeds along streams in well-shaded areas and is the vector for *T. brucei gambiense.* Humans are the only source of blood used by *G. palpalis.* In East Africa, the tsetse fly *Glossina morsitans* transmits *T. brucei rhodesiense* between its reservoirs (humans, antelopes, and wild hogs) and humans.

The trypanosomes replicate in the midgut of the insect for about 10 days before they migrate forward to infect other organs, including the salivary glands. Humans are inoculated with the trypanosomes present in the fly's salivary gland when the tsetse fly takes a blood meal. In humans, the trypanosomes replicate in the blood and lymph to cause a systemic infection. Swollen lymph nodes, especially those on the back of the neck, are known as **Winterbottom's sign** and are diagnostic of African sleeping sickness. Eventually, the trypanosomes infect the central nervous system, causing the clinical symptoms of apathy, somnolence, and malaise. Over a period of several months, the disease progresses to coma and death.

Sleeping sickness can be diagnosed by the presence of trypanosomes in the blood (Figure 28–17) or in specimens from swollen lymph glands. African sleeping sickness can be treated with organic arsenicals, suramin, and pentamidines. Suramin and pentamidines can be given in combinations and are effective in the early stages of the infection. Control of this disease remains a problem of eradicating the tsetse fly from areas inhabited by humans.

SUMMARY

Single-celled animals are classified in the phylum Protozoa. They have complex organelles, which they use for food acquisition, locomotion, and reproduction. The protozoa are classified into four taxonomic groups according to their motility: Sarcodina (pseudopodia), Mastigophora (flagellates), Ciliophora (cilia), and Sporozoa (gliding motility, if present). Protozoa reproduce asexually by binary fission, and many have complex life cycles with both asexual and sexual reproduction. Both free-living species and symbiotic species of protozoa are known. Parasitic protozoa cause widespread diseases in vertebrates, including humans, especially in the tropics.

Malaria is caused by species of *Plasmodium,* which are transmitted between humans by the anopheles mosquito (Table 28–3). The sporozoites replicate asexually in the human liver and then in erythrocytes. Malaria is characterized by recurrent chills and fever that correspond to the release of merozoites from infected cells. These symptoms recur every 48 or 72 hours depending on the reproduction cycle of the infecting species of *Plasmodium.* Malaria is diagnosed by the presence of the malaria parasite in the blood and is treated with chloroquine or a combination of quinine and other drugs.

Entamoeba histolytica causes amebiasis. Humans are infected when they ingest cysts of *E. histolytica* that grow and cause dysentery in the human colon. This ameba causes extraintestinal amebiasis when it infects the liver and lungs. *Naegleria* is often responsible for amebic meningoencephalitis. This is a rare, but usually fatal, disease of young people who have a history of swimming in freshwater. *Balantidium coli* is a common intestinal ciliate of swine that causes human dysentery. It is the only ciliate known to cause human disease.

Trichomoniasis of the urogenital tract is a venereal disease caused by *Trichomonas vaginalis.* Women suffer vulvovaginal soreness and vaginal discharge; infections in men are usually asymptomatic. Trichomoniasis is treated with metronidazole. Another

TABLE 28–3
Summary: Protozoan Diseases

Disease	Etiological Agent	Reservoir-Vector (Transmission)	Distribution	Treatment
Malaria	*Plasmodium* sp. (four species)	Human-mosquito	Tropical	Chloroquine, quinine, sulfonamide, pyrimethamine
Amebiasis	*Entamoeba histolytica*	Water, food (fecal-oral)	Worldwide	Tetracycline, diloxoanide, diiodohydroxyquin
Amebic meningoencephalitis	*Naelgeria* sp.	Freshwater (swimming)	Only 100 known cases	Metronidazole (Flagyl), amphotericin B
Balantidiasis	*Balantidium coli*	Swine (fecal-oral)	Worldwide	Tetracycline, diiodohydroxyquin
Trichomoniasis	*Trichomonas vaginalis*	Human (venereal)	Worldwide	Metronidazole
Giardiasis	*Giardia lamblia*	Human, beaver	Worldwide	Atabrine, metronidazole
Leishmaniasis	*Leishmania* sp.	Human, dog, cat, gerbil-sandflies	India, Asia, Africa, tropical America	Organic antimonials, aromatic diamidines
Trypanosomiasis	*Trypanosoma* sp.			
Chagas' disease	*T. cruzi*	Human-Reduviidae	Tropical America	Nifurtimox
African sleeping sickness	*T. brucei gambiense*	Human-*G. palpalis*	Western Africa	Organic arsenicals, suramin, pentamidine
	T. brucei rhodesiense	Human, antelope, wild hogs-*G. morsitans*	Eastern Africa	

flagellate, *Giardia lamblia,* causes giardiasis, which is characterized by foul-smelling diarrhea. Humans are infected when they ingest waterborne cysts of this protozoan. Atabrine and metronidazole are used to treat human giardiasis.

Leishmaniasis and trypanosomiasis are caused by arthropod-borne flagellates. Leishmaniasis is caused by species of *Leishmania,* which are geographically restricted by the distribution of their reservoirs (humans, dogs, cats, rodents) and their vectors (sandflies). The clinical symptoms of leishmaniasis vary geographically and may appear as kala-azar, cutaneous leishmaniasis, or mucocutaneous leishmaniasis. *Trypanosoma cruzi* causes Chagas' disease in South and Central America. Chagas' disease is transmitted by species of the family Reduviidae known as the "assassin bugs" and affects children living in primitive dwellings. African sleeping sickness is caused by trypanosomes that are transmitted to humans by tsetse flies. In West Africa, humans are believed to be the only animal reservoir for the causative agent, *T. brucei gambiense.* In East Africa, humans, antelopes, and wild hogs are reservoirs for *T. brucei rhodesiense.* African sleeping sickness is a devastating disease that is responsive to chemotherapy in its early stages.

QUESTIONS AND TOPICS FOR STUDY AND DISCUSSION

Questions

1. Name the methods of motility used by the protozoa and give an example of each. How is motility used in the classification of the protozoa?
2. How do pseudopodia function in motility and food acquisition?
3. Define or explain the following.

cytostome	zygote
schizont	trophozoite
kinetoplast	undulating membrane
encystment	merozoite
axoneme	sporozoite

4. Diagram the life cycle of *Plasmodium,* and label the stages of development.
5. What causes the chills and fever cycle of human malaria? Is the duration of the cycle always constant? Explain.
6. If *Entamoeba histolytica* were unable to form cysts, would it still cause human disease? Explain.
7. How can human amebiasis be prevented and treated? How is this disease differentiated from bacillary dysentery?
8. Describe the human disease that is caused by a ciliate.
9. Describe human trichomoniasis. How is this disease transmitted, prevented, and treated?
10. Discuss the epidemiology of giardiasis. Are you safe from this parasite if you drink water from a mountain stream? Explain.
11. What is the worldwide distribution of leishmaniasis? Describe the manifestations of this disease in humans.
12. Describe the life cycle for the protozoa that cause African sleeping sickness.

Discussion

1. Discuss the economic impact of the parasitic protozoa on the underdeveloped countries.
2. Malaria is diagnosed among persons living in the United States. What groups of people do you think are involved?

FURTHER READINGS

Books

Beck, J. W., and J. E. Davies, *Medical Parasitology,* 3rd ed., Mosby, St. Louis, 1981. A well-illustrated paperback textbook that covers protozoa, helminths, and the medically important arthropods involved in disease transmission.

Schmidt, G. D., and L. S. Roberts, *Foundations of Parasitology,* 2nd ed., Mosby, St. Louis, 1981. An introductory college textbook in parasitology.

Sleigh, M., *The Biology of Protozoa,* Arnold, London, 1973. An introduction to the biology of the single-celled animals.

APPENDIX 1

THE TWENTY AMINO ACIDS FOUND IN MOST PROTEINS

Polar

Glycine (gly)

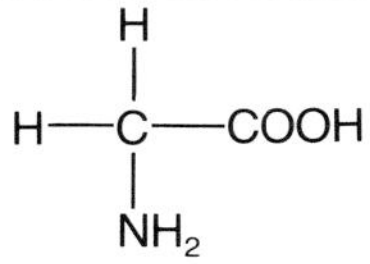

$$H-\underset{\underset{NH_2}{|}}{\overset{\overset{H}{|}}{C}}-COOH$$

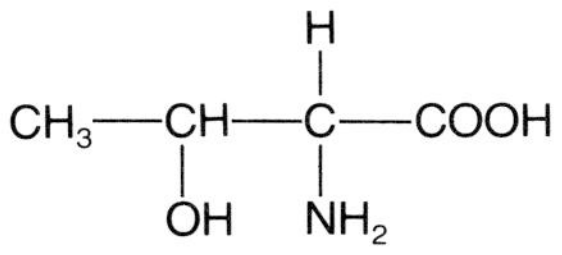

Cysteine (cys)

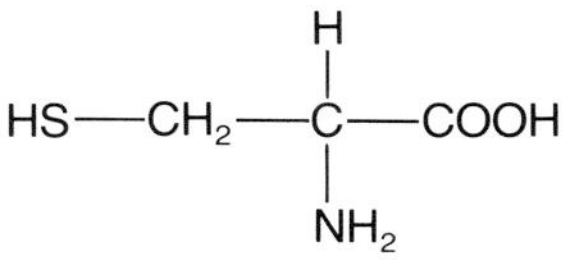

$$HS-CH_2-\underset{\underset{NH_2}{|}}{\overset{\overset{H}{|}}{C}}-COOH$$

Serine (ser)

$$HO-CH_2-\underset{\underset{NH_2}{|}}{\overset{\overset{H}{|}}{C}}-COOH$$

Lysine (lys)

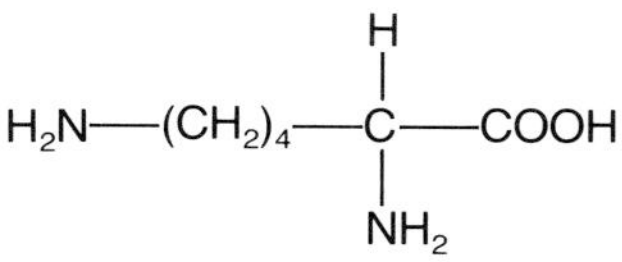

$$H_2N-(CH_2)_4-\underset{\underset{NH_2}{|}}{\overset{\overset{H}{|}}{C}}-COOH$$

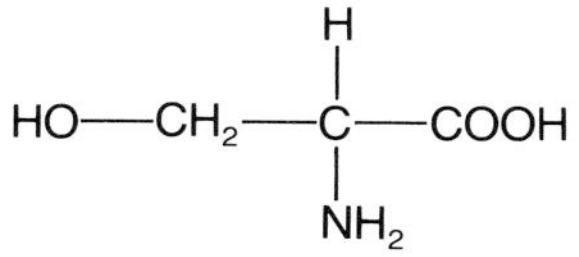

Tyrosine (tyr)

$$HO-\langle\bigcirc\rangle-CH_2-\underset{\underset{NH_2}{|}}{\overset{\overset{H}{|}}{C}}-COOH$$

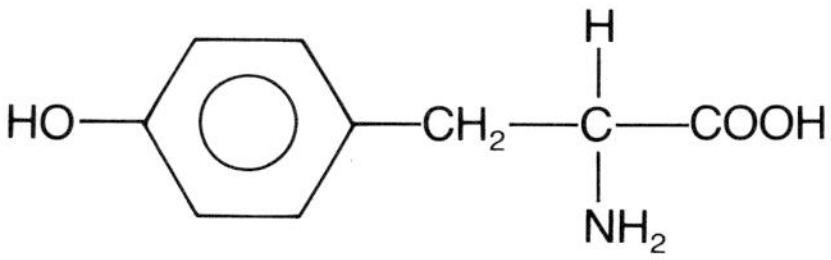

Aspartic acid (asp)

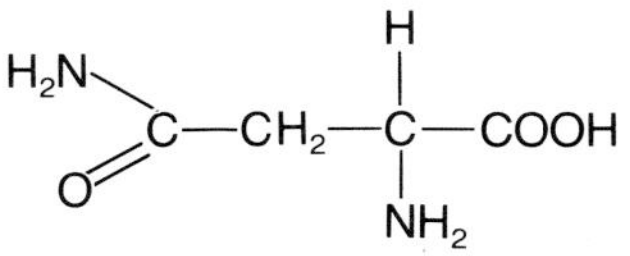

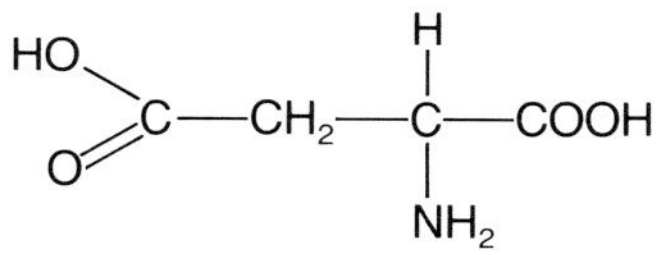

$$\underset{O}{\overset{HO}{>}}C-CH_2-\underset{\underset{NH_2}{|}}{\overset{\overset{H}{|}}{C}}-COOH$$

Asparagine (asn)

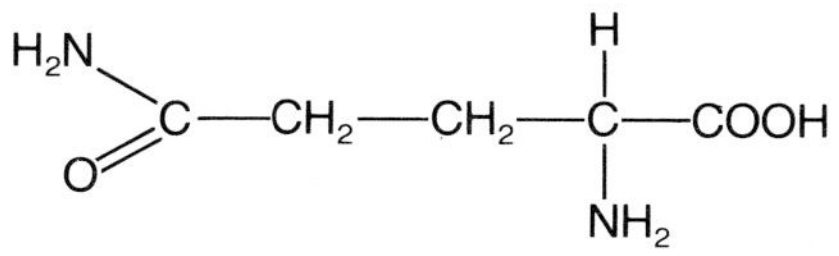

$$\underset{O}{\overset{H_2N}{>}}C-CH_2-\underset{\underset{NH_2}{|}}{\overset{\overset{H}{|}}{C}}-COOH$$

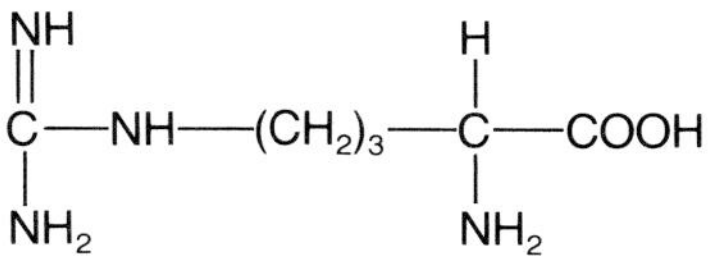

Glutamic acid (glu)

$$\underset{O}{\overset{HO}{>}}C-CH_2-CH_2-\underset{\underset{NH_2}{|}}{\overset{\overset{H}{|}}{C}}-COOH$$

Glutamine (gln)

$$\underset{O}{\overset{H_2N}{>}}C-CH_2-CH_2-\underset{\underset{NH_2}{|}}{\overset{\overset{H}{|}}{C}}-COOH$$

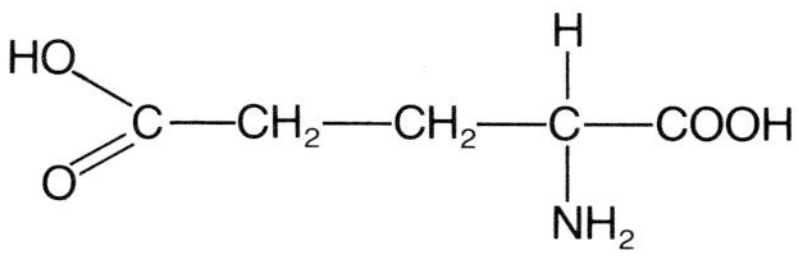

Histidine (his)

Arginine (arg)

$$\underset{NH_2}{\overset{NH}{\underset{|}{\overset{||}{C}}}}-NH-(CH_2)_3-\underset{\underset{NH_2}{|}}{\overset{\overset{H}{|}}{C}}-COOH$$

Threonine (thr)

$$CH_3-\underset{\underset{OH}{|}}{\overset{\overset{H}{|}}{C}H}-\underset{\underset{NH_2}{}}{C}-COOH$$

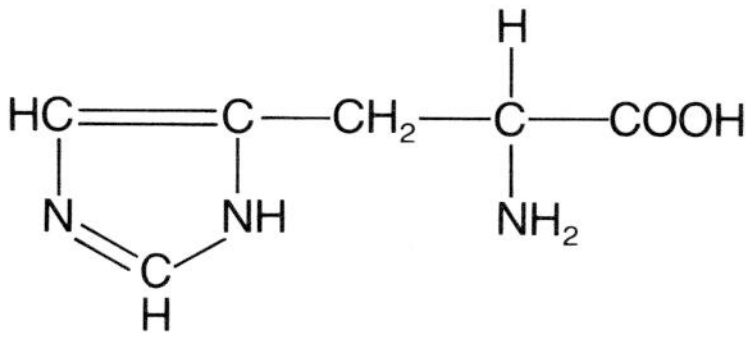

Nonpolar

Alanine (ala)		Methionine (met)	
Valine (val)		Phenylalanine (phe)	
Leucine (leu)		Tryptophan (trp)	
Isoleucine (ile)			
Proline (pro)			

APPENDIX 2

THE STRUCTURE OF OXIDIZED AND REDUCED NICOTINAMIDE ADENINE DINUCLEOTIDE (NAD)

NAD$_{oxidized}$ $\xrightarrow[2e^-]{2H^+}$ NAD$_{reduced}$ + H$^+$

APPENDIX 3
GLYCOLYSIS

Glycolysis is the anaerobic process for the metabolism of glucose that yields lactic acid. The net overall reaction is

$$\text{Glucose} \rightarrow 2 \text{ Lactic acid} + 2 \text{ ATP}$$

This process uses the Embden-Meyerhof pathway. The first part of the pathway uses two molecules of ATP to produce fructose-1,6-diphosphate from glucose. Fructose-1,6-diphosphate is then split into 2 three-carbon molecules, dihydroxyacetone-phosphate and glyceraldehyde-3-phosphate. Dihydroxyacetone-phosphate is converted to glyceraldehyde-3-phosphate. The remainder of the pathway involves the metabolism of two molecules of glyceraldehyde-3-phosphate to yield two molecules of pyruvic acid. In addition to pyruvic acid, two molecules of $NADH_2$ and four molecules of ATP (a net yield of two molecules) are produced. Pyruvic acid serves as the terminal electron acceptor when it is reduced to lactic acid. The metabolism of glucose to two molecules of lactic acid and two molecules of ATP is a fermentation.

In aerobic organisms, the pyruvic acid produced in the Embden-Meyerhof pathway is converted to acetyl-CoA, which is metabolized in the Krebs cycle. Acetyl-CoA, CO_2, and $NADH_2$ are products of the decarboxylation of pyruvic acid.

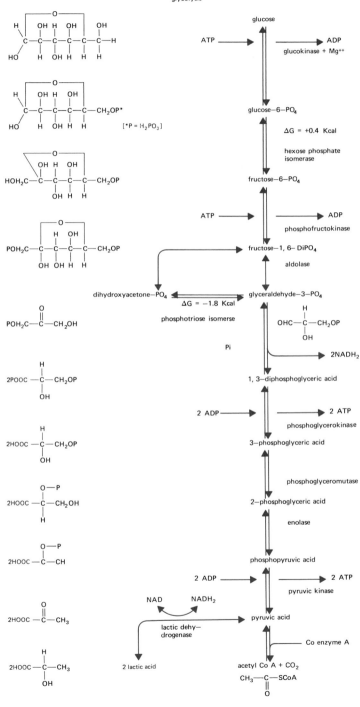

glycolysis

APPENDIX 4
THE KREBS CYCLE

The Krebs cycle (tricarboxylic acid cycle) is a major pathway for the metabolism of acetyl-CoA. The products of this cycle are two molecules of CO_2, one molecule of GTP, one molecule of $FADH_2$, and three molecules of $NADH_2$ for each molecule of acetyl-CoA metabolized. The GTP can be converted directly into ATP. In aerobic organisms, the $FADH_2$ is oxidized by components of the electron-transport chain to yield two molecules of ATP, whereas $NADH_2$ is similarly oxidized to yield three molecules of ATP. Therefore, when the Krebs cycle is coupled to an electron-transport chain, 12 ATPs are produced for each acetyl-CoA molecule metabolized.

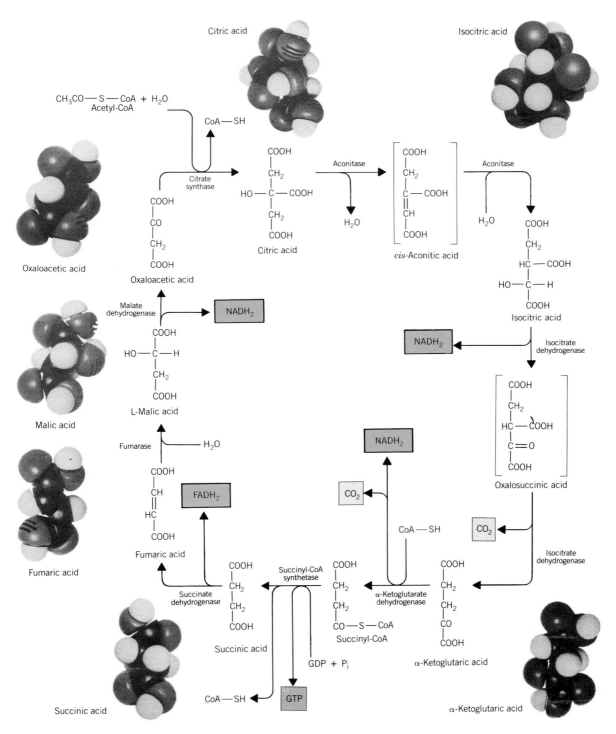

Citric acid

Isocitric acid

CH_3CO—S—CoA + H_2O
Acetyl-CoA

CoA—SH

Citrate
synthase

COOH
|
CH_2
|
HO—C—COOH
|
CH_2
|
COOH

Citric acid

Aconitase

H_2O

COOH
|
CH_2
|
C—COOH
‖
CH
|
COOH

cis-Aconitic acid

Aconitase

H_2O

COOH
|
CH_2
|
HC—COOH
|
HO—C—H
|
COOH

Isocitric acid

Oxaloacetic acid

COOH
|
CO
|
CH_2
|
COOH

Oxaloacetic acid

Malate
dehydrogenase

NADH$_2$

COOH
|
HO—C—H
|
CH_2
|
COOH

L-Malic acid

Malic acid

Isocitrate
dehydrogenase

NADH$_2$

COOH
|
CH_2
|
HC—COOH
|
C=O
|
COOH

Oxalosuccinic acid

Fumarase

H_2O

COOH
|
CH
‖
HC
|
COOH

Fumaric acid

Fumaric acid

FADH$_2$

NADH$_2$

CO$_2$

CoA—SH

CO$_2$

Isocitrate
dehydrogenase

Succinate
dehydrogenase

COOH
|
CH_2
|
CH_2
|
COOH

Succinic acid

Succinyl-CoA
synthetase

COOH
|
CH_2
|
CH_2
|
CO—S—CoA

Succinyl-CoA

α-Ketoglutarate
dehydrogenase

COOH
|
CH_2
|
CH_2
|
CO
|
COOH

α-Ketoglutaric acid

Succinic acid

GDP + P$_i$

CoA—SH

GTP

α-Ketoglutaric acid

APPENDIX 5

CLASSIFICATION OF BACTERIA

Bergey's Manual of Determinative Bacteriology is the major reference for bacterial systematics. The procaryotic cells are divided into two groups: the cyanobacteria are assigned to Division I and the bacteria are assigned to Division II. *Bergey's Manual* presents the classification of Division II, which is divided into 19 parts. The classification of bacteria is constantly being revised through the compilation of new data and the establishment of new relationships between species of bacteria. One should not view this classification as absolute: it should be used as a guide for categorizing bacteria into groups of organisms possessing similar characteristics. Selected bacterial genera are listed here.

PART 1 PHOTOTROPHIC BACTERIA (18 GENERA)

Rhodospirillum
Chromatium
Chlorobium
Rhodopseudomonas
Thiocapsa
Pelodictyon

PART 2 GLIDING BACTERIA (27 GENERA)

Myxococcus
Beggiatoa
Cytophaga
Leucothrix

PART 3 SHEATHED BACTERIA (7 GENERA)

Sphaerotilus
Leptothrix

PART 4 BUDDING AND/OR APPENDAGED BACTERIA (17 GENERA)

Hyphomicrobium
Caulobacter

PART 5 SPIROCHETES (5 GENERA)

*Treponema**
*Leptospira**
Cristispira
*Borrelia**
Spirochaeta

504

PART 6 SPIRAL AND CURVED BACTERIA (6 GENERA)

Spirillum†   *Campylobacter†*

PART 7 GRAM-NEGATIVE AEROBIC RODS AND COCCI (20 GENERA)

*Pseudomonas**   *Brucella**
*Bordetella**   *Francisella**
Azotobacter   *Rhizobium*
Halobacterium   *Gluconobacter*

PART 8 GRAM-NEGATIVE FACULTATIVELY ANAEROBIC RODS (26 GENERA)

*Escherichia**   *Salmonella**
*Shigella**   *Klebsiella**
*Enterobacter**   *Serratia**
*Proteus**   *Yersinia**
Erwinia   *Vibrio**
Photobacterium   *Hemophilus**

PART 9 GRAM-NEGATIVE ANAEROBIC BACTERIA (9 GENERA)

*Bacteroides**   *Fusobacterium**
Desulfovibrio

PART 10 GRAM-NEGATIVE COCCI AND COCCOBACILLI (6 GENERA)

*Neisseria**   *Acinetobacter†*

PART 11 GRAM-NEGATIVE ANAEROBIC COCCI (3 GENERA)

Veillonella†

PART 12 GRAM-NEGATIVE CHEMOLITHOTROPHIC BACTERIA (17 GENERA)

Nitrobacter   *Nitrococcus*
Nitrosomonas   *Nitrosococcus*
Thiobacillus   *Sulfolobus*

PART 13 METHANE-PRODUCING BACTERIA (3 GENERA)

Methanobacterium   *Methanosarcina*

PART 14 GRAM-POSITIVE COCCI (12 GENERA)

*Staphylococcus**   *Streptococcus**
Leuconostoc   *Micrococcus*
Sarcina

PART 15 ENDOSPORE-FORMING RODS AND COCCI (5 GENERA)

*Bacillus**   *Clostridium**
Sporolactobacillus   *Sporosarcina*
Desulfotomaculum

PART 16 GRAM-POSITIVE, ASPOROGENOUS ROD-SHAPED BACTERIA (4 GENERA)

Caryophanon   *Lactobacillus*

PART 17 ACTINOMYCETES AND RELATED ORGANISMS (39 GENERA)

*Corynebacterium**   *Mycobacterium**
*Nocardia**   *Actinomyces**
Streptomyces   *Arthrobacter*
*Propionibacterium**

PART 18 RICKETTSIAS (18 GENERA)

*Rickettsia**   *Coxiella**
*Chlamydia**

PART 19 MYCOPLASMAS (4 GENERA)

*Mycoplasma**   *Acholeplasma*

*Medically important genera discussed in this text.
†Other medically important genera beyond the scope of this text.

APPENDIX 6

PRONUNCIATION OF SCIENTIFIC NAMES AND TERMS

Pronunciation Key

a	*as in*	**a**dd, m**a**p	o	*as in*	**o**dd, h**o**t
ay		**a**ce, r**a**te	oh		**o**pen, s**o**
ai		c**a**re, **a**ir	oo, yoo		r**u**le
ah		f**a**ther	oy		b**oi**l
aw		d**aw**n	ow		**ou**ch
eh		**e**nd, p**e**t	u		p**u**t
ee		**e**ven	ch		**ch**eck, cat**ch**
e		t**e**rm	sh		ru**sh, s**ure
g		**g**o, lo**g**	th		**th**in, bo**th**
i		**i**t, g**i**ve	zh		fi**ss**ion
y, eye		**i**ce, wr**i**te			

Scientific Names and Terms	Pronunciation
Actinomyces israelii	ak-tin-oh-my′sees is-ray′lee-eye
Actinomycosis	ak-tin-oh-my-koh′sis
Adenosine	a-dehn′uh-sin
Adenovirus	a″dehn-oh-vy′rus
Aedes aegypti	ah-ee′deez ee-jip′tee
Aedes triseriatus	ah-ee′deez try-ser-ee-aht′us

Agar	ah′gerr
Ajellomyces	ah-jel-oh-my′sees
Allosteric protein	al-oh-steer′ik proh′teen
Alphavirus	al″fa-vy′rus
Ameba	ah-mee′bah
Amino acid	ah-mee′noh acid
Anaerobic	an-air-oh′bik
Anamnestic response	an″am-nes′tik
Anopheles	an-of′el-eez
Antigen	ant′i-jen
Arenaviridae	a-ree″nah-vir′i-dee
Arthrobacter	ar-throh-bak′ter
Ascus	ask′us
Aspergillus flavus	as-per-jil′us flay′vus
Aspergillus fumigatus	A. foo-mi-gah′tus
Auxotroph	ox′oh-trohf
Avirulent	ay-veer′yoo-lent
Bacillus anthracis	bah-sil′us an-thray′sis
Bacillus polymyxa	B. pol-ee-miks′ah
Bacillus subtilis	B. sut′il-is
Bacillus thuringiensis	B. thur-in-jee-en′sis

Bacteriocin — bak-teer-ee-oh′sin
Bacteriophage — bak-teer′ee-oh-fayj
Bacteroides fragilis — bak-te-roi′deez fra′jil-is

Balantidium coli — bal-an-tid′ee-um koh′lee

Barophiles — bair′oh-fyls
Binary fission — by′ner-ee fizh′en
Blastomyces dermatitidis — blas-toh-my′sees der-mah-ty′ti-dis

  (*Ajellomyces dermatitidis*) — (ah-jel-oh-my′sees)

Bordetella parapertussis — bor-deh-tel′ah pa-ra-per-tus′sis

Bordetella pertussis — B. per-tus′sis
Borrelia hermensii — bor-rel′ee-ah her-men′see-eye

Borrelia recurrentis — B. ree-kur-ren′tis
Borrelia turicatae — B. tu-ri-kah′tee
Borrelia venezuelensis — B. ve-ne-zway-len′sis
Brucella abortus — broo-sel′ah a-bor′tus

Brucella canis — B. kay′nis
Brucella melitensis — B. meh-lih-ten′sis
Brucella suis — B. soo′is
Bunyaviridae — bun″ya-vir′i-dee

Candida albicans — kan′did-ah al′bih-kans

Capsid — kap′sid
Capsomere — kap′soh-meer
Carcinogenesis — kar″sin-oh-jen′eh-sis
Catalase — kat′a-lays
Catarrh — kah-tahr′
Cephalosporium — sef-ah-loh-spohr′ee-um
Chancre — shang′ker
Chlamydia psittaci — klah-mih′dee-ah sit′tah-see

Chlamydia trachomatis — C. trah-koh-mah′tis
Chlamydiales — klah-mih″dee-ah′lees
Chlamydospore — klah-mid′oh-spohr
Chloramphenicol — klor-am-fen′i-kol
Cilia — sil′ee-ah
Ciliophora — sil″ee-oh-for′ah

Cladosporium carrionii — klad-oh-spohr′ee-um kar-ee-on′ee-eye
Clostridium botulinum — klaw-stri′dee-um bot-choo-ly′num

Clostridium novyi — C. no′vy-ee
Clostridium perfringens — C. per-frin′jens
Clostridium septicum — C. sep′ti-kum
Clostridium tetani — C. te′tan-ee
Coccidioides immitis — kok-sid-ee-oi′deez im′i-tis

Coenocytic — sin′oh-sit-ik
Coliform — koh′lee-form
Conidiospore — kon-id′ee-oh-spohr
Conjunctiva — kon-junk-ty′vuh
Coronavirus — ko-roh″nah-vy′rus
Corynebacterium diphtheriae — kor-eye″nee-bak-teer′ee-um dif-theer′ee-eye

Coxiella burnetii — kahks-ee-el′ah ber-net′ee-eye

Coxsackievirus — kahk-sak″ee-vy′rus
Cristispira — kris-ti-spy′rah
Cryptococcus neoformans — kryp″toh-kok′us nee-oh-for′manz

  (*Filobasidiella neoformans*) — (fi″loh-ba-si-dee-el′ah)
Culex tarsalis — koo′leks tahr-sahl′is
Culiseta melanura — kul-y-set′ah mel-ahn-ur′ah

Cyanobacteria — sy-an-o-bak-teer′ee-ah
Cytochrome — syt′o-krohm
Cytomegalovirus — sy-toh-meg″ah-loh-vy′rus

Dalton — dawl′ton
Daphnia — daf′nee-ah
Dengue virus — deng′ee vy′rus
Deoxyribose — dee-ox″see-ry-bohs
Dermacentor andersoni — der-mah-sen′tor an-der-soh′neye

Dermacentor variabilis — D. vair-ee-ah′bi-lis
Desulfotomaculum — dee-sul-foh″toh-mah′koo-lum

Diaminopimelic acid — dy-ah-meen″oh-py-may′lik acid

Dimorphic	dy-mohr′fik
Diploid	dip′loid
Echovirus	ek″oh-vy′rus
Eczema	ek′se-mah
Encephalitis	en-sef-ah-ly′tis
Entamoeba histolytica	en-tah-mee′bah his-toh-li′ti-kah
Enterobacter aerogenes	en-ter-oh-bak′ter ai-rah′jen-eez
Epidermophyton	ep-i-der-moh-fy′ton
Episome	ep′i-sohm
Epstein-Barr virus	ep′styn-bahr vy′rus
Erythromycin	e-rith-roh-my′sin
Escherichia coli	esh-er-i′kee-ah koh′lee
Eucaryotic	yoo-kar-ee-ah′tik
Euglena	yoo-glee′nuh
Filobasidiella	fi-loh-ba-si-dee-el′ah
Flagellum	flah-jel′um
Flavivirus	fla″vee-vy′rus
Francisella tularensis	fran-sis-el′ah too-lah-ren′sis
Fusobacterium	fyoo-soh-bak-teer′ee-um
Gastroenteritis	gas″troh-en-te-ry′tis
Genus	jee′nus
Giardia lamblia	jee-ahr′dee-ah lam′blee-ah
Glomerulonephritis	gloh-mair″yeh-loh-neh-fry′tis
Glossina morsitans	glos-ee′nah mor′si-tans
Glossina palpalis	G. pal-pal′is
Glycosidic bond	gly-koh-sid′ik bond
Gonyaulax catanella	gon-ee-aw′lax ka-tan-el′ah
Halobacterium	hah-loh-bak-teer′ee-um
Hapten	hap′ten or hap′teen
Hemagglutination	hee-mah-gloot-in-nay′shun
Hemolysin	hi-mol′is-in
Hemolysis	hi-mol′i-sis

Hemophilus aegyptius	hee-mah′fi-lus ee-jip′tee-us
Hemophilus ducreyi	H. du-kray′ee
Hemophilus influenzae	H. in-floo-en′zee
Hepatitis A virus	hep-ah-ty′tis
Herpes simplex virus	her′peez sim′pleks vy′rus
Herpetoviridae	her-pet″oh-vir′i-dee
Heterotroph	het′er-oh-trohf
Histamine	his′tah-meen
Histoplasma capsulatum	his-toh-plas′mah kap-soo-lah′tum
Histoplasma duboissii	H. doo-bois′ee-eye
Humoral	hyoo′mor-ahl
Hyaluronic acid	hy-al-yoo-ron′ik acid
Hypha, pl. hyphae	hy′fah, hy′fee
Icosahedral	eye-koh-sah-hee′dral
Immunofluorescence	im-yoon″oh-flohr-es′ence
Immunoglobulin	im-yoon″oh-glob′yoo-lin
Impetigo	im-pah-ty′goh
Influenza	in-floo-en′zah
Interferon	in-ter-feer′on
Jaundice	jawn′dis
Klebsiella ozaenae	kleb-see-el′ah oh-zee′nee
Klebsiella pneumoniae	K. noo-moh′nee-eye
Klebsiella rhinoscleromatis	K. ry-noh-sclee-roh′mah-tis
Lactobacillus acidophilus	lak-toh-bah-sil′us a-si-dah′fi-lus
Legionella pneumophila	lee-jah-nel′ah noo-mah′fi-lah
Leishmania braziliensis	leesh-may′nee-ah bra-zil-ee-en′sis
Leishmania donovani	L. don-oh′van-eye
Leishmania mexicana	L. meks-i-kahn′ah
Leishmania tropica	L. trop′ik-ah
Leptospira biflexa	lep-toh-spy′rah by-fleks′ah

Leptospira interrogans	*L.* in-ter'ah-ganz	Osteomyelitis	os"tee-oh-my-e-ly'tis
Leptotrombidium	lep"toh-trom-bid'ee-um	Otitis	oh-ty'tis
Leukocyte	loo'koh-syt		
Lipopolysaccharide	lip'o-pohl-ee-sak'ah-ryd	Papillomavirus	pap-e-loh"mah-vy'rus
		Papovaviridae	pap-oh"vah-vir'i-dee
Lymphocyte	lim'foh-syt	*Paracoccidioides*	par-ah-kok-sid'ee-oi-deez bra-sil-ee-en'sis
Lysogenic	ly-soh-jen'ik	*brasiliensis*	
Lysozyme	ly-soh-zym	Parainfluenza	par"ah-in-floo-en'zah
Madurella mycetoma	mah-door-el'ah my-see-toh'mah	*Paramecium multimicronucleatum*	par-ah-mee'see-um mul-tee-my-kroh-noo-klee-ah'tum
Malaise	mal-ayz'	*Paramyxoviridae*	par-a-miks"oh-vir'i-dee
Mastigophora	mas"ti-go'for-ah	Parvoviridae	par"voh-vir'i-dee
Meiosis	my-oh'sis	Pasteurization	pas-tyoor"i-zay'shun
Meningitis	men-in-jy'tis	Pathogenesis	path-oh-jen'eh-sis
Merozoite	mer-o-zoh'yt	*Pediculus humanus*	ped-ik'oo-lus hoo-mahn'us
Microsporum	my-kroh-spoh'rum		
Mitosis	my-toh'sis	*Pediculus vestimenti*	*P.* ves-ti-men'tee
Mortierella	mort-ee-rel'ah	*Penicillium griseofulvum*	pen-i-sil'ee-um gri-see-oh-ful'vum
Mucor	moo'kor		
Mus musculus	mus mus'kyoo-lus	Permease	per'mee-ays
Mutagen	myoo'ta-jen	*Petriellidium boydii*	pet-ree-el-i'dee-um boy'dee-eye
Mycelium	my-see'lee-um		
Mycobacterium bovis	my-koh-bak-teer'ee-um boh'vis	Phage	fayj or fahzh
		Phagocytosis	fag"ah-sy-toh'sis
Mycobacterium leprae	*M.* lep'ree	*Phialophora verrucosa*	fy-ah-lo'fo-rah ver-ah-koh'sah
Mycobacterium tuberculosis	*M.* too-ber-kyoo-loh'sis		
Mycoplasma pneumoniae	my-koh-plaz'mah noo-moh'nee-eye	*Phlebotomus*	fle-bot'e-mus
		Phylum, pl. phyla	fy'lum, fy'lah
Naegleria	ny-glee'ree-ah	Picornaviridae	pi-korn"ah-vir'i-dee
Nasopharynx	nay-zoh-fair'inks	Plaque	plak
Necrosis	ne-kroh'sis	Plasma	plaz'mah
Neisseria gonorrhoeae	ny-see'ree-ah gon-or-ree'eye	*Plasmodium falciparum*	plaz-moh'dee-um fal-si-pahr'um
Neisseria meningitidis	*N.* men-in-jy'ti-dis	*Plasmodium malariae*	*P.* mah-lair'ee-ee
Neurospora crassa	nur-ah'spor-ah cras'a	*Plasmodium ovale*	*P.* oh-vah'lee
Nocardia asteroides	noh-kahr'dee-ah as-ter-oi'deez	*Plasmodium vivax*	*P.* vy'vaks
		Poliovirus	poh"lee-oh-vy'rus
Nosocomial	noh-soh-koh'mee-ahl	Polyeen	pol-ee-een'
Oncogenesis	on-koh-jen'eh-sis	Polymorphonuclear	pol-ee-mor-foh-noo'klee-er
Organelle	or-gah-nel'		
Ornithosis	or-ni-thoh'sis	Poxviridae	poks-vir'i-dee
Orthomyxoviridae	or-thoh-miks-oh-vir'i-dee	Procaryotic	proh-kar-ee-ah'tik
		Prophage	proh-fayj or proh-fahzh

Propionibacterium acnes	proh-pee-on″ee-bak-teer′ee-um ak′neez
Protease	proh′tee-ays
Proteus mirabilis	proh′tee-us mi-rah′bi-lis
Proteus vulgaris	*P.* vul-gah′ris
Protista	proh-tis′tah
Pseudohyphae	soo-doh-hy′fee
Pseudomonas aeruginosa	soo-doh-moh′nas ai-roo-jin-oh′sah
Pseudopod	soo′doh-pod
Pyogenic	py′oh-jen′ik
Reduviidae	red″yoo-vy′i-dee
Reoviridae	ree″oh-vir′i-dee
Reticuloendothelial system	ri-tik″yew-loh-en-doh-thee′lee-uhl
Retroviridae	re″troh-vir′i-dee
Rhabdoviridae	rab′doh-vir′i-dee
Rhinovirus	ry″noh-vy′rus
Rhizopus arrhizus	ry′zoh-pus ah-ry′zus
Rickettsia prowazekii	ri-ket′see-ah prow-ah-zee′kee-eye
Rickettsia rickettsii	*R.* ri-ket′see-eye
Rickettsia tsutsugamushi	*R.* soo-soo-ga-moo′shee
Rickettsia typhi	*R.* ty′fee
Rotovirus	roh″toh-vy′rus
Rubella	roo-bel′ah
Saccharomyces cerevisiae	sak-ah-roh-my′sees se-ri-vis′ee-eye
Salmonella cholerae-suis	sal-mohn-el′ah kol-er-ay-soo′is
Salmonella enteritidis	*S.* en-ter-it′id-is
Salmonella schottmulleri	*S.* shot-mul′er-eye
Salmonella typhi	*S.* ty′fee
Salmonella typhimurium	*S.* ty-fi-mur′ee-um
Salmonellosis	sal-mohn-el-oh′sis
Saprophyte	sap′roh-fyt
Sarcina ventriculi	sahr-sy′nah ven-trik′yoo-leye
Sarcodina	sahr-koh-dy′na
Serratia marcescens	ser-ah′tee-ah mahr-ses′ens
Shigella dysenteriae	shi-gel′ah dis-en-tair′ee-eye
Spirochaeta plicatilis	spi-roh-kee′tah pli-kah′ti-lis
Sporangium	spohr-an′jee-um
Sporolactobacillus	spohr-oh-lak-to-bah-sil′us
Sporosarcina urea	spohr-oh-sahr-sy′na yoo-ree′uh
Sporothrix schenckii	spohr′oh-thriks shen′kee-eye
Sporozoan	spohr-oh-zoh′ahn
Sporozoite	spohr-oh-zoh′yt
Staphylococcus aureus	staf-i-loh-kok′us aw′ree-us
Staphylococcus epidermidis	*S.* e-pi-der′mi-dis
Streptococcus faecalis	strep-toh-kok′us fee-kahl′is
Streptococcus lactis	*S.* lak′tis
Streptococcus mutans	*S.* moo′tans
Streptococcus pneumoniae	*S.* noo-moh′nee-eye
Streptococcus pyogenes	*S.* py-ahj′en-eez
Streptococcus salivarius	*S.* sa-li-vair′ee-us
Streptomyces nodosus	strep-toh-my′sees noh-doh′sus
Streptomyces noursei	*S.* nor′see-eye
Sulfolobus	sul-foh-loh′bus
Symbiosis	sim-bee-oh′sis
Syncytial	sin-sish′al
Tetracycline	tet-rah-sy′klyn
Titer	ty′ter
Togaviridae	toh″gah-vir′i-dee
Treponema carateum	tre-poh-nee′mah kah-rah′tee-um
Treponema pallidum	*T.* pal′li-dum
Treponema pertenue	*T.* per-ten′yoo-ee
Trichomonas vaginalis	trik-oh-mohn′as va-jin-al′is
Trichophyton	trik-oh-fy′ton
Trophozoite	trof-oh-zoh′yt
Trypanosoma brucei gambiense	try-pan-oh-soh′mah broo′see-eye gam-bee-ens′ee

Trypanosoma brucei rhodesiense	*T.* broo'see-eye ro-dee-si-ens'	*Vibrio cholerae*	vib'ree-oh kol'er-eye
Trypanosoma cruzi	*T.* kruz'ee	Virion	veer'ee-on
Tyndallization	tin-dahl-i-zay'shun	*Vorticella*	vor-ti-sel'ah
		Yersinia pestis	yer-sin'ee-ah pes'tis
Vaccinia	vak-sin'ee-uh		
Varicella-Zoster	var-i-sel'uh zohs'ter	Zygote	zy'goht
Variola	vah-ree-oh'lah		

GLOSSARY

Abiogenesis *See* Spontaneous generation.

Acid-Fast The binding of a basic dye, such as carbofuchsin, that is not washed out with acidified alcohol.

Acids Substances that increase the concentration of hydronium ions (H_3O^+) in the liquid to which they are added.

Acne An eruptive skin disease occurring mainly on the face, chest, and back.

Acquired Immunity Resistance to a specific infectious agent developed by an individual in response to a disease (natural) or following an injection of a specific antigen (artificial).

Actinomycin D An antibiotic produced by a species of *Streptomyces* that inhibits transcription in eucaryotic cells.

Actinomycosis A bacterial infection caused by *Actinomyces israelii* or *A. bovis*, which are opportunistic pathogens of warm-blooded animals.

Active Transport The energy-dependent movement of molecules across a semipermeable membrane mediated by a carrier protein. The molecules are moved from a location of low concentration to one of high concentration against a diffusion gradient.

Aerobic Requiring free oxygen for respiration.

Aerobic Respiration The process of transforming the chemical energy in organic compounds into ATP, which employs the pathways of glycolysis, the TCA cycle, and the electron-transport chain and uses free oxygen as the final electron acceptor.

Allosteric Enzyme An enzyme that has a specific regulatory site located at a point that is physically removed from the catalytic site.

Alopecia Hair loss.

Ames Test A screening assay for carcinogenic compounds that measures the ability of a compound to cause reverse mutations in histidine-requiring strains of *Salmonella*.

Amino Acid An organic compound containing a carboxyl ($-COOH$) and an amino ($-NH_2$) functional group.

Anaerobe An organism that grows in the absence of oxygen.

Anaerobic Respiration An energy-yielding process utilizing an electron-transport system in which an inorganic compound (nitrate, nitrite, sulfate, etc.) other than oxygen serves as the terminal electron acceptor.

Analogues Compounds that have similar chemical structures but different biochemical functions.

Anamnestic Response The accelerated formation of antibody on the second and subsequent exposures to an antigen. *Also* called the memory response.

Anaphylactic Shock Trauma resulting from a direct injection of an allergen into a sensitized individual.

Anexic Culture A culture that contains only one species of organism.

Anion An element able to accept one or more electrons into its outer shell to become a negatively charged ion.

Antibiotic A substance synthesized by one organism that kills or inhibits the growth of another organism.

Antibody A protein produced by an animal in response to a foreign substance (immunogen) that will specifically react with that substance in a demonstrable way.

Anticodon The sequence of three nucleotide bases in tRNA; it is complementary to a sequence of bases (codon) on the mRNA.

Antigen Foreign substance, usually a large protein or polysaccharide, that reacts specifically with an antibody molecule. Many antigens are also immunogens.

Antigenic Drift The slow, sequential change in the antigenic nature of one or more viral surface proteins.

Antigenic Shift A major change in the viral antigens that creates a new, serologically distinct virus.

Antiseptics Chemicals with low human toxicity that destroy microorganisms capable of causing contamination or disease.

Arthrospores Asexual fungal spores produced within a hypha separated by a cross wall (septum).

Ascospores Fungal spores produced by sexual reproduction in the subdivision Ascomycotina.

Aseptic In the absence of contaminating organisms and/or infectious agents.

Aseptic Meningitis An inflammation of the meninges characterized by the absence of bacteria from the cerebrospinal fluid.

Asexual Reproduction Production of progeny without the joining of two nuclei.

Asthma A disease resulting from hypersensitivity to inhaled allergens. Symptoms include wheezing and difficulty in breathing.

Atomic Number The number of protons in the nucleus of an element.

Atomic Weight The number of protons plus the number of neutrons in the nucleus of an element.

Autotrophy The ability of an organism to grow on a completely inorganic medium with carbon dioxide as a carbon source. *See* also chemolithotroph, photolithotroph.

Auxotrophs Mutants requiring nutritional supplements in their growth medium.

Bacteremia The presence of bacteria, which are not multiplying, in the blood.

Bactericidal Able to kill bacterial cells.

Bacteriocins Bacterial proteins that are toxic to closely related bacteria and whose genes are carried by *col* plasmids.

Bacteriodaceae The family of anaerobic, Gram-negative rod-shaped bacteria.

Bacteriolytic Able to kill bacterial cells through lysis.

Bacteriophage A bacterial virus.

Bacteriostatic Able to prevent bacterial growth.

Bacteriurea An infection of the urinary tract diagnosed by the presence of 100,000 or more bacteria per milliliter of urine.

Balanced Growth Condition in which all the components of the cells in a culture are changing at a constant rate.

Barophiles Organisms that preferentially grow at high hydrostatic pressures, often certain marine bacteria from the deep ocean.

Base A substance that on dissociation releases hydroxyl (OH^-) ions. In pure neutral solvents, it produces a pH of more than 7.

Basidiospores Fungal spores produced by sexual reproduction in the subdivision Basidiomycotina.

Binomial System of Nomenclature The naming of organisms by the assignment of a genus and a species name.

Bivalence The property of antibodies that allows them to react with two separate, but identical, antigenic determinants.

Blastospores Asexual spores that are formed by budding.

Brill-Zinsser Disease A mild disease resembling typhus fever and caused by a latent infection of *Rickettsia prowazekii*.

Broad-Spectrum Antibiotic An antibiotic that is effective against both Gram-positive and Gram-negative bacteria.

Buffer A compound that chemically resists major changes in pH by neutralizing either acids or bases.

Burst Size The increase in the number of virions (infective centers) produced during a one-step growth experiment.

Capsid The protein coat surrounding the viral nucleic acid.

Capsule The diffused accumulation of material adhering to the cell wall.

Carbohydrate An organic compound having the chemical formula $(CH_2O)n$.

Carcinogen Any compound that causes cancer in animals.

Carrier An individual infected by a pathogen without showing the symptoms of the disease.

Cation An element that gives up one or more electrons from its outer shell to become positively charged ions.

Cell Cycle The sequence of steps through which a eucaryotic cell undergoes division. The steps include mitosis, gap I, synthesis, and gap II.

Cell Theory The theory that living organisms are composed of membrane-limited units called cells.

Central Nervous System The brain, spinal cord, cranial nerves, and the spinal nerves.

Chancre A lesion or hard sore caused by *Treponema pallidum* during the primary stage of syphilis.

Chemiosmotic Coupling A hypothesis that explains how electron transfer results in the formation of energy-rich phosphate bonds.

Chemolithotroph An organism that can gain all its energy needs from the oxidation of inorganic compounds.

Chemoorganotroph An organism that oxidizes organic compounds as its source of energy.

Chemotaxis Movement of cells toward chemical attractants or away from chemical repellents.

Chemotherapeutic Drug A chemical used to treat a disease.

Chloramphenicol An antibiotic that prevents translation by binding to the 70S bacterial ribosome.

Chloroplast A membrane-bound, chlorophyll-containing plant cell organelle that is the site of photosynthesis.

Cholecystitis An inflammation of the gallbladder.

Chromatic Aberration The distortion of an object visualized through a lens caused by the lack of correction for different wavelengths of light.

Chromatin The complex of DNA and histones in the eucaryotic nucleus.

Chromosome The DNA macromolecule that contains essential cellular genes.

Cilia Proteinaceous protrusions from eucaryotic cells that beat with a rhythmic motion.

Ciliophora The taxonomic group of the Protozoa containing the unicellular ciliates.

Clone A group of cells all arising from the same parent cell.

Coccus (pl. cocci) The general name given to a spherical microorganism.

Codon Any sequence of three nucleotide bases in mRNA that are read by transfer RNA.

Coenocytic Having many nuclei in the same cellular compartment.

Coenzyme A small, reusable organic molecule that plays an accessory role in one or more enzymatic reactions (NAD, FAD, and CoA are common coenzymes).

Cold Agglutinins Antibodies that agglutinate type O human blood cells at 4°C, but not at 37°C. They are often present in patients infected with *Mycoplasma pneumoniae*.

Coliform A general term that describes the nondisease-producing, Gram-negative, rod-shaped bacteria that inhabit the human intestine.

Colony A visible accumulation of microorganisms that usually arises from the growth of a single cell.

Complement A nonspecific, heat-labile group of at least fourteen serum proteins that act in concert with one another, with antibody, and with membranes to cause cell lysis.

Complement Fixation When complement binds to an antigen-antibody complex, complement is said to be "fixed." Unbound complement can be detected by its ability to lyse sensitized red blood cells.

Congenital Rubella A disease of human infants caused by the rubella virus after it infects a fetus.

Congenital Syphilis The disease of human infants caused by *Treponema pallidum* passed from the mother to the fetus.

Conidium (pl. conidia) An asexual spore formed by a fungus.

Conjugation The transfer of genetic information from a donor to a recipient cell while the two cells are physically joined together.

Conjunctivitis Inflammation of the mucous membranes that line the eyelid.

Constitutive Protein A protein that is synthesized continuously by growing cells.

Contact Dermatitis Delayed hypersensitivity to small molecules that contact the skin.

Contact Inhibition The property of animal cells whereby they stop dividing when touching adjacent cells in a monolayer.

Coryza Inflammation of the mucous membranes of the nasal passages; also known as a head cold.

Covalent Bond The attractive force between two atomic nuclei that are sharing an electron.

Coxsackieviruses A group of enteroviruses belonging to the Picornaviridae family; they are named for Coxsackie, New York.

Cutaneous Mycoses Fungal infections of the keratinous structures found in human hair, nails, and epidermis.

Cyst A resting form of a cell that is more resistant to chemical and physical stress than the vegetative cells from which it is derived.

Cystitis An inflammation of the urinary bladder.

Cytoplasm The material surrounded by the cytoplasmic membrane exclusive of the nucleus.

Dalton A measure of mass equal to the weight of a hydrogen atom (atomic weight = 1.007).

Dane Particle An object possessing the HBs antigen found in the serum of serum-hepatitis patients. These particles are composed of a nucleocapsid (25 nm) surrounded by an outer envelope (42 nm).

Decapsidation The process by which an animal virus's nucleic acid is released from its capsid once the virion is inside its host cell. *Also* called uncoating.

Defined Media Growth media in which the known concentration of each chemical constituent is known.

Densensitization The injection of allergens into the muscle of a patient in an attempt to elicit the formation of IgG against the allergens.

Dermatophytes Fungi responsible for cutaneous mycoses.

Differential Media Any medium that selectively changes in response to the presence and growth of specific organisms.

Dimorphism The morphological property of a fungus that causes it to grow as yeasts in tissue (37°C) and as hyphae at room temperature.

Diphtheria An intoxication caused by the protein toxin produced by lysogenized strains of *Corynebacterium diphtheriae*.

Disease Any departure from the normal state of health of an organism that causes damage.

Disinfectant A chemical that will inhibit the growth of, or destroy, an organism (but not necessarily spores).

DNA Hybrid A double-stranded DNA molecule formed by annealing single-stranded DNA originating from different organisms.

Echoviruses A group of enteroviruses belonging to the Picornaviridae family. Their name is short for their original name, *e*nteric *c*ytopathic *h*uman *o*rphan viruses.

Eclipse The time interval following bacteriophage infection when no complete virions are present in the host cell.

Efficacy The combined qualities of a compound that contribute to its value as a chemotherapeutic agent.

Electronegativity The relative attractiveness possessed by an atomic nucleus for its electrons.

Electron-Transport Chain The membrane-bound components that participate in those oxidation-reduction reactions that result in the formation of energy-rich phosphate bonds.

Element One of the 93 naturally occurring atomic substances that have an invariant nucleus.

Elementary Body The infectious form of Chlamydiae.

Endemic The type of disease that persists in a geographical location, causing illness in the indigenous population at a low but constant rate.

Endergonic Reaction An energy-utilizing reaction; it is expressed as a positive ΔG.

Endocarditis An inflammation of the endocardium, which lines the chambers of the heart.

Endoflagella The spirochetal structures that lie outside the cell wall and beneath the cell envelope that are responsible for motility in spirochetes.

Endoparasitic An organism that lives within a larger organism to the latter's disadvantage.

Endospore A resting form of a bacterium that is formed within (endo) a vegetative cell.

Endosymbiont An organism that lives within a larger organism to the mutual benefit of both.

Endotoxin A poisonous substance that is a structural component of bacterial cell walls (especially of the outer cell wall of Gram-negative bacteria).

Enterics Bacteria belonging to the genera of the Gram-negative, facultative-anaerobic organisms of the intestinal flora.

Enterobacteriaceae The family of oxidase-negative, facultative-anaerobic, Gram-negative rod-shaped bacteria.

Enterotoxin The heat-stabile toxin responsible for staphylococcal food poisoning.

Enzyme Induction The specific formation of the series of proteins necessary to metabolize a substrate. The substrate often serves as the inducer.

Epidemic Any illness caused by a specific disease that occurs in a large proportion of a population.

Epidemiology The study of the factors involved in the occurrence of disease in a population.

Erythrogenic Toxin The toxin produced by group-A streptococci that is responsible for the red rash in scarlet fever.

Eucaryotes The large group of organisms (plants and animals) that are composed of cells possessing a membrane-bound nucleus (Gr. *eu,* true; *karyon,* nucleus).

Eumycetoma The true mycetomas caused by fungi. Actinomycetomas are caused by bacteria (*Nocardia* sp. and *Streptomyces* sp.).

Exergonic Reaction An energy-releasing reaction; it is expressed as a negative ΔG.

Exonuclease An enzyme that cleaves bonds at the free ends of single-stranded or double-stranded nucleic acids.

Exponential Phase The growth phase during which a microbe attains the maximum growth rate (minimum generation time) for a given set of growth conditions.

F' Strain A cell containing an extrachromosomal F^+ plasmid that was formed by the excision of the F plasmid from the chromosome of an Hfr cell.

Facultative Anaerobe A microbe that is able to grow in either the presence or the absence of oxygen.

Feedback Repression Inhibition of the formation of specific enzymes in a metabolic pathway caused by the accumulation of the end product(s) of that pathway.

Fermentation An anaerobic, energy-yielding process in which one or more products of the substrate are used as the terminal electron acceptor; the products are neither more oxidized nor more reduced than the substrate.

Fimbriae Proteinaceous protrusions, from the bacterial cell wall, involved in helping bacteria to adhere to inert surfaces.

Flagellum (pl. flagella) The external, thin proteinaceous structure involved in bacterial motility.

Fomite Any inanimate object that can participate in the transfer of infectious agents.

Gamont The gamete formed in the asexual reproduction of sporozoa.

Gastroenteritis An inflammation of the mucous membrane of the stomach and the small intestine.

Gene The sequences of nucleotides in DNA that are transcribed into RNA. Most genes are translated into one polypeptide; the genes for rRNA and tRNA make only RNA molecules.

Generalized Transduction The random transfer of small pieces of host-cell DNA by defective bacteriophages.

Generation Time The interval between divisions of a growing microorganism.

Genetic Engineering The biochemical manipulation of genes to create an organism with genetic information it would not naturally have.

Genome All the genetic information possessed by a cell or a virus.

Genus (pl. genera) A taxonomic grouping of closely related species.

Glucose Effect The preferential use of glucose by cells through the repression of inducible enzymes. *Also* called catabolic repression.

Glycolysis A sequence of enzymatic reactions by which glucose is metabolized to 2 moles of pyruvic acid, 2 moles of ATP, and 2 moles of NAD_{red}.

Gummas Soft lesions caused by *Treponema pallidum* during the tertiary stage of syphilis.

Halophiles Organisms that require 12 percent or higher concentration of NaCl to grow.

Haptens Foreign molecules that function as antigenic determinants, but that are too small to elicit antibody formation.

Hemagglutination The clumping of red blood cells caused by an antibody or a virus.

Hematuria Blood in the urine.

Hemolysin One of a number of bacterial protein toxins that lyse red blood cells.

Herpes Labialis A human disease characterized by lesions (cold sores) on the lips caused by herpes simplex virus type 1.

Heterophile Antibodies Antibodies that react with erythrocyte antigens found on red blood cells in many mammals. These antibodies are present in the serum of most (90%) patients with infectious mononucleosis.

Hfr Strains Cells that contain a fertility plasmid integrated into their chromosome.

Humoral Antibodies Antibodies in fluids of the body including the blood and lymph.

Hydrolase An enzyme that cleaves a covalent bond through the addition of a water molecule.

Hydrolysis The process of cleaving a covalent bond with the concomitant addition of water to the reactant(s).

Hydrophilic Water-attracting.

Hydrophobic Lacking affinity for water.

Hypersensitivity A state characterized by immunological reactions that cause harmful effects to the host.

Hypha (pl. hyphae; Gr. *hyphe*, web) A tubular filament containing protoplasm that is surrounded by the fungal cell membrane and cell wall.

Icosahedron A symmetrical structure composed of 20 equilateral triangles enclosing a central space.

Icterus Jaundice caused by liver disease.

Immunity An individual's or a population's increased resistance to an infectious disease.

Immunogen A substance capable of provoking an immunological response.

Immunoglobulins A class of globular animal proteins that function in reactions of immunity and hypersensitivity.

Infectious Disease A departure from the normal state of health of an organism that is caused by an invading organism or virus.

Innate Immunity The repertoire of defenses, both immunological and nonimmunological, that exists prior to the individual's exposure to environmental antigens.

Interferons A class of eucaryotic, cellular proteins that protect other cells from viral infection.

Intoxication A disease caused by a toxic substance; poisoning.

Invasive Disease Damage to a host caused by microorganisms and the products they produce during their multiplication within the host.

Ionic Bonds The attractive forces between atoms caused by dissimilar charges.

Ionizing Radiation Electromagnetic waves with sufficient energy to alter the structure of atoms.

Isomerase An enzyme that catalyzes geometric or structural changes within one molecule.

Isotope An atom with an unequal number of protons and neutrons in its nucleus.

Karyoplasm The material located within the nuclear membrane of eucaryotic cells.

Kinetodesma The interconnecting fibers between the basal bodies of cilia.

Kinetoplast The dense-staining, DNA-containing structure on protozoan flagellates that gives rise to the mitochondria.

Kilocalorie The amount of heat required to raise 1 liter of water 1°C.

Lag Phase The growth phase during which a microbe adapts to a new medium.

Leptospirosis The disease caused by *Leptospira interrogans*. *Also* called Weil's disease or infectious jaundice.

Leptotrombidium A red mite that lives on rodents and acts as the vector in scrub-typhus fever.

Lethal Dose 50 Percent (LD_{50}) The amount of toxin, or the number of bacteria, which will cause death in 50 percent of a population of susceptible animals.

Leukocytes The white cells present in an animal's blood, lymph, and/or lymph tissue.

Ligases The class of enzymes that catalyze the joining of two molecules coupled with the hydrolysis of ATP.

Light Repair The light-activated enzyme system that repairs UV damage to DNA.

Limulus Lysate The material from amebocytes of *Limulus polyphemus* (horseshoe crab) that coagulates when mixed with minute concentrations of endotoxin.

Lopotrichous Flagellation Tufts of flagella located at the pole of a cell.

Lyase An enzyme that cleaves covalent bonds in the absence of an oxidation-reduction reaction and without the addition of water.

Lymphadenopathy Swelling of the lymph nodes.

Lymphocytes Leukocytes involved in antibody production (B lymphocytes) or in cell-mediated immunity (T lymphocytes).

Lymphocytosis Increased number of lymphocytes in the blood caused by a disease.

Lymphokines A large group of animal cell products, primarily glycoproteins, that affect other cells. They are involved in the inflammatory response and in cellular defense mechanisms.

Lyophilization The process of drying frozen biological material under vacuum.

Lysogenic Describes a bacterium that carries a prophage in its genome.

Lysosomes Vesicular structures, formed in the Golgi body, that contain degradative enzymes.

Lytic Cycle The viral replication that results in the lysis of the host cell and the release of virulent virions.

Macrophage A phagocytic white blood cell, derived from a monocyte, that is present in animal tissue spaces.

Maculopapular Skin Rash Spotty blemishes with raised inflamed centers.

Mast Cells Granulated cells present in tissues that are directly involved in reactions of immediate hypersensitivity.

Mastigophora The taxonomic group of Protozoa containing the unicellular flagellates; these organisms are either zooflagellates or phytoflagellates.

Mastitis An inflammation of the female breast.

Meninges The membranes surrounding the brain and the spinal cord.

Meningitis An inflammation of the membranes surrounding the brain and the spinal column.

Merozoites The progeny of schizogony (asexual reproduction by Protozoa).

Mesophile An organism that grows between the temperatures of 20 and 50°C.

Mesosomes The bacterial membranes associated with the cell septum.

Metachromatic Granules Inclusion bodies composed of polyphosphate.

MIC Minimum concentration of an antibiotic that will inhibit the growth of a microorganism (*m*inimum *i*nhibiting *c*oncentration).

Microaerotolerant A microbe that grows in low concentrations of oxygen.

Microtubules Hollow proteinaceous filaments that are structural components of centrioles, eucaryotic flagella, cilia, and the cytoplasm of eucaryotic cells.

Mitochondrion (pl. mitochondria) The membrane-bound organelle of a eucaryotic cell that is the site of aerobic respiration.

Mitosis The process of nuclear division in somatic eucaryotic cells in which the chromosomes are duplicated and distributed to daughter cells.

Mole The gram-molecular weight of a substance.

Morbidity The incidence of both fatal and nonfatal disease in a population.

Multiple Sclerosis A progressive degenerative disease of the central nervous system in which the loss of certain brain and spinal cord functions are lost.

Mutagen A chemical or physical agent that increases the rate of mutation above the spontaneous rate.

Mutation An inheritable change in a cell's normal complement of DNA.

Mycelium (pl. mycelia) An extensive, multibranched, interwinding mat of hyphae.

Mycology The study of fungi.

Myopericarditis An inflammation of heart muscle (myocarditis) and the pericardium (pericarditis).

Negri Bodies An aggregation of rabies virus particles in the brain tissue of a rabid animal.

Neuraminidase An enzyme localized on the surface of certain enveloped virions that cleaves the bond joining sialic acid to cell receptor molecules.

Nocardiosis Infection of the human lungs caused primarily by *Nocardia asteroides* and, rarely, by *N. brasiliensis*.

Nosocomial Infection An infectious illness acquired during a hospital stay.

Nuclear Region The area in the cytoplasm of a procaryotic cell that contains the cell's complement of DNA.

Nucleocapsid The protein-bound nucleic acid complex of an enveloped virus.

Nucleolus Dark-staining area of the karyoplasm containing ribosomal precursors.

Nucleotide A compound composed of a nitrogenous base, a sugar, and a phosphate group; nucleotides are the basic units of RNA and DNA and are also used in forming some coenzymes.

Nucleus The membrane-bound structure of eucaryotic cells that contain cellular DNA.

Numerical Aperture The property of an objective lens defined by $N \sin \alpha$ where N is the refractive index.

Obligate Parasite An organism that requires a host cell for growth and that causes damage to that host.

Oncogenic Virus A virus that induces tumor formation in animals.

Oophoritis Inflammation of the ovaries.

Oospore A fungal spore produced by sexual reproduction in the division Mastigomycotina.

Operon A sequence of genes, controlled by a regulator protein, that codes for proteins involved in a specific cellular function.

Opportunistic Parasites An organism that can, but does not necessarily, cause a diseased state; they are often members of the normal flora of their host.

Orchitis Inflammation of the testes.

Organelle Any membrane-bound cytoplasmic structure that performs a specialized function.

Osmophile An organism that is able to grow in media containing a high solute concentration.

Osmosis The movement of water molecules across a semipermeable membrane in a direction that will equalize the concentration of solute molecules on both sides of the membrane.

Osmotic Pressure The pressure necessary to prevent the movement of water across a semipermeable membrane because of the differences in solute concentrations.

Otitis An inflammation of the ear.

Oxidation The loss of an electron by an atom.

Oxidation-Reduction Reaction A two-substrate reaction in which one compound donates one or more electrons and the other accepts the electrons.

Oxidative Phosphorylation The formation of energy-rich bonds in ATP by an oxidative process involving the electron-transport chain.

Oxidoreductase An enzyme that catalyzes an oxidation-reduction reaction.

Pandemic An infectious disease that spreads around the world.

Parturition The act of bringing forth young; childbirth.

Passive Immunity Resistance to a specific infectious agent developed in another individual and transferred to the patient. Acquisition of this immune state can be by natural or artificial means.

Pasteurization Preservation of food materials by heating them at temperatures that do not alter the quality of the food.

Pathogen A microorganism capable of causing an infectious disease.

Pediococcus Spherical organisms that divide in two planes to form tetrads.

Peptidoglycan The sugar-peptide polymer found in many bacterial cell walls.

Periplasmic Space The area between the cytoplasmic membrane and the cell wall of Gram-negative bacteria.

Peritonitis An inflammation of the membrane that lines the human abdominal cavity.

Peritrichous Flagellation Flagella dispersed around the outside of a cell.

Pertussis A severe cough.

Phage Conversion Alterations of a host cell's phenotype resulting from the expression of one or more genes on a prophage.

Phagocytosis The process by which white blood cells engulf unwanted matter from tissue spaces.

Photolithotroph An organism that grows in inorganic medium and uses light as a source of energy.

Phototaxis Movement of cells in response to light.

Phototrophs Organisms that use light as a source of energy.

Plankton   Drifting animals and plants in open water.

Plaque   The clear spot in a lawn of growing cells resulting from the viral-induced lysis of infected cells.

Plaque Reduction   The decreased ability of a virus to form plaques when an interfering substance (interferon) is present.

Plasma   The liquid part of blood that remains after the cells have been removed.

Plasmids   The self-replicating, extra-chromosomal DNA molecules found in bacteria.

Plasmolysis   The collapse of a cell because of the high external solute concentration.

Pleomorphism   The existence of different morphological forms in the same species or strain of microorganism.

Plus RNA   Single-stranded RNA that serves as mRNA and as a template for making a replicative (minus) RNA strand.

Pneumonia   A disease of the lungs in which the tissue is inflamed, hardened, and watery.

Polyhydroxybutyric Acid   A polymer of a lipidlike substance that is present as an inclusion in the cytoplasm of certain bacteria.

Polymorphonuclear Granulocytes (PMN)   Circulating phagocytic leukocytes characterized by a multilobed nucleus and numerous cytoplasmic granules.

Polyribosomes   A complex of mRNA and two or more ribosomes engaged in translation.

Postpartum   After childbirth.

PPLO   A group of bacteria now classified in the genus *Mycoplasma* (*pleuropneumonia-like organisms*)

Procaryotae   The kingdom of organisms that contains the cyanobacteria and the bacteria.

Procaryotes   The large group of organisms (bacteria) whose nucleic acid is found in a nuclear region (no nucleus is present).

Propagated Epidemic   An illness in a population characterized by a gradual change in the person-to-person transmission of the infectious agent.

Prophage   The genome of a temperate phage when it is integrated into its host cell's DNA.

Protista   The third kingdom proposed by Haeckel to include all the microorganisms. In Haeckel's scheme, the bacteria belong to the lower protists, whereas the eucaryotic microorganisms belong to the higher protists.

Protoplast   An experimentally produced wall-deficient bacterial cell.

Prototroph   The parent cell, either the wild type or a mutant strain, from which a mutant is derived.

Protozoa   The single-celled animals.

Pseudohyphae   Yeast cells growing together to form a septated tubular protoplasm.

Pseudomonales   The family composed of the aerobic, Gram-negative, rod-shaped bacteria.

Pseudopodium   A temporary cytoplasmic protrusion from an ameboid cell that functions in locomotion and feeding.

Psychrophiles   Organisms that grow at low temperature, between $-5°$ and $20°C$.

Puerperal Fever   An infection of the female reproductive tract, occurring postpartum, that is caused by streptococci or staphylococci.

Pure Culture   A culture that is grown from a single cell. *Anexic cultures* contain only one type of organism. Often these terms are used interchangeably.

Purpura   Hemorrhages in the skin.

Pyelonephritis   An inflammation of the kidney.

Radiation   Emission and propagation of energy through space or through a substance in the form of waves.

Reagin   *See* Wasserman antibody.

Recombinant DNA   A molecule of deoxyribonucleic acid containing genes from two or more different organisms.

Reduction   The gain of an electron by an atom.

Relapsing Fever   A human disease caused by tickborne or louseborne *Borrelia* and characterized by alternating febrile and recovery stages.

Reservoir   A healthy animal that harbors an infectious agent capable of causing disease in other animals.

Resolution   The distance between two objects that can be visualized by the human eye.

Restriction Endonuclease   A bacterial enzyme that cleaves double-stranded DNA at specific sites in the middle (as opposed to the ends) of the molecule. They function to destroy DNA that is foreign to the cell.

Reticulate Body   The intracellular form of chlamydiae that is capable of growth and division.

Reticuloendothelial System   An animal's total complement of macrophages.

Ribosome   A cytoplasmic complex composed of RNA (60%) and protein (40%) that functions in protein synthesis.

Rickettsiae   Bacteria that are obligate parasites of eucaryotic cells.

Rifamycins   Antibiotics that inhibit transcription by binding to DNA-directed RNA polymerase and prevents mRNA formation.

Rise Period   The time interval between the release of the first and the last infected bacterium in a one-step growth experiment.

Rod   The name given to a microorganism that is longer than it is wide.

Saddle-Back Fever   A biphasic fever with an initial peak, remission, and then another peak.

Sarcina   A spherical organism that divides in three planes to form packets of eight cells.

Sarcodina   The taxonomic group of the Protozoa containing the single-celled animals that produce pseudopodia.

Schick Test   The use of a small quantity of active diphtheria toxin to measure a person's immunity against diphtheria.

Selective Enrichments   A culture established to enable the desired microbe to outgrow other microbes in an inoculum.

Septicemia   The presence of multiplying microorganisms in an animal's blood.

Septum (pl. septa)   The structural division between two adjoining cellular compartments.

Serology   The study of the properties and reactions of blood serum.

Serum   Blood minus all the cells and the clotting components.

Serum Sickness   The formation of soluble immune complexes in the blood following passive immunization or an inappropriate transfusion.

Schizogony   In protozoa, the asexual reproduction of trophozoites in host cells resulting in progeny known as merozoites.

Signal Hypothesis   A hypothesis to explain how membrane proteins are manufactured, positioned within the membrane, and/or transported through the membrane.

Slime Layer   Materials extending from the cell wall in a diffused arrangement.

Specialized Transduction   The bacteriophage-mediated transfer of host-cell genes that are located on the chromosome adjacent to the integration site of a prophage.

Species   One kind of microorganism.

Species Name   The specific epitaph that when modified by the genus name describes an organism; one part of the binomial system of nomenclature.

Species Resistance   Absence of susceptibility to infectious disease possessed by an entire group of animals or plants.

Spherical Aberration   The inability of a lens to focus on the entire field.

Spherule   The thick-walled structure that surrounds the endospores produced by *Coccidioides immitis*. Its presence is diagnostic for coccidioidomycosis.

Spirillum (pl. spirilla)   A curve-shaped bacterium possessing polar flagella.

Spirochetes   Helical organisms possessing an endoflagella.

Spontaneous Generation   The theory (incorrect) that living organisms can arise from nonliving matter. *Also* called abiogenesis.

Spontaneous Mutations   Inherited alterations in a cell's DNA that occur in the absence of a mutagenic agent.

Spores   Resting, resistant forms of microorganisms.

Sporozoa   The taxonomic group of Protozoa containing the nonmotile, parasitic, single-celled animals.

Sporozoite   The progeny produced from a zygote after it undergoes meiosis.

Spotted Fever Group—Rickettsiae   The bacteria that cause rickettsialpox and Rocky Mountain spotted fever in humans.

Stationary Phase   The growth phase of a culture where the number of cells dividing is equal to the number of cells dying.

Sterile   Devoid of all living things.

Sterilization   The process by which all living things are killed.

Strain   A designation that indicates a specific isolate of an organism.

Streptococci   Spherical bacteria that grow in chains.

Streptokinase   A streptococcal enzyme that breaks down plasminogen to plasmin.

Streptolysins   Hemolysins of blood cells produced by streptococci.

Subacute Sclerosing Panencephalitis   A chronic degenerative neurological disease.

Subcutaneous Mycoses   Fungal infections of the skin, subcutaneous tissue, connective tissue, and bone.

Substrate-Level Phosphorylation An enzymatic reaction that catalyzes the attachment of inorganic phosphate (H_3PO_4) to an organic compound; this phosphate is later transferred to ADP to form an energy-rich phosphate bond.

Superoxide Oxygen that has accepted an additional electron (O_2).

Svedberg Unit A measure of the relative size of a macromolecule as determined by ultracentrifugation.

Symbiosis The relationship between organisms that mutually benefit from cohabitation.

Syphilis A venereal disease caused by *Treponema pallidum.*

Systematics The organization of organisms into groups according to their evolutionary relationships.

Systemic Mycoses Fungal infections of the internal organs.

Temperate Bacteriophage A bacterial virus that either causes a replication cycle that lyses its host cell or exists in a genetic form (prophage) that is passed on to the host's daughter cells.

Therapeutic Index The ratio of the minimum dose of a drug that is toxic to the host divided by the minimum dose required for antimicrobial activity.

Thermophiles Organisms that require temperatures above 45°C to grow.

Tinea Capitis Ringworm of the head.

Tinea Corporis Ringworm of the body.

Tinea Cruris Ringworm of the groin (jock itch).

Tinea Pedis Ringworm of the foot (athlete's foot).

Titer The reciprocal of the highest dilution of serum that will bring about a demonstrable antibody-antigen reaction.

Toxigenic Disease Damage to the host caused by the presence of a toxic substance.

Toxin A natural substance that acts chemically on tissues to cause disease.

Toxoid A chemically inactivated toxin that still retains its antigenicity.

TPI *Treponema pallidum* immobilization test for syphilis.

Transcription The cellular process by which the code contained in DNA is chemically rewritten into RNA.

Transduction The viral-mediated genetic transfer of markers from a host cell to a recipient cell.

Transferase An enzyme that takes a chemical group bound to one molecule and attaches it to another molecule.

Transformation The transfer of naked DNA from the environment to a competent recipient cell.

Transformed Animal Cell A cell that grows in an unrestricted manner because it has lost the property of contact inhibition.

Translation The process of forming a polypeptide using the information contained in messenger RNA.

Transovarian Passage Transfer of an infectious agent from an adult vector to its progeny through the infection of its eggs.

Tricarboxylic Acid Cycle The enzymatic process for the oxidation of acetyl-CoA to two molecules of CO_2, GTP, and the production of reduced coenzymes.

Trophozoite The vegetative form of a sporozoan.

Tubercule The histological structure formed in response to the cells and the growth products of *Mycobacterium* sp.

Tuberculin An extract of *Mycobacterium tuberculosis* that is injected into a patient's skin for the tuberculin test.

Tuberculosis (miliary) A mycobacterial disease characterized by the presence of tubercules throughout the body.

Tuberculosis (pulmonary) A progressive, destructive disease of the lungs caused by *Mycobacterium tuberculosis* and, to a lesser extent, by *Mycobacterium bovis.*

Typhus Group Rickettsiae that cause endemic, epidemic, and scrub typhus fever in humans.

Urethritis An infection of the urethra.

Vaccination An inoculation with a specific vaccine to lessen or prevent the effects of an infectious disease.

Vaginitis Inflammation of the vagina.

Variolation Inoculation of patients with material from a smallpox lesion to produce immunity against smallpox.

VDRL Venereal disease research laboratory flocculation test for syphilis; it detects the presence of serum antibody.

Vector An agent that is capable of transferring a pathogen from one animal to another.

Venereal Disease Any disease that is transmitted primarily by sexual intercourse.

Vibrio A curve-shaped organism.

Vibrioaceae The family of oxidase-positive, Gram-negative, facultative anaerobic bacteria that are curved or rod-shaped.

Viral Envelope The outer layer of certain animal viruses that contains lipids derived from the host cell's membrane.

Virion A single virus particle.

Viropexis The engulfment of an adsorbed animal virion by the formation of a vesicle derived from the host cell.

Virulence The relative ability of an infectious agent (microorganism or virus) to cause disease.

Virus A complex macromolecular form of life that uses its genetic information, encoded in either DNA or RNA, to produce replicas of itself in its host cell.

Wasserman Antibody An antibody substance produced during infections by treponemas and other pathogens that react with cardiolipid. *Also* called reagin.

Weil's Disease *See* leptospirosis.

X and V Factors The blood components required by *Hemophilus* for growth. X can be replaced by hematin or hemoglobin and V can be replaced by NAD.

Yaw The open primary lesion in the skin disease (yaws) caused by *Treponema pertenue.*

Yeast A fungus that grows as individual cells (may reproduce by budding) and produces moist to pasty colonies.

Zoonoses Infectious diseases that occur primarily in animals; humans are occasionally infected.

Zygospores Fungal spores produced by sexual reproduction in the division Zygomycotina.

Zygote The product of sexual reproduction brought about by the fusion of two gametes.

INDEX

Throughout the index the following special notations are used: **bold face** numbers indicate tables; *italicized* numbers indicate figures.

Abiogenesis, *see* Spontaneous generation
Abortive poliomyelitis, 436
Absidia:
  mucormycosis, 470
  sporangiospore, 460
Acetaminophen, 424
Acetyl transferase, 196
Acid-fast stain, 40
  Mycobacterium leprae, 314
  Mycobacterium tuberculosis, 310
Acids, 26
Acinetobacter:
  genitourinary tract, **210**
  respiratory tract, **206**
Acne, **211**
Acquired immunity, 234
Acridine orange, 118
Actinobacillus, **206**
Actinomyces, 304
  respiratory tract, **206**
Actinomyces bovis, 315
Actinomyces israelii, 315
Actinomycetes, 153
Actinomycin D:
  antiviral activity, 198
  protein synthesis, 100
Actinomycosis, **206,** 315
  treatment, 316

Active transport, 44
Acute infantile diarrheal disease, 431
Acute respiratory illness, 398
Acyclovir, herpes, 414
Adenine, 29, *83*
Adenine arabinoside, 391
  antiviral activity, 198
Adenosatellite virus, *374*
Adenosine monophosphate, *68*
Adenosine triphosphate, **66, 67, 68.** *73*
Adenoviridae, 396, **337**
Adenoviruses, *274, 297*
  antigenic types, **395**
  cytopathic effects, *397, 398*
  diseases caused by, 398
  respiratory infection, 396
  structure, *379*
Adenylate cyclase, 292
Adenyl transferase, 196
ADP-ribose, 306
Aedes, 444
Aedes aegypti, 447, 448
  yellow fever vector, 449
Aedes triseriatus, 444
Aerobic bacteria, classification of, 152
Aerobic respiration, *76*
Aflatoxin, 470
African sleeping sickness, 494

Agar, 129
Age:
  resistance to disease, 225
  tuberculosis and, 312
Agglutination reaction, 248—249
  latex test for fungi, 464
  titers, 248
Agglutinins, **236**
Agriculture, U.S. Department of,
    tuberculosis control, 313
Airborne diseases, 265
  diphtheria, 308
Air conditioning, disease transmission,
    369
Ajellomyces, 466
Ajellomyces capsulatum, 466. *See also*
    Histoplasma capsulatum
Alcohol dehydrogenase, 70
Alcohols, 183—**184**
Algae, 12
Algaecide, copper sulfate, 185
Alimentary tract, viral disease, 422
Allodermanyssus sanguineus, 350
Allosteric enzymes, 104
Alphaviruses, 445
  characteristics of, **444**
Amantadine, 391
  antiviral drug, 198, 402